OXFORD MEDICAL PUBLICATIONS

Oxford Desk Reference
Major Trauma

Oxford Desk Reference
Major Trauma

Edited by

Jason Smith

Consultant in Emergency Medicine
Derriford Hospital, Plymouth,
Senior Lecturer in Pre-hospital and Emergency Medicine
Academic Department of Military Emergency Medicine, Birmingham

Ian Greaves

Consultant and Professor of Emergency Medicine
James Cook University Hospital, Middlesbrough

Keith M Porter

Consultant Trauma Surgeon
University of Birmingham NHS Trust, Birmingham,
Professor of Clinical Traumatology
University of Birmingham, Birmingham

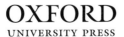
OXFORD
UNIVERSITY PRESS

OXFORD
UNIVERSITY PRESS

Great Clarendon Street, Oxford OX2 6DP

Oxford University Press is a department of the University of Oxford.
It furthers the University's objective of excellence in research, scholarship,
and education by publishing worldwide in

Oxford New York

Athens Auckland Bangkok Bogotá Buenos Aires Cape Town
Chennai Dar es Salaam Delhi Florence Hong Kong Istanbul Karachi
Kolkata Kuala Lumpur Madrid Melbourne Mexico City Mumbai Nairobi
Paris São Paulo Shanghai Singapore Taipei Tokyo Toronto Warsaw

with associated companies in Berlin Ibadan

Oxford is a registered trade mark of Oxford University Press
in the UK and in certain other countries

Published in the United States
by Oxford University Press Inc., New York

© Oxford University Press, 2011

The moral rights of the author have been asserted

Database right Oxford University Press (maker)

First published 2011

British Library Cataloguing in Publication Data

Data available

Library of Congress Cataloguing in Publication Data

Data available

ISBN 978-0-19-954332-8

10 9 8 7 6 5 4 3 2 1

Typeset in GillHandbook
by Glyph International, Bangalore, India
Printed in the UK
on acid-free paper by
CPI Antony Rowe, Chippenham, Wiltshire

Foreword

As the National Clinical Director for Trauma Care in the Department of Health charged with the implementation of Regional Networks for Major Trauma in the National Health Service in England, I have read this text with considerable interest. We are at last moving to a system where patients with serious injuries will be managed within a coordinated structure that delivers them with priority promptly to a unit that can deliver their definitive care. There will be a clear need for reference material relating to the numerous clinical issues that may arise from initial assessment through to rehabilitation. The *Oxford Desk Reference: Major Trauma*, successfully fulfils that need and is most timely in its release as Regional Trauma Networks are being planned and implemented across England through 2010-2012.

I found this resource well structured, easily searchable, and succinct.

The text is comprehensive and appropriately draws on the more recent military medical experience gained in Afghanistan and Iraq relating to patient retrieval, assessment, trauma team performance, resuscitation, massive transfusion, coagulopathy, and of course, blast and penetrating trauma.

I would expect this resource to become a popular contemporary point of reference at the start of this new era of trauma care in the UK.

Keith Willett
National Clinical Director for Trauma Care
Department of Health

Brief contents

Detailed contents

Abbreviations

0, 2-0, 3-0, 4-0, 5-0, 6-0	relate to size of suture material
6P's	painful, pale, pulseless, paraesthetic, paralysed and perishingly cold
AAGBI	Association of Anaesthetists of Great Britain and Ireland
AAST	American Association for the Surgery of Trauma
ABCDE	**A**irway, **B**reathing, **C**irculation, **D**isability, and **E**xposure
ABG	arterial blood gases
ABI	acquired brain injury
ABPI	ankle-brachial pressure index
ACCOLC	ACCess OverLoad Control
ACS	Abdominal Compartment Syndrome
AD	adjustment disorders
ADH	antidiuretic hormone
ADI	atlanto dens interval
AG	anion gap
AIC	Ambulance Incident Commander
AIS	Abbreviated Injury Scale
AKI	acute kidney injury
AKP	anterior knee pain
ALI	acute lung injury
AMPDS	Advanced Medical Priority Dispatch System
angio suite	angiography suite
AnP	anatomic profile
AP	anterior posterior
APACHE	Acute Physiology and Chronic Health Evaluation
AP-C	activated protein C
APC	anterior-posterior compression
APL	adjustable pressure-limiting
APRV	airway pressure release ventilation
APTT	activated partial thromboplastin time
ARDS	Adult Respiratory Distress Syndrome
ARF	acute renal failure
ARS	Acute Radiation Syndrome
ASA	American Society of Anaesthesiologists
ASB	assisted spontaneous breathing
ASCOT	A Severity Characterization of Trauma
ASIA	American Spinal Injuries Association
ASIF	Association for the Study of Internal Fixation
ASR	acute stress reaction
ATC	air traffic control
ATLS	Advanced Trauma Life Support
ATN	acute tubular necrosis
ATP	adenosine triphosphate
AVPU	alert; verbal; pain; unresponsive
BAI	blunt aortic injury

BAL	British Anti-Lewisite
BAT	Burns Assessment Team
BATLS	Battlefield Advanced Trauma Life Support
BETTS	Birmingham eye trauma terminology system
BIPAP	biphasic positive airway pressure
BIPP	bismuth iodoform paraffin paste
BM	Blood glucose measurement, BM stix
BMI	Body Mass Index
B-mode	brightness modulation imaging
BMP	bone morphogenic protein
BOAST	British Orthopaedic Association Standards for Trauma
BP	blood pressure
BPF	bronchopleural fistulas
bpm	beats per min
BTS	British Thoracic Society
C2, C6	cervical vertebrae 2, cervical vertebrae 6
<C>ABCDE	control of external haemorrhage, airway, breathing, circulation, disability, exposure
CaO	cardiac output
CARS	compensatory anti-inflammatory response
casevac	casualty evacuation
CAVR	continuous arteriovenous rewarming
CBF	cerebral blood flow
CBRN	chemical, biological, radiological and nuclear
CCC	Civil Contingencies Committee
CDC	Centre for Disease Control and Prevention
CISD	critical incident stress debriefing
C-ISS	Cervical Injury Severity Score
CK-MB	creatine kinase
CMRO$_2$	cerebral metabolic requirement for oxygen
CMT	cardiomediastinal thoracic
CMV	controlled mandatory ventilation
CNS	central nervous system
CO	carbon monoxide
COBR	Cabinet Office Briefing Room
COPD	chronic obstructive airways disease
CPAP	continuous positive airways pressure
CPK	creatinine phosphokinase
CPP	cerebral perfusion pressure,
CPR	cardiopulmonary resuscitation
CRAMS	Circulation, Respiration, Abdominal/Thoracic, Motor and Speech Scale
CRASH	corticosteroid randomization after significant head injury
CRM	crew resource management
CRPS	Complex Regional Pain Syndrome
CSF	cerebrospinal fluid
CT	computed tomography
CTA	computed tomography angiography

CTLSO	cervico-thoracolumbosacral orthosis		GFR	glomerular filtration rate
CTO	cervical-thoracic orthosis		GTN	glyceryl trinitrate
CvO	cervical orthosis		HART	Hazardous Area Response Teams
CVP	central venous pressure		HAS	human albumin solution
CVR	cerebral vascular resistance		HAT	Health Advice Team
CVVH	continuous veno-venous haemofiltration		HazMat	hazardous materials
CXR	chest X-ray		HBOC	haemoglobin-based oxygen carrier
DAI	diffuse axonal injury		HBOT	hyperbaric oxygen therapy
DALY	Disability Adjusted Life Years		HD	haemodialysis
DCR	damage control resuscitation		HEMS	Helicopter Emergency Medical System/Service
DCS	damage control surgery		HES	hydroxyethyl starches
DD	dissociative disorders		HF	hydrofluoric acid
DFSD	dry fibrin sealant dressing		HFOV	high frequency oscillatory ventilation
DIC	disseminated intravascular coagulation		HIC	high income countries
DJ	duodenojejunal		HIT	head injury trials
DM	diabetes mellitus		HLS	helicopter landing sites
DMS	Defence Medical Services		HME	heat and moisture exchange
DMSA	dimercaptosuccinic acid		HR	heart rate
DP	dorsalis paedis		HS	hypertonic solutions
DPL	diagnostic peritoneal lavage		IAH	intra-abdominal hypertension
DSA	digital subtraction angiography		IAP	intra-abdominal pressure
DVT	deep venous thrombosis		IASP	International Association of the Study of Pain
ECA	external carotid artery		ICA	internal carotid artery
ECG	electrocardiogram		ICD	International Classification of Diseases
ECMO	extracorporeal membrane oxygenation		ICoD	intercostal drain
ECP	emergency care practitioners		ICP	intracranial pressure
ED	emergency department		ICU	intensive care unit
EGDT	early goal directed therapy		ID	internal diameter
EMDR	eye movement desensitization and reprocessing		IIS	Injury Impairment Scale
EMS	Emergency Medical Services		ILO	International Labour Office
EMT	emergency medical technicians		ILV	independent lung ventilation
EOC	Emergency Operations Centre		im	intramuscular
EPAP	expiratory positive airways pressure		IMA	inferior mesenteric artery
EPC	enduring personality change		IMF	inter-maxillary fixation
EPL	extensor pollicis longus		IMV	intermittent mandatory ventilation
ERG	electroretinography		IOFB	intra-ocular foreign body
ET	endotracheal		IOP	intra-ocular pressure
ETT	endotracheal tube		IPPV	intermittent positive pressure ventilation
EUA	examination under anaesthetic		IPV	Interpersonal violence
EWA	early walking aids		ISS	Injury Severity Score
FAQ	frequently asked questions		iv	intravenous
FAST	focused assessment with sonography for trauma		IVC	inferior vena cava
FB	foreign body		IVU	intravenous urogram
FCI	Functional Capacity Index		JHAC	Joint Health Advisory Cell
FES	fat embolus syndrome		LC	lateral compression
FFP	fresh frozen plasma		LMA	laryngeal mask airway
FNHTR	febrile non-haemolytic transfusion reactions		LMIC	low/middle income countries
G6PD	glucose-6-phophate		LOC	level of consciousness
GBD	global burden of disease		LPS	lipopolysaccharides
GCS	Glasgow Coma Score		LSD	lysergic acid diethylamide
			LSI	life-saving intervention

LSO	lumbosacral orthosis		PCC	prothrombin complex concentrate
LVEDP	left ventricular end diastolic pressure		PCI	percutaneous coronary intervention
MACA	Military Aid to the Civilian Authority		pCO_2	partial pressure CO_2
MACC	Military Aid to the Civil Community		PCT	procalcitonin
MAP	Mean Arterial Blood Pressure		PCWP	pulmonary capillary wedge pressure
MARCH	**M**assive haemorrhage, **A**irway, **R**espiration, **C**irculation and **H**ead Injury		PDGF	platelet derived growth factor
			PEEP	positive end expiratory pressure
MARS	mixed antagonist response syndrome		PEP	post-exposure prophylaxis
MCA	Maritime and Coastguard Agency		PFC	perfluorocarbons
MCT	medial canthal tendon		PI	performance indicator
MDCT	multi-detector computed tomography		PICC	peripherally inserted central catheter
MDF	myocardial depressant factors		pO_2	partial pressure of oxygen
MIC	Medical Incident Commander		PPE	personal protective equipment
MICC	Major Incident Co-ordination Centre		PPV	positive predictive value
MILS	manual in-line stabilizaton		PRC	packed red cells
MIPPO	minimally invasive percutaneous plate osteosynthesis		PrT	prothrombin time
			PSIS	posterior superior iliac spine
MMMF	man-made mineral fibres		PT	see PyT
MMT	Mobile Medical Team		pT	pneumothorax
MNBV	mean normal blood volume		PT	posterior tibial
MODS	multiple organ dysfunction syndrome		PTA	post-traumatic amnesia
MOF	multi-organ failure		PTFE	polytetrafluoroethylene
MPI	mass psychogenic illness		PTS	post-traumatic seizures
MRI	magnetic resonance imaging		PTSD	post-traumatic stress disorder
MSC	mesenchymal stem cells		PVD	peripheral vascular disease
MTOS	Major Trauma Outcome Study		PvO_2	partial pressure of oxygen
MUS	medically unexplained symptoms		PyT	physical therapy
MVC	motor vehicle collision		qds	four times daily
NAI	non-accidental injury		RAPD	relative afferent pupillary defect
NG	nasogastric		RBC	red blood cell
NIBP	non-invasive blood pressure		RBF	renal blood flow
NICE	National Institute for Clinical Excellence		RCA	riot-control agents
NIMS	National Incident Management System		RCCC	Regional Civil Contingencies Committee
NIPPV	non-invasive positive pressure ventilation		RCT	root canal treatment
NISS	New Injury Severity Score		RDD	radiological dispersal device
NIV	non-invasive ventilation		RDH	rapid deployment haemostat
NMDA	N-methyl-D-aspartic acid		rFVIIa	recombinant factor VIIa
NOM	non-operative management		rhAPC	recombinant human activated protein C
NPV	negative predictive value		ROM	range of movement
NSAID	Non-steroidal anti-inflammatory drug		ROTES	Report of Trauma and Emergency Services
NTDB	National Trauma Data Bank		RR	respiratory rate
ODC	oxyhaemoglobin dissociation curve		RRT	renal replacement therapy
OECD	Organization for Economic Cooperation and Development		RSI	rapid sequence induction
			RTA	road traffic accident
OLIV	one lung independent ventilation		RTC	road traffic collisions
OM	occipitomental		RTS	Revised Trauma Score
OPG	orthopantomogram		RVP	rendezvous point
ORIF	open reduction and internal fixation		SAE	systemic air embolism
PA	postero-anterior		SAH	sub-arachnoid haemorrhage
$PaCO_2$	partial pressure of carbon dioxide		SAR	search and rescue
PACS	picture archiving and communication systems		SARS	Severe Acute Respiratory Syndrome
PAW	peak airway pressure		SBP	systolic blood pressure
PCA	patient-controlled analgesia			

SCD	short circuit device		TBD	tracheobronchial disruption
SCG	Strategic Co-ordinating Group		TBI	traumatic brain injury
SCI	spinal cord injury		TEDS	thromboembolic deterrent stockings
SCIWORA	spinal cord injury without radiographic abnormality		TFCBT	trauma-focused cognitive behavioural therapy
SCM	sternocleidomastoid muscle		TGF-ß	transforming growth factor ß
SDD	selective decontamination of the digestive tract		THA	topical haemostatic agents
			THAM	tris buffer
SEB	staphylococcal enterotoxin B		TL-ISS	Thoracolumbar Injury Severity Score
SFH	stroma-free haemoglobin		TLIV	two lung independent ventilation
SIC	self-intermittent catheterization		TLSO	thoraco-lumbosacral orthosis
SICU	surgical intensive care unit		TMJ	temporomandibular joints
SID	strong ion difference		TOE	transoesophageal echocardiogram
SIG	strong ion gap		TPN	total parenteral nutrition
SIMV	synchronous intermittent mandatory ventilation		TRALI	transfusion-associated acute lung injury
			TRiM	trauma risk management
SIRS	Systemic Inflammatory Response Syndrome		TS	Trauma Score
SMA	superior mesenteric artery		TTE	transthoracic echocardiogram
SMS	sms text messaging		UTI	urinary tract
SMV	superior mesenteric vein		VAP	ventilator-associated pneumonia
SNOM	selective non-operative management		VATS	video-assisted thoracoscopic surgery
SOMI	sterno-occipital mandibular immobilizer		vCJD	variant Creutzfeld-Jakob disease
SpO_2	partial pressure oxygen		VF	ventricular fibrillation
SSC	Surviving Sepsis Campaign		VHF	very high frequency
SSRI	selective serotonin reuptake inhibitor		VILI	ventilator-induced lung injury
STAC	Science and Technical Advisory Cell		VQ	ventilation perfusion
START	simple treatment and rapid triage		VrHF	viral haemorrhagic fevers
STEP	safety triggers for emergency personnel		WADEM	World Association for Disaster and Emergency Medicine
SvO_2	mixed venous oxygen saturation		WHO	World Health Organization
SVR	systemic vascular resistance		WP	white phosphorous
SVR	systemic vascular resistance		WSACS	World Society of the Abdominal Compartment Syndrome
TAC	temporary abdominal closure			
TAI	traumatic aortic injury		ZF	zygomaticofrontal
TARN	Trauma Audit and Research Network			

Contributors

Dr Karim Ahmad
Specialist Registrar in Emergency Medicine
Department of Emergency Medicine and
Pre-Hospital Care
The Royal London Hospital
London, UK

Professor David Alexander
Director
The Aberdeen Centre for
Trauma Research
Faculty of Health and Social Care
The Robert Gordon University
Aberdeen, UK

Dr Cino Bendinelli
Deputy Director of Trauma
Department of Surgery
John Hunter Hospital,
Newcastle, NSW, Australia

**Surgeon Commander
Steven Bland Royal Navy**
Consultant in Emergency Medicine
Defence Medical Services, and
Emergency Department
Queen Alexandra Hospital
Cosham
Portsmouth, UK

Dr Steven Bonner
Clinical Director Critical Care
Department of Anaesthesia and
Intensive Care Medicine
James Cook university Hospital
Middlesbrough, UK

Ms Erica Caldwell
Trauma Nurse Coordinator
Department of Trauma
Liverpool Hospital
New South Wales, Australia

Dr Dane Chalkley
Specialist Registrar in Emergency Medicine
Department of Emergency Medicine and
Pre-Hospital Care
The Royal London Hospital
London, UK

Dr Otto Chan
Consultant Radiologist
The London Independent Hospital
London, UK

Colonel Jon Clasper L/RAMC
Defence Professor Trauma &
Orthopaedics
Royal Centre for Defence Medicine
Birmingham, UK, and
Consultant Orthopaedic Surgeon
Frimley Park NHS Foundation Trust
Frimley, UK

Dr Scott K D'Amours
Consultant Trauma Surgeon
Director of Trauma
Department of Trauma Services
Liverpool Hospital
The University of New South Wales
Sydney, Australia

Mr Dan Deakin
Specialist Registrar in Trauma and
Orthopaedic Surgery
University Hospital Birmingham
NHS Trust
Birmingham, UK

**Lieutenant Colonel Jeff Garner
RAMC**
Consultant Surgeon
Defence Medical Services UK, and
Department of Colorectal Surgery
Rotherham NHS Foundation Trust
Rotherham, UK

**Wing Commander
Andrew Gibbons RAF**
Consultant in Maxillofacial Surgery
Defence Medical Services, UK, and
Department of Oral and
Maxillofacial surgery
Peterborough Hospitals NHS Trust
Peterborough, UK

Dr Geertje Govaert
Trauma Fellow
Department of Trauma and
General Surgery
Maastricht University Medical Centre
Maastricht, The Netherlands

Colonel Ian Greaves L/RAMC
Defence Consultant Advisor in
Emergency Medicine
Defence Medical Services, UK,
Professor of Emergency Medicine
Teesside University, and
Consultant in Emergency Medicine James
Cook University Hospital
Middlesbrough, UK

Dr Henry Guly
Consultant in Emergency Medicine
Emergency Department
Derriford Hospital
Plymouth, UK

**Surgeon Lieutenant Commander
Dan Henning Royal Navy**
Specialist Registrar in Emergency Medicine
Defence Medical Services, UK, and
Emergency Department
Derriford Hospital
Plymouth, UK

Lieutenant Colonel Jeremy Henning RAMC
Consultant in Anaesthesia and Intensive Care Medicine
Defence Medical Services UK, and
Departments of Anaesthesia and Intensive Care Medicine
James Cook university Hospital
Middlesbrough, UK

Dr Ian Higginson
Consultant in Emergency Medicine
Emergency Department
Derriford Hospital
Plymouth, UK

Lieutenant Colonel Simon Horne RAMC
Consultant in Emergency Medicine
Defence Medical Services UK, and
Emergency Department
Derriford Hospital
Plymouth, UK

Dr Fiona Hunt
ACCS Anaesthesia Trainee
Northern Deanery, UK

Major Paul Hunt RAMC
Specialist Registrar in Emergency Medicine and
Intensive Care Medicine
Visiting Lecturer, Emergency Medicine and Critical Care
Defence Medical Services and Northern Deanery, UK

Dr Ian Hunter
Consultant in Anaesthesia and Intensive Care Medicine
Department of Anaesthesia and Intensive Care Medicine
James Cook University Hospital
Middlesbrough, UK

Lieutenant Colonel Steve Jeffery RAMC
Consultant Plastics and Burns Surgeon
Royal Centre for Defence Medicine
Birmingham, UK

**Surgeon Lieutenant Commander
Mansoor Khan Royal Navy**
Specialist Registrar in General Surgery
Defence Medical Services, UK

Dr Susan Klein
Reader in Trauma Research
The Aberdeen centre for Trauma Research
Faculty of Health and Social Care
The Robert Gordon University
Aberdeen, UK

Lieutenant Colonel Neil Mackenzie RAMC
Consultant in Maxillofacial Surgery
Maxillofacial Unit
Queen Alexandra Hospital
Cosham
Portsmouth, UK

Mr Michael McCarthy
Spinal Fellow
Musgrove Park Hospital
Taunton, UK

Dr Scott McGregor
Associate Specialist
Department of Anaesthesia and
Intensive Care Medicine
James Cook University Hospital
Middlesbrough, UK

Professor Paul Middleton
Associate Professor
Director of Research
Ambulance Research Institute, and Medical Director,
Ambulance Service of New South Wales, Australia

Lieutenant Colonel Alan Mistlin RAMC
Head of Medical Division and Consultant in
Rheumatology and Rehabilitation
Defence Medical Rehabilitation Centre
Headley Court
Epsom, UK

Mr Matt O'Meara
Trauma Fellow
University Hospital Birmingham NHS Trust
Birmingham, UK

Professor Keith Porter
Professor of Clinical Traumatology
Royal Centre for Defence Medicine
Birmingham, UK

Major Arul Ramasamy RAMC
Specialist Registrar in Trauma & Orthopaedic Surgery
Academic Department of Military Surgery and Trauma
Royal Centre for Defence Medicine
Birmingham, UK

Mr Imran Raza
Clinical Research Fellow
Trauma Clinical Academic Unit
The Royal London Hospital
London, UK

Dr James Ryan
Consultant in Anaesthesia and Critical Care
Department of Anaesthesia and
Intensive Care Medicine
James Cook University Hospital
Middlesbrough, UK

Wing Commander Robert AH Scott RAF
Defence Consultant Advisor in Ophthalmology
Academic Department of Military Surgery and Trauma
Royal Centre for Defence Medicine
Birmingham and Midland Eye Centre
University Hospital Birmingham NHS Foundation Trust
Birmingham, UK

**Surgeon Commander Jason Smith
Royal Navy**
Consultant in Emergency Medicine, Emergency
Department, Derriford Hospital,
Plymouth, UK, and Senior Lecturer, Academic
Department of Military Emergency Medicine, Royal
Centre for Defence Medicine
Birmingham, UK

Miss Stella Smith
Specialist Registrar
Department of Surgery
The Royal London Hospital
London, UK

Mr Michael Sugrue
Department of General Surgery
Letterkenny and Galway University Hospital, Ireland

Lieutanant Colonel Nigel Tai RAMC
Consultant in Vascular and Trauma Surgery
Defence Medical Services UK and
Trauma Clinical Academic Unit
The Royal London Hospital
London, UK

Professor Lee Wallis
Professor of Emergency Medicine
Division of Emergency Medicine
Stellenbosch University and University of Cape Town,
South Africa

Mr Michael Walsh
Consultant in Trauma & Vascular Surgery
Director of Trauma Services
Trauma Clinical Academic Unit
The Royal London Hospital
London, UK

Mr Darren Walter
Consultant in Emergency Medicine
Emergency Department
University Hospital of South Manchester
Manchester, UK

Mr Mark Wilson
Specialist Registrar in Neurosurgery and
Pre-Hospital Care
Departments of Neurosurgery and Pre-Hospital Care
The Royal London Hospital and The National Hospital for
Neurology and Neurosurgery
London, UK

Dr David Wise
Consultant in Emergency Medicine and Pre-Hospital Care
Department of Emergency Medicine and
Pre-Hospital Care
The Royal London Hospital
London, UK

The trauma epidemic

The trauma epidemic

Introduction

- Injuries kill 5 million people each year, equating to 9% of worldwide deaths.
- For every death there are many more people who are left disabled.
- Injuries are expected to rise in the next 20 years.
- Globally, injury mortality in males is twice that among women, with the highest rates in Africa and Europe.
- Young people between the ages of 15 and 44 account for approximately 50% of global mortality due to trauma.
- Although injury remains the leading cause of death for young people aged between 15 and 44, individual mortality and morbidity may be higher in the elderly.

Trauma is a worldwide epidemic. The dictionary definitions of 'epidemic' include 'affecting many persons at the same time' and 'extremely prevalent or widespread', and although prevalence of different mechanisms may vary from year to year, injury forms a major cause of death and disability worldwide. A predicted rise in road traffic collisions from its current ninth position (of leading causes of death) by the World Health Organization has been revised in the most recent statistics to rank as fifth in 2030 causing 3.6% of global deaths, accounting for approximating 1.2 million people in predominantly low to middle income countries. Under-reporting of deaths and injuries is widespread, particularly given the socio-economic and geographical distributions of trauma, and in many countries it is extremely difficult to obtain reliable data on, for instance, the number of road traffic fatalities that occur. It should be appreciated that although patterns of traumatic injury are being increasingly studied and understood, particularly from the public health perspective, data is often only available from high-income, developed nations. In 1990, the Harvard School of Public Health and the World Health Organization, commissioned by the World Bank, performed the Global Burden of Disease Study, which found that although registration systems capture about 17 million deaths annually, this probably comprises only about 75% of the total. Regions such as Africa only have data available for approximately 19% of countries, and therefore the true morbidity and mortality due to injury may be much greater than we imagine.

Differences are seen in both the cause and effect of traumatic injury between males and females, between geographical areas and between low, middle, and high-income countries (Fig. 1.1.). Although injury remains the leading cause of death for young people aged between 15 and 44, and children and young people under 25 accounts for over 30% of those injured and killed during road trauma, individual morbidity and mortality may be higher in the elderly. Road trauma is the second leading cause of death from ages 10–14 and from 20 to 24, but is the leading cause of death for the 15–19-year group.

Head and spinal cord injuries form a great proportion of the causes of disability in high-income countries, whereas there is an immense burden of disability in developing countries due to extremity injury alone, suggesting that relatively simple interventions such as improved orthopaedic care and rehabilitation could provide significant benefit and relief to these communities.

Trauma has severe and wide-ranging consequences, both for the individual and for society as a whole. Although acute in onset, the chronic consequences of trauma are those that have debilitating effects in the long term. Despite the obvious emotional devastation of dealing with death due to trauma, it must be recognized that for each death there are many more people who are left disabled. In the Global Burden of Disease Study the concept of Disability Adjusted Life Years (DALYs) was developed. These express not only the years of life lost to premature death, but also years lived with a disability of a specified severity and duration. One DALY is thus one lost year of healthy life, and in 1990 it was calculated that intentional and unintentional injuries caused 10% of mortality worldwide, but 15% of DALYs.

A World Bank report projected that the global road death toll will rise by 66% over the next 20 years, but importantly, this value incorporates a greater divergence between rich and poor nations in the future. An approximate 28% reduction of fatalities is anticipated in high-income countries, but 92% and 147% rises respectively, in fatalities is expected in China and India.

The traditional view that injuries are a result of an 'accident' or a random event is increasingly being challenged with the concept that most injuries are preventable. Strategic approaches have been put in place across the world to study the prevention of injuries and to implement interventions to lessen the injury-related burden of disease. Examples of these range from handgun initiatives, road and water safety education, through to trauma system development. These have been found to be powerful tools to decrease the global burden of traumatic death and disease. Disasters, however, both man-made and natural, continue

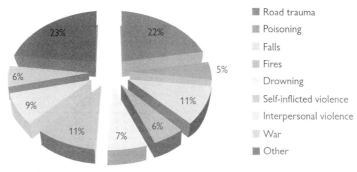

Fig. 1.1. Common causes of trauma.

- Road trauma
- Poisoning
- Falls
- Fires
- Drowning
- Self-inflicted violence
- Interpersonal violence
- War
- Other

to have profound and far-reaching effects and are clearly less amenable to prevention. Examples include the 2004 Indian Ocean earthquake and resultant tsunami whose effects spread over an immense geographical area from the east coast of Africa to Alaska, and caused approximately 230,000 deaths, and the 2008 Sichuan earthquake in China in which 69,181 were confirmed dead, including 68,636 in Sichuan province, and 374,171 injured, with 18,522 listed as missing.

Other potentially preventable factors implicated in many traumatic injuries are the use of alcohol and other drugs, which may precipitate interpersonal violence, youth violence, child and sexual abuse, elder abuse and vehicular accidents. Studies of relationships between volume of drinking and risk of injury have found risk to be positively related to increasing average levels of alcohol intake, with risk increasing at relatively low intake volumes. Other studies have shown repeatedly that alcohol consumption precedes violent events, and that the severity of subsequent violence is related to the amount of drinking. Drug intoxication has been associated with interpersonal violence, self-directed violence and vehicular trauma, although direct causality is difficult to demonstrate. In Rio de Janeiro approximately 10,000 people are involved in the drug trade, many of them children, and almost 4000 minors died of gun-related violence between 1987 and 2001.

Gender has also been demonstrated to have a substantial impact on both the incidence of traumatic injury and the mechanisms by which this occurs. Globally, male injury mortality is, in general, twice that in females, and mortality from road trauma and interpersonal violence is almost three times greater in males. There are exceptions to this rule. However. with, for instance, drowning being almost as common in female children under 4 as in male children, although above this age males form an increasingly large majority. Fire-related mortality is higher in females in some geographical areas, particularly in South East Asia and in the Eastern Mediterranean. This distribution is particularly apparent in elderly people in both areas, but is most pronounced in the Eastern Mediterranean where females have seven times the male risk for burn-related mortality.

The World Health Organization bases its statistical analyses on the concepts of six geographical regions, with the populations defined as high, middle, or low-income levels. The regions are then grouped into High Income Countries (HIC) and Low/Middle Income Countries (LMIC). In 2000, the WHO Global Burden of Disease statistics revealed that injuries accounted for a mortality rate of 83.7/100,000 population, with over 90% of deaths occurring in LMIC. Global deaths from injury rose from 5,101,000 in 1999 to 5,168,000 in 2002 maintaining a ~9% mortality worldwide.

Classification of traumatic injury

The WHO groups injuries into either Intentional or Unintentional, as demonstrated in Fig. 1.2.

Intentional injuries may include those self-inflicted and inflicted as part of an assault; examples being suicide and homicide. Unintentional injuries include traffic-related road trauma, falls, burns, poisonings, and other events that would often be referred to as 'accidents'.

Injuries may be classified according to various scales of severity, determined by anatomy, physiology, postinjuryy function, and signs and symptoms. Examples include the Abbreviated Injury Scale, the Injury Severity Score, the Anatomic Profile, the Revised Trauma Score, the Functional Independence Measure and the International Classification of Diseases (ICD) published by the WHO. This uses a wide variety of signs, symptoms, abnormal findings, complaints, social circumstances, and external causes of injury or disease for classification purposes. ICD 11 was introduced in 2008.

Injury may also be classified by mechanism, which is often an intuitive approach for clinicians, with descriptors such as motor vehicle collisions drowning and gunshot wounds.

Intentional injury

Interpersonal violence

Intentional injury accounted for almost 50% of annual mortality in 2000, with one-quarter of all deaths being due to interpersonal violence and suicides. Almost one-third of all

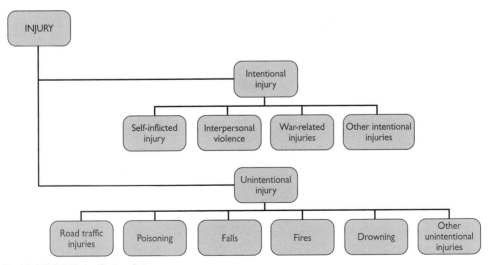

Fig. 1.2. WHO/GBD classification of injury.

deaths took place in the Americas, which also accounted for one-third of the global total DALYs lost to IPV.

The highest rates of violence are found in young males aged between 15 and 29. There are remarkable disparities in the incidence of IPV between areas with disparate income levels, with the LMIC region of the Americas having almost five times the rate of the HIC, at 27.3/100,000 versus 6.1/100,000. A similar picture may be seen in Europe with an HIC incidence of IPV of 1.0/100,000 and an LMIC incidence of 15.4/100,000.

The WHO prediction models suggest that global deaths due to intentional jury will either decrease by 5% by 2030 or increase by 13%. Certainly from 1999 to 2002 intentional injury deaths fell overall from 1689/100,000 to 1618/100,000, but these predictions do not take global population growth into account. The US Census Bureau estimated that there will be an approximate 2.3 billion person increase in global population by 2030, and this increase allows us to gain a true picture of the global trauma epidemic. In the WHO optimistic scenario just under 32 million will die of intentional injury, whereas in the pessimistic scenario there will be total deaths of just over 57 million, approximately equal to the entire population of the United Kingdom.

Homicide and violence

In 2000, males accounted for 77% of all homicides, with rates more than triple that of females, with the rate for females decreasing, but the rate for males increasing. Once again, the raw data gives a frightening picture of the impact of homicide on people and society in a global context, suggesting a decrease in female homicides over a 4-year period of just under 1 million, but an increase in male homicides of 4.25 million in the same period.

Young men characteristically feature heavily in these figures, with the highest rates of homicide seen in 15–29 year old men and the next highest in males aged 30–44, but other factors also play their part. The rates of violent death in LMIC are double that of HIC, except in the United

States of America that, unusually for an established market economy, has a high homicide rate. Although the male homicide rate stayed static at 16/100,000 from the mid-1970s to 1992, and murders using firearms peaked in 1993 to decrease to less than three-quarters of this rate by 2000, the male homicide rates for 15–24-year-old men almost doubled in the same period.

Since the collapse of communism, Russian rates of homicide have increased drastically, and in 1998 were three and a half times those in the USA. The age distribution of murder in Russia is very different to the USA however, with the peak age for victims in America being at 15–24, whereas in Russia there is a further rise to plateau between 35–55 (Figs 1.3 and 1.4).

Suicide

In 2002 the WHO declared that annual suicide numbers were greater than those for war and homicide combined, at approximately 1.5% of total global mortality. The general trend from 1999 was downwards, with a subsequent increase back to the original levels by 2002, but within this there were other disturbing details. Female deaths due to suicide decreased consistently, whereas male rates rose after 2001 to account for the overall rise. In raw figures this equates to a decrease in female deaths by 0.5 million and an increase in male deaths by 1.3 million in the same period.

Age affects suicide rates with over 50% of the global mortality occurring in people between 15 and 44, and over 40% of DALYs lost in a similar age group. Geography and economic status are also significant as there are marked disparities across countries and regions; 86% of all suicides occur in LMIC, with the Western Pacific having the greatest level of suicide deaths in the world. The highest male suicide rates are found in the European region, particularly in European LMIC, but in China the female suicide rate is double that of other parts of the world. Lithuania has the dubious honour of having the world's highest suicide rate at 51/100,000, with Russia second at 40/100,000, against a Western Europe average of 5/100,000.

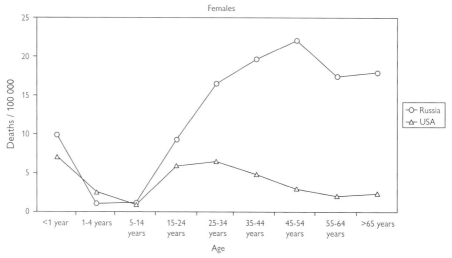

Fig. 1.3. Homicide rates in Russia versus USA among males and females.

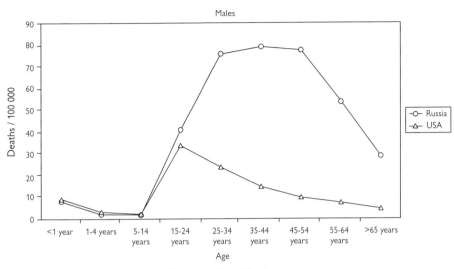

Figs. 1.3 and 1.4. Homicide rates in Russia versus USA among males and females.

War

There were, on average, 11 violent conflicts in any one year of the 1960s, 14 in the 1970s, and at least 50 in 1996. This pattern has led to 22 million people killed and approximately 60 million injured in war or violent conflict since 1945. From 1989 to 1992 only three out of 82 violent conflicts were between nation states with the rest being internal; however, contemporary warfare differs appreciably from wars in the first half of the 20th century, with the aim of modern war being to destabilize the political, cultural, and psychological foundations of the opponent, using exemplary torture, rape, and execution as social intimidation. Weapons designed to maim, rather than kill are used against civilians, as well as combatants, and the battlefield is often extended to the entire society. In the context of these changed aims of warfare it is even more remarkable that between 1999 and 2002 male warfare mortality decreased from 164/100,000 to 155/100,000 per year, but female warfare mortality dropped from 105/100,000 to 17/100,000, which translates in absolute terms to a male mortality reduction of 180,000 per year, but a female mortality reduction of over 5 million per year.

Penetrating injuries cause 90% of combat trauma compared with 20–50% in civilian settings, often caused by small arms fire and commonly from a machine gun or assault rifle, now with muzzle velocities up to 3000 feet per second (fps) and a high probability of scoring multiple hits from close range. Explosive munitions are based on the improved fragmentation principle and are essentially filled with, or composed of, preformed fragments, which cause multiple penetrating wounds.

Civilians in warfare are at escalating risk. War is increasingly being fought in towns and cities, which comprise the 'asymmetric and non-linear' battlefield of the future, rather than in large battles at well-defined fronts. In World War II approximately 50% of the casualties were civilians, in the Vietnam War 80%, and approximately 90% of casualties in modern warfare are civilians. Changes in the conduct of war have also meant that vulnerable areas, such as hospitals and health centres are targeted deliberately and health workers interned or executed. UNICEF data suggests that about 2 million children were killed in war in the 1990s, and 4–5 million were injured or disabled.

The deliberate involvement and targeting of civilian populations has been particularly seen in episodes of genocide or in wars across the world. In 1994 in Rwanda, 800,000 to 1 million Rwandans were slaughtered within 3 months; in Darfur, Sudan the United Nations has estimated that 400,000 have been killed since 2003, and before this 1.9 million civilians were reported dead by the US Committee for Refugees in the Second Sudanese Civil War.

Terrorism

Terrorism is defined as the 'systematic use of violence to create a general climate of fear in a population and thereby to bring about a particular political objective'. Global deaths due to terrorism rose to a peak in the 1980s and then diminished until September 11th 2001 when 19 terrorists linked to Al-Qaeda hijacked four passenger planes, two of which were flown into the twin towers of the World Trade Center in New York. A third plane crashed into the Pentagon and a fourth crashed into rural Pennsylvania after the crew and passengers attempted to regain control of the aircraft. A total of 2973 people were killed in the attacks.

A terrorist bombing in Madrid in 2004 killed 191 people and injured over 1700, and the London bombings of 2005 killed 52 and injured over 700. Asia has seen a consistent rise in terrorist activity in the same period with the toll in South Asia rising from 297 in 2000 to 1164 in 2005, but the Middle East, particularly Iraq, saw a rise in the same period from 62 deaths to almost 6500 in 2005. Despite the consequences of terrorism and its capability to generate publicity, the deaths must be put in context. The Organization for Economic Cooperation and Development (OECD) found over 29 countries that the annual death rate for road trauma was 390 times the annual death rate due to terrorism.

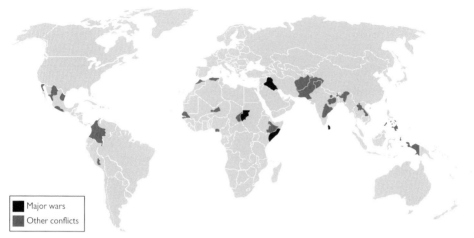

Fig. 1.5. Ongoing military conflict 2009.

Unintentional injury

Motor vehicle collisions

63 million cars were produced worldwide in 2005, and approximately 76 million babies were born, meaning there was almost one car made for each baby born. The predicted rise in motor vehicle collisions (MVCs) from ninth to fifth leading cause of death in 2030, causing approximating 1.2 million deaths in LMIC, has particular implications. Whereas experience in HIC has shown that policy initiatives such as seat belt legislation, child car seats, motorcycle helmets, enforcement programmes, alcohol control policies and traffic calming schemes may produce a rapid decline in deaths associated with MVAs, unfortunately many of these policies are not transferable to LMIC, often because the patterns of injury are different.

Under-reporting of deaths and injuries is widespread, particularly given the socioeconomic and geographical distributions of trauma, and in many countries it is extremely difficult to obtain reliable data on, for instance, the number of MVA fatalities that occur. It must be remembered that although patterns of traumatic injury are being increasingly studied and understood, particularly from the public health perspective, data is often only complete for high-income, developed nations, and only poor and incomplete data being available from the LMIC where the growth in traumatic injury is known to be occurring.

In Asia the highest rates of injury are seen in pedestrians and motorcyclists, whereas in Africa pedestrians and passengers in mass transport are the main problem. In Latin America and the Caribbean pedestrians in urban areas are the biggest concern as, together with people travelling in buses, minibuses and trucks, they have the highest injury risk in crashes, and are often male and of working age. This creates major problems as their loss has the greatest impact not only on their families, but on the country's economy. The high proportion of poor working age males involved means that vulnerable and economically disadvantaged widows and orphans are further victims of these tragedies.

Poisoning

Unintentional poisoning is the sixth most common cause of death in India and the ninth most common in China.

According to WHO data, unintentional poisoning was actually the ninth most common cause of death overall in young adults aged 15–29, with 350,000 dying worldwide in 2000; however poor data collection distorts these estimates.

An estimated 125,000 people each year die from envenomation. The WHO estimates that 2,500,000 people are envenomated each year, but it is important to realize that the mortality from envenomation is not reliant on lethality of venom alone. Mortality is a function of venom lethality combined with geography and medical service provision. Although Australia is home to 10 of the world's most venomous snakes, including the Inland Taipan, which has the world's most toxic venom, there were only 50 deaths from snake envenomation from 1979 to 1998. Vipers in various LMIC, such as Africa and Indonesia are responsible for approximately 50,000 deaths each year, which are a result of venom toxicity, snake aggressiveness, and lack of access to medical care.

Falls and domestic injuries

In 2002, falls were the second highest global cause of unintentional deaths after motor vehicle collisions a 40% rise in the 2 years since 2000. Falls have marked gender, geographical and economic distributions, with a quarter of all fall deaths occurring in HIC, but with males in the LMIC of Europe sharing the highest fall related mortality at 60% with the Western Pacific. Over 40% of fall-related mortality occurs in the over 70s, but 50% of DALYs lost worldwide due to falls are in the under 15s, often in the home.

The home is a common site of unintentional injury. Approximately 4000 victims of home accidents die in the UK every year. This is in the context of an estimated 2.6 million victims of home accident each year visiting Emergency Departments, a problem costing around 30 million annually.

A 1999 Department of Trade and industry report concluded 'Most home accidents happen when people are doing ordinary, everyday things such as going up and down stairs, cooking and gardening, or when children are playing. Only a small proportion of accidents occur when doing obviously hazardous things such as climbing ladders'. Complex interactions between social and economic circumstances, alcohol, tiredness. and safety awareness contribute to many accidents, but human behaviour appears to be the single most common cause. Low levels of income and social deprivation increase the risk of home accidents, along with lone parent households and the presence of two or more smokers. Boys are almost twice as likely as girls to be involved in home or garden accidents.

The direct causes of home accidents are also intriguing; 600,000 people attend UK EDs each year after colliding with each other, and a further 3000 people each year attend after falling over laundry baskets. Do-it-yourself tools are among the most lethal objects involved in home accidents, along with stairs, carpets and kettles of boiling water, but beanbags caused more harm than meat cleavers, and glossy magazines caused four times more accidents than chainsaws.

Occupational injuries
WHO estimates suggest that in 2005 there was a construction industry death somewhere in the world every 10 minutes. The WHO and the International Labour Office (ILO) estimated that although the work-related injury toll reached 2 million in 2005, this was predicted to continue to rise due rapid industrialization in some developing countries. Non-fatal work-related accidents causing at least 3 days if sick time reached 268 million, and the WHO estimated that approximately 4% of the world's Gross Domestic Product is lost each year to workplace accidents and illnesses.

Fires
In 2000, burns were responsible globally for almost 240,000 deaths, and more than 95% occurred in LMIC. Even in HIC burns are a significant problem, with deaths due to fires and burns being the third most common cause of fatal injury at home in the USA in 2006, and being the fifth most common cause of unintentional injury deaths overall. Although European HICs have the lowest worldwide mortality from fire, European LMICs have four times the death rates of their more prosperous neighbours. Africa and South-East Asia have higher mortality again, at over five times and over eight times the European HIC levels. In the USA someone dies from fire every 2 h and someone is injured every 30 mins. This equates, according to estimates by the Center for Disease Control, to 2% of the total cost of injuries or US$7.5 billion.

Smoking is still the leading cause of fire-related deaths, with cooking the main cause of residential fires, and as with most unintentional injuries age, ethnicity, and poverty play a large part in those injured. The young, the old, and the poor are at the most risk.

Drowning
Drowning killed 450,000 people worldwide in 2000 with 97% of deaths occurring in LMIC, rates in China being approximately three times that in Australasia. In 2002, 382,000 people died from drowning worldwide. WHO figures only include 'accidental drowning and submersion' and specifically exclude floods, transport accidents, assaults, and suicide. Drowning was identified as the second commonest cause of unintentional death in children aged 1-4 in the US, the commonest cause of injury related death in children aged 1–14 in China, and children under 5 have the highest mortality rates worldwide of any age group.

Africa, the Western Pacific, and southeast Asia account for 22, 33, and 22%, respectively, of global drowning deaths, with Europe and the USA only accounting for 6.8 and 6%.

This equates to death rates in Africa being more than eight times higher than the USA and Australia, although indigenous populations have higher drowning death rates than Caucasians in both countries.

Children under 5 have the highest drowning mortality rates worldwide, although the mechanism differs between countries, with the commonest places of drowning for Australian children being, first, the domestic swimming pool and, secondly, the bath, whereas in Bangladesh most young children who drown are between 1 and 2 years and die as a result of falls into ditches and ponds. Children account for over half the global mortality due to drowning.

Other risks for drowning are poor education, epilepsy, occupation and alcohol. Bangladeshi mothers with a primary school education alone are at significantly higher risk than better educated mothers, 10% of Swedish epileptics die from drowning, 90% of occupational mortality in Alaskan fishermen is due to drowning, and alcohol is a risk factor for drowning in adolescents and adults, being implicated in 14% of unintentional drowning deaths in Australia.

Disasters
According to data from the International Red Cross and Red Crescent Societies, and the Centre for Research on Epidemiology of Disasters, the risk of disasters is increasing, with a significant increase in the frequency of recorded disasters over the last 50 years, affecting over 2 billion people in the last 10 years. It has been proposed that these increases may be due to such diverse factors as global warming, urbanization, and civil war.

Natural disasters such as earthquakes, hurricanes, cyclones. and tsunamis inflict incalculable losses on populations, not only in terms of immediate death or injury, but in subsequent disease and starvation associated with loss of essential infrastructure. Around 90% of disasters occur in LMIC with an annual per capita income of less than US$760, and thus countries in this group have more disasters coupled with less capacity to cope, plan, and prepare, and the frequency of disasters means that there is often little time for recovery between events. In the Western Pacific there have been 127 major natural disasters described between 1999 and 2000, comprising 20% of the global total and resulting in over 41,000 deaths, almost 450,000 injuries and over 6,000,000 homeless.

Disasters display a trimodal distribution of death similar to serious trauma generally, albeit with a slightly different timescale. The Boxing Day Asian tsunami reportedly caused three phases of injury; the first occurring in the initial few minutes and causing injuries incompatible with life, the second comprising complications over the next few hours from major injury, and later complications such as infectious disease occurring over days to weeks. After the initial phase, medical care is focused on the 'golden 24-h period' during which most casualties are recovered and when most fatalities occur.

The ability of societies to plan ahead has a major influence on the effects of a disaster, which may be exemplified by the differing impacts of the Boxing Day tsunami and Hurricane Katrina. The Boxing Day tsunami occurred following an earthquake measuring 9.3 on the Richter Scale with an epicentre near Sumatra. The resulting tsunamis caused waves up to 30 m high devastating coastlines in 12 countries including Indonesia, Sri Lanka, India, Thailand, Somalia, Bangladesh, Tanzania, and Kenya. Not only did the Boxing Day tsunami kill approximately 187,000 people, but over 40,000 people went missing and an estimated 500,000 people were injured. The tsunami also destroyed infrastructure needed to treat the injured and to enable recovery, including health facilities, and a total of $37 billion was provided as aid by the rest of the world.

Hurricane Katrina was the sixth strongest Atlantic hurricane recorded and the third strongest to landfall in the USA. It devastated much of the north-central Gulf Coast of the USA including New Orleans, Louisiana, and coastal Mississippi, with winds up to175mph and storm surges breaching levees and flooding 80% of New Orleans. Due to the early warning systems developed by the USA, preparations were made that included National Hurricane Centre forecasts in Florida between 20 and 30 h before landfall, activation of a Mississippi Emergency Operations Centre, issuing of evacuation orders to 41 counties and 61 cities, and the establishment of 88 emergency shelters. 80% of the population of metropolitan New Orleans was evacuated. Because of this preparation, the death toll for Hurricane Katrina was limited to 1836 people with 705 missing, although many were injured; and despite this preparation, or perhaps also because of it, the total financial cost was estimated at US$81.2 billion.

Summary

- Injuries are expected to rise in the next 20 years, but comprise almost 10% of the world's deaths at the moment.
- Globally, injury mortality in males is twice that in women.
- People aged 15–44 account for 50% of global trauma mortality.
- Despite injury being the leading cause of death in young people, mortality and morbidity is higher in the elderly.
- Under-reporting of deaths and injury is widespread, particularly in LMIC. Regions such as Africa only have data available from one-fifth of countries.
- Despite the acute onset of trauma, the chronic consequences have debilitating effects in the longer term.

Further reading

Ameratunga S, Hijar M, Norton R. Road-traffic injuries: confronting disparities to address a global health problem. *Lancet* 2006; **367**: 1533–40.

Carrigan TD, Field H, Illingworth RN, Gaffney P, Hamer DW. Toxicological screening in trauma. *J Accid Emerg Med* 2000; **17**: 33–37.

'Casualties of the Wenchuan Earthquake', Sina.com, 8 June 2008-06-08. Retrieved on 8 June 2008-06-08. ([In Chinese),], and "'Earthquake Death Toll Rose to 69,163 as of June 13",', Sina.com, 8 June 2008-06-08. Retrieved on 8 June 2008-06-08. ([In Chinese)].

Centers for Disease Control and Prevention, National Center for Injury Prevention and Control, *Water related injuries fact sheet*. Available fromat: http://www.cdc.gov/print.do?url=http%3A// www.cdc.gov/ncipc/factsheets/drown.htm Geneva,: World Health Organization, 2002.

International Program on Chemical Safety; Poisoning Prevention and Management. Geneva: World Health Organization, 2006.

Krug EG, Dahlberg LL, Mercy JA, Zwi AB, Lozano R. *World report on violence and health. Geneva,*. Geneva: World Health Organization, 2002.

Mathers CD, Loncar D. *Updated projections of global mortality and burden of disease, 2002–2030: data sources, methods and results*. Geneva: World Health Organization, October 2005.

Mock C, Lormand JD, Goosen J, Joshipura M, Peden M. *Guidelines for essential trauma care*. Geneva,: World Health Organization, 2004.

Murray CJL, Lopez AD. Mortality by cause for eight regions of the world: global burdens of disease study. *Lancet* 1997; **349**: 1269–76.

Nantulya VM, Sleet DA, Reich MR, Rosenberg M, Peden M, Waxweiler R. Introduction: The global challenge of road traffic injuries: Can we achieve equity in safety? *Injury Control and Safety Promotion* 2003, Vol. **10**, No. (1–2): pp. 3–7.

National Center for Injury Prevention and Control. *Injury Fact Book 2001–2002*. Atlanta, GA: Center for Disease Control and Prevention; 2001.

Peden M, et al. *The world report on road traffic injury prevention*. Geneva,: World Health Organization, 2004.

Peden M, McKee K, Sharma G. *The Injury Chart Book: a graphical overview of the global burden of injuries*. Geneva, WHO, 2002.

Pridemore WA. Demographic, temporal and spatial patterns of homicide rates in Russia. *Eur Soc Rev* 2003; **19**(1): 41–59.

Sudan: Nearly 2 million dead as a result of the world's longest running civil war, U.S. Committee for Refugees, 2001. Archived 10 December 2004 on the Internet Archive. (Accessed 10 April 2007).

The Trauma Epidemic. In: Greaves I, Porter K, Ryan J, (editors.) *Trauma Care Manual,*. London: Oxford University Press; 2000. pp. 1–10.

Western Australian Department of Health. In: Chamberlain C. (ed.) *Disaster Preparedness and Management: Health Protection Group. Chamberlain C, Ed. Disaster Medical Assistance Teams: A Literature Review*. Perth, WA : WADH. April 2006. Available at: http://www.health.wa.gov.au/disaster/DMAT/index/disaster %20assistance%20teams%20literature%20review%202006.pdf (accessed April 2006).

WHO Department of Mental Health and Substance Abuse. *Global. Status Report on Alcohol 2004*. Geneva: World Health Organization, 2004.

WHO.*Number of work-related accidents and illnesses continue to increase*. Geneva: World Health Organization, 2006. Available fromat: http://www.who.int/mediacentre/news/releases/2005/ pr18/en/index.html. Accessed (accessed 12th November 2006).

Wikipedia contributors. Terrorism. Wikipedia, The Free Encyclopedia. September 30, 2006, 00:13 UTC. Available at: http://en.wikipedia.org/wiki/Terrorism. (Accessed accessed October 23, 2006).

World Health Report. *Statistical Annex*. Geneva: World Health Organization, Geneva 2008.

Pre-hospital emergency care

Pre-hospital emergency care

The provision of the pre-hospital trauma care varies greatly between different countries and across regions. However, they all share common elements in order to provide an emergency medical responder to an incident scene and to treat any casualties.

Emergency medical systems

The phrase Emergency Medical Services (EMS) reflects the evolution of the ambulance service from a purely transportation service to one that provides medical care as soon as possible on scene after a call for medical assistance has been made. In many countries, an abbreviated emergency phone number is used to call for help; this number may also be shared with other emergency services, such as fire, police, and coastguard. In the United Kingdom this is the 999 system, although the European Union uses 112.

The objectives of an EMS are:
- To provide prioritization of emergency calls.
- Allocate resources that are appropriate to the medical emergency.
- Dispatch appropriate resources.
- Provide emergency treatment on scene.
- Transport patients to the nearest or most appropriate hospital, as required.
- Handover patients to the receiving medical facility.

An EMS must have the following components to effectively operate:
- Headquarters.
- Emergency Operations Centre (EOC).
- Emergency Dispatch, usually within EOC.
- Communications infrastructure.
- Deployable units (ambulances).
- Clinical personnel [emergency medical technicians (EMT), paramedics, emergency care practitioners (ECP), nurses and doctors)].
- Support services (engineers, logistics, training, administration).
- Standard operating procedures/clinical guidelines.
- Specialist units [Hazardous Area Response Teams (HART) and specialist medical teams].

The competencies and skills mix of the emergency responders vary between countries. The US and UK models favour a deployable EMT or paramedic team, while the continental European model often deploys a physician. In the UK, there are also charity and partially state-funded pre-hospital schemes that deploy advanced medical teams with physician input. Some schemes rely on self-deployment, while others are embedded in the ambulance EOC.

Emergency planning

In addition to the management of individual casualties, EMS must be able to respond to extra-ordinary incidents, such as major incidents, including mass casualties and contingency operations. This responsibility has recently been legislated for in the UK by the Civil Contingencies Act 2004 which nominates Acute Ambulance Trusts as 'Category One Responders' with certain specific on-scene responsibilities.

Emergency medical dispatch

The allocation of finite ambulance resources requires some form of prioritization. Precise methods vary, but the systems in use widely across the UK uses a number of factors to determine the urgency of a 999 call whether a trauma or non-trauma presentation, these include:
- Type of incident (e.g. single casualty, major incident).
- Presenting complaint (e.g. chest pain).
- Age of patient (e.g. <1 year).
- Determinants (unresponsive, breathing difficulty, fitting, injury to areas of the body associated with particular risks, serious blood loss).

Computer-directed questioning and algorithms are often used with non-clinical staff asking questions of the caller making the 999 call. One system known as the Advanced Medical Priority Dispatch System (AMPDS) uses the above factors to prioritize the patient into three main categories (A, B, and C), which may then be further subdivided (see Table 2.1). EMS may then be given dispatch target timings to ensure a timely response, sometimes called ORCON. Currently urban UK ambulance services must arrive at the patient within 8 min for the highest priority cases.

Trauma call out criteria

As well as systems like AMPDS, other systems may be used to identify patients, including trauma patients that may benefit from additional clinical resources. Significant trauma cases may be difficult to identify using the criteria and algorithms, that are used more as a resource management tool for multiple calls and differing presenting complaints. Automated emergency dispatch systems lack the sensitivity and specificity for appropriate advance resource allocation. For this reason, some EMS use clinical staff embedded within the EOC, or relies on requests for additional resources once the first responders have arrived on scene. The latter has the significant disadvantage of an inherent delay.

A variety of criteria are used by a number of ambulance services to dispatch advanced medical resources. These criteria may include:
- Request by first responder(s).
- Fall from height.
- Road traffic collision with fatality.
- Road traffic collision with occupant ejected.
- Casualty under a train.

Table 2.1. Advanced Medical Priority Dispatch System

AMPDS	Definition	Category
RED 1	Actual death imminent	A
RED 2	Possible death imminent	
RED 3	Risk of death imminent	
AMBER 1	Definitely serious, not immediately life-threatening	B
AMBER 2	Possibly serious, not immediately life-threatening	
GREEN 1	Requiring assessment and/or transport	C
GREEN 2	Suitable for telephone triage and/or advice	

- Amputation above wrist or ankle.
- Penetrating injury to torso or junctional area.
- Significant head injury.
- Fall under horse.
- Hanging.
- Drowning.
- Other non-AMPDS features.

Pre-hospital team composition

The composition of pre-hospital teams, routine, or advanced, may vary depending on a number of factors. These include:
- Trauma epidemiology.
- Resources including availability of clinical staff.
- Urban or rural.
- Distance to nearest receiving hospital(s).
- Distance to nearest trauma centre.
- Ground or air transportation.
- Skills of the first responders.
- Requirement for advanced clinical skills including airway management, analgesia, and emergency thoracotomy.

Medical emergency response incident teams

These teams, also known as MERIT, have evolved from Mobile Medical Teams. Although primarily intended for use during a major incident, their skills may also be applied to any pre-hospital emergency situation. The composition of these teams may very regionally and they may be staffed by local hospitals or from pre-hospital care schemes. Skills are likely to include airway and rapid sequence induction, surgical management, and some major incident command and control training.

Air ambulances

Most UK regions utilize some form of air ambulance. The concept of the air ambulance goes back to the Korean War although the airframe used at that time required the casualties to be transported on the outside and, therefore, little in-flight medical intervention was possible. The current use of airframes for patient transportation has a number of models depending on the acute care requirements of the local population and geography. The majority of UK air ambulance services have the capacity to carry only one patient.

Generic air ambulance

This model uses paramedic staffing, although with additional aviation training. It provides remote paramedic assistance and a form of patient transport using the airframe to cover distance and arrive at the receiving medical facility in the shortest time. This is frequently used in a rural area with long distances or rugged terrain.

Helicopter emergency medical service

This aviation model uses an advanced medical team (often a physician-paramedic team). The team offer advanced medical skills including airway management, anaesthesia, and trauma care skills.

Air search and rescue (SAR)

This service has historically been provided by the Armed Forces (Royal Navy and Royal Air Force in the UK). The service covers sea or mountainous terrain with a winch capability to either extract a casualty or insert a rescuer. The provision of medical care varies between services, some using a trained medic with SAR skills, while others use a crewman with advanced first aid skills.

HM coastguard

HM Coastguard is part of the civil Maritime and Coastguard Agency (MCA). It has a responsibility for SAR over sea although this sometimes includes inland waterways, estuaries, and areas of flooding. The airframes also have a winch capability and the capacity to carry a number of casualties.

Military EMS

Current operational military EMS aims to provide advanced trauma care to the casualty as soon as possible. For planning purposes, especially in large conflicts, the concept of the 1:2:4 timeline is used. This represents the time (hours) by which a casualty should reach a higher level of trauma care.
- Battlefield Advanced Trauma Life Support (BATLS).
- Damage control surgery (DCS).
- Primary surgery.

Within the 1:2:4 timeline, there are a number of treatment algorithms which are used depending on the medical facility and the permissibility of the environment. For non-permissive environments, such as during active combat, treatment is limited to self-help and buddy aid. This focuses on the management of catastrophic haemorrhage and basic airway management (*care under fire*) (Fig. 2.1). Semi-permissive trauma care is termed *tactical field care* and reflects the limitations of pre-hospital care in a combat zone. Advanced trauma care can be provided at Role One facilities (Regimental Aid Post). The Role One facility will be manned by a medical officer with a team of combat medical technicians or medical assistants.

Role Two + medical facility

This facility will prove casualty reception, damage control resuscitation and damage control surgery. The holding capacity will be limited and it will rely on casualty evacuation to a larger Role 3 facility with greater specialty provision, or a UK Role 4 facility with full definitive care.

Military air ambulance

Current military operations use the CH-47 (Chinook) and EH101 (Merlin) airframes for casualty evacuation from the front line. In addition to carrying a senior and experienced medical team, the airframes are able to carry multiple casualties and are essentially flying casualty clearing stations. Unlike the civilian air ambulance treatment paradigm of optimization and stabilization prior to transport, treatment is generally not provided on the ground by the deployed military medical team. In-flight trauma management consist of triage, life-saving interventions, analgesia, and rapid transport to the most appropriate medical facility (which may be multinational).

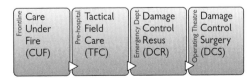

Fig. 2.1. Chain of trauma survival.

Scene safety

General safety considerations

When working within the pre-hospital setting, safety is paramount and training prior to tasking should reflect the likely hazards encountered and associated risks based upon their likelihood and consequences. In addition to specific hazards, there may be general hazards associated with most missions. The greatest risk for emergency services remains the risk of a transportation accident whether on the ground, in the air or water *en route* to an incident. Depending on the method of tasking, there is the potential for those conveying the medical team to be so focussed on the incident details that they are unable to concentrate on safe transport, and are therefore subject to so-called 'red mist'. This is associated with the combined stress of the knowledge of the incident and the driving or piloting to the scene. In these circumstances additional errors occur due to mission priority. Examples include the decision to exceed speed limits or to fly after a cut-off time determined by safe light levels.

Personal protective equipment (PPE)

In addition to safety training, pre-hospital care providers should be issued and wear appropriate personal safety equipment. Equipment includes:
- High visibility and resistant clothing.
- Clothing appropriate to the season or temperature.
- Protective footwear with metal insoles.
- Appropriate gloves (clinical contact and debris protection).
- Protective eyewear.
- Helmet.
- Torch and additional lighting.
- Stab vest with ballistic protection, as required.
- Dust mask (FFP3 specification).
- Ear protection.
- Personal alarm or radio.

Environmental factors

During any tasking, it is important to consider the ambient conditions and any specific environmental factors. During some prolonged incidents, the conditions may significantly change, and should be anticipated.

Ambient temperature

Temperatures may vary even in the same region and season. Clothing is important and additional items may need to be carried if a change in conditions is expected. Extreme temperatures may be expected in rural areas; however they do occur in urban situations as well. In some cities, underground rail systems rely on train movement to provide ventilation. When there is a failure, ambient temperature and humidity may increase rapidly.

Lighting

A torch and additional lighting should be carried in case of dark environments or night working. It will take time for vision to adapt to working in the dark, and this night vision may be lost by exposure to bright lights. Where possible, red light should be used.

Working at height

Working at height is a common pre-hospital hazard and specific training includes the use of harnesses, fall arrest devices, and specialized stretchers.

Special considerations

Part of pre-hospital training includes the recognition of specific circumstances, and the hazards and risks that are associated with them.

Road traffic collisions

There are a number of hazards that are associated with road traffic collisions. They include:
- Continuing traffic movement.
- Fuel leakage.
- Delayed airbag deployment.
- Unstable structures.
- Sharp objects, glass and debris, especially after fire and rescue extraction.
- Dangerous cargo.

Safe practices include:
- Appropriate PPE (helmet, debris gloves, goggles).
- Restricting traffic movement (police).
- Hazard management (hosing or sanding of fuel leaks).
- Isolation of car batteries (follow advice from fire and rescue).
- Deactivation of airbag system.
- Shoring and blocking of unstable vehicles.
- Look for any hazard diamonds and information if hazardous cargo.

Violent incidents

Any incident involving an alleged assault should be considered to be hazardous due to the potential for continuing and escalating violence. Stab vests with ballistic protection should be worn and a police escort or rendezvous point (RVP) sought. Patients who may appear to be the victim should also be considered as potentially hostile and checked for weapons.

Safe practices include:
- Appropriate PPE (stab vest).
- Police escort or RVP.
- Check patient for any weapons.

Psychiatric patients

Psychiatric patients, especially suicidal patients, may be hostile to medical intervention, or frankly psychotic. There is a clear duty of care to treat these patients and, in this case, consideration should be given to de-escalation or sedation using appropriate techniques. Patients should also be checked for any potential weapons and if escorted should be directed to walk in front. In the presence of a Police Officer, Section 136 of the Mental Health Act can be used in a public place. Psychosocial management should be concurrent with medical and trauma care.

Safety Triggers for Emergency Personnel (STEP) 1-2-3

The presence of hazards including harmful chemicals such as carbon monoxide should be considered, if more than one patient presents or is found with the same or unexplained presenting complaint. STEP 1-2-3 consists of:
- One casualty: Proceed as usual.
- Two casualties: Use caution and report.
- Three or more casualties: **Do not approach!**

Chemical, biological, radiological and nuclear (CBRN)

CBRN and hazardous materials (HazMat) incidents are considered in detail in Chapter 25. Scene Assessment should include looking for any hazard diamonds.

Electrical incidents

In most cases, the emergency call will suggest that there is an electrical hazard. However, there are cases of unexplained collapse, for example, in which electrocution should be considered. It is important to be aware that patients may have been thrown some distance from the electrical hazard. On assessing the scene, responders should look for any obvious electrical appliance or bare cabling. Water should be avoided. The Fire & Rescue Service may need to locate and isolate the mains supply before safe entry is permitted. Any electrical fires should be extinguished by carbon dioxide extinguishers.

Collapsed buildings

When working near a collapsed building it is important of be aware of potential hazards. These include:
- Further collapse and crush injuries.
- Fractured gas mains.
- Electrical hazards (see above).
- Asbestos and other particulate material.

  Safe practices include:
- Appropriate PPE (helmet, face mask).
- Identify fire & rescue lead.
- Identify building or site manager.
- Isolate building utilities.
- Decontaminate if possible asbestos.

Confined spaces

Confined spaces, such as sewers, may present a number of hazards and risks to first responders. In addition to the physical constraints a confined space may impose on any casualty management, confined spaces may have their own risks especially if there is more than one casualty (Think STEP 1-2-3):
- Oxygen displacement by heavier gases, such as methane.
- Toxic gases such as hydrogen sulphide.
- Flooding.
  Safe practices include:
- Seeking advice from Fire & Rescue.
- Casualties rescued by personnel in Class A (gas tight with own air supply) PPE.
- Ventilation of the confined space.
- Confirmation of the presence of breathable atmosphere, i.e. oxygen presence and absence of toxic gases.

Rail incidents

Rails incidents are common across the country, although safety issues vary depending on terrain and urbanization. Some incidents may be due to the deliberate act of a suicidal individual and involve one casualty, while other incidents may be due to derailing or collision.
  Key hazards include:
- Moving rail stock (even after loss of electrical current).
- Live rail electrical current.
- Overhead electrical current.
- Confined space if dealing with 'one-under'.
- Moving points (moving mechanisms at junctions).

  Safe practices include:
- Identify multi-agency leads, esp. rail representative(s).
- Use of similar command concepts as for a major incident, if the incident is complex and multi-agency.
- Confirming that electrical current is off both verbally and visually using short circuit device (SCD) indicators.
- Being aware of the potential hazards of parallel line working [multiple networks (regional and metropolitan line operators)].
- Being aware that a surviving one-under patient may be psychologically unwell.

Water (maritime) incidents

Incidents involving water are likely to involve environmental factors and injuries including hypothermia and near-drowning. These incidents are often associated with rescuers becoming casualties. Key agencies involved in water rescue include:
- Maritime and Coastguard Agency (co-ordination role).
- Royal National Lifeboat Institution (inland and coastal).
- RAF Search and Rescue.
- Royal Navy Search and Rescue.
- Royal Navy (at sea).
- Various lifeguard services (beaches).
- Fire and Rescue Services (inland waters/canals).

  Safe practices include:
- Avoiding becoming a secondary (rescuer) casualty.
- Use of lifelines or human chains, if essential (risk).
- Being aware of hazards associated with frozen bodies of water.
- Remembering the possibility of traumatic injuries (head and neck injuries), as well as near-drowning, especially if the casualty has fallen into shallow water or off a structure (swimming pool, bridge, pier).

Aviation safety

As many pre-hospital organizations either deploy as or work with an air ambulance, it is important to have an awareness of aviation safety.

Safe approach to helicopter

Most helicopter landing sites (HLS) will be temporary either on scene or close to a receiving hospital with few facilities having dedicated helicopter pads. Any safe HLS must have a diameter twice the diameter of the helicopter rotor disc. The site should be physically secure and clear of any potential objects that may become flying hazards in the downdraft.

  Once the aircraft has landed, it SHOULD NOT BE APPROACHED. In general, the crew will meet anyone approaching the aircraft and escort them. All aircraft have a safe route of approach, but there is significant variation with some being from the front while others are from the rear. Again, the crew will escort any responders.

Crew resource management

Safe working practices developed for the air industry (NASA) have significant application to clinical risk management for medical specialties where errors may be due to human factors and stress resulting in catastrophic consequences. Examples include obstetrics, anaesthesia, surgery, resuscitation, and pre-hospital care. In the medical context, CRM is sometimes referred to as Crisis Resource Management. Areas of practice development and training include the recognition of stress, communication skills, system design, and team work.

Air Incidents

In the event of an air crash, there are additional hazards. Some aircraft are made from man-made mineral fibres (MMMF) and following an air crash these will be a serious respiratory hazard.

Air fuel will also be a significant hazard especially during a crash during take-off where the aircraft is likely to be carrying full tanks. As with any transportation accident there may be dangerous cargo.

Scene and casualty assessment

An experienced pre-hospital practitioner should be able to assess an incident scene and, in conjunction with the clinical assessment of the casualty, identify life-threatening conditions and suspect more occult injuries. The gold standard of care within the pre-hospital environment is the timely conveyance of an optimized casualty to the most appropriate receiving hospital; this includes the treatment of any immediate life-threatening conditions. At the patient handover, one of the roles of the pre-hospital practitioner is the description and interpretation of the incident scene using verbal, written and, in some cases, photographic information.

Scene assessment

The scene assessment starts with the incident type. This is important, not only for patient management, but also personal safety. The incident type will determine the selection of appropriate PPE, as well as helping to anticipate the clinical picture.

On arrival on scene, any hazards should be sought and the scene assessed for the mechanism of injury. For each type of incident, there are important indications that may suggest significant trauma.

Road traffic collision

• Head on collision.
• Lack of seat belt use.
• Intrusion into compartment.
• Associated ejection from vehicle.
• Associated death in incident.
• Damage to steering wheel.

Pedestrian v vehicle collision

• Bulls eye to windscreen (height may also suggest speed of impact).
• Indentation into bonnet and bumper.

Other

• Fall from a height greater than 2 floors.

Some signs on scene are, however, unreliable, and should be interpreted with caution. Examples include:
• Low speed impacts that do not exclude significant trauma.
• Estimated blood loss on scene, which are often underestimated.
• Length of penetrating weapons (often poorly judged).

Patient assessment

Trauma can generally be differentiated into four main types: blunt, penetrating, blast, and burns. Each type of injury has a slightly different casualty management paradigm (see next section). Some incidents are more complex with a mixture of injury types. Examples are given below of the main incident types:
• *Blunt:* road traffic collision (RTC), fall from height.
• *Penetrating:* knife attack, shooting, impalement.
• *Blast:* explosive mechanism may include elements of blunt and penetrating injuries.
• *Burns:* fire, scalding, explosions (quaternary blast injuries), chemical burns, cold (freezing) injuries.

Blunt injuries

Blunt injuries are often associated with occult injuries especially if there is a significant transfer of energy. On comparing two road traffic collisions, one might expect high speed collisions to be associated with a relatively higher incidence of major trauma. However, in many cases the transfer of energy is over a longer period of time or distance, i.e. roll over or impact with a crash barrier at 70 mph. A relatively greater risk of significant injury may occur at lower speeds if there is a sudden impact and deceleration, for example, a head-on collision or impact into a tree at 40 mph. Road traffic collisions (RTCs) may also lead to entrapment and risk of crush injuries. Complications of blunt injuries include occult torso injuries (aortic dissection, covert bleeding, and contusions), closed head injury with reduced level of consciousness, pelvic, and spinal trauma, and long bone fractures.

Penetrating injuries

Penetrating injuries will usually have an obvious entry wound, although some can be discrete (buttock stab wound, scalp wound). Exit wounds may not be present or be mistaken for entry wounds. The main life-threatening conditions following a penetrating injury are hypovolaemia (overt or covert), tension pneumothorax and cardiac tamponade. Many penetrating injuries to the torso, especially high velocity gunshot wounds, are non-survivable. However, even in cardiac arrest some are salvageable with rapid recognition and immediate intervention (thoracocentesis, thoracostomy, and emergency thoracotomy). With rapid first aid and medical intervention, penetrating wounds to the limbs should be survivable.

Blast injuries

Blast injuries will be discussed in detail in chapter 24. The pre-hospital implications of blast injuries are the association with multiple casualties, scene safety, and the potential for the scene to be locked down as a crime scene. Casualty patterns include the full range of injuries including penetrating, blunt, and potentially burns. Key pre-hospital issues are the management of traumatic amputations, life-threatening chest injuries, and possible long extrication times and management of crush injuries.

Burns

The presence of burns patients on scene may present logistical issues, especially if critical care services are required. On scene assessment of the casualty should include an estimation of total body surface area involvement that will inform any decision on the most appropriate receiving hospital. Specialist burns beds are a finite resource within the UK and triage may need to balance the immediate clinical issues and stabilization with the long-term specialist management requirements.

Handover of scene information

Handover of the patient to the receiving hospital should include a detailed description of the scene and any useful observations. In many cases, the pre-hospital team will have had more experience of these casualty types. The interpretation of the scene and the casualty's initial injuries may help guide the further hospital management and investigation. Written handover should be given and, where possible, diagrams, or photographs of the scene.

Initial casualty management

The aims of pre-hospital trauma management are to:
- Treat any life-threatening injuries.
- Optimize oxygen delivery to vital organs.
- Prevent or anticipate deterioration or complications.
- Provide analgesia.
- Reduce on scene time to an appropriate minimum.
- Transfer and handover the patient to an appropriate receiving hospital.

Managing life-threatening injuries

The <C> ABCDE treatment algorithm should be used, encompassing control of catastrophic haemorrhage (<C>), establishment and maintenance of a patent airway with cervical spine control (A), identification and management of life-threatening chest injuries (B, breathing), assessment and management of circulatory problems (C), assessment of disability (D) and limited exposure and control of environment (E).

The following conditions are examples of life-threatening injuries that may require on scene management (some conditions are not included as they require hospital management facilitated by a rapid pre-hospital transfer):

Catastrophic haemorrhage
Catastrophic haemorrhage typically results from the disruption of a major blood vessel(s). This may be due to a traumatic amputation or penetrating injury involving a major vein or artery.

Treatment includes:
- Direct pressure to the bleeding point or amputation stump.
- Proximal control of the blood vessel either by direct pressure or a tourniquet.
- Application of novel haemostatic dressings.
- Rapid transfer to hospital and theatre.

Airway and cervical spine immobilization
Airway compromise may be due to either a problem with patency or protection. This may be due directly to an airway obstruction or indirectly due to a poor level of consciousness. Airway obstruction must be managed immediately and may require anything from a simple airway manoeuvre to definitive airway insertion. It is also important to anticipate any airway complications or deterioration, especially in cases of airway burns, reduced level of consciousness and vomiting in an immobilized patient. This is important if there is a significant transfer time to the receiving hospital. With airway management comes c-spine risk assessment and immobilization as required.

Treatment includes:
- Optimization of the airway with basic airway manoeuvres and adjuncts.
- Consideration of rapid sequence induction (RSI) of anaesthesia and intubation depending on status of patient.

Breathing and oxygen
Optimization of oxygen delivery includes the maintenance of adequate oxygenation and ventilation. Life-threatening conditions include:
- Airway obstruction.
- Flail chest segment.
- Tension pneumothorax (cardiovascular compromise also).
- Massive haemothorax.
- Open chest wound.

Treatment includes:
- Airway management (see above).
- Decompression of tension pneumothorax.
- Chest drain insertion.
- Application of one way valve dressing to open wound.

Circulation
Circulatory collapse may occur for a number of reasons—haemorrhage, pump failure including cardiac tamponade, cardiovascular obstruction (e.g. tension pneumothorax) and distributive disorder (e.g. neurogenic shock).

Treatment priorities include:
- Establishment of venous access with large bore cannulae.
- Haemorrhage control (see above).
- Judicious use of crystalloid, titrated to endpoint, such as palpable radial pulse, systolic of 90 mmHg (unless head injury in which case higher) or appropriate cerebral function. This permissive hypotension may prevent clot disruption and dilution of clotting factors.
- Rapid transport to hospital and theatre.

Disability
The main aims of pre-hospital trauma management for head and spinal trauma are to prevent secondary injuries and transfer the patient to the most appropriate hospital usually with on-site neurosurgical cover.

Treatment includes:
- Optimization of oxygenation, ventilation, and perfusion.
- Prevention of any period of hypotension, hypercapnia, or hypoxia.
- Rapid transfer to appropriate hospital with neurosurgical cover.

Scoop and run v stay and play
Rapid on-scene decision-making is vital and this is often within the first minute of assessment of the scene and casualty. In general, a patient either needs immediate transfer to hospital and surgery with optimization en route (scoop and run) or a period on scene and optimization prior to transfer. Penetrating trauma with cardiovascular compromise should fall into the former group. Patients that are likely to require and tolerate a longer transfer to a specialist unit, e.g. for head injury or burn management may need to be packaged and optimized so that the risk of deterioration en route is reduced and mitigated.

Management of traumatic cardiac arrest
The outcome of cardiac arrest in trauma is usually very poor, especially in blunt trauma. Some injuries are incompatible with life, and death is often instantaneous. However, there are a small group of patients that even in cardiac arrest are salvageable. Conditions that are rapidly reversible include:
- Airway obstruction.
- Tension pneumothorax.
- Cardiac tamponade.

For this reason, if the medical team arrives early (within 10 min of arrest) the following interventions should be considered:
- Airway management with ventilation.
- Bilateral thoracostomies.
- Consider emergency thoracotomy, if tamponade suspected.

Communications

Communication skills, both verbal and non-verbal, are important. Good skills allow for rapid passage of information between pre-hospital teams and members, as well as the receiving hospital (see Fig.2.2). Failure of communication may lead to loss of information, and at worse, clinical error and increased risk to the patient and even the pre-hospital team.

Communication may be provided by a number of modalities including telecommunications. Some organizations may also utilize remote medical advice (telemedicine) with the transmission of clinical information, digital photography, and ECGs. Advances in telecommunication have meant that there are a number of communication methods available in addition to the traditional verbal and written information. These different methods can be compared for both routine pre-hospital communication and during a major incident.

Face to face verbal

For rapid communication on scene, face-to-face verbal communication remains the mainstay. However, there may be times when there are constraints. Examples include noisy environments, such as the roadside, on board an aircraft and during a public disturbance. Additional clues to the verbal message include non-verbal signs such as lip-reading, hand gestures, and general body language. In some cases, pre-defined signals can be agreed within the team, as well as using drills for common procedures (casualty handling, analgesia dosing). This all forms part of crisis (crew) resource management.

While verbal communication is the most common form of pre-hospital communication, it does not remove the requirement to maintain good written notes. These may in the future be used to refer back to during court appearances and other medico-legal proceedings. The general adage applies that 'if it wasn't written down, it didn't happen'.

Very high frequency radio

Very high frequency (VHF) is a range of radio waves that are used widely for beyond line of sight communication. Registered frequencies are used as radio channels assigned to specific emergencies services and may reflect a role (emergency channel, major incident channel) or region of that service's response. One channel may be used to operate a number of deployed units, each with its own call-sign. While verbal communication is possible, two-way communication cannot happen simultaneously. It is therefore necessary to have voice procedures that include use of the phonetic alphabet and established etiquette to maintain an effective capability during times of high demand. The limitations of VHF are that the finite number of radio channels may become congested (jammed) during events such as a major incidents or even periods of high information exchange (complex medical cases and two-way advice).

Ultra-high frequency radio

Similar to VHF, this range of radio is used for on scene communication between services with only line of sight capability. With a reduced range, the same frequency may be used in a number of areas as long as they are a sufficient distance away. Communication is likely to be between team members of the same service. This allows for more relaxed and specific voice procedures and less risk of jamming.

Pager

Pagers work as a one-way communication device, but with greater resilience during periods of high demand. There are a number of pager networks. Some use internal transmitters within an organization and are confined to a relatively limited radius from the parent organization (hospital pager system). Other networks use national providers and have greater range. The disadvantage of most paging systems is that communication is one-way and a reply will

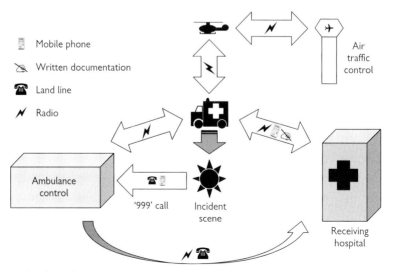

Mobile phone

Written documentation

Land line

Radio

Air traffic control

Ambulance control

'999' call

Incident scene

Receiving hospital

Fig. 2.2. Summary of pre-hospital communications.

require another communication method. There is also no formal acknowledgement that the message has either been received or acted upon.

Terrestrial telephone network

Landline telephone networks provide two-way and in some cases allow multiple (teleconference) conversations. As most lines are not shared, there is no need for rigid etiquette and two-way communication may be simultaneous (although not necessarily productive). There is no requirement for formal training in phone procedures, although phonetic spelling may still be required. Multiple phone numbers also allow for a large communication network (locally, nationally, and internationally). Landlines, however, are geographically fixed with limited mobility (~10 m).

Mobile phone

In the last decade the sophistication and miniaturization of mobile phones has led to their ubiquitous use by pre-hospital care organizations. Some organizations use mobile phones for dispatch and providing additional mission information that may not be easy or efficient to convey by radio or data communications. The chief benefits of mobile phones are relative ease of use with little training burden, two-way communication without the need for voice procedure training and additional resources such as data transmission for the uploading of pictures to the receiving hospital. Disadvantages of the mobile phone include loss of the mobile network or limitation to text messaging only. This is an area of frequent criticism of the mobile phone adding to a less resilient communications network during significant events (medical provision during New Year's Eve) and major incidents (London Bombings, July 2005). One control measure available to strategic (gold) commanders is the ACCess OverLoad Control (ACCOLC) system. ACCOLC allows specific phone networks within a localized area to be shutdown so that only ACCOLC registered phones used by the emergency services may work. Initiation of the system has significant implications for both unregistered emergency service phones, as well as public use of the mobile phone network.

SMS text messaging

SMS or text messaging is a more resilient form of mobile phone communication using less bandwidth than voice communication. During periods of high communication usage, SMS communication may be more effective for short messages or pieces of information. During routine use, SMS may be useful for passing on small data packages such as postcode or telephone numbers.

Digital radio network

Communications have remained one of the weaknesses in a major incident for decades, with many inquiries, including those for Clapham Common, Hillsborough, and the 2005 London Bombings, highlighting deficiencies. Failings include poor resilience, lack of multi-agency interoperability and poor links between the scene and the receiving hospital(s). Many forms of communication are lost once the user goes underground either into a deep basement or transportation system.

More resilient communication networks are being developed using digital technologies. If proven, advantages of the system will include voice communication either one-to-one or as a group, high bandwidth data communications and intra-operability. The network requires the establishment of the infrastructure, equipment and training.

Aircraft communications

Since many pre-hospital organizations use or liaise with air ambulances, it is important to understand the additional communications required to operate these services safely. Most air ambulances will have access to a designated ambulance dispatch channel as part of the communications array onboard. Mobile phones will usually be turned off due to potential interference.

Additional channels available to the pilot are the air band frequencies. These allow for direct communication between the aircraft and air traffic control (ATC). During a medical mission, the pilot may need to change between different air traffic controls depending on the complexity of the air space management and proximity to airfields. Additional non-verbal data communication may include navigational data especially during periods of poor visibility including at night as well as mission data depending on dispatch method. This parallels the systems used for police air services.

Written including handover

Written communication in the form of notes provides not only a continuous clinical record, but can be used to justify clinical decision-making and as evidence to support those decisions either as recorded observations or as a monitor print off. Written notes should be legible, timed, dated and signed. Written information including drawings may also be used to convey information that may not be passed effectively verbally (handover in a noisy environment). This includes scene diagrams and body maps including positions of wounds and interventions. An additional role for local written communication is as a redundancy for other communication failures during a major incident. Messages can be passed on using runners.

A handover, whether verbal or written should include mechanism of injury, injuries found or suspected, clinical observations, treatment given and any outstanding issues. For patients that are not fully conscious, or may have been sedated or anaesthetized, any medical history or allergies should also be passed on if known. An opportunity should be given for any additional questions from the receiving trauma team.

Initial assessment

Initial assessment

Why carry out an initial assessment?

Trauma is a multi-system phenomenon, which does not respect anatomical boundaries and which can involve multiple systems. While certain mechanisms of injury can suggest specific injury patterns, the unexpected should be expected. The purpose of the initial assessment is to quickly identify all significant injuries, whether obvious or occult. At the same time threats to life and limb are treated immediately, further deterioration is prevented through appropriate intervention, necessary investigations and ongoing management are instituted, and transfer to definitive care is arranged.

Anatomical and physiological injury go hand-in-hand, and both must be addressed. Obvious anatomical injury can be simple to diagnose. However, occult injury can be life-threatening, and subtle injury can be disabling in later life if not recognized early. As far as physiology is concerned, the aim should be not only to correct clinically obvious manifestations of traumatic injury such as hypoxia and gross hypoperfusion, but to anticipate and manage the more insidious problems of acidosis, coagulopathy and hypothermia. These have a critical role in late morbidity and mortality but are often already present in the pre-hospital and emergency department phases of care.

The components of the initial assessment

There are several variations on the same theme of initial assessment of the trauma patient. Current thinking supports the <C>BCDE paradigm, a development of the long established protocol espoused by the Advanced Trauma Life Support (ATLS®) course, which since its inception 30 years ago has aimed to standardize the initial assessment of the trauma patient, and give some structure to the management to avoid missing life-threatening injuries.

The primary survey and resuscitation

During this phase the patient is rapidly assessed in order to identify immediately life-threatening injuries. Treatment (the resuscitation phase) is inseparable from assessment during the primary survey, and management is initiated as the need for it is discovered.

The <C>ABCDE mnemonic is used to structure the approach to the primary survey. This does not mean that progress must be made in a linear fashion, since within team-based resuscitation the components are often assessed and treated concurrently. However, the original intention was to establish an order of priority for treatment of immediately life-threatening problems, and to offer a structure for doctors and other practitioners who might be expected to manage the seriously traumatized patient alone or with limited help (box 3.1).

The rationale for the <C>ABCDE model is that life-threatening external haemorrhage is easy to diagnose and relatively easy to treat. When it is not present, as will undoubtedly be the case in most patients, airway obstruction is the preventable mode of death likely to kill first, and it therefore should be dealt with next. Hypoxia is the next fastest mode of death and so breathing is then addressed, and on to haemorrhage control as part of circulation. This system is easily remembered and followed. In a serious trauma patient some structure is necessary to prevent major injuries being missed or diagnosed too late—the

---

> **Box 3.1.** Components of the primary survey.
> - **<C>:** control of exsanguinating external haemorrhage.
> - **A:** Airway with cervical spine immobilization.
> - **B:** Breathing with oxygen.
> - **C:** Circulation and haemorrhage control.
> - **D:** Disability.
> - **E:** Exposure and environment.
> - *History:* patient and incident.
> - Primary survey radiographs.
> - Adjuncts to the primary survey.

ease of use, recall, and simple structure of the <C>ABCDE model contributes to its popularity.

Adjuncts to the primary survey include chest and pelvic radiographs, and a FAST (focused assessment with sonography for trauma) if available.

The secondary survey

The secondary survey aims to detect injuries that may require immediate treatment, but also injuries that may require attention once life-saving interventions have been performed. A head-to-toe, left to right, back, and front approach is adopted with a detailed examination of the whole patient. It should be emphasized that patients have axillae and perineal areas that also need to be examined, particularly important in penetrating trauma.

Additional investigations (such as extremity radiographs or advanced imaging) are undertaken to define the nature of every injury detected so that appropriate plans can be made for their management in a timely fashion and with appropriate prioritization.

The secondary survey should take place once all life-threatening injuries have been dealt with, in the primary survey and resuscitation stages. In reality, parts of the secondary survey may be performed opportunistically, whilst primary survey management is ongoing, or where there are short delays in progress (waiting to go to CT scan, waiting to go to the operating theatre). The secondary survey does not take place at the expense of components of the primary survey, and should not delay them in any way.

Reassessment

Reassessment is a crucial part of the management of any trauma patient. Trends in heart rate, for example, may reveal incipient shock. It is also essential that the patient be reassessed after any intervention in order to be sure that the desired improvement in their condition has occurred.

Preparation

Preparation for dealing with trauma begins in the years and months before the patient arrives. Components include developing appropriate systems of care, education, and training, and having appropriate equipment and resources in resuscitation areas. Multidisciplinary audit is another key feature of preparation of the team.

On the day, as soon as information is received that a trauma patient is en route, preparations should begin so that reception runs as smoothly as possible. Decisions need to be made as to the make-up of the receiving team, for example whether a full trauma team should be activated, and specific roles be allocated for each member of the team (see next chapter).

When the patient arrives

The MIST handover

The handover in the resuscitation room should be given using the MIST format (Box 3.2). This should be succinct, given to the whole team and with appropriate silence from the rest of the people present so that the team can hear the information. A professional and efficient resuscitation can be carried out with the minimum of noise. There should only be two voices heard at this stage, from the team leader and person giving the handover.

The exception to this rule is if there is an emergency airway situation—in this circumstance, the airway physician and assistant at the head end need to deal with this as the rest of the team take the handover.

Before the ambulance crew departs, as much information as possible should be extracted from them, by the team leader and scribe. The history surrounding the mechanism is particularly valuable, and can give vital clues to the injuries sustained. It is also important that injuries identified by the ambulance crew or pre-hospital doctor are documented in case they are missed by the trauma team, along with any pre-hospital interventions that have been undertaken.

Unpacking the patient

Delays here translate into delays in the emergency management of life-threatening injuries and delay to definitive care, so the team needs to be practised at unpacking the trauma patient with the minimum of movement. The patient is often brought in on a long board (also known as a spinal board or extrication board), scoop stretcher, or a vacuum mattress, with the cervical spine immobilized. While they may simply be moved across to the hospital trolley with the aid of a pat-slide (see Chapter 4, The trauma team), the transfer device will often need to be moved at some point in the process, as it is not intended as a bed surface and pressure sores develop quickly in susceptible patients. It should be removed as soon as is practically achievable. Such boards are extremely uncomfortable, and so may add to the distress and agitation of patients, especially if they are already obtunded. It is common practice to remove the patient from a board as soon as possible and with a co-operative, stable patient it may occur during the initial transfer. Both log rolls and lifts are extremely manpower intensive, so this is often best achieved with the help of the delivering ambulance crew.

Most patients still have some or all of their clothing on when they arrive in the emergency department. The patient will need to be fully exposed to facilitate assessment and radiography. Two team members with trauma shears can usually undress the most well wrapped or protectively clothed patient in only a couple of minutes if given space.

Pelvic splints are indicated in all patients with a suggestive mechanism of injury who is not GCS 15 or any patient complaining of lower back, hip, or pelvic pain.

As soon as is practical, the patient should be covered and kept warm, both for their dignity and to prevent excessive heat loss (the E of the primary survey).

The airway assessment and management can take place concurrently. Essential monitoring can be applied as the patient is undressed, and as soon as a limb has been exposed venous access can be achieved. The challenge is to allow these key activities to take place as early as possible, without having a large crowd of people surrounding the trolley getting in the way. This is part of the organizational skill of a successful team leader.

AMPLET history

A brief patient history must also be obtained where possible (Box 3.3). This should include general health, medications and allergies, and also whether the patient is fasted.

Box 3.2. Pre-hospital MIST information.

- *M*echanism: mechanism of injury.
- *I*njuries: injuries apparently sustained.
- *S*igns: vital signs at scene and since.
- *T*reatment: pre-hospital treatment administered.

Box 3.3. The AMPLET history.

- **A**llergies.
- **M**edications.
- **P**revious medical history.
- **L**ast meal/drink.
- **E**xact mechanism.
- **T**etanus status.

The primary survey

Control of life-threatening external haemorrhage

In some patients a source of exsanguinating external haemorrhage will be identified. This is more common in penetrating trauma, but other causes include major compound fractures and significant combined limb injuries. Where bleeding is identified which is life-threatening, it must be immediately controlled by the application of dressings, pressure, tourniquets, or topical haemostatic agents.

The airway

An airway is essentially a hole, enabling gas to freely pass between the outside atmosphere and the alveoli of the lungs. The aim is to provide an open, protected airway. Normally, we are able to protect our own airway by exerting neuromuscular control over the muscles of the oropharynx, tongue and hypopharynx, and having an intact gag reflex. The open airway allows unimpeded gas flow and prevents hypoxia. A protected secure airway means that the patient will not aspirate blood or gastric contents leading to obstruction, or later pneumonitis or infection.

Immobilizing the cervical spine

The airway should be managed without worsening a potential cervical spine injury. The cervical spine is at risk from many mechanisms of injury and so is generally assumed to be both injured and unstable until it has been proven otherwise. Thus, control of the head and stabilization of the neck is undertaken alongside assessment of the airway.

The quickest form of immobilization is manual in-line stabilization (MILS), but this ties up one of the team at the head end of the patient. It is particularly appropriate if any airway management is necessary, as it considerably improves the view at laryngoscopy compared to when a cervical collar is in place. The cervical spine is also considered to be protected if the neck is secured in a correctly-sized cervical collar, with the addition of side blocks or sandbags, and tape running at two levels to secure to the trolley or board.

Once the neck is immobilized, no other intervention in the first phase will make any difference even if a spinal injury is present, so the priority is to move on to optimizing oxygenation, ventilation, and perfusion.

Basic manoeuvres and adjuncts

The airway is opened using manoeuvres to lift the mandible anteriorly, taking the base of the tongue forwards. The preferred technique is the jaw thrust as this minimizes movement of the cervical spine. Suction may be required and must be turned on, working, and easily accessible before any airway manoeuvres are attempted.

Various adjuncts are available to help keep the airway open. The most commonly used are the oropharyngeal and nasopharyngeal airways. Both interpose a rigid or semi-rigid tube between the anterior and posterior walls of the pharynx, keeping a patent passage to the larynx. The oropharyngeal airway is less well tolerated as it causes marked stimulation of the gag reflex. The nasopharyngeal airway may be less appropriate when there are extensive facial injuries as there are concerns that the tube could move intracranially if there is damage to the base of the skull, and insertion may exacerbate pre-existing trauma.

Both require manual airway positioning (or attention) in addition to the presence of the device.

The laryngeal mask airway is gaining popularity in some areas of practice. It allows placement of a shaped mask over the larynx, essentially moving the mask from the face (in bag-valve-mask ventilation) closer to its target. It may also offer some protection against aspiration by guiding fluids away from the epiglottis, but will not be tolerated by a patient with an intact gag reflex and should not be considered a secure airway. It is, however, more easily inserted by practitioners who are not able to intubate.

A secure airway

This provides a passage for oxygen to the lungs, and a seal within the airway preventing aspiration of stomach contents or blood from above. The definitive airway is an endo-tracheal tube with inflated cuff. Placement in trauma may be considerably more difficult than in other settings and the experienced practitioner will anticipate a difficult intubation. The oropharynx is often filled with blood, vomit, and debris including teeth. The normal anatomy may be disturbed by swelling and there is no luxury of re-adjustment of the head and neck position as there is usually a presumption of underlying unstable cervical spine fracture.

Whilst some patients are intubated by paramedics in the pre-hospital environment, most will require sedation and paralysis in order to allow laryngoscopy. Rapid sequence induction of anaesthesia and intubation in trauma is complicated by increased likelihood of cardiovascular instability, and of failed intubation. It is essential that the operator be sufficiently experienced to manage these problems.

Trauma is the most likely situation to lead to the need for an urgent surgical airway. This may be required if intubation is impossible because of severe trauma to the face, or in the *can't intubate, can't ventilate* scenario. It is possible to perform this procedure under local anaesthetic if necessary. A variety of techniques are described for performing a surgical cricothyroidotomy as an emergency procedure. Most sets work either on a puncture/dilator/introducer system, or by simple incision and then insertion of a larger tube. There is not time in these circumstances for formal tracheotomy in the resuscitation room.

The need for equipment to deal with a difficult and potentially failed airway should be anticipated and every resuscitation room that receives trauma patients should have equipment ready to deal with these problems.

Breathing

With the airway patent, and the cervical spine secure, the next stage is to optimize oxygenation by achieving the maximum FiO_2 possible, and by ensuring that ventilation is effective.

Oxygenation and ventilation

The aim is to administer the highest level of inspired oxygen possible. This is usually via a mask with reservoir bag in the spontaneously ventilating patient with adequate minute volumes. As long as the flow is sufficient, and the mask tightly fitting, then this system should provide an inspired oxygen concentration in excess of 85%. The flow into the system should be at least 15 l/min, as trauma patients may have a very high minute volume.

Supported ventilation may be required for a variety of reasons. Central respiratory drive may be diminished in the presence of severe head injury or drugs used to sedate the patient. The efficacy of spontaneous ventilation may be reduced by trauma to the chest, rendering the patient hypercapnic or hypoxic, and pain may inhibit adequate ventilation. In the UK, non-invasive ventilation is rarely used in the management of trauma, so endotracheal intubation will be required. 100% oxygen should be used in the ventilated patient.

The lung beneath chest wall injuries is likely to be contused, and patients with chest injuries are prone to the development of further, secondary problems with gas exchange. Trauma itself (as well as massive transfusion) predisposes to Adult Respiratory Distress Syndrome (ARDS) as part of the systemic inflammatory response. In anticipation of these problems, and to minimize further iatrogenic damage, high peak airway pressures should be avoided wherever possible.

Chest decompression
The next part of the assessment of breathing is whether or not the chest requires decompression by needle thoracocentesis or thoracostomy. The key to deciding which patients warrant immediate decompression and which can afford to wait for a chest X-ray lies in assessing whether the patient's physiological status is critically compromised or whether it is likely to become so imminently. If it is not, a chest X-ray should be performed to aid decision-making. Clinical clues include asymmetrical expansion, reduced air entry, and tachypnoea. In the presence of hypoxia and haemodynamic compromise, the chest should be decompressed on the side of the injury.

Chest X-ray
A chest X-ray is an extremely useful tool in aiding diagnosis and decision-making in the resuscitation room. However, it should be borne in mind that there is a considerable incidence of occult pneumothorax subsequently evident on CT, and therefore the X-ray should always be interpreted in the context of the clinical situation.

Circulation and haemorrhage control
The aim of circulatory management is to maintain end-organ perfusion. Assessment of circulation is intended to identify hypovolaemia from haemorrhage and to reveal the sources of the bleeding, either overt or occult, and allow their immediate treatment.

Haemorrhage falls into two categories in terms of immediate management—compressible or non-compressible. Compressible haemorrhage can be arrested completely with simple measures in the field or in the emergency department and, when life-threatening, is dealt with under <C>. More minor bleeding can be controlled as part of E (see below). Having been controlled, normal restoration of physiological blood pressure and perfusion may then proceed with no adverse consequences for the patient. Non-compressible haemorrhage often cannot be controlled without surgical intervention. In this situation fully normalized perfusion may not be in the best interests of the patient as this may encourage further bleeding at the site. Additional replacement will then be required with the potential for coagulopathy, cooling, reduced oxygen carriage, and other transfusion risks. A strategy of expedited surgery as an integral part of the resuscitation of these patients is increasingly common, the aim being to *turn off the tap* draining the vascular system before fully refilling it.

It is therefore critical that sufficient surgical expertise be present to make an early decision as to the need for and timing of operative intervention.

Assessment of the circulation
There are several surrogate markers of end-organ perfusion that can be quickly and easily used as part of the initial assessment. As part of the primary survey, the most useful are respiratory rate, heart rate, blood pressure, conscious level, and skin colour. Respiratory rate is an early and sensitive marker of shock. Heart rate often rises as a response to blood loss, due to physiological compensation. The response may, however, be influenced by many other factors, such as physical conditioning, β-blockers (and other rate controlling drugs), and age. Blood pressure may rise slightly as an initial response to hypovolaemia, or the pulse pressure may narrow. In younger patients blood pressure may only fall as a very late response. The level of consciousness (in the absence of brain injury) is an excellent marker of cerebral perfusion, although again deterioration may be a late sign. Skin perfusion is easily assessed both by colour, temperature and capillary refill time. The main pitfall here is that skin perfusion is reduced as a normal physiological response in the presence of hypothermia. Despite the pitfalls, a patient with a normal level of responsiveness, a good pink colour, and a normal pulse and blood pressure will usually not have catastrophic covert bleeding.

Additional measures that can be used to augment these initial evaluations include urine output, arterial blood gas analysis, and central venous pressure. Trends in all markers of circulation are generally far more revealing than single measurements and so regular reassessment is essential.

Rapid assessment of the likely sites of blood loss must take place in order to identify injuries and plan for control of the bleeding. Look for *blood on the floor and five more*-evidence of external bleeding, bleeding into the chest, abdomen, pelvis, long bone fractures, or retroperitoneum.

Circulatory support
Concomitant with assessment for signs of shock, preparations should be made for circulatory support. It is common sense to site at least two peripheral cannulae of an appropriately large gauge. Blood is drawn at the same time for cross-match and for baseline assessment (Box 3.4). Although the immediate value of some investigations may not be apparent, they may be useful later, for the management of evolving coagulopathy and renal failure, and for the assessment of pancreatic injury. The only initial test likely to change management in the resuscitation room is the serum lactate, which if raised will offer a guide to the level of potential hypoperfusion in haemorrhagic injury.

If simple peripheral access is not possible then alternatives include central access, cut-down to peripheral veins or intra-osseous access.

Box 3.4. Laboratory investigations.

- Venous gas for estimation of pH and lactate.
- Bedside glucose.
- Cross-match (type specific made available first).
- Full blood count and haematocrit.
- Urea and electrolytes.
- Clotting screen.
- Liver function and amylase.

Fluid resuscitation is controversial. Crystalloid is used in the majority of units in the UK as first line fluid for resuscitation. With the caveat of permissive hypotension, an isotonic salt solution (such as 0.9% saline or Hartmann's) is still recommended for adult patients who have signs of shock. In children, a 20 mL/kg bolus should be given and repeated as necessary. Early blood transfusion (and transfusion of blood products, such as plasma and platelets) will be required if the patient does not respond. As a rule, fully cross-matched blood is the ideal, but may take too long to be available, in which case type-specific blood is the next best. Since this only takes 10 min to prepare, it is less common for group O blood to be necessary, as long as the laboratory has prior warning and there are no delays. Initiation of a massive transfusion protocol facilitates optimal delivery of blood and blood products in appropriate patients.

In patients who do not respond to fluid resuscitation, or in whom there is evidence of ongoing blood loss, prompt surgical intervention will be required.

Stopping the bleeding

There are several means of reducing compressible bleeding. Direct pressure is very effective and can be combined with elevation of an affected extremity and even pressure over pulse points. In rare circumstances (particularly amputations) a tourniquet may be indicated to control life-threatening haemorrhage until formal surgical control can be achieved. This must be placed as distally as possible, and be kept on for the minimum time possible.

Bleeding from fractures can be decreased by reduction and stabilization of the fracture. Examples include femoral traction splintage, or pelvic binding. In some pelvic injuries external fixation may be performed early to provide basic stability allowing other more complex injuries to be addressed. A single careful palpation of the pelvis may be performed to identify instability unless imaging is immediately available.

Disability

A brief assessment of the neurological state of the patient is now required. In patients requiring intubation and, hence, paralysis and sedation, this may be the last opportunity to document gross neurology. The pupils should be examined for reactivity and size, and an estimate is made of their level of consciousness. The AVPU scale is often used for this purpose, although a formal GCS is more useful and predictive of outcome. An assessment of gross limb movement is also desirable at this stage. Gross signs of head injury or evidence of gross neurological dysfunction (such as paralysis) will usually be detected during the primary survey.

Formal neurological testing should be performed, but this is more appropriately deferred until the secondary survey when the patient's condition has been stabilized.

Exposure and environment

The patient needs to be fully undressed during the primary survey and a quick visual inspection of all the body surfaces must be carried out. This is to ensure that wounds or other clues to occult injury, such as bruising patterns are not missed, delaying important diagnoses. In order to achieve this, a log-roll should be carried out to examine the back of the patient. The exact timing of the log-roll will vary according to the patient's condition and other injuries, but will usually be delayed until primary survey radiographs have been completed.

The environment must also be addressed. The trauma patient is at risk of hypothermia through a variety of mechanisms. Hypothermia appears to be harmful in most cases of trauma, certainly when uncontrolled, and is associated with a greatly increased mortality in the general trauma population. It increases bleeding by reducing the activity of factors in the clotting cascades, as well as reducing platelet function. Efforts must be made to prevent further heat loss and they must be initiated early, preferably from the point of injury.

Patient warming is normally achieved by having the resuscitation room at an appropriate temperature, and covering the patient with a warming blanket, but may also include having a warming device under the patient on the trolley.

Primary survey radiographs

These include supine chest and pelvis radiographs. Injuries that may be found on chest X-ray are listed in Box 3.5.

Box 3.5. Injuries that may be detected on plain chest X-ray.

- Pneumothorax.
- Haemothorax.
- Pneumomediastinum.
- Fractures to ribs, clavicles, shoulders.
- Pulmonary contusion.
- Flail segments.
- Aortic dissection.
- Ruptured diaphragm.

The pelvis X-ray serves to identify significant pelvic fractures. The plain film may be able to diagnose injuries completely, or may simply highlight an area of possible concern for further investigation. Injuries to the sacrum, sacro-iliac joints, and acetabulum may be hard to detect on the initial plain film. It is worth bearing in mind that the overall sensitivity of the pelvic X-ray for significant fractures may be as low as 67% and so it cannot be relied upon to rule out significant injury in the compromised patient, particularly if a pelvic splint has been applied, as this may have re-aligned anatomy so the injury is not visible.

The lateral cervical spine view, while giving useful information, does not alter management in the resuscitation room, and, therefore, should not delay time-critical investigations or interventions. Clearly, if the patient is going to have further imaging of higher diagnostic value (computed tomography of the head and neck) then lateral cervical X-ray may not be necessary.

Other adjuncts to the primary survey

Several other investigations have an important role in the early assessment of trauma. In particular they may be used to determine the location and extent of occult bleeding, particularly in the abdomen, guiding further management. It is essential that investigations do not delay immediate surgery when indicated, although bedside ultrasound, or DPL may guide the surgical approach taken.

Diagnostic Peritoneal Lavage (DPL) is used to detect blood or contamination from hollow viscus rupture in the peritoneal cavity. It up to 98% sensitive for the detection of intraperitoneal bleeding. When negative in an unstable patient it makes it unlikely that the bleeding source is peritoneal.

However, DPL has been replaced in many units by focused assessment with sonography for trauma (FAST). FAST is rapid, portable, non-invasive, repeatable, and accurate in experienced hands. The principle role of FAST in the trauma setting is for the detection of free fluid in the abdomen, making it ideal in situations formally lending themselves to diagnostic peritoneal lavage. Its key function is to identify the abdomen as a source of bleeding in the haemodynamically unstable patient. FAST identifies fluid in any of four acoustic windows and is interpreted as being negative if none is seen. These views include the pericardium, the right and left upper quadrant, and the pelvis. FAST has a sensitivity for haemoperitoneum of around 98–99%, but this is considerably influenced by the operator skill and patient body habitus. FAST is not designed to be used as a technique for assessing intra-abdominal injury beyond asking the binary question: is there or is there not free fluid in the abdomen (or pericardium)?

CT defines head, spine, and torso injury. The increased availability of CT over the last couple of decades, and the improved technology of faster multi-slice CT scanners has made it the investigation of choice in trauma patients stable enough to undergo the investigation. In addition, because of the speed of the investigation in a modern scanner, more patients may be deemed suitable to undergo CT than previously when the scan took up to 30 min to perform. However, the CT scanner is still a potentially hostile environment. Adequate preparation should be made before taking a patient to the CT scanner, and potential problems anticipated with availability of critical care equipment in the scanner room.

CT is the imaging modality of choice for many body areas, but the main cost of these high value images is in terms of time (in time-critical patients) and radiation dose.

The secondary survey

The secondary survey allows identification of all injuries regardless of severity, not yet picked up in the primary survey. It is a thorough, systematic review of the whole patient, and it is relatively time-consuming. Since it is not performed in an order reflecting the severity of the injuries, it is essential that the secondary survey takes place once the primary survey is complete. Often, in reality, parts of the secondary survey are undertaken opportunistically during natural pauses in the primary survey, but they must never delay it.

Components of the secondary survey include:
- Top-to-toe, front and back, visual survey.
- Additional monitoring, such as urine output, central venous, and arterial pressure.
- Radiographic investigation as indicated by clinical findings, e.g. limb X-rays, CT of the head, echocardiography.
- Planning the management of each identified injury.
- Every female trauma patient must have a pregnancy test.

The scalp and head

Conventional teaching is that an isolated head injury cannot cause sufficient bleeding to cause shock, except perhaps in infants. Scalp wounds are common, however, and do bleed profusely. Usually, the bleeding can be controlled by direct pressure, but formal closure is often required. Fractures of the skull may underlie scalp wounds, and may be visible or detected on palpation. Suspected skull fracture, along with open, depressed, or basal skull fractures, is an indication for computed tomography under the current NICE guidelines even if the level of consciousness is normal. Base of skull fractures may have few clinical signs in the early stages, but rhinorrhoea and otorrhoea are usually obvious, and the eyes can be inspected for subconjunctival haemorrhage, which continues posteriorly around the globe.

Facial injuries may be far more complex than they initially appear. Lacerations may overlie serious unstable fractures. Often these injuries do not need immediate stabilization, but the swelling and bleeding that they cause may make initial airway management more difficult. CT would normally be the investigation of choice if initial plain views or evident clinical instability suggests complex fractures, but this can usually be undertaken as a lower priority investigation.

The throat and neck

The throat will have been inspected visually during the primary survey but a careful and thorough assessment is required to pick up the more subtle signs of injury. Any wounds need careful assessment. The neck should be carefully palpated for evidence of surgical emphysema (from laryngeal injury, or tracking up from a pneumothorax). The pulses should be palpated, and swelling or bruising suggestive of a vascular injury noted. The neck should be examined on all sides, so part of this visual inspection may have to wait until the log roll.

The bony skeleton will be immobilized, and will remain so. The lateral C-spine X-ray is never adequate to allow removal of immobilization. In a conscious patient with cervical tenderness and without distracting injury, with a normal neurological examination and level of consciousness,

the minimum should be a series of three views (lateral, anteroposterior, and open mouth odontoid peg X-rays). In a patient who does not meet these criteria, CT or MRI is necessary to clear the spine. MRI is the gold standard, and is preferred in many centres where it is available; although CT is adequate for recognition of bony injury, it is possible (albeit very rarely) for serious ligamentous disruption to escape detection.

The chest

The chest should have been carefully examined during the primary survey, but a repeat examination can now take place. More minor injuries, such as isolated rib fractures and bruising may be found that were missed initially. Sternal fracture may be suspected if there was an anterior compression force to the chest. An ECG may be useful. If there is any doubt about myocardial function or question of tamponade then an echocardiogram is a rapid, sensitive tool. Echocardiography gives valuable information about the myocardial function and valvular integrity, as well as some limited views of the aortic arch. It is not commonly used in the early stages of trauma assessment, but may be very helpful in the assessment of myocardial contusion.

If the patient undergoes CT chest then most major injuries should be detected. If not, then the chest X-ray from the primary survey should be reviewed and may give clues as to other injuries not dealt with as part of the initial resuscitation. Where pulmonary contusion is evident on the X-ray, it may be useful to quantify the amount of lung involved by CT; these contusions usually get worse before they improve and anticipated ventilatory compromise a few hours later may be an important determinant in the timing of surgery.

Additional cardiovascular and respiratory monitoring is important. Three-lead ECG monitoring gives early warning of increasing tachycardia and arrhythmia. Serial blood gas analysis may be useful and an arterial line is often placed to facilitate this. Central access may be useful, both to guide fluid therapy, and to give fluids and drugs.

The abdomen and pelvis

Initial assessment of the abdomen is primarily clinical, and serial examination remains the key means of assessment in the conscious patient. Increasing tenderness or the development of frank peritonism may develop over time. A thorough visual survey looking for bruising or wounds missed in the primary survey is important. Remember again that the abdomen has a back, and this needs to be thoroughly assessed during the log-roll.

Trauma patients often have distended stomachs (either from positive pressure ventilation or air swallowing) and delayed gastric emptying. These both predispose to regurgitation. Abdominal distension also reduces the functional residual capacity of the lungs and impairs gas exchange. For these reasons it is common practice to place a nasogastric catheter on free drainage. The orogastric route may be preferred if there are facial injuries.

A urinary catheter allows the urine output to be monitored (a useful marker of renal perfusion and surrogate for general end-organ perfusion) and also relieves discomfort and eases nursing of the multiply injured patient. It also allows intra-abdominal pressure to be measured; abdominal compartment syndrome is a feared consequence of major trauma (and trauma surgery). Urinalysis is a simple, sensitive marker of gross renal injury. The absence of blood in the urine makes significant urinary tract injury unlikely, although the avulsed kidney may not generate haematuria.

Rectal examination is usually performed during the log-roll and allows some assessment of the pelvis, urinary tract and neurological status. It is accompanied by visual inspection of the perineum and the genitals. Blood at the urethral meatus, peroneal bruising or clinical suspicion of pelvic fracture (high riding prostate, bony spicules or blood per rectum) may mandate additional radiography prior to catheterization.

Imaging of the abdomen involves either ultrasound (FAST) or CT. The choice of modality depends on the situation. Ultrasound is useful for demonstrating the presence of blood in the abdomen and hence confirming the need for laparotomy in the shocked patient. In many health systems ultrasound has replaced Diagnostic Peritoneal Lavage (DPL) in the diagnosis of intra-peritoneal blood. In skilled hands ultrasound can detect solid organ injury, but it is less sensitive and specific than CT. In the stable patient the latter is preferred, although CT is not without its own limitations. The need for oral contrast is debated, but there is frequently insufficient time to allow it to percolate through the gut. Hollow viscus injury is often not evident on early CT.

Ideally the pelvis should not be sprung before the primary survey X-ray shows a normal pelvic ring. Pelvic springing has a low diagnostic yield and can cause catastrophic haemodynamic collapse due to bleeding if the pelvis is unstable. Pelvic injuries can be difficult to diagnose, particularly those around the sacrum and the acetabulum. The primary survey plain film of the pelvis is a useful first line investigation, which can be augmented by CT if necessary.

The limbs

Major fractures of the long bones should have been identified in the primary survey. The secondary survey aims to identify all other injuries. These injuries are often missed, and it is common for them to be picked up later, on intensive care or even on the ward when the recovering patient complains of pain. Missed injuries can be a significant cause of morbidity.

Open fractures and soft tissue injuries such as tendon injuries are commonly missed and these can be a cause of morbidity (and litigation) later. Open fractures should be debrided and washed out early, following intravenous antibiotics, tetanus prophylaxis, and appropriate dressing and splintage in the emergency department. Any clinically suspicious areas should have at least two orthogonal plain films taken to demonstrate bony injury.

Tendon and soft tissue injuries are more difficult to assess in the multiply injured patient, but suspicions should be documented so that appropriate exploration can be undertaken later. Pulses and skin perfusion should be assessed as part of the secondary survey, and continually reassessed if there are any concerns. Doppler or angiographic studies may be required to demonstrate peripheral vascular injuries.

Neurological injuries

A formal Glasgow Coma Score must be calculated as early as possible. If the patient is intubated then the level of response prior to sedation must be noted. Gross lateralizing signs should also be documented along with pupillary reaction to light. As soon as possible formal neurological assessment must take place, although this may need to be repeated when the patient wakes in the intensive care unit.

Peripheral nerve injuries are often missed in the early stages of trauma management—an unconscious motorcyclist with a brachial plexus injury is a classic example—and these problems must be dealt with when they come to light. The earlier some form of neurological assessment can be made, and the more often it is carefully repeated, the earlier the problem will be identified.

Spinal injuries

Spinal injury is relatively common in trauma. In 10% of cases with spinal injury there is a second injury in another part of the spine. There must be a high index of suspicion of spinal injury, especially in blunt trauma, and any fracture anywhere in the spine mandates imaging of the whole of the rest of the spine.

Burns

Burns may complicate other trauma. In the initial phases the main concerns are airway management, fluid management, and analgesia. A careful assessment of burn area and depth is critical to appropriate management. Patients with burns are complex to manage and require specialized care where possible, to prevent later complications.

Further investigation and management

Decision making in the resuscitation room

Decision making in the resuscitation room is vital at different phases of care. When pre-hospital information indicates that there is a hypotensive trauma patient arriving imminently, the operating theatres should be alerted, so that when 15 min into a resuscitation, the team identify the need to go to theatres urgently, it does not come as a complete surprise to those surgical staff in the operating theatre.

Key decisions can be made before arrival (who to alert, which blood products to make available or run through), on arrival (immediate priorities), 15 min into the resuscitation (disposal to theatre, CT, or angiography) and at 30 min (confirm disposal, interventions still pending prior to transfer). An appropriate level of seniority and experience should be present in the resuscitation room to facilitate these key decisions. Ultimately, the destination of the patient will depend on the injuries sustained and their haemodynamic state. The timing of interventions will depend on the time-critical nature of their injuries. In time-critical patients, time targets may be useful to prevent unnecessary delay in management (e.g. to CT for isolated head injury within 30 min, to CT or theatre for complex multi-trauma within 45 min).

Theatre

A proportion of patients need to go to theatre urgently for initial stabilization and haemorrhage control. This should be thought of as part of the resuscitation phase. If patients require immediate surgery, their secondary survey and further investigations will need to be addressed once their physiological state has been stabilized. Often patients go from theatre to CT or angiography for further investigation and sometimes definitive treatment.

Computed tomography

Computed tomography (CT) is the principle modality for imaging the head, and the bony elements of the axial skeleton. CT of the chest may show small pneumothoraces and haemothoraces, as well as clearly demonstrating areas of collapse, contusion, and aspiration. Again, bony injuries are clearly seen. The use of intravenous contrast allows a high sensitivity for vascular injuries, particularly to the mediastinal vessels. For the abdomen, CT is the gold standard for the detection of solid organ injuries and is also able to detect free air. Under ideal conditions CT can detect injuries to the bowel (although this is less sensitive in early scans), pancreas, and diaphragm. CT is also able to visualize retroperitoneal structures. CT of the abdomen is usually undertaken with both intravenous and oral contrast, although the value of oral contrast is increasingly questioned.

CT of the pelvis can offer more detail about pelvic injury than plain films, with more detail in difficult areas, such as the sacrum and acetabulum. CT of the pelvis clearly shows disruption to the ring, as well as allowing angiography to identify bleeding areas.

The recent NCEPOD report highlights that it is preferable to scan from *top to toe*, or at least *head to hips* at the first visit to the scanner than to risk several trips for individual areas to be scanned as new problems become apparent. Such pan-scanning protocols are becoming more common, particularly in centres seeing high volumes of trauma, where teams are practised at getting patients on and off the scanner table quickly, allowing rapid definition of injury.

Magnetic resonance imaging

MRI has a very limited role in the initial assessment of trauma. Due to long scan times, in an environment that makes high dependency care extremely difficult, only completely stable patients are suitable for MRI scanning. It remains, however, the gold standard for further assessment of spinal injuries identified by other modalities.

Angiography

Angiography and angio-embolization is also an option for the management of non-compressible bleeding, and has been advocated for a variety of conditions, including pelvic trauma and intra-abdominal solid organ injury. Occasionally, patients will need immediate surgical haemorrhage control and then angiography to undergo angio-embolization techniques. The angiography suite should be equipped to deal with critical care patients, so that resuscitation can continue, while haemorrhage is controlled, similar to an operating theatre.

Again, the decision to take a patient for angiography requires senior decision makers in the relevant specialties to facilitate appropriate patient selection and timing of these interventions.

Secondary survey plain radiography

Plain X-rays are key investigations, despite the high technology modalities discussed above. Any suspected bony or joint injury identified in the secondary survey will need to be fully assessed. Unless it has already been clearly delineated by CT (in the case of spinal injuries when the torso has been scanned) then plain films are the initial investigation of choice. Good practice usually requires visualization of the joint above and below any suspected fracture. Obviously these investigations will be deferred until the patient is well enough to undergo them. They should not delay time-critical life-saving intervention.

Intensive care

Some patients will not require surgery, but will require a period of prolonged correction of physiological abnormality, or neurosurgical intensive care. Other patients will require transfer to the intensive care unit following surgery. Ideally, capacity should be available in the intensive care unit to deal with an influx of trauma patients, who by their nature are unpredictable in the timing of their arrival and nature of their injuries.

Discharge or admission to the wards

Minimally injured patients may be able to receive all the treatment that they require within the Emergency Department. However, it is still appropriate for almost all patients who have been involved in high energy collisions (or equivalent) to remain within the hospital for a period of observation. There is no perfect test for detecting injury. One of the most valuable tools available to the clinician is the ability to undertake serial examinations and physiological assessments, and to monitor changes in the patients' symptoms.

Chapter 4

The trauma team

The trauma team

Introduction

There is now good evidence to suggest the input of a multi-disciplinary trauma team improves the management and outcome of multiply-injured patients. Traditional trauma education focuses on the horizontal management of trauma patients, but with a team involved, the assessment of catastrophic haemorrhage, airway, breathing, and circulation can happen simultaneously, along with institution of monitoring, exposure of the patient, and initial trauma radiographs.

Activation of the trauma team

The pre-hospital and in-hospital phases of trauma care should be co-ordinated to ensure adequate communication between the scene of an incident and the receiving hospital so that preparations can be made to receive the patient. One suggested format for the passage of vital information is MIST (Box 4.1). This includes preparation of equipment in the resuscitation bay, and activation of an alert system that will notify the key personnel who will be needed in the management of the trauma patient (Box 4.2).

Other key areas in the hospital should also be notified that there is an in-bound trauma patient, such as laboratories (blood bank), theatres (to stop routine cases blocking the trauma theatre), and radiology (including CT and angiography). Standardized trauma team activation criteria have been proposed by the Royal College of Surgeons (Box 4.3).

Box 4.1. Pre-hospital MIST information

- *M*echanism: mechanism of injury.
- *I*njuries: injuries apparently sustained.
- *S*igns: vital signs at scene and since.
- *T*reatment: pre-hospital treatment administered.

Box 4.2. Key personnel to be informed

- ED consultant.
- ED registrar.
- General surgeon.
- Intensive care physician.
- Orthopaedic surgeon.
- Anaesthetist.
- Radiographer.
- Radiologist.
- Theatres.
- Blood bank.
- Portering staff.

Composition of the trauma team

The trauma team needs certain vital roles (Fig. 4.1). A team leader should be present, co-ordinating the management from the time the patient arrives to formal handover to another clinician in theatre, intensive care unit (ICU) or a ward. As well as being skilled in trauma resuscitation, the individual taking this role needs to have leadership qualities, communication, organizational skills, and the ability to make time-critical decisions. An airway physician, usually

---

Box 4.3. RCS trauma team activation criteria

- Airway compromise.
- Signs of pneumothorax.
- $Sp\,O_2 < 90\%$.
- Pulse >120/min.
- Systolic blood pressure < 90 mmHg in adults.
- Unconsciousness > 5 min.
- An incident with five or more casualties.
- An incident involving fatality.
- High-speed motor vehicle crash.
- Patient has been ejected from a vehicle.
- Knife wound above the waist.
- Any gunshot wound.
- Fall from >25 feet (8 m).
- A child with altered consciousness, capillary refill >3 s or pulse >130.
- A child pedestrian or cyclist hit by a vehicle.

---

either an anaesthetist or emergency physician, should be prepared to manage the airway at the head end of the bay, with an appropriately trained assistant. Another physician needs to be ready to perform a primary survey, and communicate the findings to a scribe, whose role is to document the pre-hospital and resuscitation room findings and interventions. A procedures doctor and assistant should be prepared to expose the patient, attach monitoring, gain intravenous access, draw blood for cross-matching and biochemical analysis, and perform any other emergency procedure that may be necessary. A radiographer should be standing by to perform the primary survey X-rays.

Preparation

The trauma bay needs to be prepared prior to arrival of the patient. All equipment and drugs that may be necessary should be checked and readily available. An easy way to check if all the equipment is present is to go through the primary survey <C>ABC system making sure appropriate equipment is available. For example, when thinking about airway management, basic adjuncts, suction, intubation equipment, difficult airway and failed intubation equipment, and rapid sequence induction drugs need to be prepared. Equipment should be available to decompress the chest, insert an intercostal drain, and perform a thoracostomy if necessary. Cannulation equipment and blood bottles should be at hand, warmed intravenous fluids should be run through, and a rapid infusion device prepared. Difficult access equipment including intra-osseous devices should be easily available.

Many of the interventions necessary in the resuscitation room can be anticipated prior to arrival of the patient, if there is adequate passage of information from the pre-hospital phase (Box 4.1), such as initiation of a massive trasfusion protocol.

Personal protective equipment

Every member of the team that is going to be inside the bay should wear a lead gown to enable concurrent radiography to occur alongside clinical assessment and resuscitation. Personal protective equipment should routinely include normal universal protections—gloves and eye

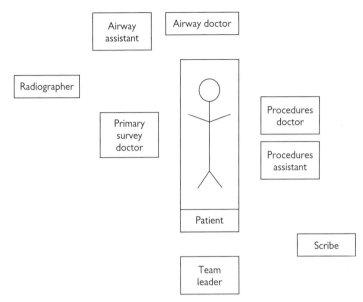

Fig. 4.1. Suggested layout of trauma bay.

protection, as well as an impermeable apron as fluid contamination is very common at trauma resuscitations.

Teamwork in action: patient handling

Patient handling is an example of when teamwork is vital. Rough handling can disrupt a fracture, dislodge a clot, and make a previously stable patient decompensate.

When the patient arrives in the resuscitation room, they will probably be on an ambulance trolley, and to get the patient onto the resuscitation trolley with the minimum of disruption requires a co-ordinated team effort.

The team leader should specify the method of transfer (Patslide®, scoop stretcher, long spinal board). For example, for a Patslide® transfer three people should be positioned along the patient's right-hand side. The airway physician takes the head, and leads the log roll. It should be explained beforehand what the call is going to be. 'We are going to log roll thirty degrees to the patient's right. I'm going to say ready brace roll and we'll roll on the 'r' of roll'. A log roll is performed, and a pat slide put under the patient. The patient is then rolled back onto the slide. The airway physician once again leads the movement of the patient, this time a move across to the resuscitation trolley. Three more are required on the left hand side of the patient. 'Ready, brace, move.' The patient is then transferred across with the minimum of movement necessary.

Environment

Several aspects of the environment in the resuscitation room can be and need to be controlled by the team leader.

Physical environment

The temperature of the resuscitation room should be as warm as is tolerable for staff, to reduce heat loss from patients exposed during the initial phase of resuscitation. The patient should also be externally warmed throughout resuscitation with appropriate warming blankets and under-patient warming devices. Good lighting is vital.

Noise levels often rise with anticipation and tension. A professional and efficient resuscitation can be carried out with the minimum of noise. Only one voice should be heard above a murmur: the team leader. Requests for drugs or equipment should be directed through one channel to avoid duplication of effort.

Overcrowding in a resuscitation room leads to inefficiency and noise. Crowd control is often a necessary element of an efficient trauma team.

Emotional environment

The emotions surrounding a resuscitation need to be controlled so that an effective assessment (and treatment) of life-threatening injuries can be made. This is most often particularly difficult in situations involving children or burns patients. Calm spreads from the top down. If the team leader is calm, the team will work effectively. However, panic can also spread from the top down.

The patient

The trauma patient is often frightened, in pain, or confused due to a head injury or hypoxia. A patient who is out of control leads to a resuscitation that is out of control. The patient needs to be reassured and given appropriate pain relief. If the situation is still out of control due to a combative patient, the team leader needs to decide the best way to safely control the situation. This may involve rapid sequence induction of anaesthesia to enable a full assessment and definition of injuries to occur safely for the patient and the team.

The trauma surgeon

The trauma surgeon plays a vital role in the initial phase of management of the trauma patient, and should be present from the outset. Different countries have a different emphasis regarding who should be leading the trauma team, and in some countries it is unusual for the trauma surgeon to be leading the team (e.g. in the UK, where it is most often an emergency physician). However, they should be present to liaise with the team leader regarding timing of surgical intervention, and often definitive haemorrhage control is achieved in the operating theatre, not the resuscitation room.

Documentation

Standardized trauma charts aid accurate documentation, and should be completed by the scribe at the time of the resuscitation. They have elements that include the pre-hospital MIST information (Box 4.1), primary survey findings and interventions, secondary survey findings and interventions, serial observations, drugs given, and the team members present. There is often also a section for a summary, which should be completed by the team leader. It should be agreed that the team leader needs to have overall responsibility for ensuring adequate and accurate documentation, even if they do not themselves complete it.

Handover

A clear handover of clinical responsibility needs to occur between the team leader and the clinician responsible for ongoing care. This may be the trauma surgeon, intensive care physician, or specialty clinician. This should be clearly documented in the patient's notes.

Further reading

Royal College of Surgeons. *Better care for the severely injured.*
London: Royal College of Surgeons, 2000.

Airway management in trauma

Airway management in trauma

Introduction and basic interventions

Airway management in trauma presents many complex challenges. The primary goal of oxygen delivery to the patient often requires the establishment of a secure protected airway, preventing obstruction by foreign bodies or external compression. The additional goal of ventilation, to remove carbon dioxide, is also vital to enable appropriate ongoing management of the patient with multiple injuries, especially if there is brain injury.

However, poor airway management is consistently noted in reports on trauma care and is a major cause of preventable deaths. In this chapter the aetiology of airway obstruction in trauma is explored, then simple manoeuvres to temporize the situation are described. Finally, the indications and processes for definitive airway care are discussed.

Aetiology

Direct trauma

Trauma to the face, larynx, or neck may cause direct airway compromise.

Maxillofacial trauma

Facial fractures from direct impact may be associated with haemorrhage, secretions, and dislodged teeth. Blood and secretions in the oropharynx may cause complete or partial airway obstruction, and limit laryngeal views obtained by direct laryngoscopy. Teeth may act as foreign bodies in the airway, either compromising the supraglottic airway, or if inhaled obstruct main or segmental bronchi contributing to hypoxia.

Laryngeal trauma

Fracture of the larynx is a rare injury, caused by blunt trauma to the anterior neck; airbag deployment is one possible cause. Laryngeal fracture can present as acute airway obstruction, indicated by a palpable fracture, subcutaneous emphysema, and hoarseness. An immediate airway assessment is required, as signs of partial or impending complete airway obstruction require rapid intubation.

Penetrating injuries to the larynx and trachea require urgent action, as occlusion of the airway with blood or soft tissue is possible.

Neck trauma

Penetrating or blunt injuries may cause disruption of the trachea or larynx. Soft tissue swelling, surgical emphysema, and haemorrhage may all lead to mass effects causing anatomical displacement and obstruction of the larynx and trachea. Penetrating injuries may involve the carotid arteries or jugular veins, and cause bleeding in or around the trachea.

Cervical spine injury may also occur, leading to increased anxiety and caution with respect to tracheal intubation.

Secondary compromise

Neurological injury resulting in a decreased conscious level may cause airway obstruction due to a decrease in tone of the upper airway musculature. A reduction in ventilatory drive may also occur.

Neurological injury may also compromise the airway by increasing the risk of aspiration of gastric contents, secondary to the loss of protective upper airway reflexes. Seizures in the trauma patient may lead to loss of airway reflexes and reduced ventilation; early intubation should be considered.

Thoracic trauma resulting in mechanical ventilatory compromise, such as flail chest or pulmonary contusion, may place a ventilatory load upon the patient that they are unable to meet: 'chest wall failure'. This may require early implementation of mechanical ventilation.

Basic airway manoeuvres

Airway obstruction during anaesthesia may occur as a result of the tongue falling back against the posterior pharyngeal wall and a reduction of local muscle tone within the soft palate and epiglottis. A similar mechanism occurs with the obtunded trauma patient, therefore, the immediate action on seeing a patient with a compromised airway must be to restore proper alignment of airway structures. However, additional concerns, such as airway soiling, laryngospasm, and foreign bodies need to be addressed in these patients; suction is a powerful and underestimated tool in these circumstances. Oxygen must also be considered a vital part of all airway manipulations.

Chin lift

The tongue is attached to the posterior part of the mandible. Lifting the chin directly forward lifts the tongue from the posterior pharyngeal wall and relieves airway obstruction. Sustained chin lift can be difficult due to poor grip and operator fatigue.

Jaw thrust

Pushing the angle of the jaw forward relieves airway obstruction by the same mechanism as the chin lift. Sustained jaw thrust is easier for the operator to maintain, although it may be very uncomfortable for the awake patient.

Head tilt

Extending neck of a patient may relieve airway obstruction by bringing the airway into a better alignment and pulling the tongue away from the posterior pharyngeal wall. This method may exacerbate any cervical spine injury and so must only be used when no concerns exist for the cervical spine in the trauma setting.

Clearing airway debris

Gurgling or noise from the airway should alert the operator to the possibility of debris within the airway. Direct suction with a rigid catheter (Yankaeur) will enable secretion clearance. It is advisable to perform suction under direct vision, e.g. using a laryngoscope as a tongue depressor, as this prevents further damage to the airway mucosa. In patients with a nasopharyngeal airway *in situ*, a soft suction catheter may be introduced to allow gentle suctioning. Removal of larger pieces of debris, such as teeth or food particles, may require the use of a laryngoscope and Magill's forceps. The ideal features of suction apparatus are given in Box 5.1.

Oxygen

All trauma patients should receive high concentration oxygen therapy, preferably via a non-rebreathe oxygen mask with a reservoir. Pain and anxiety increase the sympathetic drive of the trauma patient, increasing their oxygen requirements, whilst haemorrhage and hypovolaemia will reduce the oxygen carrying capacity and tissue oxygen delivery. In addition, a poor airway will limit tidal volume. Supplemental oxygen to improve tissue oxygen delivery is, therefore, essential.

Basic airway adjuncts

As noted, basic manoeuvres can be difficult to maintain, especially when patients are being moved, and may not clear the airway. It is important, therefore, to have a

---

Box 5.1. Requirements of a suction device

Requirements of a suction device
- Generation of enough sub-atmospheric pressure to remove viscous substances (at least −600 mmHg).
- Adequate volume displacement, i.e. the volume of air that can be moved per unit time.
- The reservoir for collection of aspirated fluid must be large enough to enable storage of large volumes of fluid, but not so large that it prevents rapid vacuum generation. A 2 L reservoir is usually adequate.

'Yankauer' suction
A rigid smooth tipped catheter is ideal for clearance of airway secretions. A side hole in the hand piece allows for more operator control, and aids flow along the suction tubing.

Endotracheal suction catheters
Soft suction catheters allow for suction of the oropharynx through an airway or endobronchial suction through an endotracheal tube. Prolonged endobronchial suction may cause alveolar collapse and hypoxia.

---

selection of simple airway adjuncts, which can be used to buy time before a more definitive airway can be established.

Oropharyngeal airways

The Guedel airway is the most commonly used oropharyngeal airway. The curve of the airway displaces the tongue forward, relieving airway obstruction. An integral bite block prevents airway obstruction secondary to involuntary biting. The central channel also allows the introduction of suction catheters to clear oropharyngeal secretions.

Oropharyngeal airways are inserted into the open mouth, either by pushing them directly backwards using a tongue depressor to displace the tongue or by inserting the airway upside down and then rotating the airway through 180 degrees when the soft palette is encountered. Care should be taken not to push the tongue backwards, worsening obstruction. A chin lift or jaw thrust may aid insertion. Rotation of the airway may cause mucosal damage, especially in children, in whom the airway should be inserted without rotation.

The Guedel airway is available in a variety of sizes from neonatal (size 00) to large adult (size 5). Airways are sized from the corner of the patient's mouth to the external auditory meatus, or alternatively the distance from the patient's incisors to the angle of the mandible may be used. Size 3 Guedel airways are usually suitable for adult female patients, size 4 for adult males.

Insertion of an oropharyngeal airway may damage teeth or dental work. Stimulation of the gag reflex may cause the patient to vomit. Coughing and laryngospasm may also be provoked. Tolerance of an oropharyngeal airway should raise concern over the overall safety of the patient's airway and the risk of aspiration; expedient tracheal intubation may be required.

Nasopharyngeal airways

Nasopharyngeal airways may be useful in patients who would be intolerant of an oral airway. They are short, soft non-cuffed tubes. The tip of the nasopharyngeal airway sits at the base of the tongue, displacing the tongue forward and providing a clear channel to the glottis. Nasopharyngeal airways are usually supplied with a prominent flange or a safety pin that should be inserted in the nasal end to prevent the airway slipping through the nose causing obstruction.

Nasopharyngeal airways are traditionally-sized by comparison with the patient's little finger, although some texts now advocate using the biggest that will easily pass through the nostril. Normally a 6.0-mm internal diameter tube is appropriate for an adult female patient and a 7.0-mm tube is appropriate for a male patient.

The nose must be assessed for the presence of any fractures, blood, polyps or foreign bodies prior to nasopharyngeal airway insertion. The suspicion of a base of skull fracture is a relative contra-indication to nasopharyngeal airway placement.

A lubricated airway is inserted into the nostril. It is then directed posteriorly along the floor of the nose; rotation may prevent the tip catching on nasal conchae. The flange of the airway should rest at the nostril.

Epistaxis is the major side effect of nasal airway insertion this haemorrhage may be enough to worsen airway obstruction.

More advanced interventions

Assisted ventilation

Assisted ventilation is an essential part of airway management. The operator should be able to support an airway and provide ventilation whilst preparing equipment for intubation.

Technique of face mask ventilation

Holding an anaesthetic facemask correctly requires practice. A two-person technique is recommended for the inexperienced operator. With the operator standing at the top of the patient, the facemask is positioned over the nose and mouth. Using the thumbs and index fingers to push the facemask down onto the nose, the other fingers are used to pull the jaw upwards into the facemask, ensuring a tight seal. An assistant can then manually ventilate the patient using either a self-inflating bag or anaesthetic circuit.

Types of facemask

A variety of facemasks are available. Adult facemasks tend to be oval or elliptical and are sized to fit the patient. Standard anaesthetic connectors will fit into the 22-mm female connection of the facemask. Small paediatric facemasks are circular to fit the facial shape of infants and toddlers.

Nasal masks have a specialist use in dental anaesthesia although they may be useful in major mandibular trauma. Newer facemask designs tend to be clear plastic and have an inflatable air cushion that may be adjusted to improve the seal obtained.

Bag and valve equipment

Bag and valve assemblies, also known as manual resuscitators, such as the Ambubag™ or the Laerdal self-inflating bag are often used to oxygenate and ventilate patients in the trauma setting. They will fit onto tracheal tubes or face masks, and allow ventilation by hand. As they will return to their starting shape (hence, the term 'self-inflating'), if oxygen supply fails it is possible to continue ventilation with room air. A uni-directional valve ensures that the patient does not breathe expired gases, by venting to them environment.

Paediatric manual resuscitators have a pressure release valve within the circuit to prevent application of high pressures to the paediatric airway, reducing the risk of barotrauma.

A heat and moisture exchange (HME) filter should be included in the system to humidify the dry medical gases before entering the patient's lungs, especially if any reusable equipment is used.

Anaesthetic circuits and the APL valve

The Mapleson Circuit is an anaesthetic system, composed of an adjustable pressure-limiting (APL) valve, a fresh gas supply and a reservoir bag connecting them to the facemask. APL valves are one-way valves that open to allow expiration, but close to prevent in drawing of air. When fully open the APL valve provides virtually no resistance to expiration, this can be varied through to complete closure allowing opening only at high pressure (60 cmH$_2$0). This allows the operator more control over the airway pressure during ventilation, and the system is usually fairly lightweight. For this reason, they are often used for the transfer of ventilated patients.

However the circuit is inefficient, requiring a gas flow 2–3 times that of the minute ventilation, therefore, more oxygen is needed and ventilation cannot occur if the gas supply fails—a clear safety problem.

Gastric insufflation

Any facemask ventilation risks insufflation of gas into the stomach, but this is a particular risk with inexperienced operators struggling to maintain an adequate airway. Children, due to greater difficulty in maintaining an airway and air swallowing whilst crying are at an additional risk. This gas insufflation will result in gastric distension, which increases the risk of regurgitation, makes ventilation more difficult due to diaphragmatic splinting and may even lead to gastric rupture.

Therefore, it is advisable to squeeze the bag with only one hand, which will limit the tidal volume that can be given and ensure only gentle ventilations (just enough to see the chest rise). Insertion of a gastric tube, either oral or nasal, is advisable after securing the airway in any trauma patient to decompress the stomach.

Advanced airway procedures

The above airway manoeuvres will undoubtedly save lives if carried out well, but they are difficult to maintain and do not provide a protected airway (aspiration of gastric contents can still occur). For this reason, a cuffed tube in the trachea is regarded as the gold standard. This is usually gained using an oral (or nasal) cuffed tracheal tube, but in some circumstances a tracheotomy may be required.

Indications for intubation

The indications for intubation can be roughly divided into those required for airway protection and oxygen delivery, and those required for ventilatory support.

Airway protection/oxygen delivery
• Coma: Glasgow Coma Score (GCS) < 9 or a significantly deteriorating conscious level.
• Severe maxillofacial, laryngeal, or neck injuries: Haematoma, fracture or foreign body obstruction risk.
• Hypoxaemia: PaO$_2$ < 9kPa (65 mmHg) on air or <13kPa (100 mmHg) on oxygen in a pre-morbidly normal adult patient.
• Loss of protective laryngeal reflexes: Risk of aspiration of blood or vomit.

Ventilatory insufficiency
• Apnoea: Unconscious patient or following administration of neuromuscular blocking agents.
• Hypercarbia: PaCO$_2$ > 6 kPa (45 mmHg). In a spontaneously ventilating trauma patient this degree of hypercarbia suggests impending respiratory failure.
• Spontaneous hyperventilation: PaCO$_2$ < 3.5 kPa (27 mmHg). Careful observation may be required as the patient may be unable to sustain this degree of respiratory drive and may rapidly fatigue. A cause for this high respiratory drive should be sought; normally it is either a compensatory hyperventilation for a metabolic acidosis or secondary to head injury.
• Respiratory arrhythmia: Abnormal respiration patterns (e.g. Cheyne-Stokes or Kussmaul) imply problems with either central respiratory drive or the need for respiratory compensation for a metabolic insult. Consideration should be given to early intubation in these patients.

• *Seizures:* Seizures may compromise the airway and venti-lation. Emergency intubation may be required in these patients. After the seizure, the post-ictal patient may not protect their airway.

Physiological effects of intubation

Intubation of the trachea is a highly stimulating procedure, due to both pharyngeal and tracheal manipulation. It may therefore have some deleterious physiological effects, which need to be weighed against the benefits of providing a definitive airway. Generally, these effects are mitigated against by only attempting intubation in the deeply uncon-scious patient or by anaesthetizing them before laryngeal manipulation.

Intracranial pressure

Normal intracranial pressure (ICP) is between 5 and 12 cmH$_2$O. In a head-injured patient ICP may be raised, sometimes to a critical point of decompensation. Laryngoscopy and endotracheal intubation cause a tran-sient rise in ICP due to a pressor response. Inadequate depth of coma may contribute, with straining in an inade-quately relaxed patient, causing a rise in ICP.

This is considered a transient response, which rarely causes lasting harm, but some authorities have recom-mended pre-treatment with short-acting β-adrenergic blockers, opioids, or lidocaine to obtund this response.

Intraocular pressure

As with intracranial pressure, intraocular pressure rises during endotracheal intubation. This may be secondary to a pressor response or patient straining. Further problems occur in the presence of a penetrating eye injury, where extrusion of vitreous from the globe is a possibility. Suxamethonium causes contraction of the extra-ocular muscles that may enhance this risk.

Urgent discussion with an ophthalmologist regarding the viability of the injured eye is advised. β-adrenergic block-ers, opioids, or lidocaine have all been suggested to reduce intra-ocular pressure. Ketamine increases intraocular pressure.

Autonomic nervous system

Direct laryngoscopy and endotracheal intubation cause a hypertensive response and tachycardia. Stimulation is via the superior laryngeal nerves, which serve sensation above the vocal cords and cricothyroid muscle, and the recurrent laryngeal nerves (sensation below the vocal cords).

The deleterious effects of this hypertension and tachy-cardia need to be considered when dealing with patients with underlying ischaemic heart disease.

Upper airway manipulation in patients with pre-existing airways disease (e.g. COPD or asthma) may result in heightened airway responsiveness and bronchospasm. In children where parasympathetic tone predominates, laryngoscopy and intubation may lead to profound bradycardia.

Anatomy of the upper airway

The upper airway is composed of the nose, mouth, pharynx, and larynx. The tongue is lifted forward by the genioglossus muscle, which is attached to the posterior part of the mandible. By placing the tip of the laryngoscope blade in the valecula at laryngoscopy the airway is brought into alignment to allow direct visualization of the glottis. This occurs by displacement of the tongue into the floor of the mouth, pulling the mandible caudally and the epiglottis anteriorly.

Grade of laryngoscopy

Approximately 1% of the population will be a difficult intu-bation in the elective scenario, but this proportion rises in the trauma patient so a difficult view at laryngoscopy should be expected. Cormack and Lehane devised a clas-sification for the view obtained at laryngoscopy (Fig. 5.1). This widely accepted classification allows ease of commu-nication when describing difficulties encountered; it is important to note this so appropriate precautions can be taken on eventual extubation.

Airway assessment

Numerous tests have been developed to allow the predic-tion of difficult intubation based upon external anatomical examination. None of these tests are highly sensitive or specific, but when used in combination they can forewarn the operator of potential difficulties. The majority of these tests require a degree of co-operation from the patient and/or the ability to move the patient's neck, neither of which may be possible in trauma. It is often wiser to just

Grade I: Complete glottis visible
Grade II: Anterior glottis visible
Grade III: Epiglottis seen but not glottis
Grad IV: Epiglottis not seen

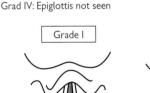 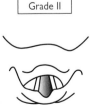 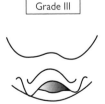 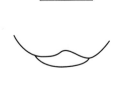

Grades III and IV are termed difficult, usually requiring additional airway interventions as outlined later in this chapter.

Fig. 5.1. The Cormack and Lehane Classification.

presume intubation will be difficult in this group of patients.

Mallampati classification

If the patient can open the mouth widely, the operator should be able to visualize the posterior pharyngeal wall. The view obtained can be described by the Mallampati classification (Figure 5.2).

Thyromental distance (Patel's test)

In an adult patient, the distance between the top of the thyroid cartilage and the tip of the chin, with the neck extended, should be more than 6 cm, 75% of difficult intubations can be predicted.

Inter-incisor distance

Mouth opening less than 3 cm (two fingers) will increase difficulty of intubation in 30% of patients.

Sternomental distance

A distance of less than 12 cm between the sternum and the chin is associated with difficult laryngoscopy.

Mandible protrusion

A co-operative patient is asked to protrude their mandible forward. For example by asking the patient to 'bite your top lip'. If the lower incisors cannot be brought forward of the upper incisors, a difficult view should be expected.

Neck flexion and extension

A normal patient should have greater than 90 degrees movement when asked to flex and extend their neck. This test is clearly contra indicated in the majority of trauma patients.

Wilson risk scoring

Wilson devised a scoring system using patient obesity, restricted head and neck movements, restricted jaw movement, receding mandible, and buck teeth. If a patient has two or more of these a difficult intubation can be anticipated.

Spinal immobilization during airway management

Cervical spine immobilization using rigid cervical collar, head blocks and straps is recognized as the gold standard of management in trauma. A well fitting cervical collar will prevent mouth opening or any significant neck movement; airway management in this situation is particularly challenging.

Indications

Cervical spine immobilization is recommended in any trauma patient with an injury (or mechanism of injury) that may involve the cervical spine, when there are distracting injuries, or in the presence of a decreased conscious level. It is, therefore, an almost universal factor during airway management of the trauma patient.

Technique

As it is practically impossible to open the mouth of a patient with a cervical collar in place, it is vital that neck stabilization during any intubation attempt is maintaining using manual in-line stabilization (MILS). This will require a team approach (Box 5.2).

Evidence for and against secondary cervical spine injury

Laryngoscopy is associated with movement of the cervical spine. Even the most carefully applied cervical spine immobilization will not prevent a small amount of movement during intubation; it may reduce head extension by 50%. Reports of catastrophic worsening of neurological function following laryngoscopy exist in the literature; closer investigation has often implicated hypotension or hypoxia as the actual causal factors. No published studies exist relating cervical spine injury to cervical spine motion during laryngoscopy.

Cadaveric studies have demonstrated fluoroscopic evidence of cervical spine motion, even with manual in-line stabilization. This motion can be reduced with the use of fibre-optic nasal intubation, although this technique may not be suitable for, or available to, the vast majority of trauma patients in the emergency department.

Class 1–soft palate, uvula, fauces and tonsillar pillars visible
Class 2–soft palate, uvula, and fauces visible
Class 3–only soft palate visible
Class 4–soft palate not visible

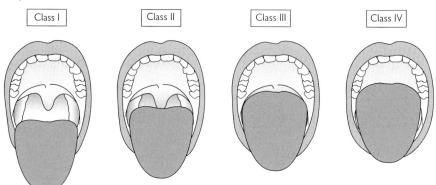

Class 3 and 4 views predict 50% of difficult intubations

Fig. 5.2. The Mallampati Scoring System.

Direct laryngoscopy remains the fastest method to enable establishment of a secure airway. A pragmatic approach where rapid airway control ensures the avoidance of hypoxia and hypotension, with an acknowledgement of the very small potential to exacerbate injury, is probably most appropriate.

Cricoid pressure

Cricoid pressure (Sellick's manoeuvre) is the application of digital pressure backwards upon the cricoid cartilage, pushing the only complete cartilage ring of the larynx and trachea against the oesophagus behind it. This is believed to occlude the oesophagus, by compression against the body of C6 vertebrae posteriorly, preventing passive regurgitation of gastric contents at induction of anaesthesia.

A force of between 20 and 40 N is applied evenly across the anterior surface of the cricoid cartilage with the fingers of one hand. In suspected cervical spine injury, a two-handed technique with the operator's other hand being used to stabilize movement behind the cervical spine, is advised.

Cricoid pressure may improve the view at laryngoscopy if applied correctly. Conversely, poorly applied cricoid pressure may worsen the view at laryngoscopy and make intubation more difficult.

If a patient is actively vomiting, compression of the oesophagus may lead to oesophageal rupture; cricoid pressure should therefore be immediately released.

Equipment

Intubation of the airway requires several pieces of specialist equipment, with which all in the team involved with need to be familiar.

Laryngoscopes

The traditional Macintosh laryngoscope is designed to afford a view of the larynx at intubation by displacing the tongue into the floor of the mouth. The laryngoscope is held in the left hand and inserted into the right side of the mouth. The shape of the Macintosh blade allows the tongue to be lifted when the tip of the blade is placed in the valecula. Operators must be careful to lift the laryngoscope, and not lever the blade, as this may cause damage to upper teeth and will worsen the laryngeal view obtained. It is available in blade sizes from 1 to 4. Size 3 is suitable for a small adult and size 4 is suitable for a large adult.

Other laryngoscope blades are available, such as the straight Miller blade. Their use is mainly for specialist work or paediatrics, and they have little role outside of specialist hands in trauma.

The McCoy laryngoscope blade has a cantilevered tip, which allows the operator to lift the epiglottis and may improve the laryngeal view, especially when the neck is fixed by MILS. The presence of a McCoy blade on the airway trolley is highly recommended (see Fig. 5.4).

Endotracheal tubes

The cuffed endotracheal tube (ETT) provides the definitive airway in trauma. A tube is sized in relation to the internal diameter (ID) in millimetres. A 7.0-mm ID ETT is suitable for a small female patient, 8.0-mm ID ETT is suitable for a

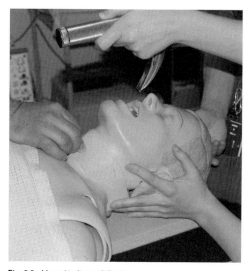

Fig. 5.3. Manual in-line stabilization.

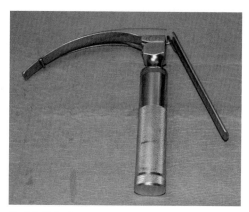

Fig. 5.4. McCoy laryngoscope.

large female or small male patient and a 9.0-mm ID is suitable for a large male patient.

Endotracheal tubes above 6.0 mm ID come with cuffs that are inflated with air when in position. Saline is used as an alternative when there is a risk of airspace expansion, such as during aero-medical transfer.

Endotracheal tubes have distance marks along their length. Length to the lips of 20 cm in a female and 22 cm in a male is usually adequate. This should be noted once the airway is secure to provide a reference should there be later movement of the tube.

Adult endotracheal tubes are supplied uncut to allow use in nasal intubation. Care must be taken to avoid placing an endotracheal tube too far into the trachea as endobronchial intubation may result. Some authorities recommend cutting the tubes to a shorter length when oral intubation is used. Care should be taken with this as it may change the manufacturer's licence for use, and should be avoided at all costs in the patient with facial burns, in whom later swelling may obscure the connections of the cut tube.

Box 5.3. Formulae used to predict tracheal tube sizes in children

- ETT size (ID mm) = 4 + child age/4 (it is advisable to have a range of tubes 0.5 ID mm larger and smaller available in case of difficulty).
- *Oral intubation:* ETT length to lips (cm) = 12 + child age/2.
- *Nasal intubation:* ETT length to nose (cm) = 15 + child age/2.

Paediatric endotracheal tubes
As the paediatric airway is circular below the vocal cords, and is more susceptible to tracheal mucosa pressure necrosis, uncuffed tubes are used in children. A small air leak should ideally be heard after intubation. The size used and the length inserted will depend on the age and size of the child. A guide to this is given in Box 5.3, but this should never detract from clinical acumen and the tube should always be checked after insertion.

Various proprietary bags and tapes exist (e.g. Broselow), which use the length or age of the child to correspond to colour-coded pouches, which contain the correct size equipment for them. These can be invaluable for the less experienced paediatric carer.

Bougies and stylets
The gum elastic bougie is an essential piece of equipment and should be available during all intubations. It is a thin malleable rod approximately 60 cm long with an upturn at one end. If the larynx is only poorly visualized during laryngoscopy the bougie may be more easily placed through the vocal cords than a thicker endotracheal tube. The bougie may also be inserted blindly and it should demonstrate characteristic clicks as the end rubs along the tracheal rings. The operator will eventually be unable to advance the bougie further as it comes to a halt in a lobar bronchus. If the bougie is in the oesophagus no clicks will be felt and it will not demonstrate hold up.

Once the bougie is in place, an endotracheal tube can be 'rail-roaded' over the bougie. Continued rotation during advancement will ensure that the tube does not get caught at the level of the vocal cords, but enters the trachea.

Stylets are shorter, more rigid introducers that can be used to stiffen endotracheal tubes and place angles within the tube to facilitate difficult intubations.

Rapid sequence induction of anaesthesia and intubation

If intubation can be performed in a trauma patient without the use of drugs, the prognosis for the patient is poor. Studies have demonstrated a survival of between 0.2% and 8% for those patients intubated in the pre-hospital arena without anaesthesia. It has been noted that attempting to intubate the airway of any patient who is not deeply unconscious leads to deleterious physiological consequences. In the less comatose patient it has also been shown that the incidence of poor views at laryngoscopy and of failed intubations is markedly increased, unless formal anaesthesia is induced.

Rapid sequence induction (RSI) is the technique of choice in the establishment of a secure airway in the emergency department (See Box 5.4 for the Aims). It is a complex succession of over 120 different psychomotor activities and makes use of potent anaesthetic agents, therefore personnel without appropriate prior training and experience should not undertake this technique. Even with this training it is easy to forget vital parts, and it is highly recommended that a checklist is used. An example of this is given In Fig. 5.5.

Box 5.4. Aims of rapid sequence induction

- To provide a patent airway, with a cuffed endotracheal tube in the patient's trachea, as rapidly as possible.
- To protect against aspiration of gastric contents.
- If a 'can't intubate, can't ventilate' situation is encountered, the patient should regain airway reflexes in time to allow the procedure to be abandoned.

Technique of rapid sequence induction

RSI should be a well-rehearsed process, with the use of pre-determined drug dosages and operator familiarity with alternative plans should difficulty be encountered (Box 5.7, Fig. 5.5). The benefit of gaining elective experience and practice in areas such as simulators before undertaking emergency RSI cannot be stressed too highly.

The process can be broken into six different phases, which need to be carried out in order, each of which has equal importance if it is to be carried out safely (Box 5.5). It must be noted that the actual intubation attempt is only a small part of the procedure—for this reason it is called Rapid Sequence Induction of Anaesthesia and Intubation.

Box 5.5. The 6 P's of RSI

- Pre-oxygenation.
- Preparation.
- Pre-medication.
- Paralysis and sedation.
- Passage of tube.
- Post-intubation care.

Pre-oxygenation

Pre-oxygenation is a vital part of rapid sequence induction as it allows the development of an oxygen reserve within the alveoli of the lungs and also within the circulation and tissues by displacing nitrogen with oxygen (denitrogenation). This reserve of oxygen may be crucial in sustaining the patient until resumption of spontaneous respiration in a 'can't intubate, can't ventilate' situation. It should be noted that the time bought by doing this is dependant on the patient, critical desaturation can occur within 2 min in the obese patient, whilst a fit healthy adult will take over 7 min.

Pre-oxygenation should be undertaken for at least 3 min, breathing 100% oxygen via a tight-fitting face-mask. Pre-oxygenation with high flow oxygen via a standard face-mask (or non re-breathe face-mask) may be inadequate, as these masks cannot provide 100% oxygen.

Preparation

All equipment should be checked and in good working order. Two laryngoscopes are preferable. The anaesthetic machine (if used) and ventilator should be checked pre-use. The patient should be placed on a trolley capable of tipping (reverse trendelenburg). An independent means to oxygenate and ventilate the patient (e.g. self-inflating Ambubag™) should be available. An assistant who is trained in the application of cricoid pressure and experienced in airway management is essential.

It is vital that appropriate monitoring is applied during this stage (if not before). The Association of Anaesthetists of Great Britain and Ireland have produced a minimum monitoring standard, which should be used before inducing anaesthesia on any patient. These standards are given in Box 5.6. Of note, capnography is gaining in importance and should now be mandatory, as it not only helps with confirming tube position, it also monitors adequate ventilation and gives some information on general physiology, such as blood pressure.

Box 5.6. Minimum monitoring standards for the induction of anaesthesia

- Pulse oximeter.
- Non invasive blood pressure monitor.
- Electrocardiograph.
- Airway gases: oxygen, carbon dioxide, and vapour.
- Airway pressure.

The following must also be available

- A nerve stimulator whenever a muscle relaxant is used.

- A means of measuring the patient's temperature.

During induction of anaesthesia in children and in uncooperative adults it may not be possible to attach all monitoring before induction. In these circumstances monitoring must be attached as soon as possible and the reasons for delay recorded in the patient's notes.

Airway adjuncts and failed or difficult intubation aids should be readily available. Consideration should be given to maintenance of anaesthesia and paralysis after intubation.

This stage should never be foreshortened, as once the drugs are given there is no going back—so all the equipment must be in place and working. Whilst preparations are being completed, the patient should be pre-oxygenated.

GNAAS pre-RSI challenge-response check list

1. Preoxygenation
Taking place and adequate oxygen available ....Check

2. Preparation
Baseline obs ....Check
Cannula   Connected to fluid and runs easily..................................Check
Suction   Working...Check
         Back-up suction available......................................Check
Airway adjuncts (or escape ventilation)
         Guedel airway...Check
         2 nasopharyngeal airways......................................Check
Ventilator and BVM connected to oxygen.......................................Check
Emergency airway kit..Check
Tape or tie (of appropriate length)..Check
Heat and Moisture Exchange Filter (HMEF)..................................Check
Endotracheal tube
         Size chosen ....Check
         Cuff tested...Check
Drugs   Induction agent dose chosen ....Check
         Suxamethonium dose chosen ....Check
         Drug giver briefed ....Check
Angle piece or catheter mount...Check
Monitoring including ECG, NIBP, SpO_2 $ETCO_2$.............................Check
Stethoscope...Check
Elastic bougie...Check
Laryngoscopes Two sizes chosen & working...................................Check
Syringe 10mls for cuff..Check

3. Premedication if required...Check

4. Paralysis and sedation
In-line immobiliser briefed...Check
Cricoid pressure person briefed...Check

5. Passage of the tube $ETCO_2$?...Check
6. Post intubation management ABCDEF.....................................Check

Fig. 5.5. An example checklist for RSI. GNAAS pre-RSI challenge-response check list. Reproduced with permission from Great North Air Ambulance.

Pre-medication
Consideration must be given to giving the patient pre-medication. These are drugs used to counteract the possible deleterious effects of procedure. Specifically, children may require atropine and the head-injured patient a potent opiate. These are discussed in more detail later.

Paralysis and sedation
At this stage the anaesthetic drugs are given, once there has been a final check to ensure everyone is ready. Drugs should be given to a pre-determined dose, based on a presumed weight of the patient. Cricoid pressure should be started once the sedative agent has been given.

Passage of tube

Once the anaesthetic drugs have been given the actual intubation attempt may proceed. It is important to give the drugs time to work; usually this is heralded by the lower jaw relaxing.

The actual technique of laryngoscopy is no different to intubating without drugs; however, there has to be particular emphasis on confirming the tube has entered the trachea. The gold standard has to be seeing the tube pass through the cords; however, this may not be possible. Feeling and listening to the chest for bilateral air movement is vital, as is seeing a waveform of expired CO_2 on the capnograph.

If the view is inadequate, it is reasonable to have a second attempt—so long as oxygenation is maintained, and something different can be done to improve the view. However, it is important not to have repeated efforts and to call a failed intubation drill before it is too late and the patient is critically desaturating.

Post-intubation care

A detailed discussion on post-intubation care is outside the scope of this chapter. Unless this is done well, the patient will deteriorate markedly and lose all the benefit of having a definitive airway. Specifically, attention should be given to ensuring ongoing sedation and muscle relaxation. Ventilation must be checked to ensure good oxygenation and an end-tidal CO_2 within the normal range (3.5–4.5 kPa), and blood pressure maintained.

Box 5.7. Summary of acceptable practice

- Operator checks all equipment (monitoring, laryngoscope, endotracheal tube, alternative method of ventilation available, tipping trolley, suction, difficult intubation aids).
- Patient is appropriately positioned—pillow under head if there is no concern over cervical spine.
- Operator begins pre-oxygenation
- Operator checks assistant is happy to continue and able to apply cricoid pressure appropriately.
- Operator/assistant gives pre-determined (or titrated) dose of induction agent, muscle relaxant, and opiate if required.
- When muscle relaxation established, direct laryngoscopy, and intubation undertaken
- Cuff of endotracheal tube inflated and position checked before cricoid pressure released.
- Ongoing sedation/anaesthesia established.
- If difficult/failed intubation encountered refer to algorithms.

Adapted from Royal College of Anaesthetists Initial Test of Competence (RCoA 2003).

Drugs in rapid sequence intubation

Outlined below is a selection of the anaesthetic agents that may be available in the emergency department. The major factor in the safe use of these agents is detailed familiarity with their effects and side effects. Familiarity with only one or two agents in each section is recommended.

Induction agents

Thiopentone

A thiobarbiturate, thiopentone probably remains the drug of first choice for the emergency RSI. Thiopentone is reconstituted in 20mL sterile water to give a solution of 25mg/mL. The recommended elective dose of 3–5 mg/kg may be too high in a hypovolaemic trauma patient, leading to considerable hypotension. A more cautious 1–2 mg/kg will induce anaesthesia with less cardiovascular instability in this situation.

Due to the onset of action within one arm-brain circulation it may be possible to titrate the dose to effect in a conscious patient. For instance by asking the patient to count, with loss of verbal contact being a cue for muscle relaxant administration.

Thiopentone reduces cerebral metabolic rate and therefore can reduce intra-cranial pressure. It may induce a crisis in patients with porphyria. Thiopentone should not be used by infusion for anaesthesia outside specialist neurosurgical indications.

Propofol

Propofol is currently the most commonly used elective anaesthetic induction agent. Propofol is a phenol derivative (2,6-diisopropylphenol) constituted in a soybean and egg phosphatide emulsion at 10 mg/mL (1%).

The recommended elective dose of 1–3 mg/kg may be too high in a hypovolaemic trauma patient. Profound hypotension and cardiovascular collapse may occur on induction of anaesthesia with standard doses. Operators must be familiar with this agent prior to its use in the emergency situation.

The onset of action of propofol is between 30 and 90 seconds, a fact that should be considered when using rapidly acting paralysis agents, such as suxamethonium.

By continuous infusion propofol provides an excellent anaesthetic agent to facilitate transfer or ongoing care, although some degree of hypotension should be anticipated. Prolonged infusion of propofol may lead to hypertriglyceridaemia.

Etomidate

Etomidate is widely used in the induction of emergency anaesthesia, due to its perceived cardiovascular stability. It is a carboxylated imidazole derivative, presented as a clear colourless solution containing 2 mg/mL.

The recommended induction dose of etomidate is 0.3mg/kg. The onset of action is 10–65 s.

Etomidate causes only a mild reduction in cardiac output, but may cause involuntary movements on induction and is highly emetogenic. Concerns over adrenal suppression, caused by a single dose of etomidate, have existed for a number of years. Recent evidence has linked etomidate to an increased mortality in critical care patients. It is therefore becoming less popular.

Ketamine

Ketamine is a non-competitive antagonist at the NMDA receptor in the brain. Ketamine produces a state of 'dissociative anaesthesia', rather than true general anaesthesia.

Ketamine is available in 10, 50, and 100 mg/mL colourless solutions. Care must be taken when drawing it up to ensure that the correct concentration used. The recommended intravenous (IV) induction dose is 1.5–2 mg/kg administered over 60 s with an onset time of around 30 s. If no IV access is available ketamine may be used intramuscularly at a dose of 10 mg/kg.

Ketamine causes sympathetic stimulation and may result in increased cardiac output in the trauma patient. It may cause intra-cranial pressure to rise; therefore, it should be used cautiously in head-injured patients, although it is not contraindicated.

Ketamine may cause hallucinations, delirium, and emergence phenomena. Use of additional opiates or benzodiazepines may offset these problems, although the additional cardiovascular effects of these drugs will require consideration.

Midazolam

Midazolam is the benzodiazepine most used in emergency anaesthesia. It is presented as a colourless solution in either 2mg/mL or 5mg/mL. The dose for sedation is 0.07–0.1 mg/kg. In order to achieve true anaesthesia much larger doses may be needed, and the time taken to establish anaesthesia can be very variable.

The variation in dose and time of response to midazolam mean that it is too unpredictable to be recommended for use as a sole induction agent. Operators may find it useful as an adjunct to other agents such as ketamine. It can also be useful in small doses to facilitate adequate pre-oxygenation in the combative patient.

Muscle relaxants

Muscle relaxants are required to facilitate intubation of the trachea. Muscle relaxation also prevents the haemodynamic response and increase in intracranial pressure caused by coughing, facilitates emergency mechanical ventilation, and lessens the chances of accidental extubation.

Suxamethonium

Suxamethonium is the only depolarizing muscle relaxant in common use. It acts as a non-competitive agonist at the neuromuscular junction, causing prolonged depolarization.

Suxamethonium is presented as a clear colourless solution containing 50 mg/mL, requiring storage at 4°C.

The intravenous dose is 0.5–2 mg/kg. Onset of action occurs within 30 s and is seen by widespread muscular twitching in the patient. Duration of action is 3-5 min. It may be given intramuscularly at a dose of 2.5 mg/kg.

Suxamethonium provides rapid muscle relaxation and facilitates intubation conditions. A short duration of action allows the patient a chance to recover spontaneous respiration should a 'cannot intubate, cannot ventilate' situation develop.

It is metabolized by plasma cholinesterase, but approximately 5% of the population are deficient in this enzyme. These patients demonstrate a variable delay in the metabolism of suxamethonium. Due to increased muscle activity suxamethonium leads to an increased oxygen demand during fasciculation, which may result in more rapid oxygen de-saturation in at-risk patients.

Muscle depolarization causes a transient rise in serum potassium. In the emergency setting this is usually of little clinical relevance, but susceptible patients who have neuronal overgrowth, such as chronic spinal injuries, myopathies or chronic burns and patients with renal failure may be at risk of life threatening hyperkalaemia. Suxamethonium is safe to use in the first 24 h following a major burn.

Suxamethonium is a trigger agent for malignant hyperthermia.

Non-depolarizing muscle relaxants

All non-depolarizing agents act as competitive antagonists at the nicotinic (N2) receptors in the post-synaptic membrane of the neuromuscular junction.

The choice of individual agents is best made based upon operator familiarity. All facilitate endotracheal intubation and controlled ventilation.

Atracurium

Atracurium is a benzyl isoquinolinium ester, presented as a clear colourless solution containing 10 mg/mL. The normal intubating dose is 0.3–0.6 mg/kg giving satisfactory conditions for intubation in 90 s.

Atracurium has an intermediate duration of action with reversal occurring usually between 25 and 35 min. It is metabolized by Hoffman degradation, making it independent of both renal and hepatic function. It should be stored at 4°C.

Atracurium may cause histamine release on injection. This histamine release may result in flushing, hypotension, and bronchospasm in susceptible patients.

Rocuronium

Rocuronium is an aminosteroid. It is presented as a clear colourless solution containing 10 mg/mL. The normal intubating dose is 0.6 mg/kg. Satisfactory conditions for intubation occur in less than 60 s.

Rocuronium has an intermediate duration of action with a single dose lasting 30–45 min. The rapidity of onset has led to its use as a sole muscle relaxant in the technique of modified rapid sequence induction. A recent Cochrane review found that rocuronium gave equivalent intubating conditions to suxamethonium when used with propofol for rapid sequence induction.

The duration of action of rocuronium means that should a 'cannot intubate, cannot ventilate' situation be encountered, the operator can not rely on spontaneous neuromuscular blockade reversal to ensure patient recovery.

A novel rocuronium binding agent has recently been released; sugammadex offers the possibility of rapid reversal of neuromuscular blockade in the 'cannot intubate, cannot ventilate' scenario.

Vecuronium

Vecuronium is a bis-quaternary aminosteroid. It is presented as a powder that is diluted in water prior to use to yield a clear, colourless solution containing 2 mg/mL. The normal intubating dose is 0.08–0.1 mg/kg, producing satisfactory conditions for intubation within 2 min.

Vecuronium has an intermediate duration of action with a single dose lasting approximately 40 min. It has minimal cardiovascular effects and anaphylaxis is very rare.

Opiates

Opiates may be used during rapid sequence induction—an additional modification to the classical induction with thiopentone and suxamethonium. Their use reduces the cardiovascular response to laryngoscopy and may allow some dose reduction of induction agent. They are also useful as adjuncts to ongoing sedation.

Alfentanil

Alfentanil is a rapidly acting, potent opioid. It is presented as a clear solution containing 500 μg/mL. The normal intravenous dose is 10–50 μg/kg, giving a peak effect within 90 seconds and a duration of action of between 5 and 10 min.

The pharmacodynamic profile of alfentanil, closely matches that of thiopentone and suxamethonium making it a suitable adjunct in a modified rapid sequence induction.

Fentanyl

Fentanyl is a rapidly acting, potent opioid. It is presented as a clear solution containing 50 μg/mL. The normal intravenous dose is 1 μg/kg, giving peak effect within 5 minutes and duration of action of 20 min.

In order to completely obtund cardiovascular response, doses up to 100 μg/kg are used; this higher dose requires very little additional anaesthesia, but has a very long duration of action. Fentanyl accumulates with prolonged infusion.

Morphine

Morphine is the most commonly available opiate. It is available in numerous formulations. The initial adult dose of morphine is between 5 and 20 mg. Much larger doses may be required for adequate analgesia in poly-trauma patients.

Morphine has a peak analgesic effect 30–60 min after administration and duration of action of 3–4 h. Due to response variability, morphine is not recommended for use in a rapid sequence induction technique.

Remifentanil

Remifentanil is a very rapidly acting, very potent opioid, usually given by infusion. It is presented as a clear colourless solution that is usually diluted to produce a 50 μg/mL or 100 μg/mL solution.

When given by infusion, remifentanil provides profound analgesia and cardiovascular stability within 1–3 min. The metabolism of remifentanil by pseudocholinesterases means that its offset is rapid and predictable.

Remifentanil use in the emergency department is limited by cost and familiarity. Bolus administration of remifentanil (and to a lesser extent fentanyl and alfentanil) may result in chest wall rigidity, causing extreme difficulty with ventilation. It is however very useful for maintaining sedation.

Other pharmacological adjuncts

Lidocaine

The intracerebral pressure rise in response to laryngoscopy may cause secondary injury in patients with head injury. As an alternative to the use of opioids to obtund the pressor response, lidocaine 1 mg/kg IV bolus at induction has been recommended (e.g. 7 mL 1% lidocaine solution for a 70 kg patient).

Maintenance of anaesthesia and sedation

Standard theatre maintenance of anaesthesia with volatile agents is very difficult in the emergency department without dedicated anaesthetic machines, and transferring patients with volatile maintenance is almost impossible.

Alternative means for maintaining anaesthesia are therefore required. Traditionally, drugs given by intravenous infusion are used in-hospital, although intermittent techniques are often used pre-hospital.

The use of an infusion of propofol (2–10 mg/kg/h) or midazolam (2–10mg/hr) is acceptable; higher doses may be required prior to interventions being performed.

Continuous infusions or bolus administration of both opioids (e.g. alfentanil or fentanyl) and muscle relaxants (e.g. atracurium or vecuronium) are also effective. Mechanical ventilation is mandatory if muscle relaxants or potent opioids are used. It is important to note that there are several deleterious effects of positive pressure ventilation, which are summarized in Box 5.8.

Box 5.8. Deleterious effects of positive pressure ventilation

Reduction of venous return

Unlike spontaneous ventilation during which a patient will generate a negative intra-thoracic pressure, mechanical ventilation requires the generation of a positive intra-thoracic pressure. This positive pressure impedes venous return to the heart and may cause hypotension due to a decrease in venous pre-load. In elective surgical patients this reduction may be mild or even unnoticed, but in the hypovolaemic trauma patient it may contribute significantly to worsening hypotension.

Pneumothorax

In the presence of blunt chest trauma an undiagnosed simple pneumothorax may be converted into life-threatening tension pneumothorax with the application of a positive intra-thoracic pressure.

Traumatic pneumothoraces require insertion of a large intercostal drain prior to intubation, or at least the availability of staff who can site an intercostal drain rapidly should it be required. Any deterioration in respiratory or haemodynamic status following intubation should raise the suspicion of a tension pneumothorax, the diagnosis of which is based upon clinical signs.

Alternative airway techniques

Numerous other airway techniques have been described for use in the trauma patient Especially if the airway is predicted to be difficult or if an intubation attempt has failed. Some can also be used to temporize the situation if experienced airway specialists are not immediately available.

Supraglottic airway devices

Supraglottic airway devices sit within the oropharynx and provide a path for airflow between the mouth and the laryngeal inlet. They are anatomically designed to fill the oropharynx. Some of the devices have an in-built suction port that sits in the upper oesophagus to allow aspiration of regurgitated stomach contents. These devices do not provide a definitive airway, as the absence of a protective cuff within the trachea allows flow of gastric fluid and secretions into the lungs. They will, however, protect the airway from contamination from above, for example, as a result of facial bleeding.

Laryngeal mask

The most popular supraglottic airway in the UK, the laryngeal mask airway (LMA), is available in a range of sizes. Size 3 is suitable for a small female, size 4 for a small male and size 5 for a large male. The LMA is inserted with direct pressure backwards over the tongue; a rotational insertion method similar to a Guedel airway can be used if difficulty is encountered. When the cuff is inflated the LMA rises slightly out of the patient's mouth and should fit snugly.

Newer variations on the LMA such as the 'pro-seal' LMA, which has a built in suction port, the i-Gel™, and the intubating LMA are all available to aid the operator in the event of a difficult intubation (Fig. 5.6).

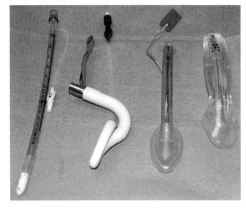

Fig. 5.6. Various LMAs.

Combitube

The combitube comprises a two-lumen (upper and lower) tube with air cuffs on both lumens. It is not strictly a supraglottic airway as it is inserted blindly and may allow intubation of the trachea with inflation of the appropriate cuff. If the main tube comes to rest in the oesophagus, inflation of this cuff allows a seal with ventilation through the upper lumen.

Fibreoptic intubation

Fibreoptic intubation is an attractive alternative to rapid sequence induction in the trauma patient. A fibre-optic laryngoscope pre-loaded with an endotracheal tube is required. The procedure is usually performed awake (through the nose) with local anaesthesia to the airway. Local anaesthesia can be provided by either a spray-as-you-go technique using 1-mL aliquots of 4% lidocaine, or with topical nerve blocks—see section on local anaesthesia for the airway. Fibre-optic intubation can also be performed under general anaesthesia, although the risk of airway obstruction due to anaesthesia is a real threat.

Fibreoptic intubation may be difficult in the grossly soiled airway as a small amount of blood will degrade obtained images and the suction capabilities of the fibre-optic laryngoscope are poor. Direct airway trauma may lead to gross derangement allowing the operator no chance of identifying anatomical landmarks. Only the experienced operator should undertake fibre-optic intubation in the trauma patient.

New airway equipment incorporating fibre-optic technology is constantly being developed. The C-Trach™ LMA is an intubating laryngeal mask airway fitted with a video screen to allow direct visualization of the vocal cords. The Airtraq® is a laryngoscope blade with a camera and video screen mounted on the end, which is designed to be inserted directly into the oropharynx, aiding intubation. The use of such devices in the difficult trauma airway has yet to be validated.

Retrograde intubation

A flexible guide wire is passed in a retrograde direction through a cannula placed in the cricothyroid membrane. The end of the guide wire is retrieved from the mouth and threaded through the Murphy's eye of an endotracheal tube. The endotracheal tube is then advanced over the guide wire until it contacts the cricothyroid membrane. The guide wire is then removed and the endotracheal tube advanced further into the trachea. Adequate local anaesthesia is required for this procedure in all but the most obtunded patient.

Inhalational induction

In circumstances where airway loss is a potential danger, consideration should be given to an inhalational induction. Theoretically if a spontaneously ventilating patient develops airway obstruction, secondary to the loss of airway tone during induction of anaesthesia, by being unable to breath in more volatile agent they will awaken before complete airway obstruction has developed.

The lateral, head down position allows drainage of any regurgitated gastric contents during inhalational induction. This position is not possible with the majority of trauma patients, so a supine position must be adopted, with operator vigilance for the need for oro-pharyngeal suction. Traditionally, the volatile agent halothane has been used for paediatric and adult inhalational induction due to its pleasant smell and lack of airway irritation. The newer agent sevoflurane is equally well tolerated and has fewer cardiovascular side effects, and as such has become the current agent of choice. Inhalational induction requires patience to ensure adequate depth of anaesthesia; the experience of the operator is the key to success.

Blind nasal intubation

A skilled operator may be able to place a nasal endotracheal tube blindly through the nose of a spontaneously ventilating patient, by listening (and feeling) for maximal breath sounds and manipulating the tube as it passes through the nasopharynx. Local anaesthetic spray or laryngeal nerve block may be required to facilitate passage of the endotracheal tube through the vocal cords. Nasal intubation in trauma should be undertaken cautiously as both the risks of anatomical disruption and further airway soiling are ever present. It is not recommended for the inexperienced.

Local anaesthesia for the airway

A number of the techniques outlined above rely upon adequate local anaesthesia of the upper airway. Nasal anaesthesia should be accompanied by vasoconstriction. Traditionally topical 10% cocaine solution has been applied. Alternatively phenylcaine, a mixture of phenylephrine and lidocaine, is becoming more widely available.

The posterior third of the tongue and oropharynx is anaesthetized with 5–10 sprays from a metered dose 10% lidocaine spray.

Superior laryngeal nerve blocks offer an approach to anaesthetizing the vocal cords. Pledgets soaked in 4% lidocaine may be placed in each pyriform fossa using Krause's forceps; this may be difficult in un-cooperative patients. Alternatively, the superior laryngeal nerve may be anaesthetized by injecting 2–3 mL of local anaesthetic deep to the thyrohyoid membrane bilaterally, at a point one-third between the midline and the tip of the superior cornu of the thyroid cartilage.

Anaesthesia below the vocal cords is provided by puncture of the cricothyroid membrane with a 22G cannula and injection of 2 mL 4% lidocaine, after aspiration of air confirms position. This will cause the patient to cough and spread local anaesthesia across the underside of the vocal cords and upper trachea. An almost painless alternative is the use of a 27G dental needle for the injection if available.

A spray as you go technique is popular with many operators when using a fibre-optic laryngoscope. Aliquots of 4% lidocaine are either injected down the suction port of the laryngoscope with intermittent advancement, or an epidural catheter is threaded down the suction port to allow more precise placement of the lidocaine.

Nebulized 4% lidocaine provides an alternative, or addition, to all of the above techniques, but its efficacy is variable.

The surgical airway

Cricothyroidotomy is a technique of last resort in the management of the difficult airway. Due to the unpredictable nature of airway management it is essential that all operators have a detailed knowledge of the technique and have continued practice on models. When faced with a failed airway the response from the operator must be timely and appropriate, as at this stage seconds may make a great difference to patient outcome. Two basic methods of cricothyroidotomy exist; the cannula cricothyroidotomy and the surgical cricothyroidotomy.

Anatomy

The cricothyroid membrane is easily palpated in the anterior neck. It lies between the thyroid cartilage (Adam's apple) and the cricoid cartilage (see Fig. 5.7). By extending the patients neck, if possible, and applying traction to the soft tissues of the neck the membrane becomes fixed to allow instrumentation.

Indications

If a 'can't intubate, can't ventilate' situation develops emergency access to the trachea is required. Cannula cricothyroidotomy is simpler to perform than surgical cricothyroidotomy.

Cannula cricothyroidotomy allows oxygenation and limited ventilation, but this may be adequate to allow more definitive airway management to be undertaken.

Surgical cricothyroidotomy allows the insertion of a small tracheostomy tube facilitating both oxygenation and ventilation. The risk of airway injury and bleeding are higher with the surgical approach.

Cannula cricothyroidotomy

Two alternative methods may be used, depending upon available resource. The intravenous cannula-over-needle technique uses readily available equipment in the

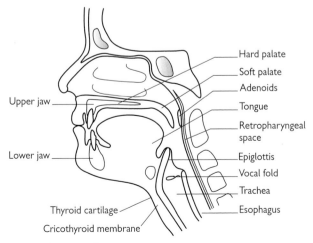

Fig. 5.7. Simple anatomical drawing of anterior neck.

Hard palate
Soft palate
Adenoids
Tongue
Retropharyngeal space
Epiglottis
Vocal fold
Trachea
Esophagus

Upper jaw
Lower jaw

Thyroid cartilage
Cricothyroid membrane

emergency room. The formal cannula cricothyroidotomy technique is more secure and may allow improved ventilation, but needs specialized equipment. Both methods require a connection to an oxygen supply.

Intravenous cannula over needle technique
- Clean the skin over the cricothyroid membrane.
- If the patient is conscious, a small amount of local anaesthetic may be injected into the subcutaneous tissue.
- Attach a 10-mL syringe containing 3–4 mL 0.9% NaCl to a large bore intravenous cannula (14–16G).
- Tense the skin over the cricothyroid membrane and advance the cannula and syringe through the skin and cricothyroid membrane in a slightly caudal direction (approximately 60-degrees to the skin). Aspirate on the syringe as the cannula progresses. When air bubbles appear in the syringe, advance the cannula a few millimetres further forward and then slide the cannula over the needle.
- Remove the inner needle when the cannula is fully advanced. Position of the cannula is checked by the free aspiration of air into the 10 mL syringe.
- Secure the cannula against kinking.

Risks/complications
Patients must have a patent passageway through the glottis to allow for exhalation; barotrauma or pneumothorax may result if the patient is unable to exhale. Kinking of the cannula may lead to complete obstruction. Surgical emphysema may result from displacement of the cannula; this may be massive and further worsen airway management.

Ventilation using the cannula over needle technique
Attaching the cannula to an oxygen supply is often fraught with difficulty so it is recommended that preparation for this be made before the technique is required.

The simplest oxygen attachment is to use a length of oxygen bubble tubing to attach the cannula to the wall oxygen flowmeter delivering 15 L/min O_2, which will produce a flow rate of 400 mL/s through a 14G cannula. A small hole should be cut in the side of the tubing, which when occluded will cause insufflation. A ratio of 1-s insufflation to 4 s expiration (side hole open) should allow expiration and prevent barotrauma. Three-way taps and Y-connectors have been used instead of the cut hole in the side of the tubing to facilitate this technique.

Formal cannula cricothyroidotomy
Commercial kits are available for cricothyroidotomy, such as the Melker or Patil (Cook Ltd, UK) sets. Both of these sets use a Seldinger technique, where a needle is placed within the trachea as previously described. A guide wire is then advanced through the needle and the needle removed.

A larger cannula, mounted on a dilator, is then placed into the trachea by inserting over the guide wire.

Alternatively, the Quiktrach (VBM Medizintechnik GmbH, Germany) set uses a premounted cannula on a Verre's needle, which is placed through the cricothyroid membrane after a small horizontal skin incision. The Verre's needle allows the anterior tracheal wall to be breached, but prevents further needle advancement through the posterior tracheal wall.

Risks/complications
As with the needle over cannula technique, patients must have a patent passageway through the glottis to allow for exhalation. Bleeding is a greater problem due to the size of the cannula. Kinking of the cannula is rare due to the size and reinforcement of the purpose made equipment.

Ventilation using the formal cannula cricothyroidotomy
Commercially available kits allow the connection of the patient to a standard anaesthetic circuit via a 15-mm connector. Due to the size of the cannula, only limited expiration via the cannula is possible, so barotrauma remains a risk if there is glottic obstruction. Oxygen jet injectors may also be attached via suitable luer lock connectors.

The surgical cricothyroidotomy
- Identify the cricothyroid membrane.
- Clean the skin over the area and insert local anaesthetic if required.
- Using a short, rounded scalpel (e.g. no. 20 or Minitrach scalpel), make a stab incision through the skin and membrane. Enlarge the incision with blunt dissection using forceps, NOT the scalpel handle.
- Providing cephalad skin traction with the non-dominant hand insert a lubricated 6.0- or 7.0-mm tracheostomy tube with obturator *in situ*.
- Remove obturator and connect to a low pressure ventilation source.
- Verify tube position with auscultation and capnography. Inflate cuff and secure tracheostomy.

Risks/complications
Haemorrhage into the airway, damage to underlying structures, misplacement, and surgical emphysema are risks of this technique.

Ventilation using a surgical cricothyroidotomy
The surgical cricothyroidotomy allows placement of a formal tracheostomy tube into the trachea, therefore, facilitating formal ventilation with normal equipment. It must, however, be seen as a short-term measure due to the risks of stenosis and laryngeal injury with long-term placement.

The failed airway

It is important to anticipate that any of these techniques, may fail. This in itself is not too much of a problem so long as oxygenation is assured. It is therefore vital to have a well-rehearsed drill that will maintain patient safety whilst alternative plans are made.

> With any failed intubation plan, maintaining patient oxygenation is of paramount importance

Early in the drill it is important to note whether it is possible to ventilate the patient or not. It is the 'can't intubate, can't ventilate' scenario that is of most concern—these patients will rapidly run into trouble unless an airway can be quickly secured by some means.

An example drill from the Difficult Airway Society is presented in Fig. 5.8; it is highly recommended that these become second nature through frequent simulator practice.

Why is the trauma airway difficult?

Every trauma patient brings individual challenges. The unique nature of the injuries, combined with the co-morbidities of the patient, and the unpredictable presentation all add to difficulties with the trauma patient's airway. It is, however, worth noting some of the more common issues, which make it especially challenging. These can be divided into patient factors and environmental factors.

Patient factors

Fasting state and aspiration risk

All trauma patients must be assumed to have a full stomach until proven otherwise. Guidelines from the American Society of Anaesthesiologists (ASA 1999) recommend that clear fluid requires a fasting time of 2 h to ensure gastric emptying, whereas a light meal requires a fasting time of 6 h. It is uncommon to encounter a patient who has not eaten within 6 h of an injury.

Opioids, anxiety, pain, head injury, alcohol, and metabolic derangement all cause a significant delay in gastric emptying.

Poorly performed bag-mask-valve ventilation may insufflate gas into the stomach and increase the risk of regurgitation. This is a particular risk during the prolonged intubation attempts of the difficult airway.

Aspiration of 30–40 mL of gastric contents into the lungs can cause significant pulmonary damage. This damage usually takes the form of a chemical pneumonitis, secondary to direct acid injury to the pulmonary endothelium. Occasionally, microbial flora of the upper gastrointestinal tract will colonize the lungs leading to aspiration pneumonia, although this tends to be a later presentation.

No pharmaceutical prophylaxis (e.g. H_2 antagonists, proton pump inhibitors, antacids or gastric motility agents) has been proven to have a role in the trauma patient in preventing this aspiration risk.

Co-morbidity

As the general population ages, more patients with significant co-morbidities will become victims of trauma. Examples of conditions with a direct influence upon the airway in trauma include diabetes mellitus, obesity, and rheumatoid arthritis.

Pregnancy

A number of factors combine to make the management of the airway in the later stages of pregnancy more difficult. Increasing intra-abdominal pressure makes gastric reflux more common. Airway anatomy in late pregnancy changes due to upper airway and vocal cord oedema.

Breast enlargement may make direct laryngoscopy more difficult. The left lateral tilt required to prevent aorto-caval compression will alter the view at laryngoscopy.

The beard

Although beards are often worn for fashion or religious reasons, some men wear them to disguise a receding chin. Caution should be taken when approaching the airway management of a bearded patient as not only is facemask ventilation more difficult, due to the inability to obtain a tight seal, but laryngoscopy may reveal further anatomical problems.

Patient anxiety

The trauma patient will be anxious. They may not cooperate with pre-oxygenation. An exaggerated loss of sympathetic drive at induction of anaesthesia may well be reflected in a propensity to cardiovascular collapse.

Anxiety slows gastric emptying making the aspiration of gastric contents more likely.

Environmental issues

The emergency department resuscitation room is usually a busy area of the hospital, with many members of staff accessing the same patient at once, and there are often multiple patients with competing demands. Contrasting this environment with the controlled atmosphere of a theatre anaesthetic room, where the individual patient's airway is the only priority, gives an insight into some of the environmental issues facing the operator attempting to manage the airway in trauma.

Operator and assistant experience

Failed intubation rates decline with increasing operator experience. Junior medical personnel need exposure to the difficult airway in trauma for training, but experienced help must be available in case difficulty is encountered.

Skilled assistance is invaluable in managing the difficult intubation, from correct application of cricoid pressure through to suggestions for alternative equipment in the failed intubation scenario. The Association of Anaesthetists of Great Britain and Ireland recommends the presence of an appropriately trained assistant during the induction of anaesthesia.

Skill maintenance

Operators undertaking intubation in the emergency department need to maintain an adequate level of airway skills.

Unfamiliar surroundings and equipment

Medical staff called to assist in the management of trauma in the emergency department may be faced with an array of equipment different from that used in the operating theatre. Medical staff may also find themselves subject to different protocols and rules. These factors may combine to increase the difficulty encountered with the trauma airway.

Unanticipated difficult tracheal intubation - during rapid sequence
induction of anaestheia in non-obstetric adult patient

Direct
laryngoscopy   ➡   Any
problems   ➡   Call
for help

Plan A: Initial tracheal intubation plan

Pre-oxygenate
Cricoid force: 10N awake → 30N anaesthetised
Direct laryngoscopy - check:
  Neck flexion and head extension
  Laryngoscopy technique and vector
  External laryngeal manipulation -
  by laryngoscopist
  Vocal cords open and immobile
If poor view:
  Reduce cricoid force
  Introducer (bougie) - seek clicks or hold-up
  and/or Alternative laryngoscope

succeed ➡ Tracheal intubation

Not more than 3
attempts, maintaining:
(1) oxygenation with
    face mask
(2) cricoid pressure and
(3) anaesthesia

Verify tracheal intubation
(1) Visual, if possible
(2) Capnograph
(3) Oesophageal detector
"If in doubt, take it out"

failed intubation

Plan C: Maintenance of
oxygenation, ventilation,
postponement of
surgery and awakening

Maintain
30N cricoid
force

Plan B not appropriate for this scenario

Use face mask, oxygenate and ventilate
1 or 2 person mask technique
(with oral ± nasal airway)
Consider reducing cricoid force if
ventilation difficult

succeed

failed oxygenation
(e.g. SpO$_2$ < 90% with FiO$_2$ 1.0) via face mask

LMA^{TM}
Reduce cricoid force during insertion
Oxygenate and ventilate

succeed ➡

Postpone
and awaken patient if possible,
or continue anaesthesia with
LMA^{TM} or ProSeal LMA^{TM} -
if condition immediately
life-threatening

failed ventilation and oxygenation

Plan D: Rescue techniques for
"can't intubate, can't ventilate" situation

Fig. 5.8. Insert failed intubation drill. (Reproduced with permission from the Difficult Airway Society).

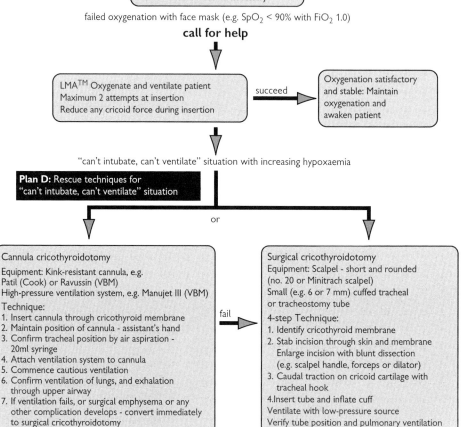

Failed intubation, increasing hypoxaemia and difficult ventilation in the paralysed anaesthetised patient: Rescue techniques for the "can't intubate, can't ventilate" situation

failed intubation and difficult ventilation (other than laryngospasm)

Face mask
Oxygenate and Ventilate patient
Maximum head extension
Maximum jaw thrust
Assistance with mask seal
Oral ± 6mm nasal airway
Reduce cricoid force - if necessary

failed oxygenation with face mask (e.g. SpO_2 < 90% with FiO_2 1.0)

call for help

LMA™ Oxygenate and ventilate patient
Maximum 2 attempts at insertion
Reduce any cricoid force during insertion

succeed →

Oxygenation satisfactory and stable: Maintain oxygenation and awaken patient

"can't intubate, can't ventilate" situation with increasing hypoxaemia

Plan D: Rescue techniques for "can't intubate, can't ventilate" situation

or

Cannula cricothyroidotomy

Equipment: Kink-resistant cannula, e.g. Patil (Cook) or Ravussin (VBM)
High-pressure ventilation system, e.g. Manujet III (VBM)

Technique:
1. Insert cannula through cricothyroid membrane
2. Maintain position of cannula - assistant's hand
3. Confirm tracheal position by air aspiration - 20ml syringe
4. Attach ventilation system to cannula
5. Commence cautious ventilation
6. Confirm ventilation of lungs, and exhalation through upper airway
7. If ventilation fails, or surgical emphysema or any other complication develops - convert immediately to surgical cricothyroidotomy

fail →

Surgical cricothyroidotomy

Equipment: Scalpel - short and rounded (no. 20 or Minitrach scalpel)
Small (e.g. 6 or 7 mm) cuffed tracheal or tracheostomy tube

4-step Technique:
1. Identify cricothyroid membrane
2. Stab incision through skin and membrane Enlarge incision with blunt dissection (e.g. scalpel handle, forceps or dilator)
3. Caudal traction on cricoid cartilage with tracheal hook
4. Insert tube and inflate cuff
Ventilate with low-pressure source
Verify tube position and pulmonary ventilation

Notes:
1. These techniques can have serious complications - use only in life-threatening situations
2. Convert to definitive airway as soon as possible
3. Postoperative management - see other difficult airway guidelines and flow-charts
4. 4mm cannula with low-pressure ventilation may be successful in patient breathing spontaneously

Fig. 5.8. (Cont'd)

Special circumstances

Airway burns

The supra-glottic airway is susceptible to obstruction as a consequence of exposure to heat. The larynx protects the sub-glottic airway. Assessment of the airway in burns is fraught with difficulty, as deterioration due to airway oedema may be rapid.

Clinical indicators of a serious inhalational injury include:

- Facial burns.
- Singed eyebrows or nasal hairs.
- Carbon deposits in the oropharynx.
- Carbonaceous sputum.
- Hoarseness.
- Impaired conscious level especially after fire in an enclosed space.
- Carboxyhaemoglobin level >10%.

Due to airway swelling secondary to direct injury and fluid resuscitation in burns, many authorities advocate a nasal intubation in preference to the standard oral approach. The lips of a burned patient may swell forward, displacing a secured endotracheal tube. The tip of the nose of a burned patient will not swell therefore allowing secure endotracheal tube placement.

The potential gross airway oedema that may occur means that any burned patient whose airway may be at risk requires intubation prior to transfer to definitive care. Intubation may be much more difficult or impossible after a transfer with ongoing resuscitation.

Direct airway injury

There is very little in the literature as to the best way to care for a direct airway injury, mainly because it is surprisingly rare. Even in penetrating trauma to the neck, it is only present in 15% of cases.

Essentially the goal has to be to bypass the injury and ensure the cuff of the tube ends up distal to the leak. In small injuries there is little distortion to the airway anatomy, so normal anaesthetic techniques can be used. Larger injuries will require other techniques. If possible awake fibre-optic techniques should be used, but it may be an indication for a semi-elective surgical cricothyroidotomy under local anaesthesia. Clearly, if the trachea can be seen through the wound it should be intubated under direct vision through the wound. If the injury is more distal a double lumen tube may have to be used. This is an area of expertise well outside the normal practise of most traumatologists.

With regards to the failed intubation drill, supra-glottic airway devices are clearly contra-indicated, as positive pressure above the wound will only serve to worsen it.

Base of skull fracture

Cerebrospinal fluid (CSF) otorrhoea, or rhinorrhoea, peri-orbital ecchymosis (raccoon or panda eyes), retroauricular ecchymosis (Battle sign), VIIth and VIIIth nerve palsies may all indicate a base of skull fracture.

Any clinical indication of a base of skull fracture should indicate that only the oral route be used for insertion of endotracheal or gastric tubes. There is a risk of direct penetration of the skull base and injury to brain with nasal instrumentation. If the nasal route must be used, careful fibre-optic-guided instrumentation may be an option, but this is very dependent on operator experience and fraught with difficulty due to distorted anatomy and airway secretions or blood obscuring the view.

Pre-hospital

Numerous recent reports have shown that pre-hospital airway support often leaves room for improvement. It has also been shown that most trauma patients in the UK do not get to an emergency department for at least 30 min after the incident. The Golden Hour is therefore, in the main, a pre-hospital event. For this reason, many doctors have taken their skills out of the emergency department and into this very demanding arena.

Complex airway control can be maintained in a quality pre-hospital system to the benefit of the patient. However, if done badly, it will clearly worsen the outcome.

Conclusions

The trauma airway can be very demanding. Its management is a vital part of the resuscitation of every trauma patient. Skilled teams must be available to manage the airway. These teams must regularly work together under agreed protocols and practise uncommon events on simulators.

It is, however, ultimately a very satisfying part of trauma care when it is done well, and will save lives.

Further reading

Aitkenhead A, Smith G, Rowbotham D. *Textbook of Anaesthesia*. London: Churchill Livingstone/Elsevier.

Arrowsmith JE, Robertshaw HJ, Boyd JD. Nasotracheal intubation in the presence of frontobasal skull fracture. *Canad J Anaesthesia* 1998; **45**(1): 71–75.

Association of Anaesthetists of Great Britain and Ireland. *The Anaesthesia Team (rev edn)*. London: AAGBI, 2005.

Brimacombe J, Keller C, Kunzel KH, et al. Cervical spine motion during airway management: a cinefluoroscopic study of the posteriorly destabilized third cervical vertebrae in human cadavers. *Anaesth Analg* 2000; **91**: 1274–1278.

Crosby ET. Airway management in adults after cervical spine trauma. *Anaesthesiology* 2006; **104**: 1293–318.

Ford P, Nolan J. Cervical spine injury and airway management. *Curr Opin Anaesthesiol* 2002; **15**: 193–201.

Henderson JJ, Popat MT, Latto IP, Pearce AC. Difficult Airway Society guidelines for management of the unanticipated difficult intubation. *Anaesthesia* 2004; **59**: 675–94.

Himmelseher S, Durieux ME. Revising a dogma: ketamine for patients with neurological injury? *Anesth Analg* 2005; **101**: 524–34.

Jewett BS, Shockley WW, Rutledge R. External laryngeal trauma analysis of 392 patients. *Arch Otolaryngol Head Neck Surg* 1999; **125**: 877–80.

Lockey D, Davies G, Coats T. Survival of trauma patients who have prehospital tracheal intubation without anaesthesia or muscle relaxants: observational study. *Br Med J* 2001; **323**: 141.

Morris C, McAllister C. Etomidate for emergency anaesthesia; mad, bad and dangerous to know? *Anaesthesia* 2005; **60**(8): 737–40.

NCEPOD. *Trauma: Who Cares? National Confidential Enquiry into Patient Outcome and Death*. London: NCEPOD, 2007.

Sprung CL, Annane D, Keh D, et al. CORTICUS Study Group. *Hydrocortisone therapy for patients with septic shock*. *N Engl J Med* 2008; **358**(2): 111–24.

Whitten C. *Anyone Can Intubate*. San Diego: Medical Arts Productions, 1997.

Wilson W, Grande C, Hoyt D. *Trauma Vol 1*. Abingdon: Informa Healthcare, 2007.

Assessment of breathing—thoracic injuries

Assessment of breathing—thoracic injuries

Accurately assessing the multi-trauma patient for significant thoracic injuries can be challenging. There is no single assessment tool that achieves reliable and accurate diagnosis of all possible chest injuries in a way that allows prompt intervention. Hence, a multimodal approach must be used in assessing all but the most minor of injuries.

The vast majority of patients will be assessed using a combination of:
- History of events and symptoms.
- Physical examination of the chest.
- Measurement of vital signs.
- Anterior posterior (AP) supine chest X-ray.
- ECG.

In addition to these basic assessment tools, a number of advanced tools are commonplace in emergency departments receiving trauma patients. These include focused chest ultrasound and multi-slice CT scanning. Some centres will also have the option of formal transthoracic echocardiography, transoesophageal echocardiography, bronchoscopy, angiography, and video-assisted thoracoscopy.

The practical approach to assessing the chest

Each assessment tool has advantages and limitations. In combination, they can allow accurate and timely diagnosis of thoracic injuries. In choosing assessment tools, two factors must be considered. First, what are the injuries that require diagnosis or exclusion; and secondly, what are the limitations placed on the patient's assessment by their clinical condition.

Life-threatening injuries
The most important life threatening thoracic injuries are:
- Pneumothorax, simple, open, or tension.
- Flail chest.
- Pulmonary contusions.
- Haemothorax.
- Tracheobronchial injury.
- Cardiac tamponade.
- Blunt cardiac injury.
- Traumatic aortic disruption.
- Traumatic diaphragmatic injury.

Each of these injuries needs to be considered and excluded. The experienced practitioner will have an index of suspicion of each diagnosis based on the initial information received regarding the mechanism of injury and the patient's preceding physiological status. For example, treating a patient with a single stab wound to the right lateral chest wall, arriving in the emergency department tachypnoeic and hypoxic, the clinician will have a high index of suspicion for a right-sided tension pneumothorax, haemopneumothorax, or mediastinal injury, including cardiac tamponade. The subsequent choice of diagnostic tool and interpretation of the result will be influenced by this index of suspicion.

The patient's clinical status

This will guide the urgency of intervention and the choice of investigation. For example:
- Is the patient able to communicate symptoms reliably, or at least react to examination to reveal clinical signs?
- Is the patient breathing spontaneously or are they being assisted with positive pressure ventilation?
- Is it possible for the patient to sit upright or are they limited by injury or immobilization in the supine position?
- Is the patient's physiological status stable enough to allow transfer from the relative safety of the resuscitation area to a remote assessment tool, such as CT scan and back again?

Each of these factors limits both the application of assessment tools and how subsequent findings are interpreted. For example, it may be extremely difficult to diagnose a haemothorax on a supine chest X-ray, but if the patient is able to sit up for an erect chest X-ray the diagnosis of haemothorax becomes relatively simple.

It is of paramount importance to recognize the patient in whom life-saving intervention cannot be delayed pending accurate diagnosis. The classic example of this is the patient with suspected tension pneumothorax with respiratory or cardiovascular collapse, in whom chest decompression should not be delayed in order to get a diagnostic chest X-ray.

Individual assessment tools

History of events
A history of the mechanism of injury is a valuable tool in predicting injuries. The history should cover whether the injury is blunt or penetrating, what order of energy transfer may have occurred and the site and direction of energy transfer. A simple summary, such as 'a fall from 10m onto concrete, landing on his back', maximizes the impact of this part of the history without unnecessary embellishment.

In penetrating trauma the type of weapon should be noted, remembering that the weapon's length is of greater importance than its width. A long screw driver, for example, can penetrate the left ventricle, leading to quickly fatal cardiac tamponade, whilst leaving the most inconspicuous of external wounds.

Symptoms
Shortness of breath (or difficulty in breathing) is a sensitive, but not specific symptom of chest injury. Chest pain may help to localize the area or side of the injury. The type of pain should be noted. The majority of injuries will produce pleuritic pain. Non-pleuritic pain may indicate rarer pathologies, such as aortic dissection, oesophageal tears, or concurrent myocardial infarction.

Examination
Maximum information from the examination is achieved by following the principles of inspection, palpation, percussion, and auscultation.

Inspection
This phase of examination is perhaps the most sensitive for picking up significant chest injuries. It is vital that the examiner inspects the chest from the end of the bed, bringing the line of sight down to the level of the patient's chest. This position allows a clear view of the movement of the chest throughout the respiratory cycle.

The patient must be assessed for:
- Symmetry of expansion.
- Mobility of the hemi-thoraces. Subtle ipsilateral hyper-expansion and reduced mobility with contralateral hyper-mobility of the chest may be the only signs of significant pneumothorax or tension pneumothorax.

- Abnormal or paradoxical chest movement. For example, diaphragmatic breathing with loss of thoracic cage movement from spinal cord injury below C5.
- Respiratory rate and work of breathing.

A further inspection of the chest should be undertaken from the bedside looking for early bruising and swelling overlying possible fractures, areas of paradoxical movement from flail segments and skin wounds suggesting penetrating injuries. The axillae and back should be examined.

Palpation

Gentle and systematic palpation should be performed covering the clavicles, the anterior and lateral chest wall, and the axillae. This may illicit crepitus from surgical emphysema, which is said to feel like subcutaneous 'rice crispies'. It will localize areas of tenderness and may reveal gross bony deformities, such as sternoclavicular dislocation, if not already picked up in the inspection phase.

Percussion and auscultation

In the noisy emergency room percussion and auscultation are relatively insensitive and may not pick up even gross abnormalities. In order to maximize sensitivity, the chest must be percussed and auscultated over the posterior aspect of the lateral chest wall (where blood will pool), as well as over the anterior chest wall (where air will collect) making careful bilateral comparisons.

It has been reported that positive findings on percussion and auscultation are reliable for diagnosing pneumothorax with a specificity of 97%. This figure may be lower in the intubated patient where inadvertent intubation of a main stem bronchus may mimic pneumothorax in the contralateral side. In terms of excluding pneumothorax, auscultation, and percussion lack the required level of sensitivity.

During auscultation of the anterior chest the examiner should listen to the heart specifically for muffling of the heart sounds associated with cardiac tamponade, and murmurs associated with disruption to the heart valves (however both of these signs are very difficult to illicit in the resuscitaion room). While neither of these signs is sensitive or specific, noting their presence may at least serve to heighten the index of suspicion for these injuries and lead to further focused investigations.

Vital signs

Abnormalities in pulse, respiratory rate and SpO_2 are sensitive indicators of thoracic injuries. Tachypnoea, tachycardia, and hypoxia identify the presence of pneumothorax far more reliably than ipsilateral, decreased air entry and hyper-resonance. Continuous measurement of vital signs demonstrates clinical deterioration and can give an immediate assessment of the physiological response to treatments such as chest decompression. They are, however, non-specific. While a low SpO_2 is an extremely sensitive finding in significant chest injury the routine application of high flow oxygen often masks this sign.

Changes in blood pressure are much less sensitive and even less specific for chest injuries than tachypnoea and hypoxia. Hypotension from chest injuries is a most serious finding.

Chest X-ray

The vast majority of chest X-rays taken for trauma patients will be antero-posterior (AP) supine films, rather than the preferred postero-anterior (PA) erect film. This has major consequences for the utility of the chest X-ray in diagnosing chest injuries. When taking chest X-rays in the resuscitation room, the team leader should ensure that the radiographer receives adequate assistance in optimizing patient positioning and the removal of unnecessary artefacts from the exposure field to facilitate the production of good quality films.

The main advantage of the chest X-ray is its accessibility. A well organized trauma reception should be able to produce a chest X-ray result within a few minutes of a patient's arrival. The main difficulty is that the majority of blunt trauma patients will have to have a supine AP chest X-ray. For example, the sensitivity of PA erect chest X-ray in identifying pneumothorax is generally thought to approach 100%, but some series have found the sensitivity of supine chest X-ray to be as low as 75% or less. A similar trend is true for haemothorax. In addition, the magnification effect of an AP film on the mediastinum often causes difficulty in interpreting the mediastinum.

Ultrasound (the eFAST)

A standard focused assessment by sonography in trauma (FAST) scan can allow an assessment for haemothorax and haemopericardium using abdominal windows into the hemithoraces and the mediastinum. Increasingly, an extended FAST (the eFAST) technique is employed adding specific intercostal windows to assess for pneumothorax.

Haemothorax

This is usually identified during the abdominal assessment of the perisplenic and perihepatic areas. The presence of haemothorax can be seen as fluid above the diaphragm outlining the lung edge, which may look like the tip of a sail floating in the anechoic (black) fluid. Volumes of 150 mL and above may be readily identifiable.

Haemopericardium

A subxiphisternal window allows visualization of the pericardium through the liver. Haemopericardium is seen as an anechoic (black) stripe between the moving ventricular wall and the stationary echogenic pericardium.

Pneumothorax

Windows through the second intercostals space in the mid-clavicular line are examined, normally with a high frequency linear probe. In the normal lung the movement of the visceral pleura against the parietal pleura produces a number of characteristic ultrasound appearances. The most frequently used of these are lung sliding and comet tails. The absence of these findings is used to diagnose pneumothorax.

Multiple studies have demonstrated that ultrasound identification of pneumothorax has a sensitivity of over 90% (compared with supine chest X-ray sensitivity of 70–80%).

The place of ultrasound in clinical decision making is evolving. Currently, portable ultrasound devices have proven useful in the pre-hospital care environment remote from radiological facilities and as an adjunct to plain supine AP chest X-ray in patients too unstable for immediate transfer for CT.

Computed tomography

CT scanning is the gold standard diagnostic tool for most chest injuries. The main drawbacks of CT are the logistical difficulties in transferring a potentially unstable patient to and from the scanning facility and the radiation dose that is required. The limitations of the other assessment tools have provoked many centres to routinely CT scan patients that have suffered a significant mechanism of injury.

Aortogram

Aortography has largely been superceded by high resolution CT except in a small number of patients where CT is equivocal or does not provide an adequate assessment of the exact location and length of a defect.

Blood gas analysis

Arterial blood gases (ABG) should be measured in any patient with a reduced level of consciousness or any sign of respiratory distress or insufficiency. ABG analysis allows an accurate assessment of both oxygenation and ventilation. ABG or venous blood gas can also be used as an adjunct to the assessment of perfusion.

Cardiac markers

Serum troponin levels lack sensitivity for significant myocardial injury and add little to the findings of an ECG. As such they are not routinely used in clinical practice. The same is true of creatine kinase (CK-MB).

Twelve lead ECG

A 12-lead ECG should be performed in all patients suffering blunt chest trauma. Blunt myocardial injury may manifest in a number of ECG changes, most commonly arrhythmias, conduction abnormalities and ST segment changes. Patients with a normal ECG are unlikely to have clinically significant blunt cardiac injuries.

Transthoracic echocardiogram

A transthoracic echocardiogram (TTE) can help identify pericardial effusions and tamponade, valvular abnormalities, and disturbances in cardiac wall motion. TTEs should be performed in patients with possible blunt myocardial injuries and abnormal ECG findings.

Transoesophageal echocardiogram

The transoesophageal echocardiogram (TOE) is a sensitive and specific tool in assessing injuries of the thoracic aorta.

Oesophagoscopy and contrast oesophagram

The combination of oesophagoscopy followed by contrast oesophagram in assessing for oesophageal injury has a sensitivity approaching 100%.

Bronchoscopy

Used mainly for assessing tracheobronchial injuries, bronchoscopy is both sensitive and specific for these injuries.

Do we need to decompress the chest prior to chest X-ray?

The key to deciding which patients warrant immediate decompression and which can afford to wait for a chest X-ray lies in assessing whether the patient's physiological status is critically compromised or whether it is likely to become so imminently. When presented with a chest X-ray showing a massive tension pneumothorax, the standard answer is to say it should never have been taken. However, clinical reality is that, whilst it may be true that a proportion of cases of tension pneumothorax will rapidly deteriorate without intervention, there is good evidence that many cases of tension pneumothorax will not deteriorate in the time it takes to perform an X-ray in the modern resuscitation department. Indeed, it is not uncommon for a chest X-ray to reveal a pneumothorax with radiological signs of tension in a stable patient in whom tension pneumothorax was not suspected. This is especially true of the self-ventilating patient.

It should be remembered that the treatment of tension pneumothorax requires emergency placement of an intercostal chest drain, which is associated with significant morbidity and even mortality. The United Kingdom's national patient safety agency received reports of 12 deaths and 15 cases of serious harm relating to chest drain insertion between January 2005 and March 2008. [National Patient Safety Agency (NPSA), 2008]. This is in addition to the less serious, but more common morbidities that are associated with chest drain insertion, and it is likely that other cases have occurred unreported.

Some retrospective analyses of chest decompression, undertaken on the basis of clinically suspected pneumothorax, reveal a significant number of cases where no evidence of tension pneumothorax was subsequently found (suggesting that decompression was not necessary). To decompress the chest of every patient in whom a tension pneumothorax is suspected, but not confirmed is to unnecessarily put a number of patients through a procedure associated with a risk of death. The morbidity and potential mortality associated with unnecessary chest decompression and use of intercostal chest drains cannot be ignored.

So why do unnecessary chest decompressions occur? Clinical detection or exclusion of tension pneumothorax can be very difficult, especially in the unstable, multi-injured patient, in whom tension pneumothorax is just one of many possible causes for physiological instability. This difficulty is compounded by a high level of anxiety that exists among doctors involved in treating trauma patients around missing tension pneumothorax. This is perhaps brought about by the way trauma is taught to junior doctors. Trauma courses nearly always present tension pneumothorax as a rapidly progressive disease that will lead to inevitable cardio-respiratory arrest within minutes if not treated immediately. In light of this it is perhaps not surprising that there is a tendency to decompress the chest as soon as the possibility of tension pneumothorax is even suggested.

Leigh-Smith and Harris, in their 2005 review of tension pneumothorax, make recommendations regarding when a suspected tension pneumothorax in a self-ventilating patient should be decompressed immediately:
- Chest X-ray not immediately available
  and
- SpO_2 < 92% on oxygen.
- Systolic blood pressure <90 mmHg.
- Respiratory rate <10.
- Decreased level of consciousness on oxygen.
- Cardiac arrest.

It must be remembered that tension pneumothoraces in patients receiving positive pressure ventilation behave more aggressively than in self-ventilating patients, and are far more likely to rapidly progress to a state of critical physiological compromise. Any decision to delay chest decompression in a ventilated patient should be taken with a much greater level of caution if it is considered at all.

In addition to considering the patient's physiological condition, the actual availability of chest X-ray must also be taken into account. A modern resuscitation department with mobile X-ray equipment and a radiographer attending as part of a trauma team should be able to gain a chest X-ray within minutes of a patient's arrival. A patient who deteriorates unexpectedly on the ward may have to wait sometime before a portable chest X-ray can be made available to the treating physician. If a chest X-ray is not going to be available in a timely fashion it may be preferable that chest decompression should be undertaken on clinical grounds.

In any case, where the decision is made to await chest X-ray confirmation of diagnosis prior to chest decompression, the patient must be continuously monitored and the clinician ready to decompress the chest immediately should the patient deteriorate. It is unlikely that this can be safely done whilst transferring the patient to an X-ray department and portable X-ray equipment should always be brought to the patient.

For patients remote from X-ray facilities, primarily in the pre-hospital arena, the application of chest ultrasound with portable machines has been used to exclude pneumothorax in unstable patients in an attempt to reduce the number of unnecessary chest decompressions. The place for the wider application of this technique, for example on intensive care units, is yet to be fully established.

Assessing the need for assisted ventilation

The wave of optimism associated with the initial application of positive pressure ventilation to trauma patients in the 1950s was muted by the recognition that mechanical ventilation is associated with a significant level of morbidity and mortality independent of the patient's original injury. The most common respiratory complication of invasive ventilation is infection, with some series reporting rates of pneumonia as high as 50% in ventilated patients with chest trauma. Other significant respiratory complications include ventilator associated lung injury and sub-glottic tracheal stenosis. In the context of trauma patients the negative haemodynamic effects of intermittent positive pressure ventilation can be significant.

The evolution of more sophisticated ventilation techniques has ameliorated some of the ventilator associated morbidity but it still represents a significant challenge.

When to intubate and mechanically ventilate

The decision to intubate and ventilate a patient is, as with any other medical intervention, a balance between the possible risks and benefits.

Intubating a patient seeks to achieve one or more of the following objectives:

- To modify the balance between tissue oxygen demand and oxygen delivery. Intubation and ventilation attempts to do this by increasing blood oxygen levels and reducing oxygen demand primarily from the respiratory muscles and the sedated brain.
- To control blood carbon dioxide levels and, hence, respiratory acidosis, optimizing conditions for cellular respiration, as well as controlling the other effects of deranged carbon dioxide levels.
- To prevent the development of a pneumonitis secondary to soiling of the airway from regurgitated gastric contents.

Indications for intubation and ventilation

Airway obstruction

Obstruction of the airway results in hypoventilation, leading to hypercarbia and hypoxaemia. In addition, where there is vigorous ventilatory effort against an obstruction, the patient may suffer from a number of idiosyncratic complications, such as negative pressure pulmonary oedema and blood vessel rupture. Where the obstruction cannot be removed or bypassed, or is likely to reoccur, intubation is indicated for as long as the risk of obstruction persists. Where the obstruction cannot be bypassed by orotracheal or nasotracheal intubation, a surgical airway is indicated.

Obstruction in the obtunded patient, as a result of failure to maintain their own airway, is usually due to a loss in the tone of the upper airway musculature. Apart from immediately reversing the cause of the problem, this must always be managed by intubation and ventilation. Simple airway adjuncts should only be used until a definitive airway can be secured with a cuffed endotracheal tube.

Loss of airway protective reflexes

The trauma patient should always be treated as if they have a full stomach. The physiological stress response to trauma reduces gut motility and increases stomach emptying time. All trauma patients should be assessed for their ability to protect their airway.

As a general rule, patients with a GCS of less than 8 are unlikely to be able to protect their airway. It should be remembered, however, that simply having a GCS of 8 or more does not automatically mean that the patient can protect their airway. Every patient who is not able to talk should be observed for the subtle signs of airway compromise. The most reliable signs will be pooling of secretions at the back of the oropharynx and a lack of active swallowing of oral secretions.

Respiratory failure

Respiratory failure occurs for a number of reasons in trauma patients:

Ventilatory failure

This can be due to depression of central respiratory drive, a decrease in lung and chest wall compliance or simply due to chest wall pain (e.g. multiple rib fractures). The primary effect of hypoventilation is to cause an increase in blood carbon dioxide levels resulting in a respiratory acidosis. Hypoxaemia also occurs, but may be a later finding or obscured by the application of supplemental oxygen. The decision to ventilate must be made after alternatives for correcting hypoventilation have been considered. Inadvertent opiate overdose may be reversed by an antagonist, but this should be used with caution as it may leave the patient in considerable pain with few options for further analgesia. Chest wall pain is a remedial cause of hypoventilation; effective pain relief can prevent the need for intubation.

Ventilation perfusion (VQ) mismatch

This primarily results in hypoxaemia. Its causes are numerous—pneumothorax, haemothorax, small airways obstruction, fat embolism, and pulmonary contusions. Some of the causes are obviously reversible, for example with the placement of an intercostal drain. Others may benefit from chest physiotherapy to encourage alveolar recruitment and the clearing of respiratory secretions. The application of non-invasive positive end expiratory pressure (PEEP) in the form of Bi-Level ventilation or continuous positive airways pressure (CPAP), can be successful in recruiting otherwise unventilated areas of lung.

Impaired pulmonary gas exchange

Impaired gas exchange at the level of the alveolar basement membrane results in impaired transfer of respiratory gases to and from the blood. As with VQ mismatch, disruption of the respiratory surface primarily causes an oxygenation defect. However, hypercapnia will occur when the fault affects such a large area of the lung that it cannot be compensated for by hyperventilation. Management strategies are primarily based around optimizing unaffected areas of lung and preventing further lung damage. Both these objectives can be achieved by non-invasive ventilation techniques. Other strategies are based around judicious fluid, blood and blood product administration.

It is unlikely that any one of these mechanisms will occur in isolation and the majority of patients who develop respiratory failure will have a combination of all three. Achieving adequate oxygenation and elimination of carbon dioxide without intubation and ventilation requires a sophisticated and individualized approach to care, but can result in a reduction in morbidity and mortality. A good example of this is in the approach to multiple rib fractures and associated pulmonary contusions. A combination of meticulous pain relief, careful fluid management and the use of non-invasive ventilation in selected patients has been shown to be effective.

There are no absolute hypoxia or hypercapnia threshold values that mandate intubation of trauma patients with respiratory failure. The trend is more important than the absolute figures.

Anticipated clinical course
The condition of trauma patients can change quickly. The likely trend in the first few hours is downwards. Therefore, a patient who has borderline indications for intubation early in their course is likely to eventually succumb. Intubation may be undertaken pre-emptively in patients undergoing transfer to the CT scanner or other remote areas.

The combative patient
The combative patient may pose a threat to themselves and others, and can only be optimally managed by induction of anaesthesia, intubation, and ventilation. The alternative options of physically restraining the patient, or sedation without airway protection are impractical and dangerous.

Humanitarian reasons
Patients with severe pain, severe burn patients, or patients with significant disfiguration, may be intubated primarily for humanitarian reasons.

Tension pneumothorax

When discussing trauma, tension pneumothoraces are afforded a disproportionate amount of attention relative to their incidence, although not without reason. Tension pneumothoraces have the potential to cause rapid deterioration into severe respiratory and cardiovascular compromise, eventually resulting in complete cardio-respiratory collapse and death. Such deaths are avoidable since tension pneumothoraces are entirely treatable (there are reports of life-saving procedures being carried out with simple household objects). In short, the trauma patient who dies from a tension pneumothorax dies a preventable death.

The exact incidence of tension pneumothorax is not clear, with reported cases varying between 0.7 and 30% of general trauma patients. Rates are higher in patients suffering major trauma and significantly higher still in ventilated patients.

Definition

Tension pneumothorax can be described physiologically as the state of positive pressure in a pneumothorax throughout the respiratory cycle. A breach in the pleura allows air into the intra-pleural space via a one-way valve mechanism. This initial pneumothorax expands until the normally negative intra-pleural pressure becomes positive at the end of expiration. This is described as an expanding pneumothorax. The intra-pleural pressure becomes positive for a progressively longer period, eventually encompassing the inspiratory, as well as the expiratory phase of the respiratory cycle.

The most useful clinical definition of tension pneumothorax is a pneumothorax causing significant respiratory or cardiovascular compromise, where the patient's physiological status rapidly improves after the pneumothorax is decompressed. This definition focuses the clinician on a pneumothorax that requires decompression to achieve improvement in the patient's condition, rather than the somewhat academic discussion as to whether a pneumothorax is a massive pneumothorax, a tensioning pneumothorax or a true tension pneumothorax.

Pathophysiology

The intra-pleural space is a potential space between the visceral pleura covering the lung and the parietal pleura lining the hemi-thorax. During quiet breathing the pressure in the intra-pleural space remains negative in comparison to airway pressure throughout the respiratory cycle. A tension pneumothorax occurs when the visceral pleura is breached in such a way that a one-way valve is created. Air enters the pleural space during inspiration and is unable to escape during expiration. This pneumothorax progressively enlarges resulting in collapse of the ipsilateral lung.

The normally negative intra-pleural pressure changes, with the increasing size of the pneumothorax, to become positive. At first this is only at the end of expiration, but then, as the pneumothorax expands, the intra-pleural pressure becomes positive throughout the entire respiratory cycle. This is the point at which the patient's condition can be described physiologically as a tension pneumothorax.

Air continues to enter the pleural space for as long as the pressure in the airway is greater than the intra-pleural pressure at any point in each respiratory cycle. For a spontaneously breathing patient the airway pressures are proportionate to the atmospheric pressure throughout the cycle of respiration. When patients are ventilated, the airway pressure during inspiration is higher due to the applied inspiratory pressures, and the pressures during expiration are proportional to atmospheric pressures (except where positive end expiratory pressure PEEP is applied). Therefore, there is potential for a pneumothorax to expand quicker and to greater pressure in the ventilated patient.

The effects and severity of a tension pneumothorax are further modified by the mobility of the mediastinum. With a more compliant mediastinum, more shift will occur per volume of gas in the pleural space. This results in a lower intra-pleural pressure for a given volume, allowing greater expansion with each breath of the lung alongside the growing pneumothorax. The cost of this is the compression of the contra-lateral lung and possible compromise of cardiac venous return from pressure on the vena cava.

As a result of this complex interplay of factors, a pneumothorax in the spontaneously breathing patient develops at a slower rate than it would in a ventilated patient. Furthermore, spontaneously breathing patients are more likely to suffer progressive respiratory deterioration (to the point of respiratory arrest) before the onset of any direct cardiovascular effects. This is not so in the ventilated patient, in whom cardiovascular collapse may be the predominant factor.

As discussed previously, correct diagnosis of a tension pneumothorax presents a significant challenge. Postmortem studies have shown undiagnosed tension pneumothorax to be the cause of death in up to 3.8% of some trauma populations. Conversely, studies have shown significant numbers of patients in whom chest decompression has been performed, where subsequent investigations have shown no evidence of a tension pneumothorax.

Clinical features

In a patient who is breathing spontaneously a tension pneumothorax may not present with the classic signs and symptoms of:

- Chest pain.
- Dyspnoea.
- Hypoxia.
- Hypotension.
- Tracheal deviation.
- Ipsilateral hyper-resonant percussion note.
- Decreased air entry.

In their review, Leigh-Smith and Harris (2005) highlight the frequency of symptoms and signs of tension pneumothorax in awake and ventilated patients (Tables 6.1 and 6.2).

This confirms a consistency in the pattern of diagnostic signs and symptoms.

Reliable and early findings in awake patients

- Pleuritic chest pain.
- Respiratory distress.
- Tachypnoea.
- Tachycardia.
- Falling SpO_2.
- Agitation.

Table 6.1. Frequency of findings in case reports of tension pneumothorax in awake patients

Chest pain	100%
Respiratory distress	100%
Tachycardia	50–75%
Ipsilateral decreased air entry	50–75%
Low SpO$_2$	<25%
Tracheal deviation	<25%
Hypotension	<25%
Cyanosis	10%
Hyper-resonance	10%
Decreasing level of consciousness	10%
Ipsilateral chest hyperexpansion	10%
Ipsilateral chest hypomobility	10%
Acute epigastric pain	10%
Cardiac apical displacement	10%
Sternal resonance	10%

Table 6.2. Frequency of findings in case reports of tension pneumothorax in ventilated patients

Subcutaneous emphysema	100%
Tachycardia	95%
Decreased breath sounds	87%
Hyper-resonance	85%
Systolic BP<90mmHg	81%
Cyanosis	75%
Low PaO$_2$	70%
Tracheal deviation	60%

Reliable and early findings in ventilated patients
- Immediate decrease in SpO$_2$.
- Decrease in blood pressure (BP).
- Tachycardia.
- Increased ventilation pressure.
- Surgical emphysema.

Investigations

The difficulty in diagnosing tension pneumothorax clinically and the acceptance that an immediate chest X-ray (CXR) may be taken, means that the condition may be diagnosed radiologically where tension pneumothorax is suspected but the patient isn't significantly compromised.

Chest X-ray
- Lung collapse towards the hilum.
- Depressed diaphragm especially if left-sided.
- Increased rib separation.
- Increased thoracic volume.
- Ipsilateral flattening of the heart border.
- Contralateral mediastinal deviation.

It is rare, but not impossible for a tension pneumothorax to exist without apparent lung collapse on a supine chest X-ray. This occurs when the air collects posteriorly or anteriorly collapsing the lung against the opposite chest wall, rather than towards the hilum. The presence of a pneumothorax may still be identifiable from a number of radiological signs.

Supine chest X-ray
- Deep sulcus sign.
- Sharp hemidiaphragmatic border.
- Sharp mediastinal border (the Halo sign).

Management

The management of tension pneumothorax is chest decompression. This is ideally done by the placement of an intercostal tube using an aseptic technique, but this takes time in preparation and execution. Where a patient is compromised, immediate decompression should be carried out. In the self-ventilating patient this should be attempted by needle thoracocentesis using either a specifically designed device, or a large bore cannula placed above the 3rd rib (the 2nd intercostal space) in the midclavicular line. In ventilated patients decompression should be achieved by open thoracostomy. Both these techniques should be followed by the earliest possible placement of an intercostal tube using an aseptic technique.

Successful decompression may be associated with a rush of air as the pleural space is breached and confirms that a pneumothorax was under tension. Any attempt at decompression of the chest must be followed by a clinical reassessment of the patient. Needle decompression may frequently be unsuccessful due to simple failure of the needle to penetrate the chest wall and enter the intra-pleural cavity.

Failure to achieve apparent clinical improvement must prompt both a reattempt at decompressing the chest and consideration of possible alternative causes for the patient's condition. Once the chest has been successfully decompressed a level of vigilance must be maintained as a tension pneumothorax can reoccur. This is most likely to occur with needle decompression, but may occur even after intercostal drain placement.

Where a recollection is suspected after open thoracostomy, a gloved finger sweep can be used to reopen the thoracostomy (taking care to avoid self-injury on sharp surfaces of rib fractures).

Massive haemothorax

Haemothoraces can result from blunt or penetrating trauma and small haemothoraces are common. The incidence of haemothorax or haemopneumothorax is as high as 30–40% of patients with blunt injuries and 70–90% in penetrating injuries.

The source of bleeding in the pleural cavity depends upon the mechanism of injury, but includes lung laceration, intercostal or internal thoracic artery injury and great vessel tears. Parenchymal lacerations generally involve low-pressure bleeds and so tend to stop bleeding spontaneously; however, the involvement of major hilar or great vessels will be more likely to lead to continued haemorrhage and will commonly necessitate early surgical intervention.

Each hemithorax can potentially hold approximately 50% of the circulating blood volume so it is easy to see how unchecked intrathoracic bleeding can cause significant haemodynamic implications. The physiological insult of hypovolaemia from blood loss is compounded by hypoxia caused by the presence of blood.

Massive haemothorax is defined as the initial drainage of 1000–1500 mL of blood on insertion of a chest tube, or a drainage rate of 200–250 mL/h over next 3–4 h.

Clinical features

The primary survey should identify massive haemothorax especially when used in conjunction with FAST.

History: key points
- Suggestive mechanism.
- Chest pain.
- Dyspnoea.
- Haemoptysis.

Examination: key points
- Low SpO$_2$, tachycardia, tachypnoea.
- The trachea may be deviated away from the haemothorax.
- Neck veins may be flat due to severe hypovolaemia or distended because of the mechanical effects of intrathoracic blood.
- Evidence of penetrating injury or significant blunt trauma (haematoma, crepitus, tenderness, emphysema).
- Decreased expansion, stony dullness to percussion and decreased or absent breath sounds on the affected side.

Haemothoraces containing 500–1500 mL of blood may cause clinical signs and symptoms such as dyspnoea, decreased breath sounds to the affected area, and mild tachypnoea and tachycardia.

When examining hemopneumothoraces caused by blunt trauma, auscultation has been shown to have a sensitivity of 100% and a specificity of 99.8% with similarly high NPVs and PPVs. Less sensitive are pain or chest tenderness, and tachypnoea, with figures of only 57 and 43%, respectively. The sensitivity of detection by auscultation when caused by penetrating wounds drops to 51%, but specificity remains high—clinical judgment is good at ruling in.

Investigations

Supine CXR
The diffuse opacity of a haemothorax (massive or not) may be confused with a contralateral pneumothorax (Fig. 6.1).

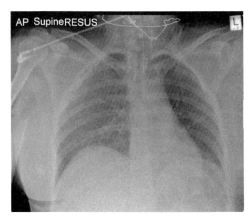

Fig. 6.1. Supine plain radiograph showing diffuse opacity in right lung field from underlying massive haemothorax.

There will be no meniscus and as the blood will lie posteriorly throughout the chest, vascular lung markings may still be visible.

Erect CXR
- An erect chest radiograph may be taken in penetrating trauma.
- Approximately 400 mL of blood is needed to obscure the costo-phrenic angle. As much as 1000 mL of blood may go undetected.

FAST
- FAST can detect smaller haemothoraces, but in the presence of air (such as a pneumothorax or subcutaneous emphysema), may be inaccurate or difficult to interpret.

On visualizing the upper quadrants during FAST examination fluid can usually be identified above the diaphragm in the pleural space. Ultrasound has the advantage of being able to be performed rapidly, making it a useful diagnostic tool for the early diagnosis of haemothorax. However, it cannot replace the chest radiograph as many other injuries can be shown on plain radiography that cannot be demonstrated by ultrasound.

Compared with the supine CXR, ultrasound is more sensitive at detecting haemothorax, and is at least as specific and accurate. The sensitivity of ultrasound has been found to be 92% with a specificity of 100%. This equates to a positive predictive value of 100% and negative predictive value of 98%.

Management

Haemothorax development (including massive bleeding) may be delayed in 2–4% of blunt chest trauma and may relate to rib fractures. The onset of new pleuritic chest pain (on the background of other pain) should warrant close attention even in the presence of normal admission radiology. Thoracostomy and chest tube insertion constitutes the initial treatment for haemothorax. If bleeding stops with no haemodynamic compromise and limited blood drained, then no further interventions may be needed. Drainage allows the two layers of pleura to appose aiding haemostasis, but also increases available lung for oxygenation. Chest tube placement should be early and, if possible, before haemodynamic compromise when large percentages of circulating volume may have been lost into the chest. Small haemothoraces that are not visible on plain films have questionable significance and their management is not entirely clear. Simultaneous restoration of volume depletion is imperative as massive haemothorax implies potential severe haemodynamic compromise. Auto-transfusion devices can be used successfully if available.

The indication that thoracotomy may be required is the drainage of sufficient blood to fulfil the diagnosis of a massive haemothorax. In the presence of haemodynamic instability this should be expedited as soon as the patient's condition and resources allow. The colour of blood in the drain does not affect the decision for thoracotomy as it is the volume lost that indicates potential circulatory collapse.

In the majority of trauma cases requiring chest exploration, the bleeding source is from the chest wall (most commonly intercostal or internal mammary arteries). Once identified, these can be easily controlled with suture ligatures in most cases. After control of obvious bleeding and evacuation of clot and blood, a rapid, but thorough exploration of the entire chest cavity should be performed. If bleeding continues in the stable patient then video-assisted thoracoscopic surgery (VATS) has been shown to control haemorrhage in up to 82% of patients.

Open pneumothorax

This uncommon injury is usually caused by a penetrating object that transects the chest wall. Occasionally blunt injuries can result in a substantial chest wall deficit resulting in an open pneumothorax. When a wound in the chest wall is approximately two-thirds of the diameter of the trachea or more, air may preferentially be drawn in through the open Pneumothorax, rather than the trachea, preventing normal gas exchange and oxygenation.

As intrathoracic pressure increases in inspiration, air moves into the intrapleural space, but may not be expelled completely during expiration. This is sometimes termed a sucking chest wound. The consequence may be the development of a tension pneumothorax through the deficit in the chest wall and further deterioration in oxygenation. This chest injury requires immediate attention before definitive treatment.

Clinical features

History: key points
- Mechanism suggestive of injury.
- Sharp chest pain.
- Dyspnoea (increasing as tension approaches).
- Anxiety.

Examination: key points
- Clinical features of pneumothorax or tension pneumothorax (see section on 'Tension pneumothorax').
- Wound or chest wall deficit, possibly bubbling with respiration.

Investigations

The development of a tension pneumothorax through a sucking chest wound should be treated clinically if cardiorespiratory compromise is present. Plain radiograph will help identify other injuries as part of the primary survey, but should not delay treatment of an open pneumothorax (as with a tension pneumothorax). If further imaging is required (e.g. CT) then this can be obtained once the patient is resuscitated, the chest wall defect attended to, lung inflated, and respiratory function stabilized.

Management

The management has three components:
- Treating the pneumothorax.
- Preventing further accumulation of air.
- Definitive management of the wound and associated injuries.

If tension pneumothorax is present then this should take precedence. Positioning of the chest tube via thoracostomy should be distinct from the wound causing the open pneumothorax.

The sucking wound itself should be treated with a flutter valve dressing—a sterile dressing that allows air to escape from the intrapleural space on expiration, but prevents further accumulation of intra-pleural air on inspiration. The optimal dressing is a chest seal with a one-way valve (e.g. Asherman® or Bolin®). If these are not available, a sterile dressing can be placed over the wound and taped on three sides. The chest wall needs to be clean and dry and can be shaved to allow adhesion. Alternatively, when the patient is continuously monitored, the hole may be covered by an occlusive dressing, but this must be removed if clinical deteriolation occurs.

With more significant size wounds a large non-permeable dressing can be applied. If a small hole is made in the centre then the chest seal can be placed over this.

Placement of a dressing over the defect may be problematic due to size of wound, site of wound, and the presence of fluids such as blood preventing adhesion. If this is the case, and the wound is amenable to temporary closure, then this should be considered early on in the management.

Definitive management of the chest wall wound will depend on the size, deficit, and damage to underlying tissues, but will usually involve surgical debridement and exploration. Intubation and ventilation should be considered in the case of further deterioration in respiratory function, or when operative management is needed.

Flail chest

Flail chest is an injury where the thoracic cage is compromised by two or more rib fractures in two or more places, or when ribs become disarticulated from sternal attachments. Its presence indicates a substantial amount of energy transfer and has a high correlation with underlying pulmonary injury. Overall mortality has been found to be 10–25% (higher in the over 65s). This is rarely attributed to an isolated flail, but often to additional extra- (or intra-) thoracic injuries.

An Israeli series of 11,966 chest injuries showed mortality in isolated unilateral flail injury to be not more than 6%. This rose to 34% for traumatic brain injury with flail, and to 61.1% with traumatic brain injury and other major injury. Road traffic collisions account for most flail injuries and elderly victims have a higher risk of chest wall injuries. The remainder result from falls, crush, and blast injuries.

Clinical features

Diagnosis relies on having a high index of suspicion, and pre-hospital accounts of mechanism are important.

History: key points
- Pain.
- Dyspnoea.
- Haemoptysis (if pain will allow cough).

Examination: key points
- Tachypnoea with shallow breathing, tachycardic, hypoxic, and hypercapnoeic.
- Inspection: ipsilateral decreased chest wall movement (from splinting), haematoma, and possible bony deformity.
- Visible flail segment.
- Palpation: may reveal crepitus and subcutaneous emphysema.
- Auscultation: wheezing, coarse breaths sounds, or decreased air entry

A flail segment is classically described as a fragment of chest wall with independent and paradoxical movement compared with the rest of the thoracic cage, although this may not be present. During spontaneous inspiration, intrathoracic pressure decreases relative to atmospheric pressure on the surface of the chest and this pushes the flail segment in. During spontaneous expiration the pressure within the chest increases and the segment moves outward. The flail segment as an entity does not tend to cause problems (unless by direct bony injury to lung or pleura), but is an indicator of severe underlying lung injury, and can cause hypoventilation secondary to pain.

Investigation

CXR

Plain chest radiograph is important revealing rib fractures, pulmonary contusion, emphysema, Pneumothorax, and other related or unrelated injuries. Injuries such as pneumothoraces should be treated as they are found in the context of the primary survey.

CT

The radiological changes associated with underlying lung injury are often delayed and contusions may appear significantly larger on CT scan (Fig. 6.2). Sensitivity of plain radiograph may be as low as 70% when compared with the gold standard of CT. Plain radiographs do not take into account the three-dimensional nature of contusions and there is evidence that the volume of the contusion relates directly to the risk of developing significant sequelae such as ARDS.

Especially if fractures of the first or second ribs are identified, the implication is that major force has been delivered. This should always prompt a search for other significant intrathoracic issues, such as aortic, tracheobronchial, and mediastinal injuries.

Pulmonary contusion

Flail chest is often associated with underlying pulmonary contusion (up to 90%). Respiratory problems are common after pulmonary contusion, with hypoxaemia and hypercapnoea greatest after 72 h. Pulmonary shunting, interstitial oedema, lack of surfactant and parenchymal haemorrhage may all contribute to alveolar collapse and consolidation.

Subsequent ventilation-perfusion mismatch is compounded by decreased compliance of the affected lung and reduction in functional residual capacity, which leads to an increase in work of breathing and physiological demand.

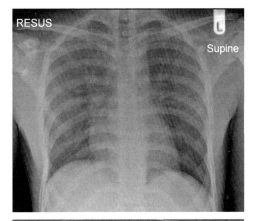

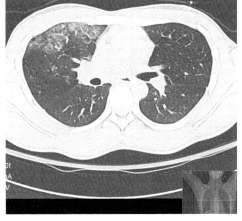

Fig. 6.2. Plain chest radiograph vs. CT chest in same patient. Significant pulmonary contusion is more evident on CT.

It is also evident that lung injury from pulmonary contusion has inflammatory components, and within 24 h inflammatory cells and cellular debris has collected.

The morbidity resulting from pulmonary contusion varies widely, ranging from mild dyspnoea to the necessity for prolonged mechanical ventilation, pneumonia, and organ failure, i.e. Acute Respiratory Distress Syndrome (ARDS). Patient age, premorbid condition and intercurrent health problems may add to the likelihood of developing severe illness. The number of ribs fractured does not appear to relate to morbidity and outcome.

Management
Pain
Pain control is vital in the conscious patient to allow adequate ventilation and pulmonary hygiene. Initial treatment will often involve intravenous opiate analgesia, but this should be followed quickly by thoracic epidural placement if comprehensive analgesia is not achieved. Bupivacaine and fentanyl have both been used as epidural agents with improvements in lung compliance, functional residual capacity and PaO$_2$. Intercostal nerve blocks may be used, but require recurrent placement with risk of pneumo- or haemothorax with each attempt. Patient controlled intravenous analgesia is an effective alternative.

Oxygen delivery
Oxygen delivery is the primary goal in management of pulmonary contusions. Treatment options include non-invasive (mainly CPAP) and invasive ventilation, high-frequency jet ventilation and differential lung ventilation, extracorporeal membrane oxygenation (when ventilation options are exhausted) and surfactant.

If patients are managed outside the ICU, respiratory parameters such as pulse oximetry and respiratory rate should be measured frequently, with any deterioration prompting repeated examination. Arterial blood samples should be used to monitor acid-base status, pO$_2$, and pCO$_2$.

CPAP can be applied by facemask immediately after the diagnosis of flail and pulmonary contusion is made. Levels should be set to reduce work of breathing without causing adverse haemodynamic effects. Application of CPAP should not be delayed for several hours, while the pulmonary contusion evolves and gas exchange deteriorates.

Endotracheal intubation and positive pressure ventilation may be required for those developing impending respiratory failure. The choice of controlled mandatory ventilation (CMV), intermittent mandatory ventilation (IMV), or airway pressure release ventilation (APRV) has been debated with the latter potentially providing better V/Q match at the level of the alveoli. Some evidence suggests that non-invasive CPAP with PCA compared with intubation and mechanical ventilation, may lead to lower mortality and a lower rate of pneumonia, but not to a decrease in length of ICU stay.

Fluids
Administration should be judicious in the presence of flail and contusion. There is debate over the use of crystalloids. Evidence that they increase the size of pulmonary contusion and amount of associated pulmonary oedema is not established. To achieve adequate resuscitation and not further the likelihood of iatrogenic lung injury, it may be necessary to monitor invasively in the intensive care setting.

Flail
Fractured ribs may undergo progressive displacement whilst healing if treated conservatively. This may lead to deformity, volume loss, and collapse of the affected lung. In survivors of flail chest, chronic pain, sensations of chest tightness, and disabling dyspnoea associated with abnormalities in functional residual capacity are common at 6-month follow-up. Surgical stabilization of rib fractures is a source of controversy. Several potential advantages have been reported including reduced duration of mechanical ventilation and subsequent shortened ICU and hospital stay, decreased likelihood of long-term respiratory problems and less chest wall deformity. The value of these procedures versus more conservative measures remains uncertain.

Other factors
Chest physiotherapy is presumed to be of benefit. Patient positioning with the injured side down can help stabilization of the chest wall, but this is likely to be contraindicated in polytrauma.

There is no evidence supporting the use of corticosteroids for pulmonary contusion and it is possible that they may worsen outcome.

Penetrating chest injuries

A global rise in knife and gun crime has resulted in a significant increase in the frequency of penetrating chest injuries. Patients with penetrating chest injuries have a high proportion of life-threatening injuries requiring immediate or urgent treatment. In the USA, it is estimated that 20–25% of trauma deaths are from chest injuries and that penetrating injuries occupy a significant proportion. World-wide, 90% of patients with these injuries are male.

General considerations
A thorough clinical assessment should be made quickly. The incidence of haemothorax, pneumothorax, or haemopneumothorax has been reported to be as high as 55% after chest penetration with a bullet or knife. A rapid evaluation should pay particular attention to these and injuries that require immediate intervention (open haemothorax, tension pneumothorax, massive haemothorax, cardiac tamponade).

The initial inspection should include a comprehensive examination of both axillae, and front and back of the torso. This ensures that any occult injury or wound is not missed. Penetrating neck and upper abdominal wounds can easily breach the chest cavity and cause significant injury. Note should be made of the number and location of wounds, haematomas, and sucking wounds (where bubbling at the surface is evident) and consideration should be given to structures deep to wounds. The seriousness of an injury to the chest cannot be evaluated by simple examination of the wound and establishing the extent of injuries always requires full assessment.

Injury to the great vessels or heart may be less apparent in the initial assessment of the uncompromised patient, but a high index of suspicion should be maintained and the patient fully re-evaluated should any deterioration occur.

The majority of patients with penetration to the chest require no more than a chest tube, oxygen, and fluids. The requirement for intervention can often be assessed with no more than a full examination and plain chest radiograph.

Investigations in general
Patients with penetrating chest wounds and a normal examination require a routine chest radiograph. The incidence of haemopneumothorax, pneumothorax, and haemothorax in the absence of clinical findings is significant and they should always be sought out. This is especially true with gunshot wounds to the chest. Haemothorax and haemopneumothorax are the most likely entities to be missed by examination and cannot be ruled out by auscultation alone. The converse is true, with a high PPV, if auscultation is abnormal.

The management of patients with a negative erect plain radiograph on initial presentation is less clear. A period of observation as an inpatient is advised. This should be coupled with regular observations, repeated examinations, and further radiology as needed.

Penetrating cardiac injury
These injuries have a very high mortality and are often fatal in the pre-hospital setting with autopsy studies showing that as few as 20% of patients reach hospital. Many of these deaths are a result of exsanguinating injuries, rather than from cardiac tamponade. Having reached hospital alive there is still a very high mortality with gunshot wounds to the heart (~80%), but less so with stab wounds (~20%).

The ventricles are the most likely structures to be penetrated—the right more commonly due to its anterior location in the chest. This is true of the coronary arteries with the left anterior descending and the right coronary more likely to be injured.

Cardiac tamponade
This is more common with penetrating chest trauma than blunt chest trauma. As little as 60–100 mL of fluid in the pericardial space can cause clinical manifestations.

Clinical features
- Beck's triad: muffled heart sounds, distended neck veins, and hypotension.
- Signs of haemodynamic compromise (including pallor, sweating, tachypnoea, and agitation or confusion).

If the diagnosis is made, emergency thoracotomy is required, but severe hypovolaemia and noisy emergency departments may hamper identification of these signs. They are non-specific and may indicate tension pneumothorax or other serious injury.

Investigations
- Chest radiograph: this is often unreliable.
- ECG: ST, T wave or rhythm disturbances, but has been shown to be abnormal in as few as 33% of patients.

Management
Anaesthesia of these patients should be undertaken very cautiously with preloading and gentle induction. Resuscitative thoracotomy is discussed elsewhere and is considered if there is a possibility of tamponade and absence of cardiac output for less than 10 min.

Subxiphoid needle pericardiocentesis has little if any place in the diagnosis or management of penetrating cardiac injury as it is extremely unlikely to alleviate tamponade. Pericardial blood is often clotted and will therefore not be removed by cannula placement. The needle can easily penetrate the ventricles or coronary arteries giving a false positive and causing further harm. The best method for investigating pericardial effusion in a stable patient is echocardiography, and the treatment of choice in the unstable patient is thoracotomy.

Pulmonary laceration
The lung parenchyma occupies most of the chest by volume and is therefore especially prone to injury by penetration. Lacerations can occur anywhere from the visceral pleura to the hilum and can involve any structures in the path of penetration. Therefore vessels and air passages can easily be disrupted causing significant pneumothoraces or haemothoraces.

In the presence of a defect in the chest wall and disruption of the pleura then a pneumothorax will probably follow, but especially if the chest wall defect remains patent. This may result in tension pneumothorax or open pneumothorax.

Clinical features
- Pain.
- Dyspnoea.
- Haemoptysis.

Clinical examination, as mentioned, has a high positive predictive value for pneumothorax and haemothorax, but lower negative predictive value.

Investigation
- *CXR:* necessary with any penetrating injury to the chest. An erect film should be taken if possible.
- *FAST:* may reveal pneumothorax (by anterior assessment of the chest wall) or haemothorax (by assessment of the posterior costophrenic angles during abdominal examination).

Management
Most cases of isolated pulmonary laceration that require drainage of air or blood from the pleura will require no further measures after closed tube thoracostomy. Admission to a ward that can manage closed chest tube systems and assessment for any change in physiology is mandatory. This should be combined with regular clinical reassessment to ensure no significant deterioration from continuing air leak or blood loss.

Any subsequent deterioration in respiratory or haemodynamic status should be investigated and treated aggressively. A high index of suspicion for other significant pathology and consideration of thoracotomy should always be retained.

Tracheobronchial injury
Potentially devastating injuries to the airways should be suspected once any penetrating wound to the neck or chest has been identified. Significant injuries of the airway and bronchial tree are more common after high energy blunt trauma and airway intervention, but are also relevant after penetrating injury. Penetration of the trachea or bronchial tree carries a very high mortality if the patient survives the scene of the injury.

Clinical features
- Respiratory distress.
- Tachypnoea.
- Haemodynamic compromise possible.
- Signs of airway obstruction.
- Pneumothorax (possible tension).
- Subcutaneous emphysema around the chest or neck.

Investigation
Plain chest radiograph may reveal pneumothorax, pneumomediastinum, and subcutaneous emphysema.

Treatment
Further investigation and treatment of tracheobronchial injuries is discussed with 'other chest injuries' and related to blunt trauma.

Systemic air embolism
Disruption of lung parenchyma, air spaces, and vessels can result in an abnormal communication between airway and pulmonary vasculature resulting in systemic air embolism (SAE). This unusual complication of penetrating and blunt chest trauma and blast injuries was initially described in the 1970s and more frequently recognized since. 70% are from penetrating injury, but it probably occurs more often in the presence of blunt chest trauma and goes unrecognized due to the presence of other significant injuries.

Systemic air emboli can be rapidly fatal, but have been treated successfully when recognized quickly. Air in the pulmonary circulation can embolize to the left heart, or to cerebral and coronary arteries with rapidly fatal results.

Clinical features
- Sudden deterioration followed by cardiac arrest unresponsive to conventional resuscitative measures.
- *Bubbles:* may be seen in retinal vessels, and during arterial puncture or cannulation.
- Seizure without head injury.
- Haemoptysis or foaming blood in a chest tube.
- More commonly noted soon after the start of positive pressure ventilation (PPV).

In the spontaneously breathing patient the pressure in the pulmonary venous circulation is higher than the airways, but this can be reversed with PPV. Consequently, air can gain access to the circulation through bronchovenous fistulae caused by trauma. This conduit is more likely in the hilar regions where pulmonary veins and bronchi are in closer proximity. High pressures are required to embolize through the pulmonary arteries, although this is possible.

The combination of hypotension, hypovolaemia and PPV is suggested to be the optimum conditions for developing SAE; however, circulatory collapse after intubation and ventilation may also result from hypovolaemia, tension pneumothorax, and cardiac tamponade and due to the presence of co-morbidities.

Investigation
Investigation and diagnosis of suspected SAE is infrequently undertaken.
- Plain chest radiograph or CT demonstrates pneumothorax, pneumomediastinum, pneumatocoele, interstitial air, or emphysema (none of these are specific to SAE).
- *TOE:* small bubbles can be detected, but its use in penetrating trauma may be limited by oesophageal injury.

Findings at thoracotomy identifying SAE include finding air in the coronary arteries, left heart, or aorta.

Management
If SAE is suspected air pressure should be decreased and fluid resuscitation started to attempt to maintain venous pressure. However, this may be a significant challenge when weighing up other effects of fluid use on clotting, haemostasis and ARDS development. Ideally, the patient should be self-ventilating, but in the intubated patient pressures and volumes should be kept to a minimum.

Oxygen bubbles will dissolve faster in blood than nitrogen so high concentrations of oxygen should be used. Nitrous oxide will increase bubble volume and should be avoided. High frequency ventilation may be of benefit. Single lung ventilation (of the unaffected side) can be achieved with a double lumen endotracheal tube if the patient is stable enough. In the absence of this device then sliding an uncuffed tube into the right main bronchus is an alternative assuming this is the side required to ventilate. If airway measures improve the clinical picture by cessation of the leak then conservative management can be considered, but ultimately the management of SAE is often surgical.

Clamping of the ipsilateral hilum, aspiration of air from coronary arteries, ventricles, and aorta are all aimed at reducing further air entering the systemic circulation. Pulmonary resection may be required if repair of damaged vessels and airways cannot be achieved. Emergency thoracotomy for SAE has a mortality of greater than 90%.

Cerebral air embolism has been treated successfully with hyperbaric oxygen therapy (HBOT), and can be considered once the cause has been treated and the patient is stable. Identification is challenging as other causes of neurological deterioration (e.g. hypovolaemia. drugs, head injury) may have to be considered first. Cerebral emboli have been identified on CT brain. Neurological outcome has been shown to be improved by using HBOT in cases of air embolism from other causes and from venous air emboli.

Venous air embolism

This can also arise from penetrating chest wounds and can arise from injuries to the subclavian veins. These are generally better tolerated than SAE.

Oesophageal injury

Identifying the true incidence of oesophageal perforation in penetrating chest trauma is confounded by a high rate of other co-existing serious injuries. The thoracic oesophagus is relatively protected in comparison to the cervical oesophagus and is less often affected when compared with penetrating neck trauma.

Clinical features

Symptoms are often non-specific but relate to oesophageal and gastric contents entering the mediastinum:
- *Severe retrosternal pain:* this may be localized to the side of the perforation as oesophageal contents spill onto the pleura on the affected side.
- *Dyspnoea:* perforation of the mediastinal pleura.
- *Hypotension:* sequestration of fluids compounding early sepsis.
- *Fever:* early in 50%.

Unless a strong suspicion is maintained for digestive tract perforation, then the clinical picture is more likely to suggest a respiratory or haemodynamic issue. Signs are obscured by other injuries. Other signs (expanding haematoma, subcutaneous crepitus, or emphysema) are not specific to an organ and may not even indicate serious injury.

Investigation

CXR
- May be normal if taken soon after injury.
- Mediastinal emphysema may take an hour to develop.
- Mediastinal widening.
- Pleural effusions.
- Later radiographic signs include hydropneumothorax and mediastinal air-fluid levels.

CT
- Extraluminal air may occur in 90% of cases.
- Other findings may include pneumomediastinum, pleural effusions, and mediastinal air-fluid collections.

Contrast oesophagography
- Requires a conscious, alert and haemodynamically stable patient. May be performed by nasogastric tube.
- Sensitive in up to 93% of cases.

Gastrograffin
More false negatives than barium but less likely to cause mediastinal fibrosis.

Flexible oesophagoscopy
- Safe and rapid.
- Awake or intubated patients.

Pleural fluid analysis
pH lower than 6, food particles or raised amylase.

Management

There is a choice of aggressive conservative management versus early surgical intervention for iatrogenic or spontaneous cases. However, little evidence is available regarding the treatment of oesophageal injury resulting from chest penetration. The aim is to maintain function whilst reducing further harm from the septic focus. Diagnostic delay increases morbidity and mortality caused by oesophageal-related complications. The choice of therapeutic procedure depends on the size and location of injury, and time between injury and intervention.

In the stable patient a primary repair with wide drainage is preferable. This allows for early preservation of oesophageal function and will reduce the need for recurrent surgery. The use of a buttressing flap is advocated for thoracic injuries if the trachea is involved as this may prevent fistula formation. Procedures should include mediastinal and pleural drainage after debridement, and thorough irrigation of all tissues involved.

Conservative management strategies for contained disruptions or those draining back into the oesophagus have been suggested. It should be noted that 20% of these patients develop significant early complications and require surgery.

The unstable patient should be treated along damage control principles with placement of a jejunostomy if possible and drainage of the pleura. All patients require aggressive antibiotic therapy and treatment of the effects of sepsis.

Vascular injury: great vessels

Injury to the great vessels from penetrating chest trauma is uncommon due to the protective effects of bony structures. If these vessels are injured and the patient reaches hospital alive then the chance of survival is low. Survivors are likely to have a stab, rather than a gunshot wound.

Clinically

Gross haemodynamic instability Non-specific and not amenable to identification on clinical grounds alone.

Investigation
- *CXR:* the CXR may demonstrate abnormality but is not sensitive.
- Contrast CT and angiography.

Management

Surgical management is required after initial resuscitation. The role of interventional radiology strategies for treatment has not been fully elucidated by may come into prominence in the future. Management strategies are based on CT findings. Careful blood pressure control using beta-blockade or calcium channel antagonists will be required post-operatively.

Venous injuries can also result in significant mortality and the venous phase should therefore be examined when contrast is given during angiography.

Vascular injury: subclavian

Penetration to the periclavicular region provides a significant diagnostic challenge to ensure that vascular injuries are not missed. Subclavian artery injuries have a high mortality and many do not reach hospital alive.

Clinically
- Expanding haematoma.
- Distal vascular compromise.
- Visible haemorrhage.

- Neurological deficit has a strong positive predictive value.

The arm and shoulder has extensive collateral vascular supply with the result that external signs may be hidden. Angiography should be considered based on location of wounds independent of the presence or absence of clinical features. However, a normal chest radiograph and normal examination is reassuring when considering subclavian and axillary artery injury. The presence of a haemothorax on chest radiograph adds to the possibility of a subclavian or axillary artery injury, although other causes are common.

Diaphragmatic injury

A diaphragmatic injury is more likely with gunshot wounds below the 4th intercostal space anteriorly, 6th intercostal space laterally or 8th intercostal space posteriorly. It is possible for abdominal contents to herniate into the chest (more often on the left) with resultant lung collapse and mediastinal shift.

Clinically

- Chest (and shoulder) pain.
- Dyspnoea.
- Deviated trachea.
- Absent breath sounds.
- Audible bowel sounds in the chest.

Respiratory compromise may be profound with tachypnoea and cyanosis.

Investigation

The diagnosis can be made with a plain chest radiograph (Fig. 6.3), but ultrasound and CT are useful. Deflation of a

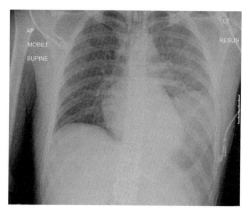

Fig. 6.3. Plain chest radiographic demonstrating ruptured diaphragm with haemothorax and bowel gas shadowing in the chest.

herniated stomach by the placement of a nasogastric tube may ease symptoms and be identified on the plain chest radiograph.

Treatment

All diaphragmatic injuries (penetrating or blunt) should be managed surgically with repair of the defect. The diaphragm should be examined for occult injury if laparotomy is indicated for other injuries.

Other chest injuries

Blunt aortic injury

Blunt aortic injury (BAI) is the second largest cause of trau-matic death after head injury. It occurs after significant deceleration injury or crush and the majority occur as a result of a motor vehicle collision (~80%). Frontal, lateral, and oblique impacts causing compartment intrusion are the commonest characteristics. Falls from height consti-tute the second largest group.

BAI is often complicated by other serious injuries as a high degree of energy is transmitted. 85% of patients with BAI from motor vehicle collisions die at scene. Older patients have a decreased survival rate due to decrease in vessel compliance and elasticity, making vessels less toler-ant of shear and compression.

Classification

The commonest site of injury is at the aortic isthmus (85–93%) just distal to the left subclavian artery, due to tethering of the ligamentum. Other sites include the descending aorta (4–5%), ascending aorta (3–5%), and arch (3–4%).

The lesions are divided into three histological types:
- Minor: Grade 1: an intramural haematoma or limited inti-mal flap.
- Major: Grade 2: a subadventitial rupture or change of aortic geometric shape.
- Major: Grade 3: aortic transection with active bleeding or aortic obstruction with ischaemia.

If these lesions remain undetected and the patient survives, progression to chronic thoracic aortic aneurysm or pseu-doaneurysm may occur in the course of several months to many years.

Clinical features

There are no specific signs or symptoms for BAI and diagnosis may be obscured by other significant injuries. Pseudocoarctation and intrascapular murmurs are unlikely to be identified in the setting of a resuscitation room.

Investigation

CXR Classically the plain radiographic features of BAI are:
- Widened mediastinum (>8.0 cm or upper mediastinum to chest ratio >0.25).
- Indistinct aortic knob.
- Left pleural effusion.
- Left paraspinous line displacement.
- Apical cap.
- Tracheal deviation to the right.
- Depressed left main bronchus.
- 'Calcium sign' – displaced calcium ring in aortic knob.
- Nasogastric tube deviation.

A widened mediastinum occurs in up to 85% of patients with BAI (Fig. 6.4), but plain radiographs have also been shown to have a high false negative rate (supine projection and lipomatosis associated with pulmonary contusions) and combinations of signs used in parallel have not proved to be greater than 90% sensitive. Erect PA films are rarely possible in this clinical situation.

Contrast CT
- Para-aortic haematoma or haemomediastinum.
- NPV of up to 100%.

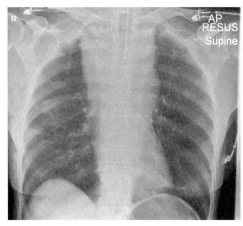

Fig. 6.4. Plain chest radiograph showing widened mediastinum in presence of blunt aortic injury.

Arch aortography

This was the gold standard imaging for BAI until recent CT advances, it is still useful for ascending injuries not classifi-able on CT.

Transoesophageal echo (TOE)

Differentiates Grade 1 from Grade 2 and 3 lesions. The trachea and left main bronchus interfere with assessment of the aortic arch.

Improved imaging means that fewer than 10% of patients will now have aortography as a first step and CT is the imaging of choice. 'Soft signs' do not help surgical planning and up to 10% may go on to have aortography.

Management

Prior to 1997 open repair was the only surgical treatment option but endovascular repair is evolving into the first-line treatment of choice, with good success rates, shorter hospital stays, and low mortality rates compared with open surgery. Patients do not require thoracotomy, aortic cross clamping or single lung ventilation and complication rates of endovascular versus open procedures have been shown to be significantly lower. Not needing to cross-clamp the aorta decreases spinal cord ischaemia and is responsible for much of the reduction in neurological morbidity. Lesions that extend into the aortic arch can be treated, whilst placing the patient on extra-anatomical bypass.

Long-term figures for morbidity and mortality from endovascular repair are not yet available. Medical manage-ment, utilizing vigorous control of blood pressure, should be initiated in those not suitable for surgery. Beta blockade and calcium channel blockade to a target SBP of 110 is sug-gested. This approach may also be useful for minor lesions and can be safely used for those whose definitive repair may need to wait for laparotomy, craniotomy (up to 24%) or treatment of other injuries.

Tracheobronchial disruption

Intrathoracic tracheobronchial disruption (TBD) is a rare injury from blunt chest trauma, but can be devastating due to ventilation and oxygenation difficulties. Lower airway injuries are less common than upper airway injuries, but are present in 0.5–2% of patients presenting for emergency surgery after blunt thoracic trauma.

TBD may be encountered rarely as it is thought that upwards of 80% of patients die before reaching hospital. A level 1 trauma centre may expect to see less than one case per year. Injury to the trachea and bronchi within the chest is thought to arise from three main mechanisms.

- Deceleration-torsion of the mobile pulmonary hilum against the fixed mediastinum. This tends to result in annular disruption within 2.5 cm of the carina.
- *Intrabronchial pressure increase:* chest compression against a closed glottis resulting in a pressure differential between the mediastinum and lower airway. This tends to cause main bronchus or membranous carina disruption.
- *Compression:* usually between the vertebral bodies and sternum. The result is complex disruption in the trachea and carina, and may be associated with brachiocephalic arterial injury.

Clinical features

- Progressing subcutaneous or deep cervical emphysema.
- Consistent bubbling through a correctly sited chest drain.
- Significant tracheobronchial injury will cause ventilation and oxygenation abnormalities.
- It is possible to have smaller tears and injuries without these findings.

Investigations

10% of patients with TBD may not have immediate radiographic evidence and as many as 30% may be missed initially.

CXR may show abnormal air collections:

- The *'bayonet sign'*: a tapering air filled bronchus.
- The *'fallen lung sign'*: 25% of cases (collapsed lung distal to a tear).
- *Mediastinal emphysema:* vertical air lateral to the tracheobronchial stripe.
- Continuous diaphragm sign (right and left diaphragm lines are continuous behind the cardiac silhouette).
- Naclerio's V-sign (V-shaped lucency at the junction of the lower mediastinum and the medial hemidiaphragm).

Treatment

TBD often requires surgical correction and this has been the traditional mainstay of treatment. The presence of the following features warrants surgical repair:

- Associated oesophageal injury.
- Severe dyspnoea/respiratory failure (especially requiring intubation).
- Mechanical ventilation difficulties.
- Worsening subcutaneous or mediastinal emphysema.
- Pneumothorax associated with persistent air leak through a chest drain.
- Mediastinitis.

Endoscopic assessment can help in the decision making process if conservative management is considered. Conservative management may be more effective in membranous injuries. Positive pressure ventilation will worsen the clinical picture if TBD is present and may unmask a TBD if mediastinal tissue is covering the site. The patient will probably develop a tension pneumothorax, progressive mediastinal emphysema, difficulty with ventilation, and

possible air embolism. One lung ventilation, ventilation distal to the injury, occlusion of the disruption, or formal repair are the options.

Blunt cardiac injuries

Blunt cardiac injuries may occur as a result of relatively low energy injury mechanisms. Contusions can be difficult to diagnose and the wide variation in cited incidence reflects this. The presence of other significant injuries may mask clinical features. Injury Severity Scores do not reflect the likelihood of cardiac injury.

Blunt cardiac injuries result from raised intrathoracic pressure and shear forces when the chest wall is traumatized, or from direct contact with adjacent (bony) structures. Haemorrhage occurs, myocardial cells may necrose, enzymes are released, and eventually scar tissue results.

The right ventricle is more likely to be injured as it lies anteriorly under the sternum, and the left-sided valves (aortic and mitral) are more likely to be damaged due to the higher pressures on the left side of the circulation. Valvular injuries include damage to the cusps, leaflets, chordae tendonae, papillary muscles, and annulus.

Clinical features

The presence of rib fractures, sternal fractures, pneumothorax, or other significant thoracic injuries should always alert the clinician to the possibility of a blunt cardiac injury. A conscious patient may experience severe retrosternal pain, which is difficult to manage with opiate analgesia and so may appear clinically similar to the presentation of an ischaemic myocardial event.

Depending on the lesion or injury sustained, the presentation may include features of:

- Ventricular (and other) dysrhythmias.
- Congestive heart failure.
- Pericardial effusion and tamponade (muffled heart sounds and bulging neck veins).
- Acute valvular regurgitation (new murmurs and haemodynamic instability).
- Ventricular aneurysm.

It is also possible for a significant delay to occur prior to development of complications, such as constrictive pericarditis, aneurysm formation or fistulae.

Investigations

ECG findings are varied and non-specific, but found in up to 80% of myocardial injury from trauma. Findings include conduction defects, focal ST and T wave changes, widespread ST changes (as with pericarditis), QT changes, and arrhythmias. Arrhythmias normally arise within 48 h (91%), but there does not appear to be a relationship between degree of contusion and severity of arrhythmia.

Serial cardiac enzymes measurement may show a rise in CK-MB and troponins, but enzymes are also released from skeletal muscle in the multiply-injured patient. Although it seems that CK-MB is not specific, it is possible that troponin measurement may be useful if measured serially. A significant rise in the level of troponin I within 6 h may predict development of serious cardiac sequelae, such as ventricular dysrhythmias and may be useful in the seriously-injured trauma patient.

Echocardiography may demonstrate contusions, defects in wall movement, valvular injuries, effusions, or thrombus. Although vision may be limited by the presence of chest drains it can be performed at the bedside either transthoracically or by TOE. TOE has been shown to be more sensitive and allows evaluation of other mediastinal structures, such as the thoracic aorta, but may not detect smaller contusions.

Management

The clinical significance and therefore need to identifying blunt cardiac injury (myocardial contusion) is questionable. Debate arises over the necessity of identifying these injuries as they may or may not result in significant morbidity and mortality.

Difficulties in identification, and the lack of gold standard diagnostic tests may contribute to the disparity. Identification of other cardiac injuries is necessary and they should be sought out. Those who are admitted to the intensive care setting with serious traumatic injuries will be monitored and evaluated continuously, and these patients should have myocardial injury evaluated should the clinical picture dictate. In the patient with less significant chest trauma, minimal clinical features, and normal ECG, myocardial contusion is unlikely to be a significant issue and cardiac work-up is unlikely to be required.

Thoracic cage injuries

Fractures to the thoracic cage are common after blunt chest injury. It is well recognized that fractures of the 1st and 2nd ribs and the scapulae are associated with a greater chance of serious intrathoracic injury as the amount of force required to cause such injury is significant. Any rib fracture in a child should be treated with caution for the same reason.

Sternal fractures

The incidence of fractures of the sternum has risen in the last 20 years by 100–150%. This is probably due to the significant increase in use of seatbelts. Before seatbelt legislation, the fracture was more commonly caused by the steering wheel.

Clinical features

- Pain.
- Tenderness, bruising, and swelling over the sternum.
- A step or crepitus may be palpated.

Investigations

Sternal fractures cannot be seen on AP or PA chest radiographs, and may not be obvious on lateral views, but can be readily visualized by CT. The sternum can be divided anatomically into six zones when considering fractures— manubrium, synchondrosis, proximal corpus, middle corpus, distal corpus, and xiphoid process. The seatbelt is more likely to be implicated in proximal fractures.

Fractures of the proximal sternum may be associated with higher incidence of occult spinal injury and the presence of multiple rib fractures with significant sternal depression indicates the likelihood of pulmonary injuries. There is no evidence of an association between isolated sternal fractures and lethal decelerational chest injuries (aorta, airway). The reasons for this are unknown, but it is possible that the sternum and the seatbelt absorb enough of the energy to prevent further transmission.

The association of blunt cardiac injury and sternal fractures has led to a previous blanket approach of admission and continuous ECG monitoring for all those with sternal fracture, often for an arbitrary 24 h. However, the minimally or non-displaced fracture can be safely treated symptomatically as an outpatient once significant cardiac and pulmonary injuries have been excluded. A significantly displaced sternal fracture should be treated with a higher suspicion of blunt cardiac injury and be investigated appropriately.

Dislocation of the sternoclavicular joint can be associated with significant airway compromise and reduction may be needed urgently to alleviate pressure on the trachea.

Operative repair of sternal fractures is possible if the patient experiences significant deformity, instability of the thorax, non-union or pain impairing respiratory function. This can be achieved with plating or circumferential wiring.

Rib fractures

Isolated rib fractures are the commonest injury identified after blunt chest trauma, but uncommonly represent significant injuries in themselves. The most commonly injured are ribs 5–9; normally at the posterior angle or at the point of impact. The elderly fracture ribs more often as their thoracic cage is relatively inelastic, whereas children infrequently fracture ribs due to their cartilaginous and pliable bones. Although fractured ribs are seldom thought of as significant injuries themselves, the ends of fractured ribs can cause lacerated pleura or lung, resulting in pneumothorax or haemothorax.

Clinical features

- Chest pain made worse by deep inspiration and coughing.
- Tachypnoea with shallow respiration or splinting.
- Tenderness and possibly guarding.

Investigations

In the absence of a high-energy mechanism, in the presence of normal vital signs, with normal clinical examination, no further investigation is required. The suspicion of a rib fracture (especially 5th–9th) is not an indication for imaging if there is no evidence of other injury.

Plain chest radiographs may be diagnostic for fractures in as few as 50% of cases, but are vital in identifying other injuries if clinically indicated (Fig. 6.5). CT is more sensitive for rib fracture if this mode of imaging is indicated for other reasons.

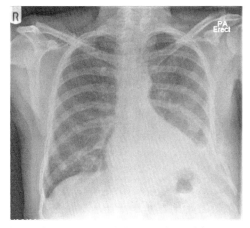

Fig. 6.5. Plain chest radiograph showing left lower rib fractures associated with clinically identified haemothorax.

Fractures of the 1st and 2nd ribs indicate a massive force has been applied to the chest wall and should raise suspicion of associated injuries; incidence of injury to the mediastinum, vessels, and brachial plexus may be as high as 15% in the presence of these fractures. They are relatively protected by the shoulder, scapula, lower neck musculature, and clavicle adding to their robustness. If there is no evidence of other injuries then further imaging is not mandatory, but CT and angiography should be considered if there are any clinical findings.

Fractures of the 10th, 11th and 12th ribs may be associated with liver, spleen, or renal injury, and these should always be considered when such fractures are found. Further imaging and investigation is imperative if clinical suspicion is aroused.

Treatment

Isolated rib fractures can be treated as an outpatient with simple analgesia and breathing exercises. The use of rib belts is now viewed as outdated and has been shown to increase risk of pneumonia and poor outcome. The main goal is adequate analgesia to improve functional vital capacity and clearance of secretions preventing atelectasis and pneumonia. Pneumonia may result from simple rib fractures in up to 6% of patients especially if co-morbidities are present.

If adequate analgesia cannot be achieved or if multiple rib fractures are present (especially in the elderly, three or more ribs), then admission may be necessary for other methods of pain relief. These include intercostal nerve block (risk of pneumothorax), opiate analgesia (titrated, PCA and nebulized have been shown some benefit), and epidural analgesia (specialist management required).

Scapula fractures

Scapula fractures are unusual and represent only 3–5% of all shoulder girdle fractures. The scapula is resilient to injury as it is shrouded in thick muscle (superficial and deep), is relatively posterior and lateral on the body, and is free to move across the chest wall. Because of this toughness, fractures of the scapula are more commonly associated with other chest injuries from high energy transmission. Many people with a scapula fracture are seriously injured and often in the presence of multisystem trauma. Isolated injuries may occur, but should always warrant serious consideration of other injuries especially if the scapula body or spine is fractured.

The body of the scapula is most commonly fractured, the neck and glenoid fracturing less often and the acromion, spine, and coracoid least frequently of all. Injuries associated with the scapula include those of the suprascapular and axillary nerves, and the subclavian and axillary arteries. The brachial plexus is also at risk.

Investigations

Plain chest radiograph taken in the context of a seriously injured patient may not show scapular fractures even if they are comminuted or displaced. The number diagnosed from the chest radiograph has been shown as low as 57% (a combination of being missed, obscured by other injuries, and not included on the film).

Dedicated scapular views can be obtained, but are unnecessary if the patient is having a CT examination of the chest.

Treatment

Fractures of the scapula are frequently treated conservatively, but operative management is more likely if there is significant displacement or rotator cuff involvement.

Diaphragmatic injury

This occurs in up to 5% of blunt chest injuries and can be difficult to diagnose. It occurs up to twice as often with penetrating injuries. A significant proportion of injuries to the diaphragm can be missed by non-invasive means (clinical examination, plain radiography, CT, and MRI), and if left untreated may result in significant morbidity. Possible sequelae include herniation of abdominal contents and resultant incarceration or strangulation.

Thoracostomy and chest drain insertion

Thoracostomy and chest drain insertion are key interventions in the treatment of pneumothorax and haemothorax. Whilst it is sometimes thought of as minor surgical procedure, significant morbidity and mortality are associated with the procedure.

Complications associated with thoracostomy and chest drain insertion

Complications include:

- Pain during and after the insertion.
- Haemothorax.
- Empyema.
- Lung contusion/perforation.
- Wound infection.
- Haemopericardium.
- Liver / spleen perforation.
- Surgical emphysema.

Such complications are often associated with poor insertion technique or inadequate supervision of junior clinicians. Prior to inserting a chest drain, it is suggested that the clinician ensure the indication is appropriate, they are competent to perform the procedure, have all necessary equipment available, and use an aseptic technique. If conditions are not optimal the procedure should be delayed unless it is an emergency. These guidelines are in keeping with recommendations from the UK National Patient's Safety Agency (NPSA 2008).

Required equipment

- Sterile gown and gloves, antiseptic solution.
- Sterile drapes.
- *Local anaesthetic:* ideally a short-acting agent (lignocaine 1.5 mg/kg) mixed with a longer-acting agent (bupivacaine 1 mg/kg).
- Using local anaesthetic plus adrenaline (1:100,000) facilitates a drier field and increases the local anaesthetic dose permissible by 2–3 times.
- 20 mL syringe with 18 and 21G needle for local anaesthetic infiltration.
- Large scalpel blade with handle and Spencer Wells forceps or similar.
- Thoracostomy tube (32–40F for adults, 24–32F for children and 18F for infants), connection tubing, and collecting bottle with under water seal.
- Hand held 0 silk suture, transparent occlusive dressing and broad adhesive tape.

Thoracostomy technique

Where possible the procedure, its indications, and common and serious complications should be explained to the patient with a frank assessment of the level of discomfort that the patient can expect. Informed consent should be gained and documented in the case notes. Large bore intravenous access is essential and SpO$_2$ and ECG must be continuously monitored. Give supplemental oxygen as required. The correct side should be confirmed by the inserting clinician.

The patient should be positioned comfortably. Ideally the patient will be supported sitting upright with the ipsilateral upper limb elevated, resting behind the head. In the supine patient the ipsilateral limb is abducted to give access to the axilla.

Time should be taken to identify the correct incision position. Ideally the thoracostomy is made in the 4th or 5th intercostal space just anterior to the mid-axillary line. This choice of space should be counter referenced against the chest X-ray, to exclude any anatomical anomalies or pathologies that might dictate alternative positioning. This space is accurately identified by finding the 2nd intercostal space just lateral to the sternal angle, counting down the intercostal space along the sternal edge and then following the space laterally to the axilla. Junior clinicians are often surprised at how high into the axilla the correct space is. In the supine male patient the 5th intercostal space at the mid-axillary line lies roughly in the same vertical line as the nipple.

Full aseptic technique should be adhered to, with the clinician wearing sterile gloves and gown. Skin should be prepared with sterilizing solution and draped to produce a sterile field.

Local anaesthetic is then generously infiltrated under the skin and along the anticipated tract of the thoracostomy down to the parietal pleura.

A 3-cm incision is made parallel to the line of the ribs in the intercostal space through the skin and subcutaneous tissue, followed by blunt dissection through the intercostal muscles and ultimately the pleura by advancing the tip of closed Spencer Wells forceps or similar, and then opening the teeth and withdrawing the instrument. This is done above the lower rib to avoid damaging the neurovascular bundle that runs in a grove below each rib.

Once down to the parietal pleura a finger is used to probe through 360 degrees to confirm that the thoracostomy penetrates the chest, that there are no anatomical structures in the way (e.g. diaphragm, colon, heart) and to sweep any adherent lung away from the thoracostomy. If a pneumothorax is under tension, a rush of air may be heard as the pleura is breached. When there is a large haemothorax, a gush of blood can be expected that may surprise the unwary.

Following thoracostomy in the self-ventilating patient an intercostal drain must be immediately placed and secured otherwise the thoracostomy may act as a sucking chest wound. In the positive pressure ventilated patient the placement of the intercostal drain may be delayed.

Chest drain insertion following thoracostomy

For pure pneumothoraces the drain should be aimed apically and anteriorly. For haemothoraces the drain is aimed posteriorly and inferiorly. Before inserting the intercostal drain the clinician should take note of the position of the fenestration (drainage hole) furthest from the drain tip. The drain should be inserted to a predetermined length to ensure that all the fenestrations are within the pleural space. The drain should not be inserted so far that it abuts the mediastinum or the costophrenic angle. If pain or resistance is felt the drain should be withdrawn 2–3 cm provided that all fenestrations remain within the thorax. Placement into the inter-pleural space will be accompanied by fogging of the drain with expiration.

The drain is then attached to an under water seal and secured by a large non-absorbable suture and dressed with a clear dressing so that the incision site can be easily monitored for signs of infection. A broad adhesive tape can be used to further secure the tube. Correct placement of the drain is confirmed by a functional assessment. There should be fogging of the drain and swinging and bubbling of the underwater seal, and the patients condition should improve.?

Once the tube has been secured a chest X-ray should be performed to confirm correct placement. The drain should be in the correct direction, with all fenestrations within the pleural space. An AP chest X-ray can only verify the position of the drain in one plane, but cannot exclude placement of the drain into an interlobular fissure, lung parenchyma or extrapleural space. These problems are often picked up on subsequent CT. Where there is significant mal-positioning of the drain, repositioning should be undertaken using an aseptic technique. It is not necessary to reposition a functioning drain simply because it is not situated apically or basally as intended. If CT demonstrates inadequate drainage of blood or air a second drain may be inserted. The thoracostomy is usually sited one space above the initial drain.

Seldinger chest drains are routinely used to drain spontaneous pneumothoraces. However, the relatively small size of these drains makes them susceptible to blocking and they are therefore unsuitable for the drainage of blood. Traumatic pneumothoraces are usually associated with a degree of haemothorax therefore the use of Seldinger chest drains in trauma is generally not thought to be appropriate.

Resuscitation room thoracotomy

Cardiac arrest following penetrating chest or upper abdominal trauma is usually caused by exsanguination. However, two pathologies are potentially survivable: tension pneumothorax and cardiac tamponade. Management of tension pneumothorax is covered elsewhere in this chapter. This section concerns cardiac tamponade.

Key points

- The most rapid way to confirm the diagnosis of cardiac tamponade is by ultrasound.
- External chest compressions will not produce effective forward flow if cardiac tamponade exists.
- If indications (below) are met, emergency thoracotomy should be performed immediately.
- Pericardiocentesis is not recommended because clotted blood cannot be effectively aspirated.
- Wherever possible, peri-arrest patients should be moved to a cardiothoracic theatre where optimal surgical expertise and facilities are available.
- If specialist cardiothoracic surgical help is not immediately available the task of performing an emergency thoracotomy will fall to a non-specialist. The technique should therefore be as straightforward as possible.
- Several procedures have been described for emergency thoracotomy. The clam-shell technique has successfully been used by non-specialists and is described below.

Emergency 'clam-shell' thoracotomy

Indication
Penetrating chest or upper abdominal trauma associated with cardiac arrest (any rhythm) of >10 min duration.

Contraindications
Definite loss of cardiac output for greater than 10 min. Any patient who has a cardiac output, including hypotensive patients.

Equipment
Gigli saw, large forceps, large scalpel, and large scissors (Fig. 6.6).

Procedural steps
Thoracotomy should not be delayed by intubation, ventilation, or intravenous access—this should ideally be performed at the same time by other members of the trauma team. Time should not be wasted on full asepsis.

- Using the same technique and landmarks as for conventional chest drains, bilateral thoracostomies are performed, the first thoracostomy on the side of the wound/s (since this is the side most likely to be under tension). **Note:** The procedure is stopped at this point if tension pneumothorax is decompressed and cardiac output returns.
- The thoracostomies are connected with a deep skin incision following the 5th intercostal space (Fig. 6.7). For forensic reasons it is important to avoid including the penetrating wound in the skin incision.
- Two fingers are inserted into a thoracostomy to hold the lung out of the way, whilst cutting through all layers of the intercostal muscles and pleura towards the sternum using heavy scissors. This is performed on left and right sides leaving only a sternal bridge between the two thoracotomies.
- The sternum, xiphoid, or xiphi-sternal joint are cut through using the heavy scissors. If the bone cannot be cut through with scissors, the Gigli saw (serrated wire) should be used by:
  - passing the large forceps under the sternum;
  - grasping one end of the Gigli saw (minus handle) with the forceps and pulling back under sternum;
  - connecting the saw handles and with smooth, long strokes cutting through the sternum from inside out.
- The 'clam-shell' is then opened using large self-retaining retractors or rib-spreader (Fig. 6.8). If this is not available, the incision can be held open manually by an assistant. The retractor should be opened to its full extent to provide adequate exposure of the chest cavity. If exposure is inadequate the wounds should be extended posteriorly.
- The pericardium is lifted ('tented') with forceps or by hand and a 2-cm midline incision made using scissors. Two fingers are inserted into the pericardial opening to protect the heart then the scissors used to cut in the midline up to the top and down to the base of the pericardium. This approach minimizes the risk of damage to the phrenic nerves, which run in the lateral walls of the

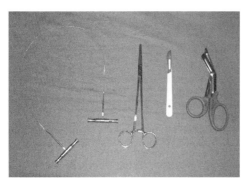

Fig. 6.6. Equipment required for resuscitation room thoracotomy.

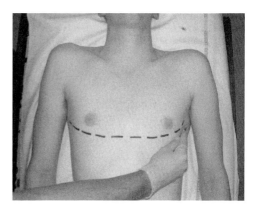

Fig. 6.7. The clam-shell incision.

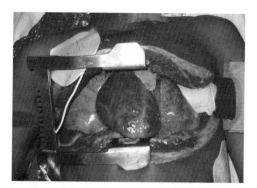

Fig. 6.8. Open chest. Rib-spreaders in situ. Central heart. In this picture the pericardium has been displaced by internal cardiac massage and lies behind the heart. A gloved hand is compressing the aorta.

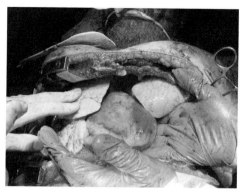

Fig. 6.9. Two-handed quality internal cardiac massage.

pericardial sac, and the heart. Making the incision too short will prevent full access to the heart.

- Blood and clot should be evacuated, and the heart inspected rapidly and systematically for the site of bleeding.

- The heart may begin to beat spontaneously with a return of cardiac output. In this situation, any cardiac wounds should be closed as outlined below.

- If the heart is asystolic or bradycardic with a markedly reduced cardiac output the cardiac wound should be closed quickly then cardiac output improved with internal cardiac massage (see below) +/– inotropic support.:

- If the heart is fibrillating (but full—see below), defibrillation is performed using internal paddles with an initial energy level of 10 J. If these are not available, the clamshell is closed and the patient defibrillated using conventional external pads. Flicking the heart is equivalent to delivering a few joules and may be successful.

- When massage is required it must be of optimal quality. Standing on the patient's left the flat right hand is placed behind the heart with the fingers pointing towards the aorta, and the flat left hand on the anterior surface of the heart pointing in the same direction as the right hand, blood is then 'milked' from the apex up (Fig. 6.9). The heart must remain horizontal during massage; lifting the apex of the heart too far out of the chest can prevent venous filling. The aorta can be compressed against the spinal column using a thumb or fingers to maximize coronary and cerebral perfusion.

- Any bleeding must be controlled.

- Holes less than 1 cm can usually be occluded temporarily using a finger or gauze swab. If this is successful no other method should be attempted.

- For larger defects, a Foley urinary catheter can be passed through the hole then inflated and gently pulled back. This technique reduces the volume of the ventricular cavity (with subsequent reduction in stroke volume), therefore, only a small volume (<10 mL) should be used in the balloon. The catheter must be clamped to prevent blood loss from it. If a catheter is used in this way, a giving set can be attached to allow rapid volume infusion directly into the heart.

- If bleeding cannot be controlled with finger, gauze or Foley catheter, it may be necessary to close the defect with large sutures, but this is a last resort as there is a risk of occluding coronary arteries.

If the procedure is successful the patient may begin to wake up so it is vital to be prepared to provide immediate anaesthesia. Restoration of circulation will be associated with bleeding, particularly from the internal mammary and intercostal vessels. Large bleeders may be controlled with artery forceps.

Further reading

Arnaud F, Tomori T, Teranishi K, Yun J, McCarron R, Mahon R. Evaluation of chest seal performance in a swine model: comparison of Asherman vs. Bolin seal. *Injury*. 2008; **39**(9):1082–8.

Asensio JA, Berne JD, Demetriades D, et al. One hundred five penetrating cardiac injuries: A 2-year prospective evaluation. *J Trauma—Injury, Infect Crit Care* 1998; **44**(6): 1073–82.

Aylwin C, Brohi K, Davies G, et al. Pre-hospital and in hospital thoracostomy indications and complications. *Annl Roy Coll Surg* 2008; **90**: 54–7.

Back MR, Baumgartner FJ, Klein SR. Detection and evaluation of aerodigestive tract injuries caused by cervical and transmediastinal gunshot wounds. *J Trauma* 1997; **42**: 680–6.

Bansal, MK, Maraj S, Chewaproug D, Amanullah A. Myocardial contusion injury: redefining the diagnostic algorithm. *Emerg Med J* 2005; **22**(7): 465–9.

Bent CL, Matson MB, Sobeh M, et al. Endovascular management of acute blunt traumatic thoracic aortic injury: A single centre experience. *J Vasc Surg* 2007; **46**(5): 920–7.

Bokhari F, Brakenridge S, Nagy K, et al. Prospective evaluation of the sensitivity of physical examination in chest trauma. *J Trauma* 2002; **53**: 1135–8.

Bokhari F, Brakenridge S, Nagy K, Roberts R, Smith R, Joseph K, et al. Prospective evaluation of the sensitivity of physical examination in chest trauma. *J Trauma* 2002; **53**(6): 1135–8.

Bonney, S, Lenczner, Eric, Harvey, EJ. Sternal fractures: anterior plating rationale. *J Trauma Injury Infect Crit Care* 2004; **57**(6): 1344–6.

Borman JB, Aharonson-Daniel L, Savitsky B, Peleg K. The Israeli Trauma Group. Unilateral flail chest is seldom a lethal injury. *Emerg Med J* 2006; **23**: 903–905.

Brooks-A, Davies-B, Smethhurst-M, Connolly J. Emergency ultrasound in the acute assessment of haemothorax. *Emerg Med J* 2004; **21**: 44–6.

Burkhart, H, Gomez, Gerardo A, Jacobson, LE, Pless, JE, Broadie, TA. Fatal blunt aortic injuries: a review of 242 autopsy cases. *J Trauma Injury Infect Crit Care* 2001; **50**:113–15.

Campione, A, Agostini, M, Portolan, M, Alloisio, A, Fino, C, Vassalo, G. Extracorporeal membrane oxygenation in respiratory failure for pulmonary contusion and bronchial disruption after; trauma. *J Thorac Cardiovasc Surg* 2007; **133**(6): 1673–4.

Casos SR, Richardson JD. Role of thoracoscopy in acute management of chest injury. *Curr Opin Crit Care* 2006; **12**: 584–9. Reviews the literature on the use of VATS in the diagnosis and treatment of intrathoracic injuries

Chen, MYM, Miller, PR, McLaughlin, CA, Kortesis, WG, Kavanagh, PV, Dyer, RB. The trend of using computed tomography in the detection of acute thoracic aortic and branch vessel injury after blunt thoracic trauma: single-center experience over 13 years. *J Trauma Injury Infect Crit Care* 2004; **56**(4): 783–5.

Coats TJ, Keogh S, Clark H et al. Prehospital resuscitative thoracotomy for cardiac arrest after penetrating trauma: rationale and case series. *J Trauma Injury, Infect Crit Care* 2001; **50**(4): 670–3.

Gasparri, MG, Lorelli, DR, Kralovich, KA, Patton, JH, Jr. Physical examination plus chest radiography in penetrating periclavicular trauma: the appropriate trigger for angiography. *J Trauma Injury Infect Crit Care* 2000; **49**(6): 1029–33.

Gomez-Caro, A, Ausin, P, Moradiellos, FJ, Diaz-Hellin, V, Larru, E, Perez, Jose A, et al. Role of Conservative Medical Management of Tracheobronchial Injuries. *J Trauma Injury Infect Crit Care* 2006; **61**(6): 1426–35.

Gunduz M, Unlugenc H, Ozalevli M, Inanoglu K, Akman H. A comparative study of continuous positive airway pressure (CPAP) and intermittent positive pressure ventilation (IPPV) in patients with flail chest. *Emerg Med J* 2005; **22**(5): 325–9.

Hamilton DR, Sargysan A, Dulchavsky SA (2004). Ultrasound of the chest. In: Brooks A, Connolly J, Chan O, (eds) Ultrasound In Emergency Care. Oxford: Blackwell, pp. 35–41.

Hans W. Schweiger, J. FCCP the pathophysiology, diagnosis and management strategies for flail chest injury and pulmonary contusion: a review. *Anesthes Analges* 2001; **92**(3S) Supplement: 86–93.

Hirose H, Gill IS, Malangoni MA. Nonoperative management of traumatic aortic injury. *J Trauma* 2006; **60**: 597–601.

Kummer C, Netto FS, Rizoli S, Yee D. A review of traumatic airway injuries: potential implications for airway assessment and management. *Injury* 2007; **38**: 27–33.

Lattin, G Jr, O'Brien, W Sr, McCrary, B, Kearney, P, Gover, D. Massive systemic air embolism treated with hyperbaric oxygen therapy following CT-guided transthoracic needle biopsy of a pulmonary nodule. *J Vasc Intervent Radiol* 2006; **17**(8): 1355–8.

LeBlang, SD, Dolich, MO. Imaging of penetrating thoracic trauma. *J Thorac Imag* 2000; **15**(2):128–35.

Leigh-Smith S, Harris T. Tension pneumothorax--time for a re-think? *Emerg Med J* 2005; **22**: 8–16.

Letting-van de Poll T, Schurink GWH, De Haan MW, et al. Endovascular treatment of traumatic rupture of the thoracic aorta. *Br J Surg* 2007; **94**: 525–33.

Marshall JC. Inflammation, coagulopathy, and the pathogenesis of multiple organ dysfunction syndrome. *Crit Care Med* 2001; **29**: 99–106.

National Patient Safety Agency (NPSA). Rapid Response Report. Risk of chest drain insertion. 2008. Available at: www.npsa.nhs.uk/patientsafety/alerts-and-directives.

Nirula R, Allen B, Layman R, et al. Rib fracture stabilization in patients sustaining blunt chest injury. *Am Surg* 2006; **72**: 307–9.

Nishiumi, N, Maitani, F, Yamada, S, Kaga, K, Iwasaki, M, Inokuchi, M, et al. Chest radiography assessment of tracheobronchial disruption associated with blunt chest trauma. *J Trauma Injury Infect Crit Care*. **202**; 53(2): 372–7.

Schmoker, JD, Lee, CH, Taylor, RG, Chung, A, Trombley, L, Hardin, N, et al. A novel model of blunt thoracic aortic injury: a mechanism confirmed? *J Trauma Injury Infect Crit Care* 2008; **64**(4): 923–31.

Schumacher H, Bockler D, Von Tengg-Kobligk H, Allenberg J-R. Acute traumatic aortic tear: open versus stent-graft repair. *Semin Vasc Surg* 2006; **19**: 48–59.

Smakman, N, Nicol, AJ, Walther, G, Brooks, A, Navsaria PH, Zellweger R. Factors affecting outcome in penetrating oesophageal trauma. *Br J Surg* 2004; **91**(11): 1513–19.

Sutyak JP, Wohltmann CD, Larson J. *Thorac Surg Clin* 2007; **17**: 11–23.

Sybrandy KC, Cramer MJ, Burgersdijk C. Diagnosing cardiac contusion: old wisdom and new insights. *Heart* 2003; **89**: 485–9.

Ungar, Todd C, Wolf, SJ, Haukoos, JS, Dyer, DS, Moore, EE. Derivation of a clinical decision rule to exclude thoracic aortic imaging in patients with blunt chest trauma after motor vehicle collisions. *J Trauma Injury Infect Crit Care* 2006; **61**(5): 1150–5.

Wise D, Davies G, Lockey D, et al. Emergency thoracotomy—'how to do it'. *Emerg Med J* 2005; **22**: 22–4.

Wright S. When to ventilate. *Trauma* 1999; **13**: 199–205.

Wu, JT, Mattox, KL, Wall, MJ, Jr. Esophageal perforations: new perspectives and treatment paradigms. *J Trauma Injury Infect Crit Care*. 2007; **63**(5): 1173–84.

Circulatory assessment

Circulatory assessment

This chapter outlines the assessment of circulation in an injured patient including the pathophysiology, recognition and management of shock. When managing an injured patient it is vital to recognize the presence of shock early, and to rapidly identify and treat the cause. Following major trauma, by far the commonest cause of shock is hypovolaemia due to bleeding.

Other less common causes of shock include cardiogenic or neurogenic shock, and these must be anticipated during the initial assessment in cases where pre-morbid conditions or other features are suggestive.

The first management priority in any patient exhibiting signs of shock should be to ensure that the airway is secure and to administer oxygen to provide the highest FiO_2 achievable (usually 85% by reservoir bag mask with a 12–15 L/min flow rate). The effort, rate and the effectiveness of breathing should also be assessed and any immediately life-threatening thoracic conditions managed as appropriate (e.g. decompression of a tension pneumothorax).

Assessment of circulation

Shock is a clinical diagnosis detected by the recognition of certain physical signs produced as a physiological response to poor tissue oxygen delivery. When assessing the injured patient, one of the primary concerns should be to ascertain an appropriate history, including the precise mechanism of injury so that attention can be focused on any specific areas of clinical concern. Enquiries should be made into any relevant past medical history, current regular medications, and drug allergies.

A 'foot of the bed' view should be taken initially and any obvious physical signs noted; for instance, the presence of pooled blood on the trolley or evidence of continued external haemorrhage. A co-ordinated trauma team approach should be followed and the patient exposed appropriately, maintaining dignity as much as possible.

Conscious level

Conscious level is a useful bedside marker of adequate cerebral perfusion and tissue oxygenation, and is often the first and most obvious thing apparent about a patient from the end of the bed. By definition, a fully alert and orientated patient must have a sufficient cardiac output to perfuse the cerebral cortex appropriately. In normal circumstances, cerebral autoregulation ensures a steady cerebral perfusion pressure with changes in blood pressure. However, this process will fail at extremes of range and is also affected by traumatic brain injury.

As cerebral hypoxia increases the level of consciousness will alter, beginning with anxiety, confusion, and agitation, and leading to aggression or combativeness and, if untreated, eventually to coma and death. Focal neurological changes, abnormal posturing, and signs of seizures may also occur.

The level of consciousness may also be affected in patients with a primary brain injury or by drugs (such as opiates or sedatives), thereby preventing further interpretation of the conscious level in relation to the presence, or absence, of shock.

Respiratory rate

The respiratory rate should be measured on arrival and at regular intervals during the initial assessment. This should be done by an observer counting the rate, as bedside physiological monitors that allow continuous respiratory rate measurement by way of transthoracic electrical impedance may give inaccurate results or fail to measure at all, especially where respiratory effort is poor or thoracic injury interferes.

The respiratory rate increases in response to reduced tissue oxygenation due to shock. In adults, a respiratory rate >20 breaths/min is considered abnormal. In children the normal range varies with age as shown in Table 7.1.

The respiratory rate can also be affected by drugs or toxins, or by intrathoracic injury. Tachypnoea may result from pneumothorax or haemothorax, as well as anxiety and pain.

Table 7.1. Respiratory rate (RR) variation with age

Age (years)	< 1	1–2	2–5	5–12	> 12
RR/min	30–40	25–35	25–30	20–25	15–20

Skin colour and capillary refill

Patients with hypovolaemic shock typically exhibit pale, cool, and clammy skin due to peripheral vasoconstriction although skin may remain warm and vasodilated in sepsis.

Capillary refill time testing is a simple estimate of skin perfusion. This is performed by gentle compression of the skin for 5 s followed by measuring the time in seconds before normal colour returns once this pressure is released. Normal capillary refill time should be less than 2 s. The test is best performed in central areas of the body such as the sternum, in order to minimize the effects of cold on the peripheral circulation.

Heart rate and pulse volume

One of the earliest signs of shock is a relative tachycardia. A heart rate above 90–100/min in an adult may represent shock. Hypovolaemic shock usually presents with a weaker, thready pulse felt as peripheral perfusion diminishes. Septic shock may present with a bounding pulse.

In children, the upper limit of normal heart rate differs with age as shown in Table 7.2.

Table 7.2. Heart rate (HR) variation with age

Age (years)	< 1	1–2	2–5	5–12	> 12
HR/min	160	150	140	120	100

However, an increased heart rate is an unreliable measure of shock. Tachycardia may have several other causes, including pain and anxiety, and is not always present in significant shock, for example, in young fit patients, those on drugs such as ß–blockers or the elderly.

Pulse points

The traditional view that various pulse points equate to certain systolic blood pressure values has a poor evidence base. However, the presence of a radial pulse does suggest that perfusion is at least sufficient to reach the peripheral circulation and, by implication, organs such as the brain, heart, and kidneys. Vascular injury, such as traumatic arterial transection may affect distal pulses and will therefore prevent any useful estimation of blood pressure in this way.

Pulse points should not be used in isolation when estimating blood pressure or for detecting the presence, or absence, of shock.

Blood pressure

Non-invasive blood pressure (NIBP) monitoring should be carried out with appropriate measurement intervals depending upon the clinical situation. An automated oscillometric system produces numerical values for the systolic, diastolic and mean arterial pressures during a microprocessor controlled sequence of inflation and deflation of the pressure cuff. Failure to measure or false readings can be caused by an incorrectly-sized cuff or by the presence of irregular cardiac rhythms, such as atrial fibrillation.

Normal blood pressure varies with age, gender, and clinical reasons such as cardiovascular drug therapy and medical conditions including hypertension. Normal systolic blood pressure in children (mmHg) can be estimated by the formula 80 + (age in years × 2).

The pulse pressure narrows in the early, compensated stages of hypovolaemic shock, and in cardiogenic shock, due to raised systemic vascular resistance from vasoconstriction. Pulse pressure generally widens in septic, anaphylactic and neurogenic shock, due to reduced peripheral vascular resistance. Postural hypotension may support the diagnosis of shock, especially due to hypovolaemia.

Non-invasive cardiac output estimation

Several non-invasive devices are available that estimate cardiac output at the bedside and may be used to help detect signs of shock. Transcutaneous Doppler, impedance cardiography and aortovelography methods used in such systems should only be relied upon to record changes in cardiac output, rather than providing reliable absolute measurements.

Technically non-invasive (although requiring sedation or anaesthesia to insert the probe), transoesophageal echocardiography (TOE) may also be utilized as a method to estimate cardiac output and demonstrate signs of shock.

Urine output

Urine output may be considered a non-invasive measure of shock in the non-catheterized patient. Failure to produce an adequate urine output may be a delayed sign of shock, although it may also be due to trauma to the urological tract, acute urinary retention due to neurological injury or from other causes of renal failure. A urine output of at least 0.5 mL/kg/h in adults, and at least 1–2 mL/kg/h in children, signifies that there is adequate renal perfusion.

Response to intravenous fluid boluses

Indirect measurement of the presence and extent of shock can be carried out by assessing the physiological response to intravenous fluid boluses. Improvement following fluid administration may support the diagnosis of hypovolaemic, neurogenic, septic, or anaphylactic shock. Deterioration following intravenous fluid therapy may be noted with cardiogenic shock.

A transient response to intravenous fluid therapy may suggest a more severe degree of shock or ongoing haemorrhage.

Causative volume loss estimates

Loss of circulating blood volume may be predictable from the apparent injuries. In addition to external haemorrhage or large open wounds, the two most important examples of apparent fluid losses are due to thermal burns and fractures. Fluid deficit from burn injury can be calculated according to the body surface area affected, and fractures also have predictable blood volume losses. For example, closed femoral fractures may lose up to 1500 mL blood and closed tibial fractures up to 500 mL in adults.

Invasive monitoring for shock

In general, invasive monitoring is required for groups of patients needing a higher level of care such as coronary, high-dependency or intensive care patients. The principle behind invasive monitoring is to enable the haemodynamic status to be more closely monitored than is possible by non-invasive techniques. Invasive monitoring involves risk that must be balanced against the benefit gained on an individual patient basis.

A variety of invasive lines are used in clinical practice including dialysis lines, Hickman lines and peripherally inserted central catheter (PICC) lines. The emphasis of this section is placed on the use of central lines and arterial lines for monitoring of the shocked trauma patient.

Bladder catheterization is not technically an invasive form of direct haemodynamic monitoring for shock; it is nonetheless 'invasive' from a procedural point-of-view. Catheterization enables close monitoring of urine output although with the associated risk of introducing infection.

Electromechanical devices: the basics

Before considering the relevant techniques and theory for invasive monitoring, it is worth summarizing how the relevant devices work and outline some of the main errors than can occur with measurements.

Manometers

The term manometer usually refers to a type of liquid column pressure measuring instrument enabling bedside pressure monitoring without the need for electronic devices. A column of fluid in direct continuation with the required line is measured in height against a scale (usually in cm of water). This technique is appropriate for central venous pressure (CVP) monitoring, but not for arterial pressure, which is usually too high to measure in this manner.

Transducers

A transducer is a device that converts energy from one form to another. Pressure transducers used for monitoring through central and arterial lines measure electromotive forces via a strain gauge variable transducer. Most pressure transducers contain four strain gauges, which form the four resistances in a Wheatstone bridge on a tiny printed circuit board and diaphragm.

Pressure transducers are connected via a column of fluid (usually sodium chloride 0.9%) at a pressure of 300 mmHg. This column of fluid moves back and forth with each pulsation causing the transducer diaphragm to move. This movement results in a change in resistance and current flow, which is measured and electronically converted in order to display pressure readings.

Common sources of error Confounding errors in measurements can arise from:
- The system not being calibrated and *zeroed*.
- Inappropriate damping of the system.
- The transducer not being at the level of the heart.
- The system not being pressurized to 300 mmHg.

Central venous lines

The CVP is the pressure found within the right atrium and great veins of thorax. Normal pressure should be 0-8 cm H_2O. Hypovolaemia and vasodilatation will result in a fall in CVP due to reduced venous return. CVP can also be used to assess the efficacy of fluid resuscitation, suggested to be adequate if a sustained rise in CVP is demonstrated following an appropriate fluid challenge.

Indications For continuous monitoring of haemodynamically compromised patients and to enable responsive replacement of circulating volume in accordance with CVP. Central venous access may also be required for inotrope and vasopressor infusions or for other drugs for which peripheral administration is not recommended.

Other indications include:
- Facilitating the insertion of pacing lines.
- Regular blood sampling, including mixed venous gases.
- Provision of renal dialysis.
- Administration of parenteral nutritional support.

Contraindications Contraindications to the insertion of central venous catheters are generally relative and related to the site of insertion and mechanism of injury. Injury to the upper thorax or neck may prevent use of the internal jugular or subclavian veins, leaving the femoral vein as the most viable option. Maintaining appropriate sterility of the femoral region is difficult, although any risk of infection must be balanced against the urgency of achieving appropriate access. Femoral lines may not truly represent right atrial pressure and must be interpreted with caution.

There is an increased risk of bleeding from the insertion site in patients with coagulopathies, or who are known to be on anticoagulation therapy. Obesity or anatomical abnormalities can make insertion of lines more problematic, and may be more risky in agitated or confused patients without the use of sedation.

Central line insertion may also be difficult in patients whose respiratory function is compromised and who cannot be laid flat. Very rapid respiratory rates may also increase the risk of air embolus from jugular or subclavian line insertion due to lower intrathoracic pressures.

Complications and limitations Central line insertion is associated with a number of potential complications, some of which are potentially life-threatening:
- Pneumothorax (pleural puncture).
- Arterial puncture or nerve damage.
- Cardiac arrhythmias (direct intravascular stimulation).
- Air embolism.
- Infection by skin commensals.
- Occlusion and thrombosis.

Normal central venous lines (triple or quad lumen) are not always the best form of access for rapid fluid administration in emergency situations as their relatively narrow gauge and longer length may restrict maximum flow rates compared with larger peripheral lines. However, insertion of larger lumen lines, such as vascular catheters (normally used for emergency dialysis) or Swan–Ganz catheter introducer sheaths can permit very rapid central infusions.

Technique of insertion The identification and cannulation of central veins may be difficult in hypovolaemic patients. The 2002 NICE guidelines recommend the use of ultrasound guidance where available to facilitate safer insertion. A standard landmark technique may still be appropriate in the emergency situation. ECG monitoring is required in case of arrhythmias.

Once the vein is located, a percutaneous Seldinger technique is used to insert the catheter. The Seldinger technique comprises the following general steps:
- A 'seeker' needle is passed into the vessel.
- A guide wire is passed through needle into vessel.
- The needle is removed leaving the guide wire in place.
- A dilator passed over the guide wire to widen skin the incision.
- The cannula is introduced into the vessel over the guide wire.
- The guide wire is removed and the catheter secured.

In case of inadvertent arterial puncture, firm pressure should be applied to the site for 5–10 min or until the site has stopped bleeding completely. The catheter position must be checked by x-ray (i.e. chest x-ray for jugular or subclavian lines, or pelvis x-ray for femoral lines), as well as to exclude a pneumothorax.

Pulmonary artery catheterization Central line access is required in order to introduce this type of catheter. A flow-directed balloon-tipped pulmonary artery catheter is floated into the pulmonary artery via the right atrium and ventricle, usually from a right internal jugular site. Pulmonary capillary wedge pressure (PCWP) is the pressure measurement at the tip of the catheter with the balloon inflated and, in most patients, represents left atrial filling pressure and, therefore, left ventricular end-diastolic pressure.

As with CVP measurements, interpretation of PCWP measurements is more useful when monitoring trends rather than single readings. The response of PCWP to fluid resuscitation may be used to indicate intravascular volume status. The use of pulmonary artery catheters is controversial in critical care, with no clear evidence of any benefit to overall morbidity or mortality.

Arterial lines

Arterial lines provide both measurements of blood pressure and a waveform, the shape of which can also provide useful information regarding the haemodynamic status of the patient. Stroke volume and cardiac output can be derived from the area under the systolic part of the curve. Myocardial contractility may be indicated by rate of pressure change over time. Hypovolaemia is suggested by a low dicrotic notch, narrow waveform, and swinging peak pressures with the respiratory cycle.

Indications The main indication for insertion of an arterial line in trauma patients is to allow continuous direct arterial blood pressure monitoring. Arterial line measurement provides a continuous reading and is more accurate than non-invasive methods. It will also enable regular arterial blood gas sampling and measurements. Arterial BP trend is often more important than single readings. Several variables can affect blood pressure readings including age and the existence of pre-morbid medical conditions. Decreased aortic compliance in the elderly may result in higher peak pressures.

Contraindications As with central lines, there may be an increased risk of bleeding from the insertion site or haematoma formation in patients with coagulopathies. Infection may also occur after insertion, with risk increasing the longer the line remains *in situ*.

Complications and limitations The potential complications of arterial line insertion are similar to those associated with central lines as listed. User error may minimize the benefit of arterial pressure measurement. Air bubbles, blood clots, a soft diaphragm, or soft tubing may cause damping of the arterial waveform signal, preventing accurate interpretation. Damping is caused by dissipation of stored energy resulting in a progressive diminution of amplitude of oscillations. Increased damping lowers the systolic pressure and elevates the diastolic pressure, although mean arterial pressure is unaltered. The transducer should be at the level of the right atrium; raising or lowering the transducer will result in errors.

Technique of insertion The common sites of insertion of arterial lines are the radial and brachial arteries. Femoral or dorsalis pedis arteries may also be used. Catheters are inserted either using a catheter over needle technique similar to peripheral venous cannula insertion [e.g. Floswitch™ (*BD*)], or by a Seldinger wire guided insertion technique similar to that used for inserting central lines [e.g. Leadercath (*Vygon*)]. Normal catheter sizes are 18–22G. Similar to central lines, the arterial line system consists of the cannula, connecting catheter, transducer and electrical monitor with appropriate connections.

Shock

In layman's terms, the word shock is commonly used in the context of a sudden surprising event or experience. From a medical point of view the term shock is used to describe a specific physiological syndrome, which can occur due to several different causes and pathological processes, although will present with similar clinical features.

The Online Medical Dictionary defines shock as:

… A condition of profound haemodynamic and metabolic disturbance characterized by failure of the circulatory system to maintain adequate perfusion of vital organs; it may result from inadequate blood volume (hypovolaemic shock), inadequate cardiac function (cardiogenic shock) or inadequate vasomotor tone (neurogenic shock, septic shock) …

Following trauma shock can occur as a result of several mechanisms, the most common of which is hypovolaemia secondary to bleeding. Hypovolaemic shock is associated with considerable mortality. In shock from other causes, such as cardiogenic or septic shock, the mortality exceeds 50%. It is, therefore, vital to recognize and appropriately manage signs of shock rapidly in trauma patients. The various consequences of shock are outlined below.

The causes of shock can be divided as follows:

- Hypovolaemic:
  - haemorrhagic;
  - non-haemorrhagic.
- Cardiogenic shock:
  - Intrinsic;
  - Extrinsic.
- Distributive shock
  - neurogenic;
  - septic;
  - anaphylactic.

The pathophysiology of shock

Shock is a systemic clinical syndrome that can be said to exist when perfusion is insufficient to meet the metabolic demands of body tissues. In severe shock this will manifest at both a cellular and organic level due to hypoxia, failure of normal cellular metabolism, and subsequent acidosis. This failure tends to represent a vicious spiral where deteriorating perfusion, metabolism, and acidosis produce further cellular and organ dysfunction, thus worsening the situation.

In order to understand the pathophysiological consequences of shock, it is important to review a number of relevant basic physiological functions and processes.

Aerobic respiration

Aerobic respiration is the normal process by which cells generate much of their energy (mainly stored in the form of adenosine triphosphate—ATP) and is dependent on oxygen. Much of this process takes place in mitochondria.

ATP, and other stored energy compounds such as phosphorylcreatine (found in muscle), are required for normal cellular functioning. Without ATP, cells will be unable to utilize available energy sources efficiently, will fatigue rapidly and may eventually die. Mitochondria are also responsible for many other cellular mechanisms, which will also fail in anaerobic conditions.

ATP production

- *Glycolysis (anaerobic step):* glycolysis involves the creation of two pyruvate molecules from one glucose molecule producing a net gain of two molecules of ATP in the process.
- *Pyruvate decarboxylation:* each pyruvate molecule is oxidized to acetyl-CoA and carbon dioxide in the mitochondria producing three ATP per pyruvate molecule. The process is also known as the transition or link reaction, by linking glycolysis to the Krebs cycle.
- *Tricarboxylic acid cycle:* the tricarboxylic acid cycle (or Krebs cycle) takes place within the mitochondrial matrix in aerobic conditions. The cycle is an 8-step sequence of reactions producing ATP molecules via the oxidative phosphorylation of associated co-enzymes in conjunction with the electron transport chain. Carbon dioxide is also created during this cycle.
- *Oxidative phosphorylation (electron transport chain):* This occurs in the mitochondrial cristae where ATP is synthesized by the ATP synthase enzyme by the phosphorylation of ADP. This process is powered by a chemiosmotic gradient (proton gradient) across the inner mitochondrial membrane from oxidation of the co-enzymes produced from the Krebs cycle.

Overall, the theoretical total yield of aerobic respiration from one glucose molecule is 36–38 ATP, assuming all reduced coenzymes are used for oxidative phosphorylation. In reality, the likely maximum is around 30 ATP per glucose molecule due to losses and some energy use throughout the various pathways.

Anaerobic respiration

When oxygen delivery is limited, such as in the case of shock, pyruvate is metabolized by anaerobic respiration. Anaerobic respiration is far less efficient at using the energy from glucose and will produce lactic acid as a waste product. This can occur in skeletal muscle and red blood cells.

As stated above, aerobic metabolism can generate a maximum yield of 36–38 ATP molecules per glucose molecule. If perfusion and oxygen delivery are sufficiently impaired by shock that cells have to rely upon the anaerobic metabolic pathway, only two ATP molecules are generated per molecule of glucose.

Oxygen delivery and consumption

The theoretical maximum carrying capacity of oxygen is 1.39 mL O_2 per g Hb, but *in vivo* measurement gives a maximum capacity of 1.34 mL O_2 per g Hb. This number is known as Hüfner's constant.

Blood oxygen content

Blood oxygen content mainly relies upon the oxygen carrying capacity of haemoglobin and its oxygen saturation level. A small amount of oxygen is also carried dissolved in plasma (unbound to Hb), which is dependent on the partial pressure of oxygen in solution. This is taken into account in the following equation to calculate the arterial oxygen content (CaO_2):

$CaO_2 - O_2$ bound to Hb + O_2 dissolved in plasma
$CaO_2 - (Hb \times S_aO_2\% \times 0.01 \times 1.34) + (0.0225 \times P_aO_2)$

Similarly, in order to calculate venous oxygen content, the values of mixed venous oxygen saturation (SvO_2) and venous partial pressure of oxygen (PvO_2) are substituted.

In shock, hypoxia or loss of haemoglobin will result in impairment of CaO_2. Total oxygen carrying capacity is diminished, thus affecting oxygen delivery.

Oxygen delivery

Oxygen delivery (DO_2) represents the amount of oxygen being delivered to the peripheral tissues per unit time. It is calculated by the product of the cardiac output (Q) and the arterial oxygen content (CaO_2). As the oxygen content of blood is calculated per 100 mL blood, the CaO_2 is multiplied by 10 in the equation, as follows:

$$DO_2 - Q \times CaO_2 \; (mL/L) \times 10 - 850{-}1200 \; mL/min$$

Oxygen consumption

Oxygen consumption (VO_2) represents the amount of oxygen utilized by body tissues per unit time. It is calculated by the product of the CaO and the difference between arterial and mixed venous oxygen content.

$$VO_2 - Q \times (CaO_2 - CvO_2) - 240{-}270 \; mL/min$$

The primary management goal in shock is to ensure adequate oxygen delivery to enable tissues to meet their metabolic demands, in turn represented by a balance between VO_2 and DO_2. The extraction ratio is the ratio of VO_2 to DO_2 and is expressed as a percentage. The normal extraction ratio is around 25%, but can double to 50% if tissue oxygen demand increases. The key to managing traumatic shock in practical terms therefore involves returning the cardiac output, oxygen saturations and haemoglobin as near to normal values as possible to maximize DO_2. This will include appropriate oxygen supplementation, fluid resuscitation and blood transfusion as required.

Metabolic (cellular) consequences of shock

Hypoperfusion and subsequent inadequate delivery of substrates and oxygen fails to meet the metabolic requirements of the tissues. Cells are not able to sustain efficient energy production via the aerobic method and respiration will occur anaerobically. This metabolic dysfunction results in production of lactic acid from anaerobic respiration resulting in systemic acidosis. In addition to acidosis, cellular metabolism will no longer be able to generate enough energy to power the vital components of normal cellular homeostasis. The cellular consequences of this include disruption of cell membrane ionic pumps with accumulation of intracellular sodium and cytosolic calcium. Hyperkalaemia occurs due to the subsequent release of intracellular constituents.

An initial rightward shift of the oxyhaemoglobin dissociation curve (ODC) will occur although sustained acidosis will eventually cause the red cell 2,3-DPG to decline and shift the ODC back towards normal. Metabolic acidosis also has negative effects on numerous protein and enzyme functions, such as the coagulation cascade. Cellular gene expression is affected causing deterioration in cell function and signalling.

Tissue injury due to trauma itself causes release of inflammatory mediators resulting in vasodilation, microvascular permeability, and increased metabolic compromise.

If anaerobic conditions continue unchecked, cells swell as water follows the rise in intracellular sodium, cell membranes break down eventually leading to cell death and subsequent organ dysfunction (see below).

Organic (macroscopic) consequences of shock

Metabolic acidosis can cause significant physiological effects, particularly affecting the respiratory and cardiovascular systems. If cellular death is widespread this can result in multiple organ dysfunction and eventual failure.

Respiratory effects

Hyperventilation (Kussmaul respiration) is the compensatory response to metabolic acidosis. Hyperventilation in the trauma patient may therefore represent severe metabolic acidosis due to shock, or a primary respiratory cause such as pneumothorax or haemothorax.

Cardiovascular effects

Acidosis will depress myocardial contractility and result in sympathetic over-stimulation, leading to tachycardia, vasoconstriction, and a decreased arrhythmia threshold. Indirect effects may result from hyperkalaemia. Other effects that may be noted include:

• Resistance to the effects of catecholamines.
• Peripheral vasoconstriction.
• Pulmonary vasoconstriction.

Sympathetic stimulatory effects and the release of catecholamines usually counteract direct myocardial depression, while plasma pH remains above 7.2. At systemic pH values less than this, direct depression of myocardial contractility usually predominates.

Physiological consequences of shock

The main physiological consequences of shock are listed below, generally in the sequence given below:

• Tachycardia.
• Hypotension.
• Metabolic acidosis.
• Oliguria leading to acute renal failure.
• Hepatic, gastrointestinal and pancreatic impairment.
• Acute respiratory distress syndrome (ARDS).
• Disseminated intravascular coagulation (DIC).

For the purposes of discussion, shock may be divided into three phases. There is no abrupt transition between them and clinical progression through these stages is variable, being dependent upon the cause, as well as individual patient factors, such as age and associated co-morbidities.

In the initial stages of shock the metabolic effects are just starting to become apparent. Following the onset of shock, several physiological mechanisms are employed in an attempt to reverse these metabolic effects.

Compensatory phase

As the signs of shock become more apparent various homeostatic mechanisms attempt to improve tissue perfusion and oxygen delivery. These consist of various neuroendocrine reflexes involving sympathetic activation and renal conservation of salt and water. Increased cardiac output is brought about primarily by vasoconstriction, tachycardia, and reduced renal fluid losses.

As blood pressure falls, arterial baroreceptors detect hypotension and trigger activation of sympathetic chain of the autonomic nervous system. The resulting catecholamine release causes tachycardia and vasoconstriction (skin, viscera, and kidneys), thus improving stroke volume and cardiac output. As a result of the underlying metabolic acidosis, hyperventilation attempts to reduce CO_2 levels and thereby raise the blood pH nearer to normal.

The renin-angiotensin axis is also activated and antidiuretic hormone (ADH) is released in order to conserve intravascular fluid. This causes vasoconstriction of the renal and gastrointestinal systems in order to redistribute blood volume to the heart, lungs and brain. Diminished renal blood flow causes the characteristic oliguria. Corticosteroid secretion also increases as part of the stress response.

Progressive (decompensating) phase

If left untreated, normal compensatory mechanisms will eventually fail, resulting in worsening perfusion, acidosis, and cellular dysfunction. Inflammatory mediators are released and further depress the cardiovascular system, particularly causing myocardial depression and inducing fluid loss from the intravascular compartment.

Hydrostatic pressure increases along with inflammatory mediator release lead to leakage of fluid and protein into the extravascular space. Arteriolar smooth muscle and precapillary sphincters relax such that blood pools in the capillaries and, as fluid is lost, blood concentration and viscosity increases, causing sludging of the micro-circulation and microvascular thrombosis.

As the gastrointestinal tract becomes ischaemic, bacteria and endotoxins (typically lipopolysaccharides, LPS) may enter the blood stream via the portal circulation, which causes further promotion of the systemic inflammatory response. Hypoperfusion-reperfusion injury may represent a second hit as the cardiovascular consequences of shock progress.

Refractory phase

This is also referred to as irreversible shock. As cardiovascular and metabolic function deteriorates further, the resulting organ damage is too severe for recovery to take place, even if appropriate resuscitation is commenced. Signs of multiple organ failure will appear and the later complications of shock may become apparent such as renal failure, ARDS or DIC.

Classes of shock

Haemorrhagic shock has traditionally been classified by the volume of blood loss and the resultant physiological signs and symptoms. However, this classification system does not take into account the multifactorial nature of shock or individual patient factors that may produce variance from these.

Despite its limitation, this classification may be useful when considering the effect of increasing volumes of blood loss on a normal, healthy adult:
- Even a rapid blood loss of up to 500 mL is likely to be well tolerated and compensated.
- By 1000 mL the initial signs of tachycardia and postural hypotension are likely to appear.
- Above 1500–2000 mL shock will definitely be apparent with signs of hypoperfusion and metabolic acidosis.

Later consequences of shock

Multiple organ dysfunction syndrome

Defined as a syndrome of organ dysfunction affecting two or more organs, this involves a severe inflammatory response and tissue injury associated with hypoperfusion. Multiple organ dysfunction syndrome (MODS) usually occurs days after sepsis or SIRS, and can also follow severe trauma, especially following massive haemorrhage and blood transfusion.

Acute lung injury and ARDS

Acute lung injury (ALI) is a syndrome of inflammation and increased permeability of lung tissue associated following severe trauma and massive blood transfusion, amongst others. It usually occurs within 2–3 days of the injury or insult. ARDS is the most severe form of ALI and distinct from this purely on the basis of the PaO_2/FiO_2 ratio.

Disseminated intravascular coagulation

DIC is a pathological process resulting in fibrin clot formation, consumption of platelets and coagulation factors with secondary fibrinolysis. It may be precipitated by shock and severe trauma.

Measuring shock

Continuous haemodynamic monitoring will be required for all trauma patients exhibiting signs of shock. In the initial stages, basic physiological parameters are likely to be sufficient in order to guide management and clinical decision making.

More accurate beat-to-beat physiological monitoring will be required in more complex or severe cases and where critical care interventions are required, such as endotracheal intubation and ventilation.

Physiological parameters

Minimum monitoring standards

Continuous pulse rate (ECG rhythm), pulse oximetry, and non-invasive blood pressure are convenient and safe to monitor and constitute the minimum monitoring standards required when dealing with a trauma patient. Signs of shock may be indicated by a rise in heart rate or fall in blood pressure without an apparent alternative cause (e.g. pain causing tachycardia). Oxygen saturation may also fall, or the signal trace may fail to pick-up properly, due to poor peripheral perfusion.

Urine output

Regular measurement of urine output, facilitated by urinary catheterization and the use of an hourly urine collector bag, can be useful as a measure of the response to fluid resuscitation in shocked patients. Maintenance of a urine output greater than 0.5 mL/kg/h would suggest adequate renal perfusion and intravascular volume.

Central venous pressure

Serial measurements of CVP in shocked trauma patients may reveal a reduced venous return due to ongoing hypovolaemia and also be useful for monitoring adequacy of fluid resuscitation when treating haemorrhagic shock.

Quantitative measures of shock

By defining shock as a syndrome of insufficient tissue perfusion to maintain adequate metabolic demands a quantitative measure of shock could be said to be that which can provide a measurement of perfusion. Changes in cardiac output or in the extraction ratio of DO_2 to VO_2 may be useful to measure shock and the response to resuscitation. Most of these are invasive techniques requiring central venous or arterial line insertion. More recently, various bedside monitoring devices have become available that may be useful in shock due to trauma.

Cardiac output measurement

A variety of techniques may be employed to measure cardiac output incorporating the Fick principle (e.g. NICO®), dilution by thermal, dye or lithium methods, Doppler, echocardiographic or impedance plethysmography. As discussed previously, accurate measurements of cardiac output are possible using pulmonary artery catheters, although this is associated with considerable risk.

Combined dilution and arterial waveform analysis systems may enable bedside monitoring (e.g. PiCCO™ or LiDCO™). Systems such as these could be used to identify trends in shock and guide ongoing fluid resuscitation of severe or complex trauma patients in emergency settings, although their use is limited by a regular need for recalibration and the risks associated with attendant lines.

DO_2 and VO_2

Obtaining accurate values for DO_2 and VO_2 can enable calculation of the extraction ratio, thus helping to guide ongoing fluid resuscitation and subsequent critical care management.

Surrogate markers of shock

Lactate level

Lactate is produced by skeletal muscle, brain, gut, and erythrocytes, and is metabolized mainly by the liver and kidneys. Raised plasma lactate levels can indicate the severity of hypoperfusion and hypoxaemia due shock. For a significant increase in blood lactate to occur, lactate must be released into the systemic circulation, and the rate of production must exceed uptake and metabolism.

Normal plasma lactate levels are 0.6–1.8 mmol/L. A rise in the level above 2.0 mmol/L may therefore indicate hypoperfusion. Lactic acidosis is characterized by persistently increased blood lactate levels (usually >5 mmol/L) in association with metabolic acidosis. Rate of change, rather than individual levels, may be more useful as a marker of shock and the response to clinical interventions and resuscitation.

Mixed venous oxygen saturation

Mixed venous blood must be obtained from the right atrium or pulmonary artery and therefore requires a central venous line. Mixed venous oxygen saturation can be used along with arterial oxygen content to estimate oxygen consumption and as an indicator of haemodynamic failure. Delivery of oxygen can be said to be at a critical level at SvO_2 of <50% (normal is 75%). Continuous monitoring may also be possible via pulmonary arterial catheters.

Gastric tonometry

The indirect measurement of gastric intramucosal pH by a balloon tonometer placed in the stomach can be used as an indicator of gastric mucosal oxygen delivery and consumption. Acidosis may indicate impaired gastrointestinal oxygen delivery or utilization, and has been proposed as a surrogate indicator of splanchnic hypoperfusion. This may prove useful as a guide to fluid resuscitation and onward critical care management in trauma, although the technique has not been accepted widely due to its cost, technical difficulty, and poor specificity.

Hypovolaemic shock due to haemorrhage

Hypovolaemia due to haemorrhage is the most common cause of shock in trauma patients, and should be anticipated and excluded before considering other potential, although less frequent, causes such as neurogenic or cardiogenic shock.

The injury mechanisms responsible for haemorrhage following trauma may be divided into four main groups:

- Capillary bleeding (generally oozing in nature).
- Arterial or venous bleeding due to vessel damage.
- Bleeding from organs due to laceration or rupture.
- Bleeding from bone marrow due to fractures.

Each of these may be subdivided into external or internal haemorrhage, depending upon the presence or absence of local open wounds. External haemorrhage is more likely in the context of penetrating injury or blunt injury causing lacerations or open fractures. Internal haemorrhage is often well concealed until the signs of shock become apparent. Pain and agitation may be the only initial features.

Significant burn injuries may also reduce circulating blood volume due to loss of plasma (although they will not reduce the haemoglobin concentration as red cells are not lost). This is unlikely to cause shock during the initial phase of assessment and management.

Haemorrhage can be classified according to the actual amount of blood lost or as a percentage of the circulating blood volume. Classification systems that rely upon physiological parameters are limited by individual patient factors and co-morbidities.

Basic physiological principles

The average fluid proportion of total body weight in lean adults is between 55 and 60%, which can be divided roughly into 2/3 intracellular fluid (ICF) and 1/3 extra-cellular fluid (ECF), of which 80% is interstitial fluid and 20% plasma.

Circulating blood volume comprises around 7% of the total body weight (70–80 mL/kg), therefore, a 70-kg person will have a total blood volume, also referred to as mean normal blood volume (MNBV), of around 5000 mL.

Cardiac output (CaO) is the volume of blood pumped per minute and is the product of the stroke volume and heart rate. The normal CaO for a fit 70-kg person is around 5000 mL/min, which therefore represents the total blood volume circulating around the body every minute. The potential for rapid exsanguination due to major blood vessel injury is therefore high.

Normal cardiac output is distributed approximately in the following proportions:

- Liver   25%
- Kidneys   22%
- Muscle   20%
- Brain   14%
- Heart   5%
- Other   14%

As can be seen, injury to the liver can be associated with considerable haemorrhage—theoretically the full blood volume in only a few minutes.

Haemostasis

Haemostasis involves a series of rapid and complex processes both at a local and systemic level. Smooth muscle constricts and endothelium becomes procoagulant at the site of vessel injury. Platelets are activated and begin to aggregate at the site, establishing a temporary plug. Following this, fibrin binds with the platelet plug to form a definitive clot. The coagulation pathway is a cascade mechanism involving many circulating factors. At the same time, various inhibitory mechanisms ensure coagulation is confined to the site of the injury.

Acquired coagulopathy may develop in severe haemorrhage due to consumption of clotting factors or dilution due to the administration of fluids or blood products. In response to blood loss, the body also tries to conserve circulating volume by shifting fluid from the extra-vascular compartment to the intravascular compartment. This may exacerbate the haemodilutional effect.

Normal haematological values

Normal values (for a 70-kg patient) are:
- Circulating volume   5000 mL
- Cardiac output   5000 mL/min
- Red blood cells $4–6.5 \times 10^{12}/L$*
- Haemoglobin   11.5–18 g/dL*
- Haematocrit   0.37–0.54*
- Platelets $150–400 \times 10^{9}/L$
- Prothrombin time (PrT)   12–15 s
- APTT   23–42 s

  *Values are generally lower in women than in men

The six compartments

The concept of compartments is useful when considering the potential sources of life-threatening haemorrhage secondary to trauma. Each compartment can be defined as a potential space into which haemorrhage may occur. This can facilitate a systematic review of the trauma patient with signs of haemorrhagic shock where the site of bleeding is not immediately apparent.

The six compartments are listed below:
- External.
- Chest.
- Abdomen.
- Retroperitoneum.
- Pelvis.
- Extremities.

External haemorrhage

External haemorrhage is usually obvious but can be concealed. Occasionally the cause of haemodynamic instability is only established once the resuscitation trolley is moved, whereby a large pool of blood is apparent on the floor. A thorough physical examination is vital to discover any external sites of bleeding.

The quantity of blood loss externally is extremely difficult to judge by observation alone. A cupful of blood goes a long way on a white floor.

Scalp wounds deserve a particular mention. They can continue to bleed profusely, despite being covered with a dressing, so early attention should be paid to closing the wounds with large sutures (which may be a temporary measure) and achieving haemostasis.

Chest

Bleeding into the chest can occur as a result of lung parenchymal injury, as well as injury to the blood vessels in the chest and the intercostal vessels.

Clinical examination may reveal bruising, pain, reduced expansion, dullness to percussion, and reduced breath sounds. Blood in the chest can be confirmed by a chest X-ray as part of the primary survey. Most thoracic bleeding can be managed with tube thoracostomy.

Abdomen

Bleeding into the abdomen is common, but not always obvious. Clinical clues may be present such as bruising to the abdominal wall, abnormal movement, involuntary muscle guarding, or tenderness to palpation, and absence of bowel sounds. However, in the majority of cases clinical examination needs to be supplemented by further investigation, commonly by ultrasound (FAST), to detect free fluid, and CT if the patient is stable enough.

Concealed intra-abdominal haemorrhage should be assumed if the patient is haemodynamically unstable without any other obvious cause following blunt trauma. Any intra-abdominal bleeding is referred to as non-compressible haemorrhage and is likely to be controlled only by surgery.

Pelvis

Injury to the pelvis should be assumed and excluded on X-ray during the primary survey. In the pre-hospital environment (or emergency department if not already done), when the mechanism of injury suggests a possible pelvic injury, a pelvic splint should be applied and left in place until significant injury is excluded.

Extremities

Significant bleeding can occur from extremity fractures, particularly if they are open or multiple. Long bone fractures should be splinted and, in the case of femoral fractures, traction splints applied to reduce bleeding. Clinical examination and X-ray confirmation give the diagnosis.

Retroperitoneal space

The retroperitoneal space contains the abdominal aorta, inferior vena cava, part of the duodenum, pancreas, kidneys, and ureters, and part of the colon. The lower part of the retroperitoneal space lies within the pelvic cavity.

The retroperitoneum is hidden from view in the resuscitation room. It can only be visualized on CT, where occult haemorrhage into the retroperitoneum is sometimes found.

Treatment of haemorrhagic shock

Uncontrolled haemorrhage accounts for around 40% of mortality in major trauma and the survival rate for trauma patients requiring massive transfusion is around 50%.

Early detection and control of haemorrhagic shock is therefore of paramount importance. The primary aim is always to restore adequate oxygen carrying capacity to meet the physiological needs of the patient, taking into account any pre-existing medical conditions.

The main objectives can be summarized as follows:
- Achieving rapid haemostasis.
- Restoring and maintaining tissue oxygen delivery.
- Restoring and maintaining adequate tissue perfusion.
- Restoring and maintaining normal clotting function.

In all cases of haemorrhagic shock, the priority is to control the source of bleeding.

The <C>ABCDE paradigm

Experience of trauma in the military setting, especially from blast and ballistic mechanisms, has resulted in changes to the way in which military personnel assess and treat patients. This new paradigm is now increasingly accepted in civilian care. The emergency treatment algorithm ABC has now been replaced by <C>ABC, where the first <C> stands for catastrophic haemorrhage.

External haemorrhage control

New methods of external haemorrhage control have been developed as a result of military medical trauma experience and include new kinds of compressive elastic dressings, the early use of tourniquets for limb trauma and topical haemostatic agents (THA).

A step-wise approach may follow:

Dressing → Pressure & Elevation → THA → Tourniquet

Direct pressure and limb elevation

Direct pressure and elevation are the first priorities for all compressible external haemorrhage. This approach is most effective for limb and extremity injuries.

Topical haemostatic agents

Increasing military experience of these agents has led to their routine, protocol-led use in situations where external haemorrhage is either non-compressible or other measures have failed to control exsanguination.

QuikClot® (Z-Medica)

QuikClot® is a granular zeolite powder derived from volcanic rock, which creates a matrix within the wound allowing the formation of clot around the damaged blood vessel. It was introduced into UK Defence Medical Services (DMS) practice in April 2004. When the material comes into contact with blood it takes up water molecules, concentrating local platelets and clotting factors, and thereby promoting natural clotting mechanisms at the bleeding point. Animal studies have demonstrated improved survival and reduced blood loss in vascular and soft tissue injury, and severe liver injury. Contraindications to its use include open head injuries, open thoracic wounds, and abdominal injury with exposed viscera.

QuikClot® is chemically inert although it will generate an exothermic reaction in the presence of water. As a result, a dry wound and surrounding skin is required to prevent thermal damage to local tissue. A sealed, porous teabag form has also been developed in order to avoid known problems associated with administering the granular form.

HemCon® (HemCon Medical Technologies, Inc.)

HemCon consists of a pliable dressing impregnated with chitosan acetate (derived from the exoskeleton of crustaceans including shrimp and crabs). The amino group in chitosan is positively charged and soluble in acidic to neutral solutions making it bio-adhesive. It readily binds to negatively charged surfaces, such as mucosal membranes. The haemostatic effect of HemCon is thought to be due principally to this muco-adhesive property. Unlike QuikClot there are no known harmful effects associated with the use of this dressing, although significant variability of adherence between the manufactured dressings has been observed. Similar dressings also include Celox® and Combat Gauze®.

Others

Two potential (future) alternatives to QuikClot® and HemCon® include the dry fibrin sealant dressing (DFSD) and rapid deployment haemostat (RDH) dressing. These have mostly attracted attention in the USA.

The DFSD is a pliable dressing primarily composed of clotting proteins purified from donated blood and plasma. The mechanism of haemostasis involves the clotting proteins dissolving in plasma and an enzymatic reaction of thrombin with fibrinogen forms a fibrin layer that adheres tightly to the injured tissue. The dressing is not currently available for clinical use, and further studies are required to investigate its efficacy and safety for FDA approval. The RDH dressing is an algae-derived dressing composed of poly-N-acetyl-glucosamine. The proposed mechanisms of haemostasis are thought to include red blood cell aggregation, platelet activation, activation of the clotting cascade activation, and local vasoconstriction via endothelial release. Although the RDH has received FDA approval in the US, it is not yet commercially available.

Tourniquets

Tourniquets are increasingly utilized in the pre-hospital environment in order to arrest bleeding distal to the point of application, although considerable controversy exists about their safety and efficacy. However, the relative risk to the limb is outweighed by the likely risk of death from severe exsanguination.

Internal (non-compressible) haemorrhage

Where haemorrhage cannot be controlled externally, initial management should include a cautious approach with regard to fluid resuscitation in order to avoid rapid rises in blood pressure that may fragment established clot and cause re-bleeding. However, signs of hypovolaemic shock must be treated in order to restore adequate perfusion. This is even more important in the presence of severe traumatic brain injury where higher mean arterial blood pressures are required to ensure adequate cerebral flow and limit secondary brain injury.

Surgery

Internal haemorrhage will almost certainly require urgent surgical intervention to achieve haemostasis. Senior clinical decision making is the key to ensuring that patients requiring rapid and safe transfer to theatre are recognized and managed appropriately. Early recognition is vital and the use of imaging techniques such as FAST (ultrasound) and CT are a vital component of this.

Fracture haemorrhage control
Haemorrhage from long bone (particularly femoral shaft) and pelvic fractures may be reduced by traction, binding or splinting. The aim is to stabilize the fracture, reduce the available volume into which bleeding can occur (tamponade) and enable the formation of a stable clot.

Angiographic embolization to control pelvic bleeding is potentially beneficial although time-consuming. An alternative technique involves extraperitoneal packing in the operating theatre.

Red cell salvage
Peri-operative red cell salvage is recommended where appropriate in order to minimize blood product use and subsequent complications.

Traumatic coagulopathy
Traumatic coagulopathy occurs due to consumption and dilution of clotting factors, hypothermia, and acidosis—the so called *lethal triad*. The risk is higher in circumstances of massive haemorrhage and transfusion. The emphasis should therefore be on attempts to predict and prevent coagulopathy, rather than treatment.

Haematological targets for the trauma patient include:
- Haemoglobin >8 g/dL (haematocrit of >35%).
- Platelets >75×10^9/L (>100×10^9/L in severe trauma).
- APTT and PrT <1.5 × normal levels.
- Fibrinogen >1.0g/L.

Recombinant factor VIIa (rFVIIa)
The use of rFVIIa has been described in a number of different clinical scenarios including traumatic or post-surgical coagulopathy refractory to conventional therapy with continued haemorrhage. Despite growing peer-reviewed clinical evidence, it is still not yet licensed in any country for this indication. It is also not an alternative to surgical control of haemorrhage and is by no means a magic bullet. Adequate clotting factors, cryoprecipitate and platelets need to be present for its full effect and both significant acidosis (pH<7.2) and hypothermia reduce rFVIIa activity.

The usual rFVIIa dose regime quoted is 90–100 mcg/kg, repeated once only within the next 2 h if required.

Trauma in the anticoagulated patient
An increasing number of patients are on regular anticoagulant therapy for prophylaxis of thromboembolic disease. Any injury that bleeds will obviously do so more in the anticoagulated patient. This is of most significance in traumatic brain injury. In the context of hypovolaemic shock due to haemorrhage, the emphasis is on rapid reversal of anticoagulation.

In all cases anticoagulant therapy must be stopped immediately and, in cases of major bleeding, prothrombin complex concentrate (e.g. Beriplex®) 25–50 U/kg (or FFP 15–20 mL/kg if PCC is unavailable) followed by vitamin K. PCC may be contraindicated in the presence of DIC and this should be discussed with a senior haematologist.

Fluid resuscitation therapy

The primary goal of fluid resuscitation in trauma is to treat hypovolaemic shock in order to ensure adequate perfusion and oxygen delivery to the tissues. Secondary goals of fluid resuscitation are to attempt to modify the immunological responses to trauma and aid haemostasis.

Permissive hypotension is a resuscitation technique that attempts to limit blood loss until haemostasis has been achieved, although the risk and benefits of tissue hypoperfusion versus further bleeding have to be assessed for each individual patient. This technique is best suited to young patients without co-morbidities, but is contraindicated in the presence of traumatic brain injury.

Resuscitation fluids, including blood, should be warmed prior to administration to reduce further heat loss. The lethal triad of hypothermia, acidosis, and coagulopathy must be avoided in severe trauma as this situation is almost universally associated with a poor outcome.

Use of blood products

Blood loss is commonly under estimated and haemoglobin and haematocrit values do not fall until several hours after acute haemorrhage.

Blood transfusion should not be used to expand vascular volume when oxygen carrying capacity is adequate. Blood transfusion is likely to be required when 30–40% of mean normal blood volume (MNBV, around 70–80 mL/kg body weight) has been lost. Blood products may also be necessary to replace deficient coagulation factors.

Transfusion protocols based upon packed red cell : fresh frozen plasma (PRC:FFP) ratios of 1:1 or 2:1, as well as PRC/FFP/platelet ratios of 1:1:1, have been suggested in situations where massive transfusion is likely on the premise that proactive transfusion management may avoid traumatic coagulopathy. Cryoprecipitate may also be required. The key to the best use of blood products in trauma is timely and effective communication with local blood bank and haematology speciality services, which works best in the presence of an established massive transfusion protocol.

Compatibility testing

Full ABO group and cross-match takes up to 45 min to complete. In urgent cases, just ABO and Rhesus group compatibility can be tested more rapidly, although this may still take up to 10–15 min. An antibody screen is then performed retrospectively. Further cross-matching is not required after replacement of one full MNBV.

In life-threatening haemorrhage, where there is established need for immediate blood transfusion before type specific or cross-matched blood is available, group O Rh D-positive blood may be used. Due to limited supplies, group O Rh D-negative blood is usually reserved for premenopausal females to avoid haemolytic disease of the newborn in future pregnancies.

Issues and possible complications

Rapid transfusion may result in hyperkalaemia, hypothermia, impaired clotting, and citrate toxicity causing hypocalcaemia. Metabolic alkalosis may occur as citrate is metabolized to bicarbonate. Bacterial contamination of donor blood may result in rapid development of severe sepsis. Elderly patients are more susceptible to fluid overload and cardiac failure, and may require diuretic therapy during, or following, blood transfusion. Stored blood will have impaired oxygen delivery characteristics due to left-ward shift of the oxyhaemoglobin dissociation curve as a result of inactivity of 2,3-DPG in the first 24 h. Red cell viability is around 70% at 24 h post-transfusion. Coagulation factor activity in PRC solution is negligible and dilutional thrombocytopenia is to be anticipated during massive blood replacement.

Transfusion reactions

Life-threatening:
- immediate haemolysis due to ABO incompatibility;
- anaphylaxis may occur rarely but can be fatal;
- transfusion-associated acute lung injury (TRALI).

Non life-threatening:
- febrile non-haemolytic transfusion reactions (FNHTR) and delayed haemolysis;
- urticarial reactions from donor plasma proteins.

Risk of infection

In the UK, donor blood is currently screened for hepatitis B, hepatitis C, HIV, syphilis, HTLV-1, and CMV (for selected recipients). Variant Creutzfeld-Jakob disease (vCJD) risks are thought to be extremely low.

Risk of transmission (per unit transfused):
- Hepatitis B = 1 in 100,000–400,000
- Hepatitis C = 1 in 200,000
- HIV = 1 in 4 000,000

Storage issues

Packed red cell (or red cell concentrate) units and platelets are stored at 2–6°C. FFP and cryoprecipitate require thawing for around 30–40 min before use. PRC units left unrefrigerated for more than 30 min should be transfused within 4 h or discarded.

Massive haemorrhage

Massive haemorrhage may be defined as:
- Loss of 100% of MNBV in 24 h.
- Loss of 50% of MNBV in 3 h.
- Loss of >150mL/min (externally or into drains).

Despite limited evidence, the early use of cryoprecipitate, FFP and platelets may be beneficial and improve survival. Improved survival in massively transfused patients is also associated with more effective and efficient rewarming techniques and aggressive resuscitation. The use of a massive transfusion protocol to activate a pre-determined sequence of events, supply appropriate blood products and monitor their use is recommended.

Intravenous fluids

In physiological terms, the most ideal resuscitation fluid to use for treating haemorrhagic shock would be fully cross-matched fresh whole blood, restoring haemoglobin, clotting factors, and plasma volume. The risk of transmitting infection means that stored blood products are generally used instead. For this reason intravenous fluids (electrolytes or plasma replacement) are generally the first choice for initial resuscitation until haemostasis is achieved and blood product administration becomes available, if required.

Intravenous fluid solutions may be broadly divided into two groups: electrolyte (crystalloid) solutions, and plasma or plasma substitutes (colloid). Hypertonic sodium chloride solutions are discussed separately. The choice of which fluid to use for resuscitation of the trauma patient remains

a highly controversial issue and depends upon several factors, logistical and clinical:
- Unit cost and shelf life.
- Potential allergenicity.
- Duration in intravascular space.
- Immunomodulatory effects.

From a research perspective, hypertonic sodium chloride solutions may offer some important immunomodulatory benefits over other fluids. Although there have been promising clinical results in head-injured patients, the role of these solutions for routine volume replacement in all trauma patients is as yet unproven.

Administration route

Isotonic solutions may be safely infused via a peripheral venous cannula. Hypertonic solutions are best infused through central venous lines, although they may still be administered peripherally in emergency situations.

The intraosseous route of administration is becoming increasingly common in trauma patients and may be considered a safe route for all isotonic solutions, including plasma and plasma substitutes. However, research into the intra-osseous route for hypertonic solutions has demonstrated a significant risk of local complications including myonecrosis in some animal models. Further research is required before hypertonic solutions are recommended for administration by the intraosseous route in humans.

Electrolyte solutions

Electrolyte solutions contain relatively small molecules that may readily pass through capillary and glomerular membranes, but not cell membranes. Cell membrane pumps subsequently alter the distribution of ions. As a result, electrolyte solutions usually remain within the intravascular space for up to 30 min, after which only around 25% of the infused solution is left.

Electrolyte solutions have advantages over plasma replacement solutions by the absence of allergenicity or coagulation dysfunction. Both electrolytes and plasmas are relatively cheap and plentiful with a good shelf life. The main disadvantages of electrolyte solutions are that they are short-lived in the circulation with risk of pulmonary and cerebral oedema from fluid overload. This fluid shift into the interstitial space is further promoted by increased capillary permeability and decreased intravascular colloid oncotic pressure seen as a result of normal physiological responses to trauma.

Most electrolyte solutions are supplied in 500- or 1000-mL bags, except for bicarbonate 8.4%.

Sodium chloride 0.9%
- Constituents:
  - 150 mmol/L sodium;
  - 150 mmol/L chloride.
- Specific indications:
  - hyponatraemia;
  - diabetic ketoacidosis.
- Cautions and complications:
  - sodium accumulation;
  - hyperchloraemic acidosis;
  - fluid overload.

Glucose 5% or 10%
- Constituents:
  - 5% solution = 50 g/L dextrose;
  - 10% solution = 100 g/L dextrose.
- Specific indications:
  - free water replacement;
  - hypoglycaemia.
- Cautions and complications:
  - peripheral venous irritation and thrombophlebitis;
  - disturbances of glucose control in diabetics.

Hartmann's/Ringer lactate solution
- Constituents:
  - 131 mmol/L sodium;
  - 111 mmol/L chloride;
  - 29 mmol/L bicarbonate (as lactate);
  - 5 mmol/L potassium;
  - 2 mmol/L calcium.
- Specific indications: water and electrolyte replacement.
- Cautions and complications:
  - requires normal hepatic function to metabolize lactate to bicarbonate;
  - fluid overload.

Sodium bicarbonate
Sodium bicarbonate is supplied in two main forms:
- 1.26% (150mmol/l each of sodium and bicarbonate).
- 8.4% (1000mmol/l each of sodium and bicarbonate).

The 1.26% form is usually supplied in either 500- or 1000-mL bags for infusion. The 8.4% solution comes in 10- or 50-mL minijet® containers and is generally reserved for slow injection in emergency situations.
- Specific indications:
  - severe metabolic acidosis (ph <7.1);
  - emergency treatment of hyperkalaemia;
  - prolonged cardiac arrest;
  - tricyclic antidepressant toxicity.
- Cautions and complications:
  - high osmolar load (8.4% solution);
  - may exacerbate intracellular acidosis.

Potassium-containing solutions
Constituents of potassium containing solutions vary depending upon the solution used with potassium concentrations being either 0.15% (20 mmol/L) or 0.3% (40 mmol/L). Pre-prepared bags of fluid are typically made up with glucose 5% or sodium chloride 0.9%.
- Specific indications: hypokalaemia.
- Cautions and complications:
  - inadvertent hyperkalaemia;
  - rapid infusion may cause cardiac toxicity.

Plasma and plasma substitutes

Plasma and plasma substitutes vary substantially in their pharmacology and pharmacokinetics. Molecules with a molecular weight of less than 50,000 D will readily pass through the glomerular membrane and be excreted, although still less rapidly than any electrolyte solutions.

Synthetic colloids are now widely accepted as an effective alternative to human albumin for volume replacement in trauma patients. Most plasma solutions are supplied in 500- or 1000-mL bags, except for human albumin solution (HAS) and Haemaccel®, which are supplied in bottles.

Human albumin solution from 4.5–25%
HAS consists of naturally occurring albumin, derived from pooled human plasma by fractionation, with a molecular weight of around 69,000 D. HAS is heated and sterilized by

ultrafiltration and is generally accepted to have a very low risk of transmission of infectious diseases.

In addition to its colloid properties, albumin also proffers some theoretical advantages from its involvement in plasma molecular carriage, coagulation, and membrane integrity, as well as being a free radical scavenger.

- Constituents:
  - 4.5% solution = 45 mg/mL human albumin.
  - 5.0% solution = 50 mg/mL human albumin.
  - 20% solution = 200 mg/mL human albumin.
  - 25% solution = 250 mg/mL human albumin.

Usually supplied in 50-, 100-, 250-, 400-, or 500-mL bottles (for isotonic solutions) and 20-, 50-, or 100-mL bottles (for hypertonic solutions).

- Specific indications:
  - replacement of plasma volume losses, e.g. burns;
  - hypoalbuminaemia.
- Cautions and complications:
  - despite its theoretical advantages, HAS is yet to be proven in clinical practice, although careful use may be beneficial in some trauma patients;
  - the incidence of serious adverse reactions following the use of HAS is around 1:30 000

Gelatin solutions

Gelatin solution is a generic term applied to the three main proprietary solutions each containing a different mixture of solutes. All gelatin solutions have an average molecular weight of 30,000 D (compared with around 69,000 D for human albumin). Although derived from beef, gelatin solutions are generally agreed to be free of risk of prion transmission.

- Gelofusine® (Braun):
  - 4% (40g/L) succinylated bovine gelatine;
  - 154 mmol/L sodium;
  - 120 mmol/L chloride;
  - 0.4 mmol/L each of potassium, calcium, and magnesium.
- Haemaccel® (KoRa):
  - 3.5% (35g/L) polygeline;
  - 145 mmol/L sodium;
  - 145 mmol/L chloride;
  - 5.1 mmol/L potassium;
  - 6.25 mmol/L calcium.
- Volplex® (Maelor):
  - 4% (40g/L) succinylated gelatine;
  - 154 mmol/L sodium;
  - 125 mmol/L chloride.
- Specific indications: plasma volume replacement.
- Cautions and complications:
  - the incidence of serious adverse reactions following the use of Gelofusine® is around 1:13,000;
  - relatively short intravascular half-life (approximately 2 h).

Esterified starches

These are high polymeric glucose compounds manufactured through hydrolysis and hydroxyethylation from >90% amylopectin. Also referred to as hydroxyethyl starches (HES).

Two main non-proprietary solutions are available, both of which are presented in sodium chloride 0.9% solution:

- Hetastarch (450,000 D) 6%.

- Pentastarch (200,000 D) 6% or 10%.

Voluven® (Fresenius Kabi) is a proprietary form of tetrastarch (130,000 D) 6% and, like the other starch solutions, is also presented in sodium chloride 0.9% solution.

- Specific indications: plasma volume replacement.
- Cautions and complications:
  - HES will accumulate, although <1% of the total dose will remain in the body after 2 weeks;
  - the incidence of serious adverse reactions following the use of Hetastarch is around 1:16,000.

Hypertonic solutions (HS)

There is an increasing enthusiasm for the use of HS in the treatment of hypovolaemic shock in trauma patients. Several cardiovascular advantages are believed to be conferred including:

- Displacement of fluid into intravascular compartment
- Vasodilatory effects on pulmonary vasculature
- Direct positive inotropic effects on myocardium

Other potential advantages include the fact that only small volumes of HS are necessary to achieve the same desired effect of isotonic solutions, thereby less chance of fluid overload and also smaller volumes needed to be carried by pre-hospital personnel.

Various concentrations of HS are available, both alone and in combination with other fluids. Individual vials of sodium chloride are also supplied in 3, 5, 7.5, and 10% strengths, and their use is generally limited to critical care management of severe head injury. The most commonly used combined hypertonic sodium chloride solutions include:

- RescueFlow® (Vitaline): 250 mL sodium chloride 7.5%, containing 6% dextran 70 (70,000 D).

Dextrans are glucose polymers available in different molecular weights preparations. Negative adverse effects of dextrans solutions include coagulation abnormalities and severe life-threatening hypersensitivity reactions.

- HyperHAES® (Fresenius Kabi): 250 mL sodium chloride 7.2%, containing 6% hydroxyethyl (tetra-) starch (200,000 D).
- Specific indications:
  - Hyponatraemia;
  - traumatic brain injury;
  - low volume resuscitation of trauma patients.
- Cautions and complications:
  - the incidence of serious adverse reactions following the use of Dextran 70 is around 1:4500;
  - effects of HS alone are reported to be transient;
  - limited number of clinical trials for high dose HS.

Future developments

Although still at an experimental stage, haemoglobin and synthetic oxygen carrier solutions may have a potential future role in the management of trauma patients.

Examples include:

- Stroma-free haemoglobin (SFH).
- Micro-encapsulated haemoglobin (neo red cells).
- Chelating agents.
- Perfluorocarbons (PFCs).

The advantages of such products include minimal infection risk, no need for cross-matching, long shelf life, and easier storage at ambient temperature. Of these, haemoglobin-based oxygen carriers (HBOCs) and PFC emulsions are the most likely candidates for general clinical use.

Summary
Overall, there is still no clear evidence to support the use of one fluid over another. Appropriate and early use of blood and blood products should be the priority in the most severely injured patients.

Other causes of shock

In the context of trauma, shock is generally the result of hypovolaemia due to haemorrhage. Other causes of shock may be directly related to trauma, or may develop following trauma. These may be recognized immediately, or may present later during the initial management of the injured patient.

Other causes of shock are:
- Non-haemorrhagic hypovolaemic shock
- Cardiogenic shock, including:
  - intrinsic cardiogenic shock;
  - obstructive cardiogenic shock;
  - distributive shock, including:
    - neurogenic shock;
    - septic shock;
    - anaphylactic shock.

Non-haemorrhagic hypovolaemic shock

Non-haemorrhagic hypovolaemic shock can occur in the injured patient and may be especially relevant where the circumstances or environment predispose to greater fluid losses, such as a lengthy entrapment or crush injury. An increase in fluid losses may be due to several medical conditions and may develop as a complication of the injury, or could even be responsible for the injury itself.

Aetiology
Non-haemorrhagic hypovolaemia can occur due to uncompensated fluid volume loss, from extravascular fluid sequestration (third spacing) of intravascular fluid or following burns. Causes of increased fluid loss include burns, crush injury, and pancreatitis.

Pathophysiology
Intravascular and interstitial compartments are usually held in equilibrium, with losses from one resulting in passage of fluid from the other. Losses of interstitial fluid volume will therefore lead to a reduction in intravascular volume and subsequent shock.

Head injury may result in a deficiency of ADH (vasopressin) production due to hypothalamic or pituitary damage. Termed neurogenic (or cranial) diabetes insipidus, this condition is characterized by excretion of large amounts of highly diluted urine, which will lead to hypovolaemia if untreated. This process may take a few days to develop and in head injury may be temporary, often recovering within a few weeks.

Third spacing of intravascular fluid may occur due to post-traumatic pancreatitis or following injury to the liver or bowel. Increased renal losses of protein from nephrotic syndrome can also lead to increased third spacing.

Specific management
The diagnosis of non-haemorrhagic hypovolaemic shock should only be made by exclusion in the injured patient.

The management of hypovolaemic shock should focus on treating the cause of the volume loss. This will usually only require the replacement of water deficit and restoration of appropriate electrolyte balance. Neurogenic diabetes insipidus can be treated with the vasopressin analogue, desmopressin, although mild cases may be managed appropriately with increased fluid intake alone.

Cardiogenic shock

Cardiogenic shock can occur in a susceptible patient due to the physiological stress of the traumatic event. Patients may also present with trauma that has occurred as a direct consequence of a primary cardiac event, such as a myocardial infarction causing arrhythmia and loss of consciousness while driving.

Aetiology
Cardiogenic shock may be divided into intrinsic or extrinsic causes and may co-exist in trauma patients. Intrinsic causes are due to insufficient ejection fraction and cardiac output despite adequate intravascular volume and cardiac filling. Relevant intrinsic causes include myocardial infarction or contusion, traumatic valvular, or ventricular defects, arrhythmias due to ischaemia or toxins, and pre-existing cardiomyopathy.

Extrinsic causes are either due to obstruction of venous return or from external compression preventing adequate cardiac filling and stroke volume. Causes include:
- Tension pneumothorax.
- Cardiac tamponade.
- Mediastinal haemorrhage or pneumo-mediastinum.
- Massive pulmonary embolus.
- Diaphragmatic hernia.
- Positive pressure ventilation.

The most important traumatic causes of cardiogenic shock include cardiac contusion from blunt thoracic trauma, cardiac tamponade from penetrating injury or tension pneumothorax.

Pathophysiology
The most common cause of cardiogenic shock is acute myocardial infarction, leading to a marked decrease in myocardial contractility, reducing the ejection fraction and thereby cardiac output. Cardiogenic shock usually involves some degree of left ventricular dysfunction. Decompensation may occur as a result of falling arterial pressure with the subsequent exacerbation of myocardial ischaemia. The heart rate usually increases to compensate for hypotension, exacerbating myocardial oxygen demand.

Direct injury to the heart may result in rupture to the ventricular wall resulting in a pericardial haematoma and cardiac tamponade, valvular rupture reducing forward flow and ejection fraction, or ventricular contusion reducing myocardial contractility.

A tension pneumothorax causes a rise in intrathoracic pressure and may reduce cardiac output. Injury to the mediastinum may result in increased pressure exerted upon the pericardial space and an indirect tamponade effect. The use of positive pressure ventilation, especially when using higher positive end expiratory pressures (PEEP), may also reduce cardiac filling due to the increase in intrathoracic pressure.

Pulmonary embolus is unlikely to present early as a result of trauma, although it may be a later complication. A large pulmonary embolus will obstruct blood flow returning to the left ventricle and thus cause a reduction in cardiac output.

Presentation
Cardiogenic shock is more likely to occur in the elderly and those with known cardiac disease. A history of

previous myocardial infarction and atherosclerotic disease increases the likelihood of developing cardiogenic shock.

All forms of cardiogenic shock lead to a fall in cardiac output and a rise in systemic vascular resistance. Central venous pressure is generally increased in cardiogenic shock, although the true CVP falls due to tension pneumothorax from reduced venous return. The CVP may appear falsely raised, reflecting the intrapleural rather than vascular pressure.

ECG complexes may appear small in the presence of a pericardial effusion large enough to result in tamponade.

Specific management
The specific management of cardiogenic shock should focus on treating the cause, particularly in obstructive shock and myocardial infarction, which may include urgent reperfusion therapy in appropriate cases.

The general approach to managing intrinsic cardiogenic shock is to optimize oxygen delivery and left ventricular filling pressures. Fluid resuscitation may be necessary where there are signs of hypotension due to poor cardiac filling. Inotropic and vasodilator therapy may be used with signs of raised left ventricular filling pressures, such as pulmonary oedema. Typical drug therapy involves the use of oxygen, opiates, nitrates, and diuretics. Inotropic agents include dobutamine, which increases myocardial contractility while reducing left ventricular end-diastolic pressure.

The approach to managing obstructive shock involves the restoration of cardiac filling and stroke volume by the removal of external compression forces (in the case of tension pneumothorax for example) or of internal vascular obstruction from pulmonary embolus. In the case of tension pneumothorax, immediate needle decompression is required initially followed by tube thoracostomy. Cardiac tamponade usually requires emergency surgical removal of clotted blood by thoracotomy.

Distributive causes of shock
Distributive shock is the term applied to shock caused by rapid shifts in fluid distribution. Hypotension occurs either as the result of vasodilatation and capillary leakage due to the inflammatory responses of sepsis and anaphylaxis, or may be due to loss of peripheral sympathetic vasopressor tone in the case of neurogenic shock.

Neurogenic shock
Of the three distributive causes, neurogenic shock must be recognized and differentiated from hypovolaemic shock as soon as possible during the management of the trauma patient. Spinal cord injury may rapidly produce hypotension due to a loss of peripheral sympathetic vasopressor tone, and an absence of the normal tachycardia response in the case of high spinal cord injury. However, signs of neurogenic shock should be initially managed as if due to hypovolaemia, as patients who have sustained severe spinal injuries often have co-existing thoracic, abdominal or pelvic injuries. Neurogenic shock may mask the normal physiological response to hypovolaemia. Associated head injury occurs in about 25% of spinal cord injury patients.

Pathophysiology
Neurogenic shock occurs in spinal injuries above the T6 level and is secondary to the loss of normal sympathetic autonomic outflow below T1. This results in a loss of systemic vascular resistance due to interruption in normal vascular smooth muscle (vasoconstrictor) tone.

The release of catecholamines immediately following a spinal injury may maintain a partial pressor response and therefore the signs of neurogenic shock may take a few minutes to hours to appear.

Presentation
The dominating presenting feature of all causes of distributive shock is due to the loss of systemic vascular resistance. Central venous pressure is often unaffected, unless there is concurrent cause for hypovolaemia, and cardiac output may remain the same or elevated. A spinal injury level above T6 is characterized by hypotension and, above T1, additionally by bradycardia, due to unopposed vagal tone.

Specific management
It is important to exercise caution when dealing with trauma patients with signs of spinal shock as there may also be evidence of hypovolaemic shock requiring urgent surgical intervention. The hypovolaemic trauma patient on ß-blocker therapy may show appearances consistent with an apparent spinal injury.

Where the injury mechanism and clinical signs suggest spinal shock, and there are no signs of a hypovolaemic cause, initial management relies on optimizing oxygen delivery and sufficient fluid volume resuscitation to fill the expanded intravascular space. Subsequent management may require use of an appropriate vasopressor, such as noradrenaline, dopamine, or phenylephrine. Regular bolus therapy with the vasopressor metaraminol may be useful while waiting for an infusion to be commenced. A haemodynamically significant bradycardia may be treated with atropine 500-mcg aliquots up to 3 mg intravenously.

Septic shock
Sepsis is a rare early cause of shock in the injured patient, although it may occur following trauma if there has been sufficient delay before presentation. Sepsis may be defined as the presence of the Systemic Inflammatory Response Syndrome (SIRS) with an established source of infection. Septic shock is defined as hypotension, or the requirement for inotropic support despite adequate fluid resuscitation associated with sepsis. SIRS criteria defined as two or more of:
- Hypothermia (<36°C) or hyperthermia (>38°C).
- Tachycardia (heart rate >90/min).
- Tachypnoea (>20/min).
- Leucopenia (<4 × 10^9/L) or leucocytosis (>12 × 10^9/L).

As can be seen, these criteria do not differentiate the process, as trauma itself will result in a SIRS clinical state. Therefore, these features cannot be relied upon alone to diagnose or exclude sepsis as a cause for shock.

Aetiology
The main causes of sepsis from trauma include translocation of bacteria and endotoxins across the gut wall into the systemic circulation either due to splanchnic hypoperfusion as a result of hypovolaemic shock or from local bowel wall perforation, wound infections, and aspiration of gastric contents.

Pathophysiology
The release of inflammatory mediators into the circulation causes a loss of systemic vascular resistance, venous pooling, reduced venous return, and thereby a fall in cardiac output. Hypovolaemia then follows, causing a further reduction in central venous pressure and cardiac pre-load

and subsequently cardiac output. Eventually, falling arterial blood pressure leads to myocardial ischaemia producing a superimposed intrinsic cardiogenic shock.

Most cases of sepsis are due to bacterial sources, traditionally due to Gram-negative organisms, such as *E. coli*, although Gram-positive organisms are increasingly being implicated (including streptococci and staphylococci). Contributory factors include a loss of immune function due to concomitant therapy or from splenectomy.

Presentation

- *Early:*
  - SIRS clinical state;
  - hyperdynamic circulation with reduced SVR;
  - metabolic (lactic) acidosis;
  - reduced oxygen extraction and utilization;
  - multiple organ dysfunction.
- *Later:*
  - acute renal and hepatic failure;
  - pancreatitis and diabetes mellitus;
  - Acute Respiratory Distress Syndrome (ARDS);
  - disseminated intravascular coagulation (DIC);
  - Cardiac failure.

Specific management

Initial management is supportive with appropriate oxygen therapy and fluid resuscitation. Inotropic and vasopressor therapy will be required in the presence of organ dysfunction secondary to ongoing hypoperfusion despite adequate fluid resuscitation. Antibacterial therapy must be instituted as early as possible and the choice of drug must be based upon the most likely causative organism and modified by the results of culture from suitable body fluid and tissue samples. Ideally, such samples should be taken before antibiotic therapy is started. Treatment may also require the use of antiviral or antifungal agents, as guided by culture results.

Early surgical care, including wound debridement and drainage of infected tissue or pus collections will be required to treat the underlying source.

The severe sepsis bundles are a distillation of the evidence-based recommendations from the Surviving Sepsis Campaign and wider critical care community. These are designed to allow medical teams to follow the appropriate timing, sequence, and goals of individual elements in the care of septic patients.

Anaphylactic shock

True anaphylaxis occurs when a pre-sensitized individual is exposed to a known allergen. Typical features are of a sudden onset and rapid progression with potentially life-threatening airway, breathing, and circulatory problems. Although not usually directly related to the mechanism of injury, anaphylaxis in a trauma patient may occur as the result of treatment administered during resuscitation. Causative agents include antibiotics, intravenous colloids and anaesthetic induction agents, such as thiopentone.

Pathophysiology

Anaphylaxis is a Type I immune reaction, which is characterized by the release of various vasoactive substances (particularly histamine) and results from an antigen-antibody reaction on the surface of mast cells. Release of these substances causes angioedema, as well as vasodilatation with increased capillary permeability and myocardial depression, resulting in shock.

Presentation

- Angioedema with pharyngeal or laryngeal oedema.
- Bronchospasm.
- Vasodilation and subsequent hypotension.
- Cutaneous erythema and urticaria.

Specific management

The specific management of anaphylaxis requires rapid recognition with airway protection and the early use of adrenaline. Triggers should be removed if possible (stop the antibiotic or colloid infusion if thought to be the cause).

Further reading

American College of Surgeons Committee on Trauma. *Advanced Trauma Life Support, Student Course Manual* (6th Ed). New York: ACS, 1997.

Bilkovski RN, Rivers EP, Horst HM. Targeted resuscitation strategies after injury. *Curr Opin Crit Care* 2004; **10**: 529–38.

Boffard K, Riou B, Warren B, Choong P, Rizoli S, Rossaint R, et al. Recombinant factor VIIa as adjunctive therapy for bleeding control in severely injured trauma patients: two parallel randomized, placebo-controlled, double-blind clinical trials. *J Trauma: Injury Infect Crit Care* 2005; **59**(1): 8–18.

Borgman M, Spinella P, Perkins J, Grathwohl K, Repine T, Beekley A, et al. The ratio of blood products transfused affects mortality in patients receiving massive transfusions at a combat support hospital. *J Trauma* 2007; **63**: 805–13.

Holcomb JB, et al. Damage control resuscitation: directly addressing the coagulopathy of trauma. *J Trauma* 2007; **62**: 307–10.

Mannucci PM, Levi M. Prevention and treatment of major blood loss. *N Engl J Med* 2007; **356**: 2301–11.

Nguyen HB, Rivers EP, Abrahamian FM, Moran GJ, Abraham E, Trzeciak S, et al. Emergency Department Sepsis Education Program and Strategies to Improve Survival (ED-SEPSIS) Working Group. Severe sepsis and septic shock: review of the literature and emergency department management guidelines. *Annl Emerg Med* 2006; **48**>: 28–54.

NICE (2002) *Central Venous Catheter—Ultrasound Locating Devices.* London: NICE.

Pinnock C, Lin T, Smith T (eds). *Fundamentals of Anaesthesia*, 2nd edn. Greenwich: Medical Media, 2003.

Smith JE, Hall MJ. Hypertonic Saline. *J Roy Army Med Corps* 2004; **150**: 239–43. Available at: http://www.survivingsepsis.org/

Spahn D. Editorial: Is recombinant FVIIa the magic bullet in the treatment of major bleeding? *Br J Anaesthes* 2005; **94**(5): 553–5.

T J Hodgetts, P F Mahoney, et al. ABC to <C>ABC: redefining the military trauma paradigm. EMJ 2006; **23**: 745-746.

W Sapsford. A role for recombinant activated factor VII in trauma? *Trauma* 2002; **4**: 117.

Yentis SM, Hirch NP, Smith GB. (eds) *Anaesthesia and Intensive Care A–Z,.* 3rd edn. Amsterdam: Elsevier, 2004.

Zalstein S, Pearce A, Scott D, Rosenfeld J. Damage control resuscitation: a paradigm shift in the management of haemorrhagic shock. *Emerg Med Aust* 2008; **20**: 291–3.

Head injuries

Traumatic brain injury (TBI) is the world's leading cause of morbidity and mortality in individuals under the age of 45. It is also an important disease of the elderly who are anatomically and physiologically predisposed to more severe injuries and worse outcomes from smaller transfers of energy. The insidious onset of pathology in the elderly can often result in the seriousness of their condition being overlooked. Whilst it is the remit of public health advisors and politicians to reduce the incidence of TBI (by enforcing speed limits and the wearing of helmets), it is the remit of clinicians to reduce the secondary brain injury that follows. One-third of patients who die from TBI will talk or obey commands between their injury and their death which implies that the primary injury *per se* is not the lethal injury.

The incidence of TBI is difficult to ascertain, however it is estimated to be 400 per 100,000 per year or roughly 1.4 million per year in the UK alone. Of these, around 10% are classified as moderate or severe. Half of those who die from TBI do so within 2 h of the injury. Approximately 30% of patients admitted to hospital with a GCS of <13 will die, and if <8, this increases to 50%. Of the 900 pedal cyclists who die each year in the US, three-quarters die primarily because of their brain injury. The morbidity outcomes associated with TBI are more difficult to calculate.

Neurological assessment

In the pre-hospital environment, assessment of disability occurs while still approaching the patient. The mechanism of injury, the bulls-eyed windscreen, and the crushed A-post all give an indication that a head injury is likely. Whilst still approaching, with the patient out of sight, the sounds of talking, fighting, or silence lend yet further clues. So while D is the fifth priority in the <C>ABCDE primary survey, it is often the first thing assessed. If a patient is talking sense in full sentences, then A, B, and C are almost certainly adequate, at least for the moment.

> There is no such thing as an isolated head injury during initial assessment. It should always be assumed that the patient has a C-spine injury as well.

There are multiple components to assessing disability and they are often done in parallel. (For information pertaining to assessment of the spine see Chapter 11, Spinal injuries). Specific areas that need assessment include:
- Conscious level.
- Pupil response.
- Limb weakness.
- Morphological evidence of injury (lacerations, bruising, signs of skull fracture).

An informal assessment of neurological state can be made rapidly by asking 'what is your name?' and 'move your arms and legs'. This quick assessment then allows either formal assessment of GCS (if the responses are inappropriate) or to a more fine assessment (Mental Test Score, lateralizing signs) if the pathology is more subtle.

If the patient is a motorcyclist, helmet removal should be performed by someone experienced in the procedure, as part of airway assessment, while maintaining in-line cervical immobilization. The sides of the helmet need to be pulled apart to remove the helmet without undue adverse movement of the neck.

Assessment of conscious level

A number of systems have been proposed for repeated assessment of conscious level, of which two have reached popular usage.

AVPU or ACDU

AVPU reflects the assessment of the patient being **A**lert, responding to **V**oice, responding to **P**ain, or being **U**nresponsive. These have been shown to correspond to median Glasgow Coma Scores of 15, 13, 8, and <6, respectively. **ACDU** is another acronym sometimes used referring to the subjective decision that the patient is **A**lert, **C**onfused, **D**rowsy or **U**nresponsive. Median GCS values are 15, 13, 10 and 6 respectively. While these scoring systems are useful for rapid assessment and for junior staff, they do not provide a clear level of detail and do not detect subtle changes.

Glasgow Coma Scale

The GCS is an internationally adopted system for repeatable monitoring of level of unconsciousness. When proposed in 1974, three separate responses (eye, voice, and motor) were scored separately. Subsequently, the medical community took to adding the three values to give a score out of 15 (originally this was 14; however, the flexion response was later divided into normal and abnormal). This addition of the three components implies equal weight to each, which is probably not the case in terms of severity of injury or prediction of outcome. Many consider the motor response to be of most significance, and for this reason, a breakdown of the GCS is more meaningful than the score alone. Referring to the responses in words, rather than numbers also conveys a clearer understanding and demonstrates that a formal assessment has truly been made. Table 8.1 explains each component.

Although the GCS was originally designed for head injury assessment, it should be remembered that conscious level can be affected by many other things. Hypoxia, hypotension, hypoglycaemia, and narcotic overdose should be reversed prior to GCS assessment in the context of trauma. Jennett and Teasdale defined coma as the inability to obey commands, to utter words and to open the eyes, and therefore 8 is a commonly quoted defining number. Reassessment of the GCS at regular intervals enables monitoring of conscious level and acts as a warning of worsening injury.

It should be clear that the patient is responding to either voice or pain, therefore the two stimuli should not be combined. It is important that each component is assessed properly and separately. Nail bed pressure is the best for assessing flexion (withdrawal), but unless the patient can move the opposite side, may not indicate localization of pain. Hence, after assessing response to voice, it is best to start with nail bed pressure on both sides and move on to supra-orbital pressure to assess response to pain (Fig. 8.1). Some clinicians use sternal pressure to illicit a response to pain.

The combative patient

It is very easy to mistakenly say that a patient who is combative is GCS 15. However, this group often have significant brain injury and this highlights the need for formal GCS assessment. Often such patients are vocalizing inappropriately (V = 4) and do not obey commands (M = 5). For ward or ICU-based clinicians, a GCS of 13 usually equates to a drowsy patient, but in this case it refers to an agitated aggressive patient. Such a patient is unlikely to be co-operative for CT scanning and, hence, may require intubation to safely

Table 8.1. GCS and a paediatric version of verbal response for the under 5s

Eye opening (E)	
Spontaneous	4
To voice	3
To pain	2
None	1

Verbal response (V)	
Orientated	5
Confused conversation	4
Inappropriate words	3
Incomprehensible sounds	2
None	1

Motor response (M)	
Obeys commands (normal movement in children)	6
Localizes pain	5
Normal flexion (withdrawal)	4
Abnormal flexion (decorticate)	3
Extension (decerebrate)	2
None (flaccid)	1

Paediatric verbal response (V)	
Best response for age (as before injury)	5
Confused or spontaneous irritable cries	4
Cries to pain	3
Moans to pain	2
None	1

define the injury. This is surprising to some as traditional teaching implies that only those with a GCS of 8 or less require intubation.

Drugs and alcohol
The presence of drugs or alcohol can make head injury assessment extremely difficult. The presence of alcohol does not exclude an underlying brain injury and, hence, although a sensible judgement (and proper examination) needs to be made, it is advisable to always assume a reduction in conscious level is due to the head injury, rather than the alcohol.

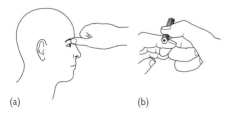

(a)   (b)

Fig. 8.1. Technique of assessing GCS motor response: apply nail bed pressure, then supra-orbital pressure.

E4,V1,M1
If a trauma patient has their eyes open, is looking around, but fails to vocalize or move their limbs then they may have a high cervical cord injury. Intubation because their GCS is 6 has the potential to worsen the cervical injury, although it may be necessary for respiratory support.

Paediatric GCS
The assessment of children with head injuries can be exceptionally difficult. The differences in verbal responses (Table 8.1) are more blurred than in adults. More attention should therefore be paid to the motor and eye responses. There are different versions of the paediatric GCS and distinction is made between under and over 5s. An example is included in Table 8.1.

Severity of head injury
The GCS is sometimes used as a marker of severity of head injury (mild = GCS 14–15; moderate = GCS 9–13; severe = GCS 8 or less). While such a classification is useful for audit and research purposes, it is worth remembering that a GCS 15 patient may subsequently die from an evolving extradural haematoma and a GCS 3 patient may walk out of hospital when he recovers from his metabolic or drug-induced coma. In a large study of mild head injury patients it was found that 13% of those with an initial GCS of 15 had positive CT findings. This increased to 40% of those with an initial GCS of 13.

Pupillary response
The eyes are often thought of as our window to the world, but they are also a window to the brain. When a patient is sedated, paralysed and ventilated, they are the only clinical guide to changes within the cranium (until Cushing's pre-terminal response).

Together with limb movement, pupillary response is referred to as a lateralizing sign (it gives an indication as to which side of the brain the pathology exists). An understanding of the anatomy and physiology of the pupillary light reflex is necessary to interpret examination findings (Fig. 8.2; Table 8.2). In the pre-hospital setting, opening both eyes and ensuring both pupils are equal and react to light takes only a couple of seconds. In the intubated patient, checking and documenting that both pupils remain small can be used for reassurance that tentorial herniation is not imminent, and that sedation and analgesia are adequate.

When light reaches the retina, fibres from ganglion cells transmit the signal within the optic nerves. The fibres decussate within the optic chiasm and continue within the optic tracts bypassing the lateral geniculate nucleus (LGN) and primary visual cortex. The fibres enter the brainstem via the brachium of the superior colliculus. They synapse within the pretectal area and are distributed to the ipsilateral and contralateral Edinger Westphal nuclei. From here efferent (parasympathetic) pupillary fibres travel on the outer aspect of the oculomotor nerve. The oculomotor nerve runs along the edge of the tentorium cerebeli, which makes it vulnerable to compression by the temporal lobe if swelling occurs (Fig. 8.3). The fibres then synapse in the ciliary ganglion. The final stage comprises short ciliary nerves which innervate the iris and ciliary body.

The sympathetic system (Fig. 8.4) also directly innervates the pupil. The pathway probably originates in the

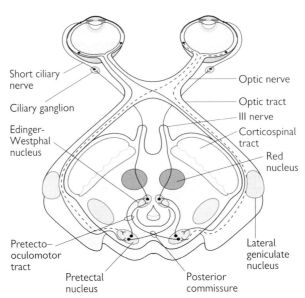

Fig. 8.2. Optic pathway demonstrating how the optic nerves, Edinger-Westphal nuclei, and oculomotor nerves contribute to the direct and indirect papillary light reflexes. (Reproduced from Sundaram et al. *Training in Opthalmology* 2009, with permission from Oxford University Press.)

hypothalamus, descending uncrossed to the level of C8–T2. From here sympathetic fibres form the perivertebral sympathetic chain, synapsing in the superior cervical ganglion. They join the carotid plexus, the ophthalmic division of the trigeminal nerve and finally reach the ciliary body and the dilator iris by via the long ciliary nerves. Optic or oculomotor nerve damage, drugs or brain stem death can therefore alter pupillary responses within the neural arch.

When evaluating the pupils dim ambient light aids examination (if the patient is on their back, they are often looking at the sun or ceiling lights). A bright torch should be used, and direct and consensual responses should be

assessed (the swinging light test—3 s of light in one eye then flick to the other over 1 s). The size of each pupil in both dark and light should be recorded.

Afferent pupillary defects

A relative afferent pupillary defect (RAPD or Marcus Gunn pupil) is seen when neither eye responds to light shone on the affected side (with a normal response on the other side). This implies injury to the retina (severe detachment), optic nerve (e.g. orbital fracture), optic chiasm, or optic tract.

Efferent pupillary defects

In the trauma setting, an efferent defect (dilatation of a pupil that is sluggish or unresponsive to either direct or consensual light) raises concerns of compression of the third nerve which is an impending sign of lateral tentorial herniation (Fig. 8.3). The assessment of a complete third nerve palsy (ptosis, reduced eye movements) is usually not possible due to reduced conscious level (although the eye may be 'down and out').

Bilateral small pupils

If pupils are extremely small, reactivity is difficult to assess. Small pupils are seen with drug (especially opiate) use, midbrain (pontine) lesions, and age-related miosis (due to autonomic degeneration).

Bilateral fixed dilated pupils

This can occur in hypoxia (when they may rapidly resolve with assisted ventilation), but can also occur with drugs (see pitfalls box) or, of course, with brain stem death.

Horner's syndrome

This comprises ptosis, miosis (small pupil) and anhidrosis. In the trauma setting cervical injury, or vertebral or carotid artery dissection disrupting the sympathetic supply should be considered.

Table 8.2. Pupillary response

Pupil size	Light response	Possible interpretation
Unilaterally dilated	Sluggish or fixed	CN III compression secondary to tentorial herniation
Bilaterally dilated	Sluggish or fixed	Inadequate brain perfusion
		Bilateral III palsy
Unilaterally dilated	Cross reactive (Marcus Gunn)	Optic nerve injury
Bilaterally miotic	Difficult to assess	Drugs (opiates)
		Metabolic encephalopathy
		Pontine lesion
Unilaterally miotic	Maintained	Sympathetic injury e.g. carotid dissection

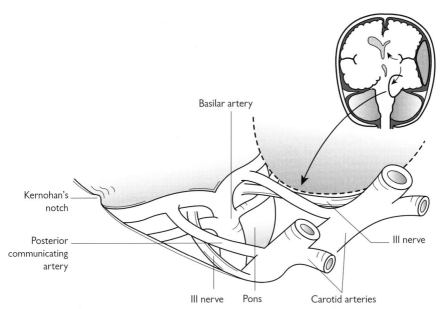

Fig. 8.3. Third nerve compression caused by medial deviaton of the temporal lobe over the tentorium cerebelli. Note the posterior cerebral artery can also become occluded leaving, in survivors, a homonymous hemianopia. (Reproduced from Lindsay *et al. Neurology and Neurosurgery Illustrated.*)

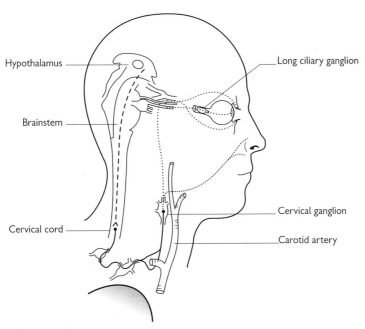

Fig. 8.4. The sympathetic innervation of the eye. The pathway probably originates in the hypothalamus. Sympathetic fibres descend into the lower cervical/upper thoracic spinal cord (C8–T2) and then exit to form the perivertebral sympathetic chain, synapsing in the superior cervical ganglion. Fibres then join the carotid artery (and are at risk in carotid dissection) and follow the ophthalmic division of the trigeminal nerve to reach the ciliary body and dilator of the iris via the long ciliary nerves.

Fundoscopy and visual field assessment (if possible) are also important parts of a neurological examination during the secondary survey following trauma.

Limb movement

A quick assessment of limb movement should be made as part of disability assessment ('wiggle your toes, squeeze my hands') as it gives information regarding the patient's conscious level (obeys commands), any lateralizing signs (weakness down one side) and any gross spinal injury. Documenting that a patient moved all four limbs on scene or in the resuscitation room is extremely important. A more formal neurological examination of each myotome and dermatome is part of the secondary survey, when possible.

Corticospinal tracts (Fig. 8.5)

From the motor cortex, approximately 90% of the descending fibres decussate in the pyramids and descend in the lateral corticospinal tract. Only around 10% travel ipsilaterally within the anterior corticospinal tract and just a few fibres descend in the ipsilateral corticospinal tract. The anterior corticospinal tract fibres subsequently decussate at a segmental level. The somatotopic arrangement within the lateral corticospinal tract is such that the legs lie most lateral and the arms most medial (hence, central cord syndrome picks off arms more than legs). Because of the cross-over, the location of a mass lesion in a head-injured patient not moving one side is most likely to be on the opposite side. For more chronic lesions (such as a subdural haematoma) a simple test is to ask the patient to left both arms up in front of their face with palms facing up, then ask them to close their eyes and look for the pronator drift as the weak side turns in and descends.

Morphological signs of head injury

Lacerations, bruising, and vault fractures

Blows to the skull vault can result in a variety of injuries from simple contusions to open depressed skull fractures, sometimes with extruding brain. While such signs are evidence of injury, absence of them does not exclude a significant brain injury. Lacerations should subsequently be thoroughly washed out and sutured as appropriate. In combination with the history and assessment of consciousness level, a low threshold should be applied for CT scanning when skull fracture or intracranial pathology is suspected.

Signs of basal skull fracture

Anterior fossa fracture:

* *CSF rhinorrhoea:* if there is doubt, a BM stix® or urine dipstick may be used to test for glucose, which if present signifies CSF rather than mucus
* *Bilateral peri-orbital haematoma* or 'racoon eyes'.
* *Subconjunctival haemorrhage:* blood under the conjunctiva that extends to its posterior limit indicates blood tracking from the orbital cavity.

Petrous fracture:

* *CSF otorrhoea or blood from the external auditory meatus:* distinguish between CSF tracking through a torn tympanic membrane and blood from a lacerated external auditory meatus.
* The ears should be examined for haemotympanum.
* Battle's sign, or bruising over the mastoid (can take 24–48 h to develop).

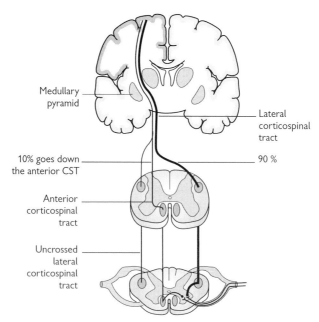

Fig. 8.5. The corticospinal tracts: Motor fibres originating from the motor cortex descend to the medullary pyramids where 90% of fibres cross to form the contralateral corticospinal tracts. Approximately 8% descend in the ipsilateral anterior corticospinal tract (with a further 2% descending uncrossed in the ipsilateral corticospinal tract). Hence, a supratentorial lesion principally causes a contralateral hemiplegia.

Pathophysiology of brain injury

Primary brain injury refers to the injury incurred at the moment of impact. Once it has occurred, there is currently little that medical management can do to effect repair.

Secondary brain injury refers to the cascade of pathophysiological mechanisms that can further damage the brain after the primary insult. For head-injured patients, it is common for a large part of their final brain injury to be secondary. For example, an extradural haematoma usually has no underlying brain injury, but the accumulating blood increases the pressure on surrounding brain, raising intracranial pressure (which can ultimately cause death).

There are a number of types of secondary injury (Box 8.1). Hypoxia, for example from an obstructed airway, is the most immediate. Ischaemia from poor cerebral perfusion (commonly due to hypovolaemia) is another. The accumulation of intracranial haematoma or oedema can raise intracranial pressure also reducing perfusion. Calcium influx due to the presence of glutamate can initiate a cytotoxic cascade.

Box 8.1. Causes of secondary brain injury

- Hypoxia (e.g. airway obstruction).
- Ischaemia (e.g. hypovolaemia, hypotension).
- Raised intracranial pressure.
- Acidosis.
- Vasospasm.
- Coagulopathy.
- Cytotoxic cascade.
- Abnormal blood glucose.

The break down of neurons and the release of their contents can also trigger a massive inflammatory response and disseminated intravascular coagulopathy which in turn can severely worsen brain injury.

The prevention and reduction of secondary brain injuries relies on a system of trauma care that enables optimal pre-hospital care and rapid transport to an appropriate centre with neurosurgical facilities. If taken to a non-neurosurgical centre, a system of rapid referral (including image linking) needs to be in place to enable subsequent rapid transfer. Within the neurosurgical centre, rapid access to appropriate radiology and theatres is vital.

In many guidelines, times are set as targets, for example, CT within one hour and surgery within 4 h are often audit standards. These numbers are arbitrary. Common sense says that faster surgical intervention to reduce brain compression will result in a better outcome. There is good Class III evidence that in patients with extradurals or subdurals, when time from injury to surgical care exceeds 2 h, the mortality rate almost doubles.

Injury at the cellular level

Mechanical pressure from a haematoma or raised ICP can damage neurons directly, but there is also a metabolic component to the injury. Impaired cerebral blood flow and metabolism result in lactic acid accumulation, which causes increased membrane permeability and oedema. ATP stores deplete, resulting in failure of energy dependent membrane pumps. There is subsequent terminal membrane depolarization with excessive release of excitatory neurotransmitters (e.g. glutamate and aspartate). These in turn open NMDA and voltage gated Ca^{2+} and Na^+ channels causing influx of these ions, which initiate catabolic processes by lipid peroxidases, proteases and phospholipases that ultimately lead to cell death.

Oxygen free radicals (and associated superoxides, hydrogen peroxide, nitric oxide and peroxinitrite) are also formed as part of the excitotoxic cascade. These saturate the endogenous antioxidant systems and induce peroxidation of cellular and vascular structures, as well as inhibition of mitochondrial electron transport. The diffuse swelling that results compromises other areas of the brain and a further cascade of injury can occur.

Cerebral blood flow

Studies have shown that hypoperfusion and sometimes hyperperfusion occur after traumatic brain injury. Both can be detrimental, although hypoperfusion is associated with a significantly worse outcome. Normal autoregulation in response to changes in cerebral perfusion pressure (related to blood pressure) is often impaired (Fig. 8.6). CO_2 reactivity is a more robust phenomenon although it can be impaired in severe brain injuries and in the early stages of trauma.

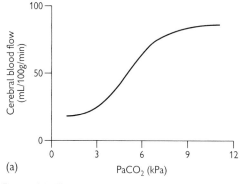
(a)

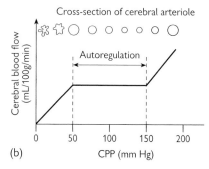
(b)

Fig. 8.6. (a,b) Effects of arterial blood pressure, the partial pressure of carbon dioxide ($PaCO_2$) and partial pressure of oxygen (PaO_2) on cerebral blood flow (CBF). (Reproduced from Gardiner et al. Training in Surgery, 2009, with permission from Oxford University Press.)

Vasospasm is thought to occur in over 30% of patients with traumatic brain injury and indicates severity of brain injury. Onset is between 2 and 15 days following injury and is thought to occur through chronic depolarization of vascular smooth muscle due to reduced potassium channel activity, reduced endothelin, and reduced nitric oxide availability. Potentiation of prostaglandin-induced vasoconstriction and free radical formation may also contribute.

Cerebral oxygenation and metabolic dysfunction

Cerebral oxygen and glucose consumption, and lactate/pyruvate ratios are commonly disrupted after TBI. The uncoupling of blood flow and metabolism may play a role in this and may contribute to secondary injury. A number of studies have now demonstrated improved outcome in TBI patients who have their cerebral oxygenation monitored either invasively or by near infra-red spectroscopy and subsequently optimized.

Oedema

Brain oedema is classified as vasogenic (leakage through a disrupted blood–brain barrier) or cytotoxic (increased intracellular volume due to disrupted cell membranes or ion pump failure; see Fig. 8.7. Both occur following TBI and raise intracranial pressure. Both cause secondary injury and, hence, strategies to treat them or prevent them occurring should improve outcome.

Inflammatory response

In combination with oedema, an inflammatory response occurs in injured brain. The release of tumour necrosis factor, interleukin 6, and transforming growth factor ß has both positive and negative effects, but importantly, can cause secondary injury.

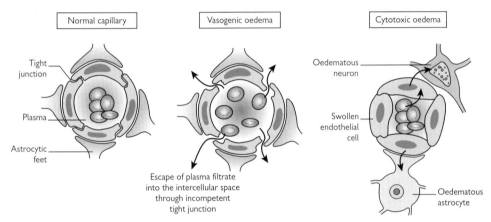

Fig. 8.7. Normal appearances of a cerebral capillary contrasted with the changes that occur in vasogenic or cytotoxic oedema. Under normal conditions, the intracellular tight junctions are intact. In vasogenic oedema, the tight junctions are not competent, allowing leakage of plasma into the interstitial space. In cytotoxic oedema, there is a primary failure of ATP-dependent sodium pump mechanism resulting in intracellular accumulation of sodium and secondarily water. (Reproduced from Rengachary and Ellenbogen *Principles of Neurosurgery*, 2005).

Classification of brain injuries

Brain injuries can be classified in a number of ways: closed or penetrating; by severity (mild, moderate, severe) and by morphology.

Skull fractures

With the increase in availability of CT, it is now rare to have to use plain X-ray to assess for fractures. When looking for fractures on CT, bone window views should be used. Vault fractures can be classified as linear or stellate, and depressed or non-depressed. If depressed with an overlying laceration, there is a significant risk of infection, especially if the dura is breached (which also increases seizure risk – see below). Such wounds will need effective debridement and cleaning. As a rough rule, if a fracture is depressed more than the thickness of the skull, it should probably be elevated.

Skull base fractures are often more difficult to distinguish, but are nearly always managed conservatively. The key is to recognise asymmetry and fluid within the sinuses or mastoid air cells. Cranial nerve function should be carefully examined.

Intracranial lesions

These can be focal (e.g. haematoma) or diffuse. There are many variations on imaging guidelines that differ between countries. In general, a lower threshold for CT scanning has prevailed in recent years with the increasing availability of CT (see Box 8.2). The UK National Institute for Clinical Excellence Guidelines can be found on the web address given at the end of this chapter. It is worth remembering that around 13% of people presenting to an emergency department with a normal conscious level following a head injury have a positive finding on CT (Fig. 8.8).

Box 8.2. Five things to look for on a head CT

- Fractures on bone window setting.
- *Obvious injury* (hyperdensity usually means acute blood): note location and size.
- *Midline shift:* measure it on the computer or, if on film, measure the bitemporal distance, halve it and measure how far the falx is deviated from the midpoint (there is a scale).
- *Signs of raised ICP:* loss of sulci over the cerebral surface. Effaced ventricles & effaced cisterns—the basal cisterns should be smiling at you.
- Loss of grey-white differentiation.

Extradural (epidural) haematomas

The incidence of extradurals is about 0.5% of all head injured patients, and 9% of those in coma following head injury. Extradural haematomas classically result from tearing of the middle meningeal artery (or one of its branches), usually in the temporal region. However, they can also occur from venous bleeding and torn venous sinuses. The classical history is of someone who is hit over the head, collapses, comes round then 'talks and dies'. This implies they have little underlying brain injury, but succumb to the secondary bleeding as it rapidly accumulates. On CT extradurals form lens-shaped convex collections. This is because the dura is normally adherent to the inner table of the skull and is especially so at the sutures, hence, blood

accumulates, peeling the dura off from the inside. Although small extradurals can be managed conservatively, neurosurgical evacuation is the normal treatment. Burr hole evacuation can be life-saving where formal neurosurgical facilities do not exist.

Subdural haematomas

Subdural haematomas are much more common (approximately 30% of severe head injuries) and usually result from tearing of bridging veins between the cerebral cortex and draining sinuses. They can also result from brain lacerations. Usually the underlying brain injury is more severe than with extradural haematoma, and the outcome is often worse. It is important to distinguish acute and chronic subdural pathologies. Although the space in which blood is accumulating is the same, a subdural presenting acutely (which appears hyperdense or white on CT) is an emergency. They often have an acute mass effect over a large area of the brain (unlike an extradural where the dura is held to the inside of the skull, below the dura blood is free to track across the surface of an entire hemisphere). An acute subdural comprises clotted blood that will not simply come out through a burr hole, and formal craniotomy is usually required. Subdurals that present chronically, on the other hand, usually affect elderly or alcoholic patients who are predisposed to the condition due to brain atrophy. Often the history is of a head injury a few days or even weeks before. Blood accumulates in the subdural space, and they may display confusion, headache, or weakness. On CT the blood is hypodense (black), and because it has liquefied, it is usually removeable through one or two burr holes. Many subdurals occur in people who are on anticoagulants (aspirin, clopidogrel, or warfarin). It is imperative that these are stopped and (unless there are overriding medical reasons) reversed if possible. Factor concentrates (II, VII, IX and X), such as Beriplex (30 iU/kg) are now commonly used in addition to vitamin K for the rapid reversal of warfarin in these circumstances.

Subarachnoid haemorrhage

Subarachnoid blood can sometimes be found on CT following a head injury. In itself, this does not require surgical treatment, but good physiological care for the injured brain. Subsequent investigation to exclude an aneursymal cause (aneursymal subarachnoid haemorrhage that subsequently results in trauma) is sometimes necessary. There is no evidence that the use of nimodipine to prevent vasospasm is of benefit in these circumstances.

Contusions and intracerebral haematomas

Contusions and intracerebral haematomas are being found more often with more liberal use of CT scanning. Common sites of injury are frontal and temporal, usually resulting from road traffic collisions, or falls. Although the two lesions can be quite distinct, there is some overlap and, over time, contusions can evolve into more well defined haematomas. The swelling associated with such lesions tends to peak between 48 and 72 h following injury. Management depends on neurological status and, if monitored, intracranial pressure. Although these injuries are little more than 'bruises' in the brain, the dramatic swelling that can occur around them and the associated rise in ICP can make them life-threatening and very difficult to treat. Steps to maintain a normal ICP, either medically or surgically, may be needed. For the conscious patient, a period of observation may suffice.

Diffuse injuries

Diffuse brain injuries comprise a spectrum of poorly understood conditions ranging from mild concussion [with or without amnesia] through to severe diffuse axonal injury (DAI); Fig. 8.9]. DAI describes a prolonged post-traumatic state in which there is loss of consciousness from the time of injury that continues beyond 6 h. DAI can be divided into mild, moderate, and severe, the severe forms commonly being the result of road traffic collisions and rendering patients comatose for prolonged periods. Decerebrate or decorticate posturing, and autonomic disturbance may result. The underlying pathology is thought to be axonal shearing resulting in microscopic retraction balls and microgial clusters. The long-term management of these patients is difficult and is usually performed in regional severe brain injury centres.

What to look for and describe on CT

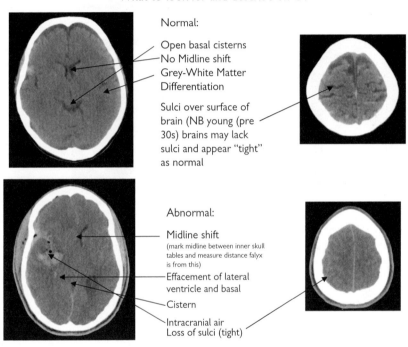

Normal:

Open basal cisterns
No Midline shift
Grey-White Matter
Differentiation

Sulci over surface of brain (NB young (pre 30s) brains may lack sulci and appear "tight" as normal

Abnormal:

Midline shift
(mark midline between inner skull tables and measure distance falyx is from this)

Effacement of lateral ventricle and basal

Cistern

Intracranial air
Loss of sulci (tight)

Fig. 8.8. Axial CT images demonstrating salient features of normal and abnormal CT scans.

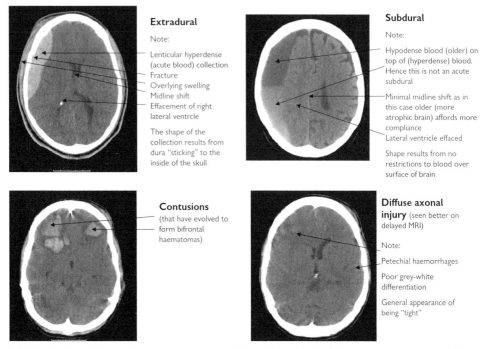

Extradural

Note:

Lenticular hyperdense (acute blood) collection
Fracture
Overlying swelling
Midline shift
Effacement of right lateral ventrcle

The shape of the collection results from dura "sticking" to the inside of the skull

Subdural

Note:

Hypodense blood (older) on top of (hyperdense) blood. Hence this is not an acute subdural

Minimal midline shift as in this case older (more atrophic brain) affords more compliance
Lateral ventricle effaced

Shape results from no restrictions to blood over surface of brain

Contusions
(that have evolved to form bifrontal haematomas)

Diffuse axonal injury (seen better on delayed MRI)

Note:

Petechial haemorrhages

Poor grey-white differentiation

General appearance of being "tight"

Fig 8.9. Axial CT images demonstrating common neurotrauma pathologies (extradual and subdural haematomas, contusions, and diffuse axonal injury).

Management of head injuries

The principal aim in the management of moderate and severe head injury is to minimize secondary injury. To achieve this, a co-ordinated approach is required from pre-hospital, emergency medicine, anaesthetic, and neurosurgical staff. Rapid controlled transfer to the most appropriate centre with subsequent rapid diagnosis and treatment is the key.

Current algorithms for the management of head injuries can be found on the National Institute for Clinical Excellence (NICE) (UK) and Brain Trauma Foundation (USA) websites (see further reading).

Pre-hospital care

The evolving field of specialist pre-hospital trauma care requires the matching of major trauma (despite being a major cause of young mortality, this is a relatively rare disease), to highly skilled paramedical and appropriately trained medical personnel (a relatively rare resource). Different services have different methods of dispatch, but a combined method that incorporates immediate dispatch with certain mechanisms of injury (fall >2 floors, ejection from vehicle, another death in vehicle, fall under train) and interrogation of the caller (the patient is unconscious) seems an appropriate way to attempt to do this. Others have suggested asking the caller to assess the motor response of the GCS, and dispatch depending on this assessment, although this is more complex and subjective.

The skill level of the pre-hospital team is also an area of controversy. An ideal system would have trained personnel who are regularly dealing with major trauma, and experienced in assessment of the need for, and ability to perform advanced procedures, such as intubation with drugs. There is no doubt that outcome in a trauma centre with neurosurgical facilities is better than outcome in a non-trauma setting (and primary transfer to such a centre avoids the delays that accompany a secondary transfer). Pre-hospital care personnel therefore need to be confident and empowered to assess and manage patient needs and transport them to the most appropriate centre. Such policies need local and regional development. In the US for example, the Brain Trauma Foundation guidelines advise that patients who are GCS 14–15 with brief loss of consciousness do not need to go to a trauma centre. Such a policy requires a system that robustly and rapidly facilitates secondary transfers for the odd patient who is subsequently found to have an evolving extradural haematoma.

Fundamentals of physiology and resuscitation for head injuries

Adequate resuscitation comprising airway protection (with cervical spine control), optimization of ventilation, and adequate blood pressure are vital before specific neurological treatments are initiated.

Airway (with cervical spine immobilization)

Obstruction of the airway due to loss of protection, from profound unconsciousness, aspiration, or local trauma, will rapidly result in acute hypoxic brain injury. In such circumstances, securing the airway with a cuffed endotracheal tube is a priority. However, often the lack of appropriately experienced personnel or the confines of the pre-hospital environment (e.g. when trapped beneath a vehicle) prevent this. In such cases the use of alternative airway adjuncts (e.g. nasopharyngeal and oropharyngeal airways)

is appropriate. The dangers of nasopharyngeal airways in patients with suspected base of skull fractures should be appreciated. If this is not suspected, the insertion of two nasopharyngeal airways and an oropharyngeal airway (a technique termed 'siloing', since it looks like the chimneys when flying over American silos) should help to optimize the airway until definitive care is reached.

Management of the aggressive or combative patient is difficult. In the presence of appropriate skills and experience, induction of anaesthesia and intubation at scene is the safest option, and facilitates passage of the patient through the resuscitation room to CT. The alternative is to risk aspiration during transfer, with suboptimal oxygenation and ventilation.

The technical procedure of passing an endotracheal tube over a bougie into the trachea is relatively easy to teach and, in most cases, straightforward. However, the neurological assessment to determine the need for intubation, and the subsequent airway management if intubation fails, is not. Intubation itself is not a dangerous procedure since it is carried out thousands of times daily across the world electively, with complications being extremely rare. However, studies have reported varying rates of success at paramedic pre-hospital intubation, ranging from 35 to 89%. Manual hyperventilation, which can be harmful to the already injured brain, is also an area of concern.

Breathing and ventilation

Diagnosing and treating chest injuries to improve oxygenation and ventilation are vital to maintaining cerebral oxygenation. If the patient is intubated, a state of normocapnia, with an end tidal CO_2 of 4.5 kPa or 30–35 mmHg should be the aim (usually requiring about 10 breaths/min). Hyperventilation, while possibly reducing ICP, also results in vasoconstriction and, hence, cerebral hypoperfusion (this has been confirmed using positron emission tomography in brain-injured patients). Chronic hyperventilation has been shown to result in a worse outcome. If the patient is rapidly deteriorating (e.g. clinically coning with a blown pupil), temporary hyperventilation could be considered simply to buy time for surgical or other medical intervention.

Circulation

Maintenance of cerebral perfusion pressure (CPP) is paramount in head injured patients (see Box 8.3). A head-injured patient may have a raised ICP that will reduce their cerebral perfusion pressure, but it is usually not possible to define this in the emergency setting. The multiply injured patient may be hypotensive from other injuries, and their CPP may be compromised both by a reduction in MAP and a rise in ICP. Strategies for management therefore comprise maintaining MAP and lowering ICP.

Box 8.3. Cerebral perfusion pressure
- CPP = MAP – ICP
  (CPP = cerebral perfusion pressure, MAP = mean arterial blood pressure and ICP = intracranial pressure). Normal CPP = 85 – 15 = 70 mmHg
- CBF = (MAP – ICP)/CVR
  (CBF = cerebral blood flow, CVR = cerebral vascular resistance). This is V = IR with the letters replaced.

Maintaining MAP

Control of haemorrhage is the first step. This may comprise direct pressure, binding of a pelvic fracture, or splinting of limb fractures. The second is correction of hypovolaemia, which is an area of controversy. Hypotension must be avoided, but a careful balance has to be struck. In the conscious talking patient, their blood pressure (whatever it is) is adequately perfusing their brain. In the unconscious patient it is a common practice to ensure that a systolic of >100 mmHg is maintained.

It has been shown that having a systolic of <90 mmHg on arrival in the emergency department increases mortality from 27% to 50% and a single hypotensive episode in the pre-hospital phase doubles mortality from traumatic brain injury. It is also worth noting that only when a patient has an adequate blood pressure is the neurological examination meaningful.

The American pre-hospital management guidelines for blood pressure in head injured patients advocate maintaining a systolic pressure of >90 mmHg, whereas European guidelines suggest a mean arterial pressure of >90 mmHg (and a systolic pressure of >120 mmHg). The evidence surrounding these guidelines is minimal, and local policy should be followed.

The correct fluid for volume resuscitation of the head injured patient is also controversial. An isotonic or hypertonic solution (such as saline) is the current recommendation. There is now evidence that hypertonic saline affords improved outcome, especially in TBI with a GCS <8. Hypotonic solutions should be avoided. Early replacement of blood products in hypotensive multiply injured patients is recommended.

Guideline targets for CPP-driven resuscitation (calculated when ICP is also measured, usually in an intensive care unit) vary from high recommendations (>70–80 mmHg), which aim to improve perfusion, to low levels (50 mmHg), which aim to minimize oedema formation. There is no class I evidence for either approach; however, class II evidence suggests a CPP of 60 mmHg is an adequate perfusion pressure for most adults with TBI. A randomized study has shown that higher CPPs reduce secondary hypotensive ischaemic insults (although not resulting in improved neurological outcomes); however, the higher CPP was associated with a 5-fold increase in adult respiratory distress syndrome (ARDS). Generally accepted CPP figures used on most ICUs are between 60 and 70 mmHg.

Control of intracranial pressure

As explained by the cerebral perfusion equation, a raised ICP will reduce blood flow to the already injured brain. A raised ICP is akin to compartment syndrome of the brain. Monro and Kellie (1874) described the skull as a closed box and, since its volume is therefore constant, if a substance (e.g. blood, swelling, or tumour) is added, another component must be displaced for pressure to remain constant. The ventricles provide much of this pressure buffer. The accumulation of a haematoma results in ventricular effacement and displacement of CSF down the vertebral canal. Further accumulation results in further displacement and possibly some displacement of venous blood (another low pressure substance). At some point, however, this buffering capacity reaches a limit and the system decompensates into a hydraulic system with a sudden and rapid rise in intracranial pressure (Fig. 8.10). At this point there is a high risk of displacing brain from within the cranial cavity, termed coning. This can be medial temporal lobe through the tentorium cerebeli or the cerebellar tonsils through the foramen magnum (Fig. 8.11).

There is no class I evidence for ICP monitoring improving outcome because a randomized trial would not be ethical. There is good evidence that ICP monitoring provides early detection of evolving mass lesions and reduces the indiscriminate use of ICP lowering treatments (which themselves have complications). When ICP targeted

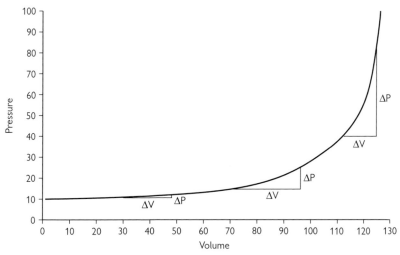

Fig. 8.10. A graph demonstrating changes in intracranial pressure with increasing volume of an additional mass. Initially, as an additional volume (e.g. extradural haematoma) accumulates, there is a period of compliance where low pressure contents (e.g. CSF and venous blood) are displaced. Once this compliance is utilised, the system becomes 'hydrolic' in nature and there is an exponential rise in intracranial pressure. This phenomenon which occurs because the skull is a 'closed box' is commonly referred to as the Monro-Kellie Doctrine [after Alexander Monro and George Kellie].

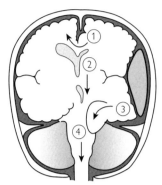

Fig. 8.11. Brain Shift: Diagram of the different types of brain herniation. (1) Subfalcine 'midline' herniation—can cause ipsilateral anterior cerebral artery occlusion. (2) Tentorial herniation—herniation of the uncus (medial temporal lobe) through the tentorial hiatus causing compression of the occulomotor nerve and brain stem. (3) Central herniation – diffuse supratentorial swelling causing vertical displacement of the midbrain through the tentorial hiatus. (4) Tonsillar herniation—a subtentorial expanding mass or greater supratentorial pressure causes herniation of the cerebellar tonsils through the foramen magnum.

treatments are used, a value of 20 mmHg is commonly considered to be a pressure at which to escalate treatment.

There are different types of ICP monitoring:
- *Intra-parenchymal monitoring:* the insertion of an ICP bolt into the brain parenchyma (usually a quiescent area such as right frontal lobe or into the side with a focal lesion) enables continuous ICP waveform monitoring. There are risks of causing both extra-axial and intra-parenchymal haemorrhage, so it is advisable that this procedure should only be performed where facilities exist to treat the complications. The monitor itself is not in any way therapeutic.
- *Intraventricular monitoring:* the placement of an extraventricular drain (Fig. 8.12) within a ventricle (to measure intraventricular ICP) is the gold standard ICP monitor, and in addition enables the evacuation of CSF which can lower ICP. The technique requires more skill than bolt placement (especially if ventricles are small) and has greater risk of concurrent brain injury and infection if left *in situ.*

Other modalities of monitoring include jugular venous saturation, brain tissue oxygen (PbtO$_2$), CBF, and microdialysis techniques. These allow further investigation of brain metabolism in the intensive care setting, but all require specialist placement and interpretation.

Techniques for reducing ICP include (see also Box 8.4):
- *Nursing with the patients head up at approx 30 degrees:* this is important for prolonged care on ICU and also in the emergency department and during prolonged transfers (note, helicopters and aeroplanes fly at different angles and this needs to be considered when loading a patient).
- *Diuretics and hypertonic saline:* mannitol is commonly used to reduced ICP acutely. Classically, it is used to buy time for the patient who is deteriorating to allow transfer for surgical intervention. Its rapid mode of action is through increasing intravascular volume, decreasing haematocrit and viscosity, and hence increasing cerebral blood flow and oxygenation. Mannitol comes in concentrations of 10 and 20%, and a dose of between 0.5 and 1 g/kg is given intravenously, repeated if necessary. It is important to ensure the patient's blood pressure is maintained, that serum osmolality does not drift much

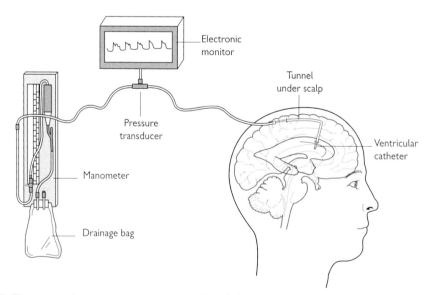

Fig. 8.12. Direct intracranial pressure monitoring using a ventricular cathether and manometer. A pressure transducer connected midway enables digital display of intracranial pressure. The advantage of this system over intraparencymal monitors is that it allows CSF drainage to reduce intracranial pressure. Disadvantages are that greater skill is required to insert the ventricular catheter (especially into compressed ventricles) and increased risk of surgical morbidity/infection. (Reproduced from Rengachary and Ellenbogen *Principles of Neurosurgery,* 2005).

Box 8.4. Simple techniques to lower ICP in pre-hospital or emergency department setting:

- Don't strangle patient with cervical collar.
- Nurse head up (30 degrees).
- Analgesia.
- Paralyse and sedate.
- Control ventilation: normocapnia and try to keep PEEP <12cmH$_2$O.
- Avoid harsh braking in transfer.
- Mannitol and hypertonic saline.

above 320 mOsm/l and they do not develop an acidosis as a result. A good guide as to whether it is working is to check for a profound diuresis of dilute urine. Repeated doses can result in mannitol crossing the disrupted blood brain barrier and worsening cerebral oedema. Some clinicians also advocate the addition of 0.3–9.5 mg/kg frusemide with mannitol, although this is not common practice in the UK. A recent Cochrane review found no evidence to support the use of mannitol in the pre-hospital care of head injured patients. Hypertonic saline (6mL/kg of 5% up to a maximum of 350 mL) has similar effects to mannitol, drawing extracellular fluid into the vascular compartment, reducing viscosity and improving cerebral blood flow. It is therefore advocated in a number of centres especially in the hypotensive head injured patient.

- *Sedation:* anaesthetic agents usually suppress neurotransmission, and in doing so, metabolic rate is reduced. This may be of benefit at a time of ischaemia. Sedation will reduce the ICP of an agitated patient. The deeper the sedation, the greater the reduction in cerebral metabolic rate and, hence, the greater the reduction in ICP. The pay-off is that most forms of sedation also reduce blood pressure (and hence CPP). Hence, a common scenario on ICU is that a patient is sedated, but given inotropic support to maintain blood pressure. The careful balance of sedation, inotropes, diuretics, and intravenous fluids needs expert care to prevent worsening of cerebral oedema. It is worth remembering that nature may often be better at maintaining ideal brain perfusion than we clinicians think we are.
- *Induction agents:* there is often debate over the best induction agent for brain-injured patients, often in conjunction with the paralytic agent of choice. The simply answer is to use what you are used to, and try to maintain normotension and normoxia during the process.
- *Propofol* depresses cerebral metabolic rate and scavenges free radicals. There is evidence of transient cerebral protection, although it reduces blood pressure which can, in turn, exacerbate ischaemia.
- *Etomidate* has less cardiovascular depressive effects than propofol, but may not offer cerebral protection. It may, by inhibiting nitric oxide synthase, intensify the ischaemic insult. It is also an adreno-supressant.
- *Ketamine* use in head injury patients would strike horror into many clinicians. This has historically been based on a few studies of its use during air ventriculograms, with a subsequent rise in ICP. However, it has the advantage of maintaining cardiovascular stability and it has neuroprotective (NMDA antagonist) properties. It is now coming back into clinical practice, being more commonly used in Australia than the UK, and with further trials it may well

become the preferred induction agent in acute head injury management.
- *Paralytic agents:* the choice of paralytic agent is usually related to the need for a short-acting agent that reverses spontaneously if intubation fails, rather than an agent specific for its neuroprotective properties. This means suxamethonium is still the agent of choice despite the transient rise in ICP that it causes.

For intra-operative management, there is good laboratory evidence that inhalational anaesthetics (sevoflurane and isoflurane) offer some degree of ischaemic neural protection.
- *Barbiturates:* barbiturates such as phenobarbitone reduce cerebral metabolic rate and have been shown to be protective in cerebral anoxia and ischaemia. They also reduce ICP. However, as with other forms of sedation, they reduce blood pressure and, in hypotensive patients, their use correlates to a poorer outcome. They are often considered a last resort in medical management, and EEG monitoring to ensure burst suppression optimizes adequate dosage.
- *Muscle paralysis:* non-depolarizing muscle relaxants reduce ICP. Their use is extremely important if a sedated patient is being cooled as they stop shivering (which can raise ICP).
- *Cooling:* cooling patients to 35°C reduces ICP, as well as possibly affording some cerebral protection. There is now good evidence that mild sustained hypothermia in survivors of out of hospital cardiac arrest affords some neuronal protection. Mild hypothermia in head injuries is thought to provide some neuroprotection, although trials are ongoing in this area. During these studies it has been clearly demonstrated that hyperthermia worsens outcome, hence temperature monitoring and treatment of hyperthermia are minimum requirements. Deep hypothermia (18–22°C) is neuroprotective, but results in circulatory arrest and hence cardiac bypass is also needed. The rapid cooling and mechanisms to maintain blood flow means that, currently, deep hypothermia is not used in brain injury.

Other considerations include:
- *Normoglycaemia:* lack of glucose in the presence of oxygen results in neuronal necrosis; however, the presence of glucose with lack of oxygen causes greater damage, possibly because the intracellular acidosis that results from the anaerobic metabolism of glucose causes amplification of the injury. Animal studies have demonstrated that hyperglycaemia causes exacerbation of most forms of cerebral ischaemia. Higher blood glucose concentrations on admission to hospital result in a poorer outcome in stroke patients and hyperglycaemia results in a more rapid expansion of ischaemic lesions. For these reasons, maintaining normoglycaemia is probably of benefit to the brain-injured patient.
- *Nutrition:* patients with severe brain injury exhibit metabolic responses similar to patients with 20–40% body surface area burns, hence early caloric and nitrogen intake via enteral (or if required parenteral) routes should be initiated.
- *Hyperoxaemia:* there is currently no good evidence either way for the use of hyperbaric oxygen. It may be beneficial in transient focal ischaemia, but appears deleterious in global ischaemia. More research is needed.

- *Steroids*: steroids, such as dexamethasone, reduce cerebral oedema associated with brain tumours. They were therefore used extensively to reduce cerebral oedema associated with TBI. In 2004, a large multi-centre prospective trial (corticosteroid randomization after significant had injury, CRASH) using high-dose methylprednisolone in head-injured patients with a GCS of 14 or less was terminated early because of the increased 2-week mortality in the steroid compared with the placebo group. Although the cause of this increase is not clear, it is now difficult to justify the use of steroids in TBI except in specific circumstances.

Surgical management

Ventricular drainage
Often a rise in ICP, from either focal or diffuse swelling, results in effacement of the lateral ventricles and CSF is displaced from them. Sometimes the ventricles still contain CSF, which becomes trapped. In some centres, it is therefore routine to pass an extraventricular drain into the ventricles to allow tapping of this CSF to reduce ICP. There are risks of brain trauma on passing the catheter and subsequent infection of the CSF.

Haematoma evacuation
If a patient has a high ICP with a surgically amenable lesion, then evacuation of that lesion will usually be appropriate (an exception to this may be where anticoagulation has not yet been reversed). Surgical technique depends on the nature of the lesion and its location. For chronic subdural haematomas (or to quickly relieve a raised ICP from an extradural before proceeding to craniotomy), one or two burr holes in the appropriate locations may be performed (Fig. 8.13). For a temporal extradural or acute subdural. a convexity craniotomy through a question mark trauma incision would be a standard approach.

The increased availability of CT over the last 20 years has meant that exploratory burr holes are rarely performed. If a hospital does not have a CT scanner, it is unlikely to have a clinician who has ever performed burr holes. Even if a CT has confirmed the diagnosis of a lesion such as an extradural haematoma, few clinicians would be comfortable performing burr holes outside a neurosurgical centre (military practice notwithstanding). However, systems of very rapid transfer of patients from such hospitals into trauma centres are often lacking, and not treating such a condition locally is akin to transferring a patient with a known untreated tension pneumothorax. It may be that, in the future, with appropriately trained personnel, emergency department treatment of amenable haematomas may be performed prior to transfer.

Burr hole technique
Figure 8.13 shows where burr holes should be placed. The procedure starts at the most likely place (if struck on the right temporal region with a dilated right pupil, start with the right temporal burr hole). After appropriate anaesthesia and skin preparation, a 3-cm incision is made at the first site down to bone. Self-retainers are used to keep the skin edges apart and the periosteum scraped off. Using a drill (either a perforator with a clutch mechanism or a Hudson Brace) a hole is made through the bone. The thin layer of bone left is then removed. This gives access to the extradural space. If the pathology is subdural, the dura can be open, but if the blood is clotted, it will be very difficult to get any useful amount out without a craniotomy.

Craniotomy or craniectomy for haematoma evacuation
A craniotomy or craniectomy (where the bone is left out at the end of the operation) is performed by creating a skin flap, a number of burr holes that are joined with a craniotome, and then removing the bone flap. This enables clotted extradural and subdural blood to be removed. Storage of the bone flap allows replacement 1–3 months later if clinically appropriate. Replacement of the bone flap helps restore normal blood flow and metabolism, and prevents development of the 'syndrome of the trephined'. Some surgeons advocate storage of the bone flap in a subcutaneous pocket in the abdominal wall. This is no longer

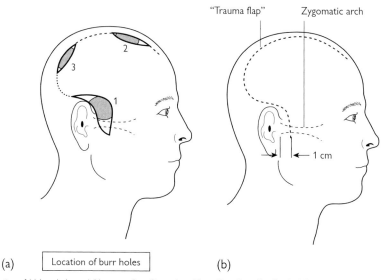

(a)   Location of burr holes   (b)

Fig. 8.13. Location of (a) burr holes and (b) trauma flap. (Reproduced from Greenberg *Handbook of Neurosurgery*, 6th edn, 2005.)

common practice due to the risk of autolysis except where patient and bone need to be repatriated (e.g. from conflict zones).

Decompressive craniectomy
Decompressive craniectomy refers to the removal of part of the cranium (e.g. bi-frontal) to allow underlying swollen brain to expand out of the constraints of the skull, or closed box. This nearly always reduces the ICP; however, it is a major procedure supported by only class III evidence. Currently, there are a number of randomized prospective trials underway to gain class I evidence. These are the Rescue ICP study (www.rescueicp.com) in Europe and the DECRA study in Australia.

Issues of evidence-based management of head trauma
There is scant class I evidence to support many aspects of brain injury management, as few people are willing to sacrifice their or their children's brains to randomized treatments and emergency neurosurgical techniques. This has resulted in a vacuum of evidence. However, this is not absence of knowledge. For example, the first recommendation of the Brain Trauma Foundation second edition 'Pre-Hospital Guidelines' states that patients should be monitored for hypoxaemia (with peripheral oxygen saturations), for which there is little supporting evidence, but ample theoretical benefit. Therefore, current clinical practice is based on theory, previous experience, and level II or III evidence. There are some areas that remain controversial and some of these are described below. Common sense should tailor care to the individual circumstances of the patient involved.

Anticonvulsants after head injury
Seizures occur in up to 25% of TBI patients in the first week after injury. A GCS of <10, cortical contusion, depressed skull fracture, haematomas, and penetrating head injuries are thought to increase the risk. A seizure increases metabolic rate and raises ICP, and should be avoided. However, while meta-analyses of trials using phenytoin and carbamezepine show a reduction in early seizures (relative risk 0.34), there is no impact on outcome or long-term seizure development. Therefore, they should be considered if the patient is thought to be high risk, but current European guidelines do not give advice on this.

Appropriate fluids for head injury resuscitation
The use of hypertonic saline as the resuscitative fluid has been shown to improve blood pressure and survival outcome slightly (with *post hoc* analysis of class II data). Most guidelines continue to recommend normal saline or other isotonic crystalloid.

Antibiotics in open fractures
Local protocols vary in the use of prophylactic antibiotics for open skull fractures, although only one trial has demonstrated that they reduce the risks of subsequent meningitis. By far the most important component of care is good wash-out and debridement of such wounds. Tetanus vaccination should be given if required.

Antibiotics in base of skull fractures
There are a couple of meta-analyses of many poor trials of antibiotic use to prevent infection in base of skull fractures with and without CSF leak. There is no evidence that they are of benefit.

Calcium channel and NMDA antagonists
A Cochrane review has failed to demonstrate any benefit of nimodipine in trauma although its benefit in aneurismal subarachnoid haemorrhage has been clearly demonstrated. The British and Finnish Head Injury Trials (HIT) have occasionally shown slight, but statistically insignificant benefit from nimodipine in traumatic SAH, but most recently no benefit has been shown. Trials of NMDA antagonists in humans have so far had disappointing results. Selfotel (CGS 19755) is a competitive NMDA antagonist. A large phase II trial was terminated early because of concerns that had arisen from a stroke trial. Cerestat (CNS 1102), a non-competitive NMDA antagonist, reduces contusion volume, hemispheric swelling, and lowers ICP in animal studies, but the phase II human trials again were cut short because of concerns in a separate stroke trial.

Magnesium
Magnesium is an NMDA antagonist and calcium channel blocker, but no benefit has yet been demonstrated.

Free radical scavengers
Tirilazad mesylate (which inhibits free radial medicated lipid peroxidation) and polyethylene glycol-conjugated superoxide dismutase (PEG-SOD—a free radical scavenger) have both had good phase I and early phase II trial results. Unfortunately, large phase II studies have failed to demonstrate any significant benefit with either.

Outcome after brain injuries

Glasgow Outcome Score

The GOS originally described outcomes as falling into five categories: death, persistent vegetative state, severe disability, moderate disability, and good recovery. Persistent vegetative state refers to the inability to communicate or follow commands. Severe disability refers to conscious patients who require assistance with basic needs such as feeding and hygiene. Moderate disability means some persistent neurological or cognitive impairment, but can manage basic needs, use public transport, and work in a sheltered situation. To increase sensitivity, the severe and moderate disability and good recovery outcomes have been divided into upper and lower categories, and so the revised GOS has an 8-point rather than a 5-point scale.

Factors predicting outcome include fixed risk factors and secondary insults.

Fixed risk factors:

- *Mechanism of injury*: penetrating worse than blunt. NAI in children and pedestrians and cyclists (compared with vehicle occupants) fare worse.
- *Age, gender, genetics*: being older affords a worse outcome, as does being female. The ε4 allele of apolipoprotein E also predisposes to a poor outcome.
- *Pupillary signs*: bilateral reactive > unilateral fixed > bilateral fixed.
- *GCS*: there is a steep relationship between GCS and improving survival between GCS 3 and 7, which becomes shallower between GCS 8 and 15.
- *CT findings*: mid-line shift, compression of basal cisterns and traumatic subarachnoid haemorrhage are associated with a worse prognosis (Marshall grading system predicts mortality, but not functional outcome).

Secondary insults:

- *Hypotension*: a single episode of hypotension between injury and resuscitation doubles mortality and morbidity (even when other injuries and hypoxaemia are accounted for).
- *Hypoxia*: (SaO_2 <90%) correlates with a poorer outcome.
- *Hyperglycaemia*: associated with a worse outcome, though this may reflect a stress response, which is proportional to severity of injury.
- *Hyper- and hypocapnia*: both are thought to result in a worse outcome, although evidence is weak.
- *Other injuries:* although improvements in trauma care have now reduced this considerably.

Summary

Traumatic brain injury is the commonest cause of death in the under 45s. A great deal can be done to reduce morbidity and mortality by reducing secondary injury. This relies on good multi-disciplinary team work, from paramedic crews, through the emergency department to the neurosurgeons and intensive care unit staff. There remains a great deal of controversy regarding many aspects of TBI care because performing randomized controlled trials is extremely difficult in this area.

Further reading

Brain Trauma Foundation. Guidelines for the Management of Severe Traumatic Brain Injury. *J Neurotrauma*, 2007; **24**(Suppl 1): S1–106.

Brain Trauma Foundation. *Guidelines for the Prehospital Management of Severe Traumatic Brain Injury*, 2nd edn. New York: BTF, 2007.

Bullock MR, Chesnut R, Ghajar J, Gordon D, Hartl R, Newell DW, et al. Guidelines for the surgical management of traumatic brain injury. *Neurosurgery* 2006; **58**(Suppl 3): S2–62.

Mokri B. The Monro–Kellie hypothesis: applications in CSF volume depletion. *Neurology*, 2001; **56**: 1746–8.

National Institute for Health and Clinical Excellence. *Triage, assessment, investigation and early management of head injury in infants, children and adults, Clinical guidelines CG56*. London: NIHCE, 2007.

Schierhout G, Roberts I. Antiepileptic drugs for preventing seizures following acute traumatic brain injury. *Cochrane Database System Rev* 2001, Issue 4.

Smith M, Mahajan RP. Clinical neuroscience: relevance to current practice. *Br J Anaesthes* 2007; **99**(1): 1–3.

Sydenham E, Roberts I, Alderson P. Hypothermia for traumatic head injury. *Cochrane Database of System Rev* 2009; Issue 2.

Valadka AB, Andrews BT (Eds). *Neurotrauma: Evidence-Based Answers to Common Questions*. New York: Thieme, 2005.

Wakai A, Roberts IG, Schierhout G. Mannitol for acute traumatic brain injury. *Cochrane Database of System Rev* 2007; Issue 1.

Radiology in trauma

Introduction

Improvement in trauma outcomes is dependent on optimizing all aspects of pre-hospital and hospital care. A multidisciplinary approach is critical in delivering optimum care for injured patients.

There have been huge technological advances in radiology in the past decade. The advent of portable ultrasound equipment, picture archiving and communication systems (PACS), digital imaging, and in particular multi-detector computed tomography (CT), has revolutionized the role of radiology in trauma.

In order to adopt these technological advances, a wholesale review is necessary and accepted practice needs to be challenged, with evidence-based change where necessary.

History of computed tomography and the arrival of multi-detector computed tomography

The CT scanner was introduced into trauma care in the 1970s and single slice detector CT scanners were the norm until the late 1990s, when 2-, 4-, 8-, and 16-slice multi-detector computed tomography (MDCT) scanners were introduced. In the past decade, there have been huge advances in computing power, in addition to the introduction of 32, 64, 128 and 256 MDCT and dual tube scanners. These scanners produce exquisite images at the touch of a button with virtual real-time multi-planar imaging.

In simple terms, a 256-slice MDCT scanner can do 256 slices every 0.5 s, so that in 1 min it can produce 35,720 ($256 \times 2 \times 60$) images. In effect, it can scan a whole body from vertex to pubic symphysis in under 10 s and display these images in any plane in real time with almost instant three-dimensional (3D) reconstruction. These same images can be manipulated or simultaneously viewed if there are sufficient monitors, showing the skeletal system, cardiovascular system, and the solid and hollow organs of the body.

There is now general acceptance that MDCT is the single biggest advance to the care of trauma patients in the past decade and good evidence that it can significantly change trauma outcome. The CT scanner should now be pivotal in the management of trauma patients if sited and used appropriately. The principle that definitive diagnosis is not necessary to treat the patient initially can now be challenged if CT is used appropriately. Clinical examination is unreliable in major trauma and it is essential that patients are not examined to death. In particular, time can be saved by using CT to define injury and aid decision-making. However, in order to maximize the potential of MDCT, it needs to be integral to the delivery of emergency services and located close to or within the resuscitation room.

Role of the radiologist in major trauma

The role of the radiologist has dramatically changed over the past decade. Radiologists should be an integral part of the trauma team management and also the trauma team in the resuscitation room with a wide-ranging set of responsibilities. These may include

- Trauma team management.
- Radiology services - 24/7/52 service.
- Acute trauma team.
- Communication with team leader.
- Providing rapid access to imaging during primary and secondary survey.
- Protocol imaging.
- Reporting all imaging.
- Decision-making.
- Interventional radiology services.
- Design of Trauma Unit.
- Education.
- Research.

Radiologist involvement at an early stage in the planning and organization of trauma care into regional systems, setting up specialist trauma centre networks, and implementation of specialist multidisciplinary trauma hospitals will lead to optimization of radiology resources locally, regionally, and nationally. A major difficulty in setting up a 24/7 trauma service is the provision of radiology services, in particular interventional trauma radiology. Trauma radiology is a neglected specialty and even pooling the expertise available may be insufficient to provide the quality necessary to staff a 24/7 service. PACS and teleradiology have been quoted as a means of providing acute cover at night and weekends, but to provide optimum care for patients, the trauma radiologist needs to be in the hospital. In addition, if MDCT is being used as part of the initial management of trauma patients, the volume of information and speed of decision-making necessary makes teleradiology an impractical solution.

Evidence-based practice for change

There is now sufficient evidence to provoke a sea change in acute trauma care, not least in the involvement of radiology. The role of ultrasound—focused assessment with sonography for trauma (FAST)—plain radiography and, in particular, MDCT has changed dramatically over the last few years. In particular, a reduction in time from admission to MDCT is seen as vital to optimizing outcome for multiply-injured patients.

This chapter will concentrate on optimizing radiology services that are available at present, and provide a framework for the future of trauma radiology.

Key points about radiology in trauma

- CT is the doughnut of life, NOT the doughnut of death.
- MDCT is the single biggest advance in trauma care in the last decade.
- Radiology needs to provide a 24/7/52 trauma service.
- Do not x-ray patients to death.

Primary survey

The main goal of pre-hospital care is to retrieve rapidly, and safely deliver a traumatized patient to the appropriate institution to provide definitive care. The aim of the primary survey is to rapidly assess and stabilize patients with a view to defining injury and providing definitive care, be that surgery, interventional radiology, or critical care. The adjuncts to the primary survey include relevant imaging during resuscitation.

In practice, individuals from the trauma team carry out the primary survey steps simultaneously.

The chest and pelvis X-rays are part of the primary survey (Fig. 9.1). These should be taken alongside the primary assessment, and ideally a report given to the team leader by the radiologist as soon as they become available. It is imperative that communication is clear and that the report is documented, in addition to a later written report.

The chest radiograph should be done as soon as it is practicably possible, preferably within the first few minutes of arrival. It should be performed with the patient fully exposed and in a non-rotated supine position in full inspiration. Failure to optimize the CXR will lead to problems with interpretation and potential failure to diagnose a life-threatening injury. The pelvis radiograph should also be done as soon as it is practically possible, paying attention to avoid rotation.

Only essential imaging should be performed at this stage. Delaying life-saving definitive care such as surgery in order to get spine or skeletal radiographs (part of the secondary survey) is not appropriate.

It is the duty of the radiographer to ensure that there is no unnecessary exposure to radiation to the trauma team and that they are all suitably protected before exposure.

In future, where MDCT is located within the resuscitation room, the role of plain radiography may diminish (Fig. 9.2).

Ultrasound machines are now so portable, that arguably the FAST examination should be performed during the pre-hospital phase, either at the scene or during transportation, so that facilities can be made available for urgent surgery if necessary. The scenarios where FAST can be life-saving are when the patient is haemodynamically unstable and fluid is detected in either the pleural space, pericardium, or in the peritoneal cavity. In these circumstances,

rapid insertion of a chest drain, open thoracotomy or an immediate laparotomy may be life-saving.

FAST may be initially negative in the presence of significant intra-abdominal haemorrhage. In addition, FAST detects fluid, not necessarily blood. Therefore, it should not always be assumed that haemorrhage is the cause of fluid detected on FAST, not least when there is a pelvic fracture and a potential bladder injury is suspected (urine) or occasionally in blunt trauma with a bowel injury (bowel contents; see Box 9.1).

FAST can be performed by any clinician suitably trained and experienced in its use. If the radiologist is present, they may either perform or supervise the examination.

> **Box 9.1.** FAST advantages and disadvantages
>
> *Advantages*
> - Cheap.
> - Portable.
> - Fast.
> - Easy (to perform).
> - High sensitivity.
> - High specificity (for fluid).
> - Repeatable.
>
> *Disadvantages*
> - Unable to localize source of bleeding.
> - Unable to differentiate fluid.
> - False negative—occasionally.
> - Compromised—obesity, surgical emphysema, previous surgery.

With a well functioning trauma team, the AP chest radiograph should be taken within 1–3 minutes, the pelvis radiograph within 5–10 min, and the FAST within 1–10 min of the patient's arrival.

MDCT (primary CT survey / CT triage)

This approach challenges many of the present established principles laid down in trauma care. There is now sufficient evidence to advocate this approach. The key to using this

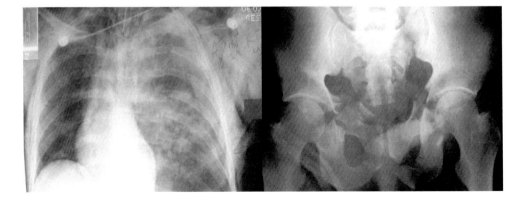

Fig. 9.1. Supine trauma chest X-ray and pelvis trauma X-ray.

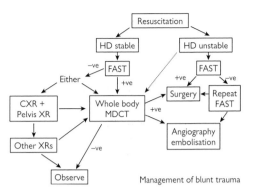

Fig. 9.2. Suggested algorithm for plain radiography, FAST and CT in blunt trauma.

approach is the design of the resuscitation room and the proximity to MDCT. The scanner should ideally be within the resuscitation room, but the alternative is that it is sited adjacent to the emergency department. With proximity and the speed of modern scanners even haemodynamically unstable patients could be imaged and their injuries defined before definitive care is instituted.

The basic concept is that the patient is directly transferred onto the MDCT table and resuscitation is initiated. The airway and breathing are addressed, IV access is obtained and a whole body CT is the next step (primary CT survey). Decisions on further management are then made based on the clinical state of the patient and the CT findings (CT triage; see Box 9.2).

> **Box 9.2.** The <C>ABCD approach
> - **<C>** control of exsanguinating external haemorrhage.
> - **A:** airway.
> - **B:** breathing
> - **C:** CT—whole body with contrast, then circulation.
> - **D:** diagnosis and definitive treatment.

This approach cuts out all the major delays to definitive treatment and is likely to be the key to future care in major trauma patients. However, units with the facility to perform CT at this stage of resuscitation are few, and until this is more commonplace traditional approaches are likely to remain.

Interpretation of the supine AP CXR
The trauma supine CXR should be interpreted by detecting the greatest threat to life first, using the ABCDE systematic assessment (Box 9.3).

The supine trauma CXR is often taken sub-optimally, with rotation, poor inspiration, over or under-penetration and artefact being common problems. All these factors can mimic pathology, make the heart and mediastinum look widened or indistinct, and it can be difficult or sometimes impossible to diagnose pathology.

Adequacy
The patient should be exposed with no overlying artefacts if possible. The name should be checked (this is extremely important, in particular in major incidents, when there

> **Box 9.3.** The ABCDE systematic assessment
> - **A:** adequacy, airway and ALL lines and tubes.
> - **B:** breathing.
> - **C:** circulation.
> - **D:** diaphragm.
> - **E:** edges.
> - **S:** spine, skeleton, and soft tissues.

may be several patients with similar injuries arriving simultaneously). There should be a side-marker. The patient should be straight and supine. Rotation can be assessed by ensuring that the spinous processes are equidistant from the medial end of the clavicles. Rotation can be a cause of misinterpretation of the CXR findings. Interpretation of the CXR in a patient with a scoliosis can be difficult and misleading. The CXR should include the apices of both lungs, and the costophrenic recesses on both sides. It should be taken in full inspiration even if the patient is ventilated.

The anterior aspect of at least 5 and preferably 6 ribs should be visible at the mid-point of the hemidiaphragms. Visualization of more than 7 anterior ribs on a supine CXR suggests large volume lungs or air-trapping. Review of the shape of the diaphragm is then necessary.

Supine CXRs are taken with a low kV technique, which allows better visualization of the bony skeleton and adequate visualization of lung and pleural pathology. In a correctly exposed CXR, the T8/T9 disc space should be visible. With digital radiography/PACS, it is usually possible to manipulate images to optimize this.

Airway
The trachea lies in the mid-line above the clavicles, but deviates slightly to the right below this. It is critical that if the patient is intubated, that the position of the endotracheal (ET) tube is checked. The tip of the ET tube should be at least 3.5 and preferably 5.5 cm above the carina on the CXR. An alternative method of assessment is that the tip of the ET tube should be at or above the level of the aortic arch.

If a collar is removed, the head goes into a more flexed position and the ET tube tip will usually migrate distally by approximately 3–5 cm. Therefore, the commonest cause of an airway problem in a trauma patient is a misplaced ET tube (usually too low). The most serious and, therefore, the most important diagnosis to make is the misplacement of an ET tube into the oesophagus. The airway should be clear and in a normal position (rarely it is possible to detect FBs, such as teeth or dentures).

Tracheal deviation may be due to ipsilateral shift related to either volume loss from collapse of the lung, surgery (lobectomy or pneumonectomy), fibrosis (either intra-pulmonary disease or radiotherapy), or contralateral shift related to the mass effect of a tension haemothorax, tension pneumothorax, or a combined tension haemopneumothorax.

All lines and tubes
All tubes and lines are radiologically visible. The vast majority have either barium impregnated into the catheter making them radiopaque or have a radiopaque tip or radiopaque line within the catheter.

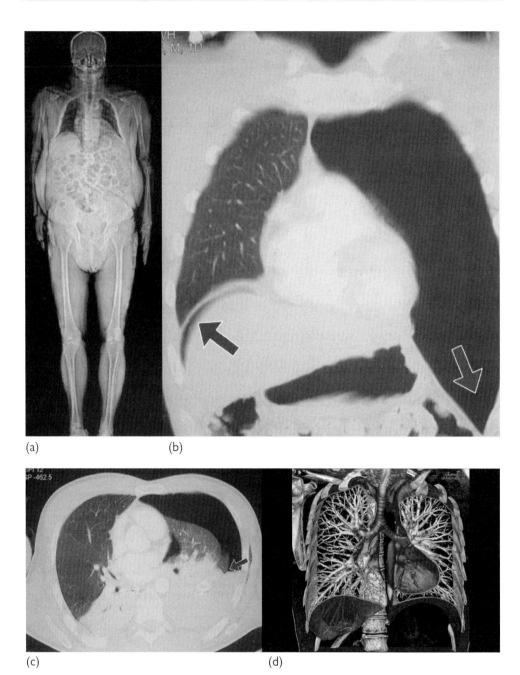

(a)   (b)

(c)   (d)

Fig. 9.3. Figure montage of CT findings with CT primary survey. (a) Whole body CT. (b) Coronal CT chest—lung windows (c) Axial CT chest—lung windows. (d) 3D CT chest. (e) 3D CT bone windows. (f) CT 2D angiogram. (g) 3D CT cervical spine. (h) 3D CT face.

The nasogastric (NG) tube tip should lie below the diaphragm and is usually easily visible. Rarely, the NG tube will be misplaced and lie in the bronchi, usually the right lower lobe bronchus or even more distal than this.

Care should be taken to check the position of the NG tube before use. The position of all central lines should be checked on a CXR. The tip of the central line should be between the lower margin of the right clavicle (start of the SVC) and above the right atrium. All central lines should lie straight below the right clavicle in the SVC, if there is bowing or a curvature within the distal part of the catheter, this would suggest that it is impinging in a vessel wall or the

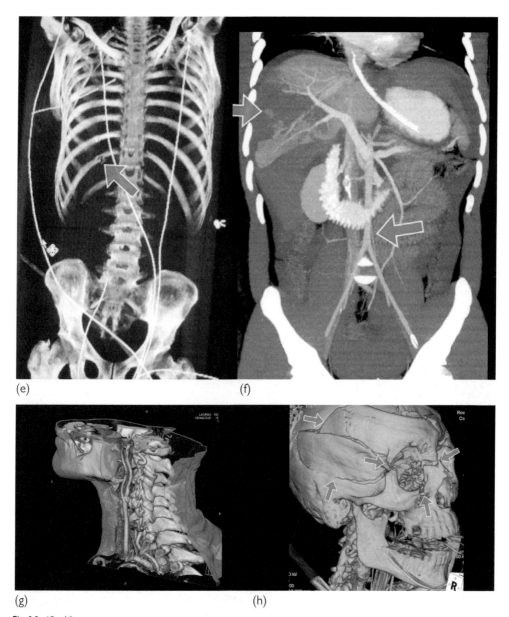

(e) (f)

(g) (h)

Fig. 9.3. (*Cont'd*)

endocardium. In this position, there is the potential that the catheter may erode through the wall of the vessel or endocardium. The ET tube that only lies just above the carina on a supine CXR will almost certainly migrate distally into the right or sometimes the left main bronchi after the CXR has been taken (Fig. 9.4).

The tip of the ET tube should be above the aortic arch or 5.5 cm above the carina on a supine CXR.

Breathing

Initially, a tension pneumothorax, haemothorax, haemopneumothorax and flail segment should be excluded. The lungs should be well aerated and clear, with no focal abnormality.

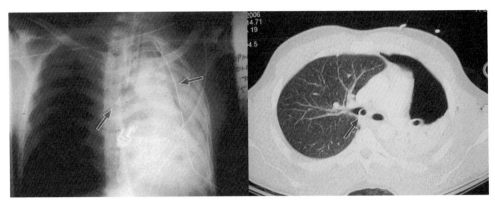

Fig. 9.4. (a) ETT too far into RMB (blue arrows). (b) CT done 1h later still shows ETT in RMB.

Circulation (mediastinum, hila, and pulmonary vasculature)

The heart size and shape, the mediastinal size, position, and contour, the hilar size, shape, position, and density and finally the symmetry of the pulmonary vasculature of the lungs should be examined.

The maximum transverse diameter of the heart is difficult to assess on a supine CXR, but the cardiothoracic ratio should be less than 0.6 (less than 0.5 on an erect PA CXR).

The left hilum is higher (by up to 1.5 cm) or the same height as the right. The normal right hilum is never higher than the left, so indicates pathology if this is the case. The mediastinum should be one-third to the right and two-thirds to the left of the mid-line. Before attributing the shift of the mediastinum to pathology, it is imperative that rotation is checked for. If the CXR is rotated, then a repeat CXR is advised. If there is mediastinal shift, ipsilateral shift indicates volume loss (due to either collapse, surgery, or fibrosis) and contralateral shift indicates tension (due to either a pneumothorax, haemothorax, or a haemopneumothorax).

Mediastinal contour should be examined for widening, blurring, loss of the contour or a change in shape of the contour, which in the context of major trauma may indicate a mediastinal haematoma (Box 9.4). In these circumstances, it is imperative that a traumatic aortic injury (TAI) is excluded using CT. It is difficult to give measurements for the mediastinum—old literature indicated that if the mediastinum measured more than 8 cm or the cardiomediastinal thoracic (CMT) ratio was greater than 0.25 (or 0.35), then this mandated further imaging. A CXR only gives indirect signs of a TAI. The indirect radiological signs for the diagnosis of a TAI are divided into the signs for a

mediastinal haematoma and those of related abnormalities (Box 9.5).

Box 9.5. TAI—associated injuries

- Fractured ribs (not just first and second)
- Left apical pleural cap
- Left haemothorax
- Left pneumothorax
- Pulmonary contusion
- Sternal fracture
- Scapula fracture
- Spine fracture

Diaphragm

The right hemidiaphragm is usually higher than the left (by up to 2.5 cm). Both diaphragms should have very well defined sharp contours throughout their course. Loss of visualization of part or the whole contour of the diaphragm in the context of trauma is indicative of lower lobe consolidation or collapse, ruptured diaphragm, or pleural pathology (haemothorax).

The area below the diaphragm should always be checked, in particular to look for free intraperitoneal air.

Edges (pleura)

The costophrenic angles should be easily visualized; if they are not, in particular through blunting of the costophrenic recesses, this usually indicates a haemothorax.

The visceral pleural edge, which is parallel to the inner chest wall, cannot be normally visualized—a visible pleural edge is diagnostic of a pneumothorax (pT, Fig. 9.5). Unfortunately, over 50% of supine CXRs do not show the classical pneumothorax appearances that are familiar from an erect PA CXR. Often small traumatic pneumothoraces are invisible on a supine CXR. The majority of traumatic pneumothoraces have subtle appearances and usually become more obvious with the signs of radiological tension, namely increased transradiancy, depression of the diaphragm, widening of the costophrenic sulcus (the deep sulcus sign) and contralateral mediastinal shift.

A further complicating factor is that traumatic pneumothoraces are often associated with haemothorax or lung contusion, giving an opaque rather than a transradiant hemithorax.

Box 9.4. TAI—mediastinal haematoma signs

- Widening of the aortic arch.
- Loss of contour of the aortic arch.
- Change in shape of the aortic arch.
- Wide right paratracheal stripe.
- Deviation of the trachea.
- Depression of the left main bronchus.
- Displacement of the NG tube.
- Wide left paraspinal line.

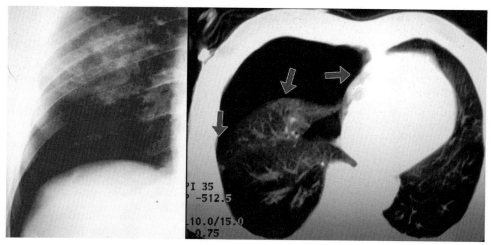

Fig. 9.5. (a) CXR—no obvious pT. (b) The same patient —CT 'tension pT' (blue arrows).

Skeleton (especially spine)

Although dedicated views of all skeletal injuries are advocated, the initial supine CXR is often the only evidence available that a patient has sustained major skeletal injuries. In addition, major trauma patients with multiple injuries often have subtle skeletal injuries, which are overlooked (including dislocated shoulders or fractured ribs, scapula, and spine). These injuries often only become apparent when the patient regains consciousness.

Rib fractures can be difficult (sometimes impossible) to identify. Every effort should be made to detect these, as they may often provide indirect evidence of the severity of the trauma and associated injuries.

The presence of rib fractures are associated with virtually any injury in the body, but certain injuries should be looked for and excluded when particular rib fractures are identified:

- *1st–3rd ribs:* great vessel and major airway injuries.
- *4th–8th ribs:* pneumothorax, haemothorax, and lung contusion.
- *9th–12th ribs:* abdominal solid and hollow viscus injuries.

The associated injuries are in some cases so common that specific investigations are indicated when these fractures are identified. A CT should be considered in all patients with low rib fractures to exclude an intra-abdominal injury (44% of splenic injuries have rib fractures and 20% of left rib fractures have a splenic injury).

The CXR is often the only clue that the patient has sustained a spinal injury. The abnormality seen on a CXR initially may be very subtle. The paraspinal lines should be examined, as these can be displaced or lost in the presence of vertebral fractures.

Scapular fractures should alert the clinician to large forces at the time of injury such that major injuries should be excluded, namely the head, spine, chest, abdomen and major vessels (in particular traumatic aortic injury). Mortality due to these associated injuries is as high as 35%. Whole body CT should be performed in these patients.

Soft tissues

The soft tissues should be reviewed specifically looking for the presence of air (surgical emphysema), asymmetry of the soft tissues (usually indicates bleeding into the tissues), and foreign bodies (from gun shot, knives, debris, surgical clips).

Interpretation of the pelvis XR

The pelvis radiograph should be interpreted using a systematic approach:

- *A:* adequacy and alignment.
- *B:* bones.
- *C:* cartilage and joints.
- *S:* soft tissues.

It is essential that all efforts are made to make sure that a good quality radiograph has been obtained, in particular that the patient is not rotated. Check that the iliac crests and the hips are included. A good AP pelvis radiograph gives a good overall assessment of most major injuries. With the advent of MDCT, there is no longer any necessity to do further views, in particular during the primary survey.

Secondary survey imaging

The conventional approach is to perform the plain chest and pelvis radiographs during the primary survey and then take the stable patient into the CT scanner. The more practical approach is for major trauma patients who need CT, to have a whole-body CT using a MDCT scanner. This will include scanning the head, chest, abdomen, and pelvis, and the whole of the spine. This obviates the need to image the spine with plain radiography, which is time consuming and has clear limitations (both in terms of adequacy and diagnosis).

The skeletal (including spine if whole body CT has not been performed) injuries are imaged as part of the secondary survey, in effect after clinical examination has been performed and potential injuries have been identified. Which X-rays are taken and in what order is dependent on the patient's clinical findings and haemodynamic status. In general, major and obvious skeletal injuries are imaged first and the whole spine is imaged at the end of the secondary survey, if deemed necessary.

With the advent of MDCT, it is now increasingly rare that plain radiography is used to image the spine in major trauma.

The 'Rules of Two' and the ABC systematic assessment

There are general principles to skeletal trauma imaging which need emphasis to avoid errors in imaging and interpretation, best summarized as 'The Rules of Two' and 'The ABC' systematic assessment.

The Rules of Two relate to what films to request, what to do with them and how to get help:

- *2 views:* one view is always one view too few. The 2 views should preferably be performed perpendicular to each other. This applies to all radiographs except the chest, abdomen and pelvis. Fractures are sometimes very subtle and only visible on one view.
- *2 joints:* the joint above and the joint below should be imaged. This relates to long bones and in particular the forearm (radius and ulna) and lower leg (tibia and fibula).
- *2 sides:* comparison with the opposite side can be helpful in difficult cases, in particular in children. However, a second opinion is important before exposing a patient to unnecessary radiation. In addition, when interpreting the CXR and pelvis XR, comparing both sides for symmetry is essential.
- *2 abnormalities:* the classic mistake is to stop looking after detecting one abnormality. It is not unusual to find multiple fractures. Furthermore, polytrauma patients may also have an incidental finding or additional pathology (such as metastatic disease) that may predispose them to sustaining an injury even after minor trauma.
- *2 occasions:* the most useful investigation in radiology is often an old X-ray. Comparison with old X-rays can be very helpful, not least with CXRs.
- *2 visits:* patients should always be re-X-rayed after a procedure, in particular if a patient has had an MUA or fixation of a fracture, or removal of a FB. A check CXR should always be performed if a patient has been intubated, had any form of intervention, such as a central line or chest drain insertion to confirm the position and to exclude a complication.
- *2 opinions:* two opinions are better than one. The radiograph should be shown to a colleague, in particular if the radiograph looks normal. As a general principle, all radiographs are best initially interpreted without the clinical information, but a report should not be provided until after the clinical information and request are made available. Radiographers are usually very experienced at looking and interpreting radiographs, so there is no excuse for not getting a second opinion.
- *2 records:* it is easy to request and look at a radiograph, but to forget to record the findings. It is essential that the initial clinical impression or interpretation is recorded in the notes.
- *2 specialists:* a radiologist ideally should also report all radiographs. This is of particular importance, if the radiograph has been deemed as normal by the clinical team.
- *2 examinations:* if the radiograph is considered normal, but the clinical suspicion is high, then further imaging is required. Either additional views or another imaging modality should be considered.

Other imaging modalities should always be considered depending on the clinical problem. There is nowadays virtually no role for plain radiography of the head. Significant head injuries should have a CT. Arguably in suspected scaphoid fractures, the initial investigation should be an MRI scan rather than a scaphoid series.

Interpretation of radiographs—ABC

All radiographs should be assessed using a systematic approach. The ABC systematic approach is a simple approach, easy to teach, easy to learn, and easy to use, which helps to avoid errors in interpretation.

Peripheral and axial skeleton
- *A:* **a**natomy, adequacy, and alignment.
- *B:* **b**ones.
- *C:* **c**artilage and joints.
- *S:* **s**oft tissues.

Abdomen
- *A:* **a**ir (exclude free intraperitoneal air).
- *B:* **b**owel gas pattern (and distribution).
- *C:* **c**alcification (normal and abnormal).
- *D:* **d**ensities (FBs, tablets).
- *E:* **e**dges (look at lung bases and hernial orifices).
- *F:* **f**at planes (bladder, psoas, kidneys).
- *S:* **s**oft tissues, skeleton and spine.

Head CT scans
- *A:* **a**irspaces.
- *B:* **b**rain.
- *C:* **c**erebrospinal fluid spaces.
- *D:* **d**ura.
- *E:* **e**yes.
- *F:* **f**ace.
- *S:* **s**oft tissues and skull.

Control of haemorrhage, angiography, and interventional radiology

The key objective when faced with a haemodynamically unstable patient is to identify and treat injuries suspected to be the major source of bleeding. The need for early identification of a suspected injury in these patients is critical and is a major cause of preventable death. These deaths are invariably due to a delay in diagnosis.

There has been much debate and controversy as to how these difficult patients should be managed over the past two decades, but there is now general agreement to most imaging strategies.

General rules
- Patients who are haemodynamically stable should have a CT.
- Patients who are haemodynamically unstable should NOT go to CT.
- Patients who are haemodynamically unstable should have a CXR, pelvis X-ray, and FAST.
- In haemodynamically unstable patients, if FAST detects fluid, then surgery is indicated.
- In haemodynamically unstable patients with a pelvic fracture with a negative FAST, angiography and embolization is indicated.

The general rule should be that haemodynamically unstable patients should not be transferred for CT. The debate arises over whether haemodynamically stable patients who have an apparent or clear indication for emergency surgery (such as free fluid on FAST or penetrating injuries) should have a CT prior to surgery. There is now sufficient evidence in the literature to advocate the use of pre-operative CT in patients who are haemodynamically stable, even in the presence of apparent indications for surgery, such as free fluid seen on FAST. These patients may be either observed or undergo angiography and embolization and obviate the need for surgery.

The trend is towards non-operative management (NOM) in blunt abdominal trauma, using CT to guide further management. Over 50% of splenic, 80% of liver, and virtually all renal injuries can be managed conservatively.

In addition, CT can be used to follow-up patients and to treat complications.

CT has a very high negative predictive value and can therefore rule out significant injuries. In addition, it has very high sensitivity and specificity for the detection of solid organ injuries and retroperitoneal injuries. CT-based grading systems have been developed, but most are of limited value, because they have limited, if any, value at predicting the success of NOM.

The single most useful sign is contrast blushes, which can represent either pseudoaneurysms (which can usually be embolized) or active contrast extravasation, either into the organ or into the peritoneum (depending on the haemodynamic presentation, these patients may need an urgent laparotomy or embolization). The presence of this sign suggests active bleeding and in the spleen over 80% fail non-operative management. Therefore, grading systems that incorporate contrast blushes are more likely to be helpful, but NOM is always dependent on the clinical state of the patient, not least the haemodynamic state and presence of other injuries (Fig. 9.6).

These patients can be transferred to the angiography suite, where selective or non-selective embolization can be performed, depending on the clinical state of the patient and the angiographic findings.

The direct CT signs of bowel injury can be very subtle and, therefore, bowel injuries are sometimes not immediately apparent. However, careful scrutiny for these subtle signs will usually detect most injuries (Fig. 9.7):
- *Free intraperitoneal fluid:* haemoperitoneum, urine, bowel contents, or ascites.
- *Free air:* direct bowel injury, penetrating trauma, or iatrogenic.
- *Laceration:* linear non-enhancing low density area.
- *Haematoma:* oval or round non-enhancing low or high density area.
- *Contusion:* ill-defined low density areas that enhance poorly.

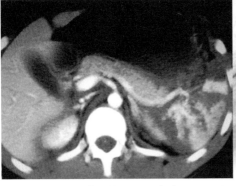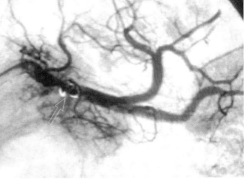

Fig. 9.6. Haemodynamically stable patient with splenic maceration on CT. Same patient treated successfully with splenic embolization. Note that splenic perfusion (and, therefore, splenic function) has been maintained.

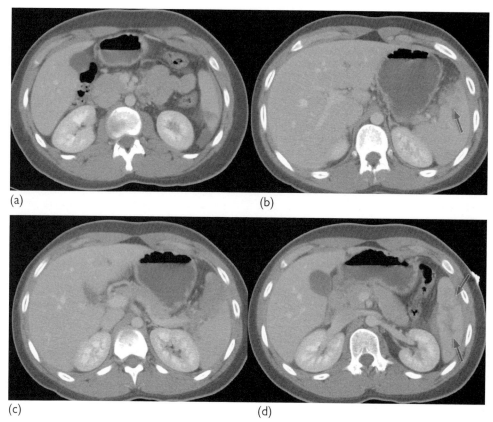

(a)   (b)

(c)   (d)

Fig. 9.7. (a) Splenic laceration. (b) Splenic contusion. (c) Splenic haematoma. (d) Splenic laceration with contrast leak.

- *Sub-capsular haematoma:* contained haematoma on the periphery of organs.
- *Pseudoaneurysm:* contrast persistent blush (usually round).
- *Active extravasation:* contrast blush that leaks.
- *Shattered or fragmented:* 3 or more enhancing fragments.
- *Devascularized:* when there is no enhancement.
- *Severe hypotension:* small aorta, flat IVC, bright adrenals, shock bowel.

In penetrating injuries, CT can be used as part of the rule-out strategy of decision-making along with clinical examination, to avoid unnecessary diagnostic laparotomies.

A major problem arises when a patient is unstable, requires massive transfusion and there is no obvious source of bleeding (occult) and the CXR, pelvis X-ray, and FAST are all apparently normal. A single negative FAST does not exclude major intra-abdominal haemorrhage. Initially, a repeat FAST should be performed by the most senior and experienced operator. If this is negative, then a decision has to be made as to whether the patient should have life-saving surgery in an attempt to gain *haemodynamic* stability, and then perform CT. This will depend on how unstable the patient is, how confident the team leader is of the likely site of haemorrhage, and the relationship of the

CT scanner to the resuscitation room. Fortunately this clinical scenario is very rare.

The presence of a pelvic fracture further complicates the management (Fig. 9.8), particularly in haemodynamically unstable patients, where morbidity and mortality is significantly higher.

The major difference in management is that in haemodynamically unstable patients with a pelvic fracture, if the

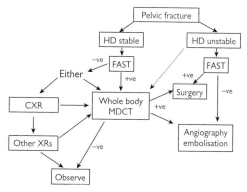

Fig. 9.8. Management of pelvic fracture.

FAST is negative, patients should undergo angiography and embolization without delay. If active contrast extravasation is seen, then initially selective embolization is recommended. If there are multiple sites of active bleeding, non-selective embolization of major vessels is advised for the sake of expediency. Rarely, in the absence of any other major cause of occult bleeding, even if there is no active extravasation seen, embolization of one or both internal iliac arteries may be necessary.

Unfortunately, patients with major pelvic fractures have sustained a huge impact and transfer of forces, to the extent that they have also invariably also injured numerous other pelvic (bladder, colon, uterus, veins, arteries) and extra pelvic (head, chest, abdomen, and skeleton) structures.

Conclusion

Early planning and organization of trauma care into regional systems, setting up of specialist trauma centres and networks, and implementation of specialist multidisciplinary trauma hospitals will lead to optimization of radiology resources locally, regionally and nationally

Improvement of trauma outcomes depends on optimizing pre- and in-hospital care using a multidisciplinary approach. The advent of new technological advances, not least MDCT, has dramatically changed the role of the radiologist in trauma. It has also opened opportunities to challenge current accepted management pathways, not least the role of conventional imaging versus MDCT and traditional primary and secondary surveys versus Primary CT Survey. The early detection, diagnosis, and treatment of life-threatening conditions are critical to improving outcome.

Further reading

American College of Radiology. *ACR Appropriateness Criteria for Blunt Abdominal Trauma.* ACR.

American College of Radiology. ACR Appropriateness Criteria®: Blunt Abdominal Trauma. Available at: http://www.acr.org/SecondaryMainMenuCategories/quality_safety/app_criteria/pdf/ExpertPanelonGastrointestinalImaging/BluntAbdominalTraumaDoc3.aspx (accessed 26 February 2010).

American College of Surgeons Committee on Trauma 2008: *Advanced Trauma Life Support Student Manual,* 8th edn. Chicago: ACS.

Anderson ID, Woodford M, de Dombal FT, Irving M. Trauma Audit and Research Network. Retrospective study of 1000 deaths from injury in England and Wales. *Br Med J* 1988; **296**: 1305–8.

Chan O. *ABC of Emergency Radiology,* 2nd edn. London: BMJ Books, 2007.

Lecky FE, Woodford M, Bouamra O, Yates DW, Trauma Audit Research Network. Lack of change in trauma care in England and Wales since 1994. *Emerg Med J* 2002; **19**: 520–3.

MacKenzie E, Rivara F, Jurkovich G, Nathens A, Frey K, Egleston B, et al. A national evaluation of the effect of trauma-center care on mortality. *N Engl J Med* 2006; **354**: 266–78.

Marmery H, Shanmuganathan K, Alexander MT, Mirvis SE. Optimization of selection for non-operative management of blunt splenic trauma: comparison of MDCT Grading Systems. *Am J Res* 2007; **189**: 1421–7.

Mirvis E, Shanmuganathan K. *Imaging in Trauma and Critical Care,* 2nd edn. Philadelphia: Saunders/Elsevier Science, 2003.

National Confidential Enquiry into Patient Outcome and Death. *Trauma: Who cares?* Report. London: NCEPOD, 2007.

Raby N, Berman L, de Lacey G. *Accident and emergency radiology a survival guide,* 2nd edn. London: Elsevier Saunders, 2005

Rogers LF. *Radiology of Skeletal Trauma,* 3rd edn. New York: Churchill Livingstone, 2002.

Royal College of Surgeons of England. *The Management of Patients with Major Injuries.* London: RCS, 1988.

Yates DW, Woodford M, Hollis S. Trauma Audit and Research Network. Preliminary analysis of the care of injured patients in 33 British hospitals: first report of the United Kingdom major trauma outcome study. *Br Med J* 1992; **305**: 737–40.

Tertiary survey

What is a tertiary survey?

The tertiary survey is a complete examination of the patient and a review of all the patient's investigations from the time of admission. This includes:

- Obtaining information on the mechanism of injury and background medical history.
- A review and confirmation of both primary and secondary survey information.
- A complete 'head to toe' examination of the patient.
- An examination and review of all patient investigations including final radiology reports.
- Documentation of survey findings.

The aim is to *reassess identified injuries, to confirm or exclude suspected injuries* and *to identify undiagnosed injuries*. The tertiary survey is regarded as an adjunct to the primary and secondary surveys, and whilst those first two assessments focus primarily on acute trauma care and managing potentially life-threatening injuries, even minor, non-lethal injuries have the potential to result in long-term discomfort or morbidity. Studies on the effectiveness of tertiary surveys show missed injuries in up to 65% of all trauma patients and an overall reduction in detecting those injuries after the implementation of a formalized tertiary survey of 36%. The difficulty in interpreting this data is that there is no uniform definition of a missed injury. Some studies regard every injury that escaped detection during the primary and secondary survey as a missed injury while others define missed injuries as injuries identified after the tertiary survey or detected more than 24 h after admission. In a prospective study of 206 trauma patients, 136 patients (65%) had 309 missed injuries (defined as an injury that escaped detection during the primary and secondary survey, and initial investigation in the resuscitation room and operating room) composing 39% of all 798 injuries seen. This high percentage of missed injuries included a significant number of external soft-tissue injuries, mostly contusions and abrasions. However, once these 48 patients were excluded the missed injury rate for the remaining group of patients decreased from 65 to 41.7%, which is still higher than reported in most other studies. Furthermore, the significance of recognizing the severity of external soft tissue injury must not be underestimated. It can lead to a high index of suspicion for underlying bony, vascular, or organ injury and should therefore be recorded. In the same study, 14.5% of all missed injuries were regarded as clinically significant. Tertiary survey was successful at detecting 56% of all early missed injuries and 90% of clinically significant injuries within 24 h, making it a valuable concept in trauma care.

The importance of the tertiary survey is underscored by a recent review of missed fractures in admitted patients at Liverpool Hospital in Sydney, Australia between 1995 and 2005. Of 10,065 patients in the major injury database during this time, 6920 patients had fractures diagnosed during their hospital stay. Of these, 6684 patients (96.6%) had their fractures diagnosed within 24 h of admission, but 236 (3.4%) had missed fractures. In a comparison of the groups of patients who had missed fractures and those who had all fractures diagnosed, patients who had trauma team activations or went from the resuscitation room directly to the operating theatre or ICU were more likely to have a missed fracture. However, those patients who had a tertiary survey were less likely to have a missed fracture than those whose tertiary survey was not done ($p < 0.0001$). Additionally, of the 236 patients with 253 missed fractures, 34.6% were to the lower extremity, 21.5% spinal, 16.3% upper extremity, and 12.5% facial. It is important to note that of these missed fractures, none resulted in permanent disability. However, as many as 39% were considered to have a mild or moderate impact; meaning that there was unnecessary (but temporary) discomfort or functional disability as a result. This demonstrates the importance of paying special attention to these specific areas during the tertiary survey both in terms of clinical examination and in the review of radiological images.

'Head to toe' clinical examination

Vital signs, pain score, lines, and devices

This includes:

- Measurement of blood pressure (on both arms), pulse rate, oxygen saturation, temperature, intra-abdominal pressure, and determine the pain score.
- Checking the integrity, position, and fixation of intravenous cannulae, central venous lines, chest drains, abdominal, and other drains, urinary catheters, intracranial pressure monitors, and regular or negative pressure dressings.
- Ensuring adequate intravenous access and removing intra-osseous needles or venous cut down lines used for initial resuscitation.

Head and neck (the collar should be temporarily removed whilst an assistant maintains manual cervical in-line stabilization):

- The scalp should be checked for lacerations and haematomas.
- Pupil size and reaction to light, visual acuity, ocular motility, integrity of globe and lens must be assessed. Hyphaema, subconjunctival haemorrhage, associated orbital swelling, hypoaesthesia of cheek or upper lip (infra-orbital nerve) and injury to the eyelids and bony orbital rim should be excluded
- Signs of traumatic asphyxia (bulging eyes, oedema, petechiae, subconjunctival haemorrhage) should be noted.
- Pain, swelling, soft tissue injuries, and instability of zygomatic arch, maxilla, mandible, and telecanthus (wide displacement of the medial canthal region suggestive for a Le Fort II or III fracture) should be excluded. The integrity of facial nerves and parotid glands is be established.
- The nasal bones are palpated and the patency of nasal ducts determined. An inspection is made for septal haematoma.
- The ears must be checked for lobe lacerations, integrity of the tympanic membranes and hearing impairment.
- The jaws and teeth are examined for normal occlusion, and the mouth for dislocated or avulsed teeth and oral lacerations or swelling.
- Difficulty breathing or stridor due to swelling, purulent sputum (aspiration), or pharyngeal or airway injuries must be excluded. The larynx is palpated for crepitus and examined for subcutaneous emphysema, deviated trachea, distended neck veins, and integrity of thyroid gland.
- Signs of vascular injury (diminished or unequal pulsations, swelling, seatbelt sign in neck (Fig. 10.1), bruit over carotids) must be sought.
- The neck is assessed for C-spine tenderness, reduced range of motion, and radiating pain.

Chest

- The chest must be examined for expansion, subcutaneous emphysema, scars from previous thoracic surgery, paradoxical breathing, seatbelt signs, soft tissue injuries, clavicle, and sternal fractures or dislocations.
- Percussion is used to identify the presence of unrecognized pneumothorax or haemothorax.

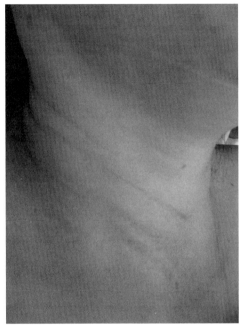

Fig. 10.1. Seatbelt signs on the neck.

- Auscultation of the chest may identify diminished breath sounds, muffled heart sounds, 'crunching' sounds over mediastinum (pneumomediastinum) and bruits.
- Chest drains must be checked for fluid output (blood, haemoserous, chylous), swinging of fluid column, and air leak.

Abdomen and pelvis

- The abdomen is inspected for seatbelt signs (consider hollow viscus injury), abrasions, and penetrating wounds.
- Abdominal tenderness, distension, and the presence of bowel sounds are assessed.
- The integrity of recent laparotomy wounds and the viability of stomata (if present) must be determined.
- The pelvic bony prominences are examined for tenderness, abrasions, contusions, and for pain on (gentle) compression. Pain on manipulation of the hip joints should be identified.
- The femoral arteries are assessed for the presence of normal pulses and abnormal bruits.

External genitalia

- The external genitalia must be inspected for ecchymosis, lacerations, swelling, or haematoma of penis, scrotum, or vulva.
- Vaginal or urethral bleeding should be sought, and the ability to void normally and the presence of normal sensation (spinal injuries) determined.

Back

- The back is examined for spinal tenderness, steps, abrasions, haematomas, flank contusions, and scapula fracture, and the sacrum and SI joints are examined.
- A rectal examination should be performed (tone, sensation, blood), and the perineum and pressure areas inspected.

Extremities

- The limbs are assessed for pain, swelling, deformity, and crepitus. Joints must be examined for instability, reduced range of motion, and active movement.
- The signs of muscular compartment syndrome should be excluded, these include:
  - pain out of proportion to any injury present;
  - swelling of involved compartment, hypoaesthesia in first web space of foot (compression of cutaneous branch of peroneal nerve);
  - increased intra-compartmental pressures.

- The shoulders and arms are examined for evidence of brachial plexus injury.
- The vascular status (peripheral pulses, ankle and brachial indices, bruits, presence of pulsatile swellings) is determined.

Neurological assessment

- The Glasgow Coma Score, pupillary size, and reactions are determined. The patient should be assessed for post-traumatic amnesia.
- Muscle strength, and the integrity of sensation and motor function are established.
- The cranial nerves are examined and the presence of CSF via nose or ears determined.

Timing of tertiary survey

The timing of the tertiary survey is institution-specific, but typically occurs within the first 24 h of admission and is repeated when the patient is awake, responsive and able to communicate any complaints. The 24-h time limit is somewhat arbitrary, but the goal is to identify all injuries as soon as possible without compromising the initial trauma resuscitation. At the same time, unnecessary delay is to be avoided; early on the day following admission is often the most convenient time. This ensures enough time for a thorough evaluation of the patient's injuries, as well as a secure environment in which good communication between the patient and the assessing doctor is enhanced.

Repeated tertiary survey

Trauma patients admitted to the Intensive Care Unit, with an Injury Severity Score $\geq$ 16, a reduced Glasgow Coma Score (GCS) or multiple fractures and patients who are pharmacologically paralysed have an increased risk of having a missed injury. One of the disadvantages of an early (<24 h post-admission) tertiary survey is that some patients have an altered level of consciousness, which may prevent them from communicating any complaints. Additionally, the non-ambulatory patient has not had an opportunity to identify decreased function or pain when mobilizing. For this group of patients the initial tertiary survey is regarded as incomplete and it therefore needs to be repeated as soon as the patient is ambulatory, extubated and/or regained consciousness.

Who should do the tertiary survey?

The person responsible for the completion of the tertiary survey is also institution-specific. In most institutions it will be the surgical trainee on the trauma team that will undertake the role. In other institutions it can be done by a dedicated Trauma Nurse Practitioner or another member of the general surgical team. The most important principle is that the person who does the tertiary survey possesses the advanced medical and diagnostic skills, the extra vigilance and the clinical experience that are required to completely reassess all available information and to combine this with a high index of suspicion based on mechanism of injury in order to reveal the otherwise overlooked injury.

Review of radiological imaging

Missed injuries

One of the easiest mistakes to make during the tertiary survey is failing to review all the previously performed radiological imagining. In the heat of the moment, findings on X-ray, ultrasound and CT can easily be misinterpreted or missed, especially since many trauma patients will arrive after-hours when less experienced staff are often on duty. Even if plain X-rays are reviewed by an experienced trauma surgeon a formalized trauma radiology round as part of the tertiary survey will identify as many as 9.7% new diagnoses. It cannot be stressed enough that every trauma service should have a system in place to repeat the review of all initial trauma radiological imaging and to obtain the formal radiologist reports as a standard part of the tertiary survey. Correlation between clinical and radiological findings can then be made by the treating team and will direct further management.

Incidental findings

As the use and the quality of CT scans in trauma increase, the revelation of incidental findings in the trauma population will also increase. In a prospective study of 1027 patients the rate of incidental findings was found to be 7.4%; most were detected by CT scans and during tertiary survey. Some of the incidental findings can be very important indicators of non-trauma related disease (e.g. adrenal masses, pulmonary nodules, aortic aneurysms). Every mature trauma service needs to have a system in place to provide further follow-up for these sorts of findings so that indicators of non-trauma-related disease are not ignored or overlooked.

Additional diagnostic procedures

Additional radiographic studies, laboratory, or other additional tests are a vital part of the completion of the tertiary survey. It is the sole responsibility of the doctor who orders the tests to have these followed-up in a timely manner and acted upon promptly. If this responsibility is handed over to someone else then both providers need to be in agreement regarding this and it has to be clearly documented in the notes who will follow-up any pending results. The tertiary survey is not completed until all results of additional investigations are officially reported upon and their interpretation and subsequent management plan documented in the patient's hospital record.

Documentation

Tertiary survey assessment form

The findings on tertiary survey should be clearly documented in the patient's hospital record. These notes should include the interpretation of old, new and suspected findings, a treatment plan and date, and time of completion of the tertiary survey. Many hospitals use a standardized form which will not only aid in the uniform performance of the tertiary survey but also identify those patients in whom the tertiary survey is still pending [see Fig. 10.2].

Medico-legal aspects of documentation

Although modern, organized trauma services have amongst the lowest medical malpractice risks of all medical and surgical specialities, medical records of trauma patients are regularly subjected to investigation for purposes of compensation. Also, trauma surgeons are often asked by insurance companies and legal representatives to provide detailed medical information regarding the nature and severity of the injuries sustained by their clients. Apart from the normal professional obligation to correctly document all relevant information in the patient's medical notes, incomplete or incorrect documentation can also lead to the release of a misleading or incomplete report. Accurate and complete documentation of the findings on tertiary survey will assist in recounting the correct information at a later date.

Communication

Communication between teams

One of the challenges in trauma care is to ensure that all teams involved in caring for trauma patients are aware of other injuries, ongoing investigations, and treatment plans.

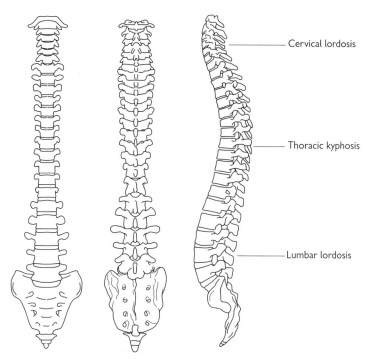

Fig. 11.1. The spinal column.

processes project horizontally. The lumbar facets are biplanar—the superior facets face posteromedially and the inferior facets face anterolaterally. This allows for flexion and extension, but limits rotation. The transition zone at the thoracolumbar junction (as with the cervicothoracic junction) is prone to injury as there is a move from kyphosis to lordosis and from a stiff thoracic to a mobile lumbar spine (Fig. 11.4).

The sacral spine

The sacrum is the mechanical nucleus of the axial skeleton. It is the both the base of spinal column and the keystone of the pelvic ring. The sacral nerve roots exit anteriorly through the sacral foramina (Fig. 11.5).

The spinal cord

The spinal cord is a continuation of the brainstem. It ends in the conus medullaris at L3 in the newborn and L1 in adults. The cord is bathed in cerebrospinal fluid which is regulated by the blood–brain barrier. It provides nutrients and protection to the central nervous system. The spinal

cord is enclosed by the meninges (the dura, arachnoid, and pia mater). The dural sac ends in the filum terminale in the sacral region and contains the spinal nerve roots of L2–S5. Given its gross appearance this region forms the so called 'cauda equina' (horse's tail).

Exiting the spinal cord on either side are the ventral and dorsal rami of the spinal nerve roots which join together to form spinal nerves at each vertebral level. The area of skin supplied by a spinal nerve is a dermatone and the muscles a myotome. The ventral rami are composed of motor neurones whose cell bodies lie in the anterior horns of the spinal cord. The dorsal rami are composed of sensory neurones the bodies of which are found in the dorsal root ganglion (Fig. 11.6).

The spinal cord has grey and white regions on gross inspection of its cross section. The grey matter is formed by cell bodies and synapses, and the white matter by myelin nerve sheaths. Within the spinal cord there are a series of highly specialized nerve tracts. The anterior and lateral corticospinal tracts arise from the motor homunculus of the cerebral cortex in the parietal lobe. They control voluntary skilled activity. The lateral tract is formed from 85–95% of the neurones, which decussate in the medullary pyramids. The remaining 5–15% of uncrossed neurones form the anterior corticospinal tract. The dorsal columns carry sensory fibres that detect proprioception, deep pain, vibration, and joint and muscle sensation. The fasciculus gracilis arises from the lower limb and fasciculus cuneatus from the upper. The neurones tend to cross in the brainstem. The spinothalamic tracts form the other major sensory tract in the spinal cord. The lateral tract transmits pain and temperature and the anterior tract, touch. The neurones tend to cross in the spinal cord at or adjacent to their level of entry.

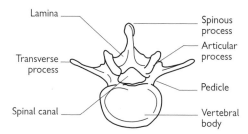

Fig. 11.2. Typical structure of a vertebra.

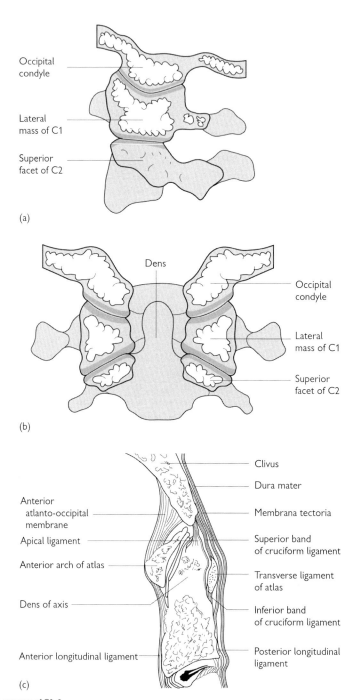

Occipital condyle

Lateral mass of C1

Superior facet of C2

(a)

Dens

Occipital condyle

Lateral mass of C1

Superior facet of C2

(b)

Clivus

Dura mater

Anterior atlanto-occipital membrane

Membrana tectoria

Apical ligament

Superior band of cruciform ligament

Anterior arch of atlas

Transverse ligament of atlas

Dens of axis

Inferior band of cruciform ligament

Anterior longitudinal ligament

Posterior longitudinal ligament

(c)

Fig. 11.3(a). The anatomy of C0–2.

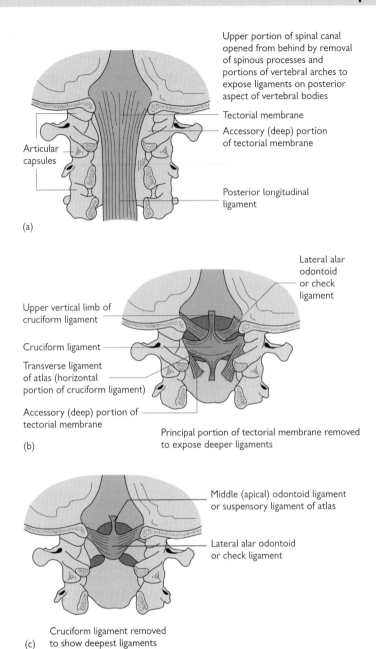

Upper portion of spinal canal opened from behind by removal of spinous processes and portions of vertebral arches to expose ligaments on posterior aspect of vertebral bodies

Tectorial membrane

Accessory (deep) portion of tectorial membrane

Articular capsules

Posterior longitudinal ligament

(a)

Lateral alar odontoid or check ligament

Upper vertical limb of cruciform ligament

Cruciform ligament

Transverse ligament of atlas (horizontal portion of cruciform ligament)

Accessory (deep) portion of tectorial membrane

(b)

Principal portion of tectorial membrane removed to expose deeper ligaments

Middle (apical) odontoid ligament or suspensory ligament of atlas

Lateral alar odontoid or check ligament

Cruciform ligament removed to show deepest ligaments

(c)

Fig. 11.3(b) The anatomy of the cervical spine. (Reproduced from *Oxford Textbook of Orthopaedics and Trauma* with permission of Oxford University Press.)

The sympathetic outflow arises from T1–L2 and the parasympathetic from cranial nerves 3, 7, 9, and 10, and from S2–4. The spinal nerve of C1 exits between the skull and the axis, C2–7 exit above their corresponding vertebra, C8 exits below C7 and above T1, and below T1 the nerves exit below their corresponding numbered vertebral pedicle. The C2 nerve exits posterior to the C1–2 facet and the rest exit anterior to the facet joints.

There are eight cervical nerves but only seven vertebrae.

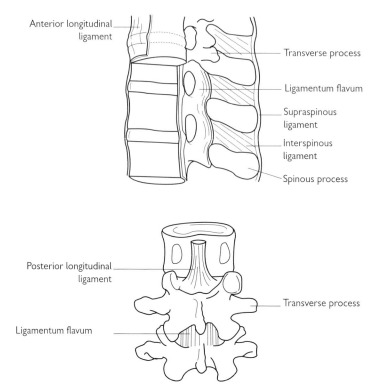

Fig. 11.4. The anatomy of the thoracolumbar spine.

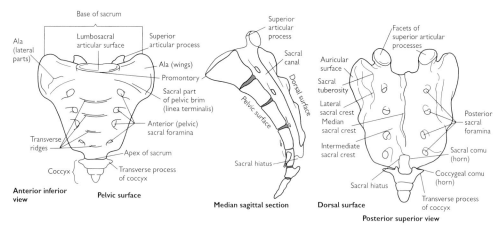

Fig. 11.5. The anatomy of the sacrum.

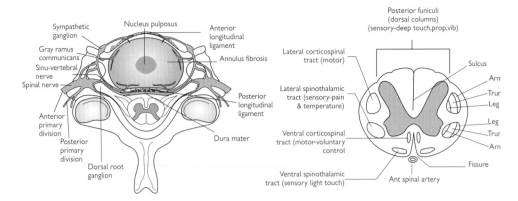

Fig. 11.6. The gross and microscopic structure of the spinal cord.

The blood supply to the spine

The vertebrae are supplied by segmental vessels arising from the aorta and vertebral arteries. The spinal cord is supplied by three longitudinal arterial trunks (one anterior and two posterior spinal arteries) and radicular vessels. The anterior artery arises from the vertebral arteries in the brainstem and supplies the whole cord anterior to the posterior grey matter bilaterally. The posterior arteries arise from the posterior inferior cerebellar arteries or the vertebral arteries in the brainstem and each supply the corresponding side of the grey and white posterior columns. A large radicular vessel is worthy of note—the

arteria radicularis magna or artery of Adamkiewicz that arises from the aorta at T8–L1 90% of the time on the left side. This reinforces the longitudinal arterial tracts (Fig. 11.7).

Spinal biomechanics

The spine can be divided into anterior and posterior columns. The anterior column consists of those elements in front of the spinal cord. It acts as a strut, which transmits the majority of body weight (>80%). In the standing position, the centre of mass of the body lies anterior to the spine and the posterior column acts as a tension band preventing forward bending (Fig. 11.8).

Anterior spinal artery

• single artery that arises from each vertebral artery at foramen magnum to run lenght of cord
• usually bigger than posterior spinal arteries but may be quite small
• supplies whole cord anterior to posterior grey columns, bilaterally

Other vessels

From vertebrals, deep & ascending cervicals, intercostals, lumbars & lateral sacrals. Note that all vessels anastomose under the pia mater in the periphery of the cord

Posterior spinal arteries

• arise at foamen magnum from posterior inferior cerebellar arteries (or vertebral)
• lie anterior & posterior to posterior rootlets
• run length of cord but poor anastomosis except at lower end of cord
• supply own side of grey & white posterior columns

Radicular (feeder) arteries

• enter via intervertebral formina and reinforce anterior & posterior spinal arteries & supply dorsal root ganglia
• variable number at variable levels but largest is arteria radicularis magna, usually at T10 or 11 (artery of Adamkiewicz)

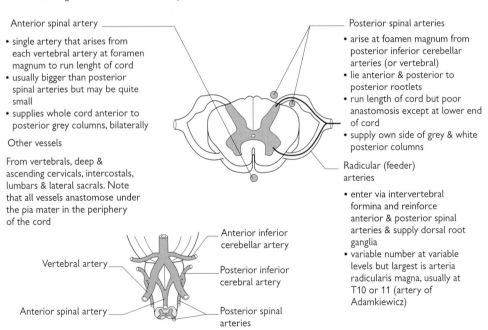

Fig. 11.7. The blood supply of the spinal cord.

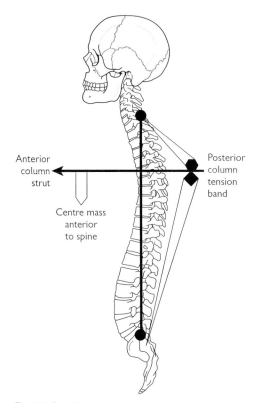

Anterior column strut

Posterior column tension band

Centre mass anterior to spine

Fig. 11.8. Spinal biomechanics.

Concept of spinal stability

Clinical instability is defined as 'the loss of the ability of the spine under physiological loads to maintain its pattern of displacement so that there is no initial or additional neurological deficit, no major deformity, and no incapacitating pain' (White and Panjabi). It is a dynamic concept and can be divided into two types:

- *Mechanical stability*: the ability to maintain alignment under physiologic loads without significant onset of pain or intolerable deformity
- *Neurological stability*: the ability to prevent neural symptoms or signs under anticipated loads. There are various clinical and radiological indicators and parameters used in assessing spinal stability that will be discussed later.

Pathophysiology of spinal cord injury

SCI occurs due to a primary mechanical insult to the cord. This can be due to:
• Rapid compression.
• Distraction.
• Shear.
• Penetration.

Subsequent secondary injury can occur due to a cascade of mechanisms which include:
• Vascular changes:
  • reduced blood flow;
  • ischaemia;
  • loss of autoregulation;
  • neurogenic shock;
  • haemorrhage;
  • loss of microcirculation;
  • vasospasm;
  • thrombosis.
• Electrolyte derangements.
• Accumulation of neurotransmitters.
• Free radical production.
• Inflammatory cascade and oedema.

Both primary and secondary mechanisms result in reduced oxygenation and perfusion of the spinal cord and subsequent ischaemia (to which nerve cells are very sensitive). A zone of partial preservation or zone of critical ischaemia arises around the site of primary injury. This zone can expand with poor oxygenation or perfusion. It is common for the level of SCI to rise by a segment or two during the first 48 h following injury. Undue ascent requires urgent investigation. The subsequent descent to the previous segmental level may take several weeks. Unfortunately, nerve cells have very little potential for recovery. Hence, the primary insult often dictates the final outcome and very little can be done to treat it. Current treatment is aimed at preventing secondary insults and damage in the zone of partial preservation.

Spinal and neurogenic shock

Spinal shock refers to the period of transient areflexia, flaccid paralysis and lack of sensation secondary to physiological spinal cord 'shut down' in response to injury. It can be considered as a neuropraxia of the spinal cord. It usually resolves within 24 h (99%) and rarely lasts longer than 48 h. Resolution is defined when the reflex arc most caudal to the injury returns. The lowest of these that can be tested clinically is the bulbocavernosus reflex (mons–clitoral reflex in women). The importance of spinal shock comes when determining whether a patient has a complete or incomplete spinal cord injury. This cannot be assessed until the reflex activity of the spinal cord returns (e.g. reflex arcs such as the knee jerk).

Neurogenic shock refers to the immediate loss of sympathetic tone that occurs after SCI. It generally occurs with cord damage at T6 or above, and the higher the level the more profound the effects. There is unopposed vagal tone (parasympathetic) resulting in:
• Hypotension due to loss of blood vessel tone with resultant venous pooling.
• Bradycardia due to reduced cardiac sympathetic input.

This bradycardia distinguishes neurogenic shock from the other types of shock (hypovolaemic, cardiac, anaphylactic and septic).

Spinal cord injury and syndromes

A complete SCI means that there is no motor or sensory function more than three segments below the neurological level of injury. In complete SCI, there is no sacral sparing. An incomplete SCI indicates there is partial preservation of sensory and/or motor function below the defined neurological level. Sacral sparing indicates that there is some continuity of long tract fibres and, hence, an incomplete SCI. The sacral structures are innervated by fibres lying most peripheral in both the posterior columns and lateral corticospinal tracts (hence, they are more resistant to ischaemic injury). The signs of sacral sparing are:
• Intact perianal sensation (S4–5 dermatome).
• Voluntary external anal contraction.
• Great toe flexor activity.

The neurological level of injury is defined as the most caudal level with bilaterally normal motor and sensory function. It frequently does not correlate with the level of skeletal injury. The suffix '-plegia' denotes paralysis, whereas '-paresis' refers to muscular weakness. Paresis implies a lesser degree of weakness than plegia, but the two terms are often used interchangeably.

Complete SCI

Complete SCI can be further classified into cervical tetraplegia, thoracic paraplegia and lumbar paraplagia. As a general rule patients with C1–4 tetraplegia have absent limb function and are ventilator dependent (C3,4,5 keeps the diaphragm alive—the phrenic nerve). The functional outcome of patients with C5–T1 tetraplegia depends on the level of the injury:
• *C5*: deltoids and biceps—limited independence with the use of feeding aids.
• *C6*: biceps and wrist extension—some upper limb control and ability to lift light objects.
• *C7*: wrist extension and triceps—ability to transfer and use a wheelchair.
• *C8*: functional hand grasp.
• *T1*: intrinsic hand function.

For patients with thoracic paraplegia there is better respiratory and trunk control the lower the lesion. Again, the functional outcome of lumbar paraplegia is very much dependent on the level of the injury:
• *L2: hip flexion.*
• *L3: knee extension—good quadriceps function required to permit ambulation.*
• *L4: foot dorsiflexion.*
• *L5: extensor hallucis longus.*
• *S1: gastroc-soleus complex.*

Incomplete SCI

Incomplete SCI occurs in a number of well-defined clinical syndromes, which are discussed below.
• *Central cord syndrome*: this is the most common incomplete syndrome. It generally occurs in older patients with pre-existing spondylosis and is due to a

hyperextension injury. Anteriorly, the spinal cord is pinched by osteophytes and posteriorly it is pinched by bunched up (sometimes hypertrophic) ligamentum flavum. Hence, the central portion of cord becomes injured. The upper extremity is affected more than the lower and the distal portion of limbs affected greater than proximal. It carries the best prognosis of the incomplete syndromes. The earliest and greatest recovery is seen in the legs followed by the bladder. Hand dexterity is the last function to recover.

• *Anterior cord syndrome:* this occurs secondary to anterior spinal artery injury. This affects the anterior two-thirds of the cord leaving the posterior column function intact. It frequently occurs due to retropulsed bone or disc material. The prognosis is poor with <20% chance of motor recovery.

• *Posterior cord syndrome:* this is rare and occurs due to injury to the posterior spinal arteries, which results in loss of proprioceptive function. Patients maintain ambulation, but rely heavily on visual input.

• *Brown-Sequard syndrome:* this is a functional hemisection of the spinal cord and usually occurs secondary to penetrating trauma. There is ipsilateral loss of motor function, proprioception, vibration, and deep pressure and contralateral loss of pain, temperature and light touch sensation. 75% regain independent ambulation, and 80% recover bowel and bladder function.

• *Conus medullaris syndrome:* there is injury to the tip of the spinal cord at the L1–2 level, which presents as a mixed picture of cord and nerve root damage. There is bowel, bladder, and sexual dysfunction, and it can disrupt the bulbocavernosus reflex. In this situation, defining the end of spinal shock can be unreliable.

• *Cauda equina syndrome:* this is defined as a spectrum of low back pain, uni- or bilateral sciatica, saddle anaesthesia, and motor weakness in the lower extremities with variable rectal and urinary symptoms. It is a lower motor neuron lesion (the nerve roots and not the cord are affected). It is most commonly caused by a central disc protrusion and emergency decompressive surgery is indicated as this is the only modifiable factor that may improve outcome. The prognosis is better than for SCI but poorer than isolated nerve root injuries.

The incidence of neurological injury is dependent on the level of injury (Table 11.1).

Table 11.1. Incidence of neurological injury with level of injury

Level of injury	Complete SCI (%)	Incomplete SCI (%)	Neurologically intact (%)
Cervical	32	41	26
Thoracic	62	26	12
Thoracolumbar	29	42	29
Lumbar	2	57	41
Sacral	0	100	0

Principles of treatment of spinal injuries

The clinician must first protect, then detect and then manage patients with spinal injuries. The goals of treatment are:

- Protect the neural elements and maintain/restore neurological function.
- Prevent or correct segmental collapse and deformity.
- Prevent spinal instability and pain.
- Restore normal spinal mechanics.
- Permit early ambulation and return to function (rehabilitation).

As with all forms of trauma, prevention is better than cure. Motor vehicle collisions are less likely to occur if speed limits are adhered to, seat belts used, and side impact systems and airbags utilized. In sports, adherence to the rules, the use of appropriate safety equipment, proper training and expert supervision have all been shown to prevent spinal injury.

Pre-hospital management

In the pre-hospital setting a spinal injury should be suspected when:

- There is high energy injury:
  - motor vehicle collision;
  - fall or jump from a height;
  - accident resulting in impact or crush injuries;
  - accident resulting in multiple injuries;
  - accident resulting in the patient losing consciousness (head injury);
- Following trauma, the patient:
  - complains of back or neck pain, and is guarding their back or neck;
  - complains of any sensory changes or loss such as numbness or tingling;
  - is unable to pass urine (normally a later sign).

The main goal of pre-hospital management is to retrieve the patient from the site of injury safely and rapidly, and deliver them to a suitable facility for assessment and stabilization prior to definitive treatment. Maintenance of oxygenation and tissue perfusion are paramount.

Patients may present without any neurological deficit. If spinal injury is suspected then the patient should be placed in the neutral supine position as soon as it is feasible. The cervical spine should be immediately immobilized at the scene either by manual in-line stabilization or 3-point immobilization with hard collar, blocks, and straps. If the patient is still in the position in which they have been injured, careful movement of the head to restore anatomical alignment of the cervical spine should be made. If resistance is met or if the patient complains of worsening pain, the attempt should be stopped, and the head and spine should be immobilized in that position until further investigation is possible. If the patient is wearing a helmet then two people are needed for its removal.

The patient should be placed on a spinal board to protect the spine during transportation. If endotracheal intubation is required then head tilt or hyperextension of the neck should be avoided. Severe bradycardia can occur during the intubation of patients with SCI (due to unopposed parasympathetic input) and this can lead to cardiac arrest. The patient should be pre-oxygenated and topical anaesthetic spray may be of benefit prior to intubation. Atropine may be required.

Immediate management and clinical assessment

The initial management of all patients with suspected spinal injury should follow standard trauma protocols (discussed in previous chapters), and all trauma patients should be assumed to have a spinal injury until proven otherwise. Specifically, secondary SCI can be minimized by mechanical immobilization, and optimization of ventilation and perfusion. Once a spinal injury is identified the patient should be discussed with the local spinal injury unit for advice and further management.

The following is a summary of measures specific to patients with spinal injuries that should be taken into account during the primary and secondary surveys.

The primary survey

Airway and cervical spine control

- The patient should be given high flow oxygen.
- For airway optimization, the jaw thrust technique should be employed and the use of naso- or oropharyngeal airways should be considered.
- Hyperextension of the neck should be avoided as this reduces the canal diameter.
- Early involvement of a clinician experienced in airway management is vital.
- As discussed above, severe bradycardia may occur during intubation and should be anticipated.
- The cervical spine should be immobilized either by manual in-line stabilization or 3-point immobilization with hard collar, blocks and straps or tape.
- If the patient is still in the position in which they have been injured, careful movement of the head to restore anatomical alignment of the cervical spine should be made. If resistance is met or if the patient complains of worsening pain, the attempt should be stopped, and the head and spine should be immobilized in that position until further investigation is possible. This is particularly important in patients with ankylosing spondylitis or pre-existing deformity.
- The anterior aspect of the neck should be examined for bruising, swelling, and tenderness.

Breathing and ventilation

- The effects of concomitant chest trauma must be considered.
- Patients with SCI may have lack of diaphragm and intercostal muscle function, be prone to fatigue of the intercostals, have paradoxical diaphragmatic breathing, be unable to cough, retain secretions, and develop basal atelectasis. Abdominal distension may worsen respiratory function by splinting the diaphragm.
- For A and B think cord oxygenation.

Circulation

- Hypovolaemic shock is the commonest cause of shock in trauma patients.
- Neurogenic shock can occur in isolation or in combination with the other causes of shock (compounding the effects).
- It may be necessary to support vital organ perfusion to prevent secondary injury to the spinal cord, using fluids and inotropes.

- The mean arterial pressure should be maintained at >85 mmHg.
- Due to the lack of sympathetic outflow, exaggerated abnormal vaso-vagal responses can occur during rapid log rolling, tracheal suctioning or intubation, passing a NG tube or performing a rectal exam.
- For C think cord perfusion.

Disability

- Neurological status should be assessed—conscious level and pupillary response—and blood glucose recorded.
- In the unconscious patient, a spinal injury must be assumed until proven otherwise.
- In the patient with cervical spine fracture and altered mental status—think head injury. If head trauma is minimal—think vertebral artery injury.

Exposure

- A rapid examination of the torso and limbs should be performed (avoiding hypothermia).
- Gross movement of the limbs should be noted.

As part of the primary survey a urinary catheter should normally be inserted. Bladder damage due to over-distension should be avoided and the catheter should be left on free drainage. Occasionally, patients with SCI exhibit priapism, in which case suprapubic catheterization is recommended.

The secondary survey

A top to toe examination of the patient should be performed. The mechanism of injury should alert the clinician to potential spinal injuries. A seatbelt mark could indicate flexion distraction of the spine (cervicothoracic and thoracolumbar injury) and intra-abdominal visceral injury (the sentinel signs being shoulder and abdominal wall bruising). A fall from a height can result in a compression force down the whole spinal column. This can result in fractures occurring anywhere down the spine—from the occipital condyles right down to the sacrum.

Neurological assessment

A careful neurological examination is critical as it can dramatically influence the outcome of patients with SCI. Repeat examination is crucial, but the best spinal cord monitor is the alert conscious patient. Extension of the lesion is not uncommon and accurate initial assessment will help detect this, and permit early investigation and intervention. In a high cervical injury, cord oedema can progress resulting in respiratory dysfunction and arrest. One must remember that the zone of critical ischaemia at the site of cord injury may expand with poor oxygenation or perfusion. In particular, poor autonomic vascular control and postural hypotension can worsen injury. The patient must be nursed flat.

Spinal pain, loss of sensation or movement in the limbs, and burning or electric shock sensations in the trunk or limbs should alert the clinician to a neurological insult. A standardized examination should be performed, and the ASIA Chart (Fig. 11.9) is recommended. Sensory dermatomes should be mapped and motor power assessed using the MRC grade. Pin prick sensation is more reliable than light touch in a trauma patient in view of distracting injuries.

The log roll

This requires a minimum of five people. One person performs manual in-line stabilization and is in control of the log roll. Three other people line up by the patient's side and place their hands over the opposite side of the body, with three hands over the torso and three hands under the opposite leg—'three over and three under'.

Instructions from the head end should be clear. The fifth person examines the back and spine and performs a rectal examination:

- Palpation should begin at the occiput to C2 (C1 is not normally felt) and then down the midline dorsal processes and ligaments to the prominent C7 and continued right down to the anus (so as not to forget the sacrum).
- In particular, the clinician should feel for gaps, steps, bogginess, crepitus, and alignment.
- Once the midline has been palpated, both paraspinal gutters should be palpated.
- The sacral segments have great prognostic significance in SCI (as discussed above) and careful examination of anal sensation, tone, power and primitive reflexes is required (anal wink and bulbocavernosus/mons-clitoral reflex).

The risk of pressure sores on long spinal boards is very high and they can develop in less than 2 h. The spinal board should be used as a pre-hospital extrication or transfer device, and should, therefore, be removed at the earliest opportunity once in hospital. The thoracolumbar spine must be protected against angulation and torsion, which can be achieved by flat bed rest. Pressure sores can be avoided by good nursing care (log rolling every 2 h) and the use of a specialized spinal bed and mattress.

Signs of spinal injury in the unconscious patient

- Diaphragmatic breathing.
- Neurogenic shock.
- Flaccid areflexia (spinal shock).
- Flexed posture of the upper limbs (loss of C6).
- Response to pain above clavicles only.
- Priapism.

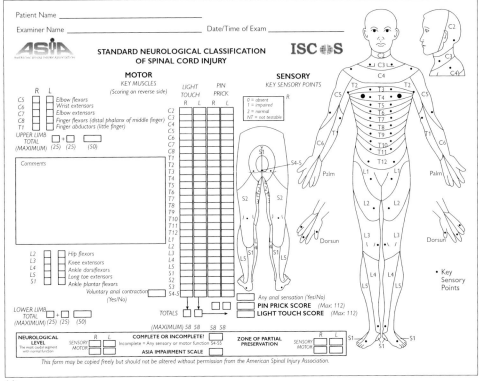

(a)

MUSCLE GRADING

0 total paralysis

1 palpable or visible contraction

2 active movement, full range of motion, gravity eliminated

3 active movement, full range of motion, against gravity

4 active movement, full range of motion, against gravity and provides some resistance

5 active movement, full range of motion, against gravity and provides normal resistance

5* muscle able to exert, in examiner's judgement, sufficient resistance to be considered normal if identifiable inhibiting factors were not present

NT not testable. Patient unable to reliably exert effort or muscle unavailable for testing due to factors such as immobilization, pain on effort or contracture.

ASIA IMPAIRMENT SCALE

☐ A =**Complete**: No motor or sensory function is preserved in the sacral segments S4-S5

☐ B =**Incomplete**: Sensory but not motor function is preserved below the neurological level and includes the sacral segments S4-S5

☐ C =**Incomplete**: Motor function is preserved below the neurological level, and more than half of key muscles below the neurological level have a muscle grade less than 3

☐ D =**Incomplete**: Motor function is preserved below the neurological level, and at least half of key muscles below the neurological level have a muscle grade of 3 or more

☐ E =**Normal**: Motor and sensory function are normal

CLINICAL SYNDROMES (OPTIONAL)

☐ Central cord
☐ Brown-sequard
☐ Anterior Cord
☐ Conus Medullaris
☐ Cauda Equina

STEPS IN CLASSIFICATION

The following order is recommended in determining the classification of individuals with SCI.

1. Determine sensory levels for right and left sides
2. Determine motor levels for right and left sides.
   Note: in regions where there is no myotome to test, the motor level is presumed to be the same as the sensory level.
3. Determine the single neurological level.
   This is the lowest segment where motor and sensory function is normal on both sides, and is the most cephalad of the sensory and motor levels determines in steps 1 and 2.
4. Determine whether the injury is Complete or Incomplete (sacral sparing).
   If voluntary anal contraction = No AND all S4-5 sensory scores = 0 AND any anal sensation = No, then injury is COMPLETE. Otherwise injury is incomplete
5. Determine ASIA Impairment Scale (AIS) Grade:
   Is injury complete? If YES, AIS=A Record ZPP

   NO ↓   (For ZPP record lowest dermatome or myotome on each side with some (non-zero score) preservation)

   Is injury motor incomplete? If NO, AIS=B

   YES ↓ (Yes=voluntary anal contraction OR motor function more than three levels below the motor level on a given side.)

   Are atleast half of the key muscles below the (single) neurological level graded 3 or better?

   NO ↓   YES ↓
   AIS=C   AIS=D

If sensation and motor function is normal in all segments, AIS=E
Note: AIS E is used in follow up testing when on individual with a documented SCI has recovered normal function. If at initial testing no deficits are found, the individual is neurologically intact; the ASIA Impairment Scale does not apply.

(b)

Fig. 11.9. The ASIA Assessment Form. (Reproduced from Gardiner *et al. Training in Surgery*, 2009, with permission from Oxford University Press.)

Investigations

Controversy still exists regarding the best way to exclude spinal injury in the patient with minor trauma, and in the obtunded polytrauma patient, at opposite ends of the spectrum. In the unconscious patient it must be assumed that the whole spine is unstable. Once one spinal fracture or column injury is identified in any patient, the entire column needs to be imaged to exclude concomitant injury (risk 3–17%).

X-ray

For any fracture the clinician must have two orthogonal views. A lateral cervical spine X-ray will detect 85% of significant cervical spine injuries, but in assessing the cervical spine a minimum of three views are required—an AP, lateral, and peg view. Approximately 5% of cervical trauma radiographs are misinterpreted and 50% of missed cervical spine fractures are due to incomplete views.

The lateral cervical spine X-ray

This is regarded as the single most important radiographic examination of the spine (although increasing availability and use of CT in trauma may replace this). The X-ray must show the occiput to the C7–T1 junction, as up to 20% of cervical spine injuries occur at this area. To facilitate this, the arms should be pulled downwards towards the feet as the image is taken. A 'swimmers' view may help to visualize the area, but ultimately a CT may be necessary to exclude an injury.

There are often problems with collar superimposition when assessing the C0–2 region. The posterior arch of C1 may be absent and there are a number of anatomical variants which may be seen. In difficult cases, or if in doubt, a specialist opinion should be requested. The ABC approach to interpretation is recommended:

- **A:** **a**dequacy and alignment;
- **B:** **b**ones;
- **C:** **c**artilage and facet joints;
- **D:** **d**isc spaces;
- **S:** **s**oft tissues.

Four lines may be drawn to check alignment (Fig. 11.10):
- *The anterior spinal line:* along the anterior aspect of vertebral bodies (anterior longitudinal ligament).
- *The posterior spinal line:* along the posterior aspect of vertebral bodies (posterior longitudinal ligament).
- *The spinolaminar line:* joins the anterior margins of the junction of the lamina and spinous processes.
- *The spinous process line:* joins the tips of the spinous processes.
- *Soft tissue indicators of injury* are:
  - pre-vertebral soft tissue swelling (at the level of C3, >7 mm; at the level of C7, >3 cm);
  - loss of normal cervical lordosis.

The open mouth (peg / dens) view

The dens should be checked for fracture and for symmetrical position between the lateral masses of C1 (checking for rotational abnormalities). The lateral masses of C1 should align over the facet joints of C2. Combined lateral mass displacement (overhang) >7 mm indicates transverse ligament rupture and instability (significant C1 injury) (Fig. 11.11).

The AP cervical spine view

The following should be assessed (Fig. 11.12):
- **A:** **a**dequacy and alignment (dorsal process malalignment is seen in facet dislocations and lateral body or pillar fractures).
- **B:** **b**ones.
- **C:** **c**artilage and joints—including the lateral masses/pillars and the uncovertebral joints of Luschka.
- **D:** **d**isc spaces.
- **S:** **s**oft tissues and swelling—is the trachea deviated?

Oblique views of the cervical spine are sometimes performed, but these are becoming less common with the increased availability of CT scanning in trauma patients.

Supervised flexion-extension views to assess stability are NOT recommended in the acute trauma setting.

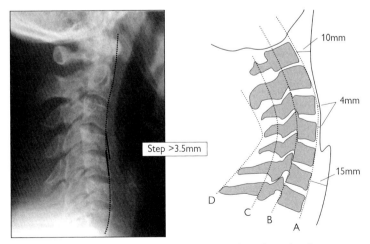

Fig. 11.10. The lateral cervical X-ray: A-anterior spinal line; B-posterior spinal line; C-spinolaminar line; D-spinous process line.

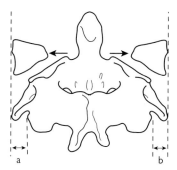

Fig. 11.11. Lateral mass overhang: a+b > 7mm suggests transverse ligament rupture .

The prerequisites of normal X-rays, normal neurology, and normal mental status are rarely fulfilled and the patient is often in too much pain to perform the examination. They are usually performed as a specialist investigation by the spinal team and are good for detecting latent instability post injury.

Thoracolumbar X-rays
AP and lateral thoracolumbar X-rays are indicated in any patient in whom there is a suspicion of spinal injury. As with the cervical spine, the ABC approach should be used to assess the films. Transitional lumbar vertebra at the lumbosacral junction are common and are seen in 20% of the normal population. The upper thoracic column is frequently not well demonstrated on plain lateral films and CT may be appropriate (especially if the patient is unconscious). The following should be assessed.

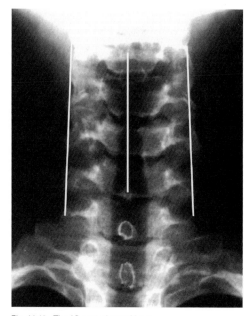

Fig. 11.12. The AP cervical spine X-ray.

Lateral X-ray
- Degree of kyphosis.
- Percentage anterior vertebral body compression.
- Posterior cortical disruption (burst).
- Vertebral body translation.

AP X-ray
- Transverse process fracture (which is associated with renal or ureteric injury, and L5 transverse process fracture is associated with pelvic or sacral fracture in 50%).
- Widened dorsal processes (may be the only sign in a flexion distraction injury).
- Widened pedicles (seen in burst fractures).
- Paravertebral haematoma.

Indicators of cervical spine instability
C0–2 instability
- >8° axial rotation C0–1 to one side.
- Powers ratio distance BC/DA > 1 (occipitoatlantal dislocation) (Fig. 11.13).
- Increased odontoid basion distance—the tip of the odontoid should be in line with basion, with the odontoid basion distance 4–5 mm adults and up to 10 mm in children.
- >1 mm C0–1 translation in flexion/extension (this is a specialist investigation, not in the acute trauma setting).
- >7 mm overhang C1–2 (total left and right—Fig. 11.11).
- >45° axial rotation C1–2 to one side.
- Atlantodens interval >5 mm (should be <3 mm) (Fig. 11.13).

C3–T1 instability
- Horizontal vertebral body translation >3.5 mm or 20%.
- Difference in intervertebral angulation between adjacent levels >11 degrees.
- Vertebral body height loss.
- Disc space >1.7 mm.
- Facet fracture, subluxation, or widening.
- Flexion teardrop–small antero-inferior body fracture.

Indicators of thoracolumbar instability
- Neurological deficit.
- Clinical posterior tenderness or deformity.
- >20–30 degrees kyphosis (segmental or combined).
- >30% loss of vertebral height (thoracic).
- >50% loss of vertebral height (lumbar).
- >50% canal compromise.
- Rotational malalignment.
- Fracture dislocation.
- Multiple adjacent fractures (combined height loss >50%).
- Scoliosis >10 degrees.

Sacral X-ray
A plain AP pelvis may show a paradoxic inlet view of the sacrum when a fracture is present. Anterior sacral foraminal disruption should be assessed on the plain film (the stepladder sign). The bony sacrum is, however, best visualized on CT and the neural structures on MRI.

Erect radiographs
These should not be routinely performed in the acute trauma setting. They can be useful in the ambulatory

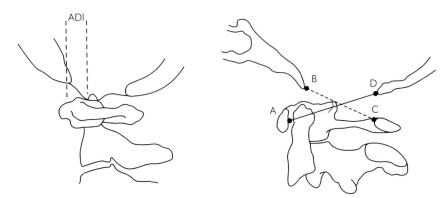

Fig. 11.13. Atlanto-dens interval (ADI) and Powers Ratio.

patient with no neurological symptoms or signs. In patients where there is suspicion of instability and potential for neurological injury (as shown on supine plain films or on CT) they are a specialist investigation and should only be performed after discussion with the local spinal injuries team. Medical supervision is often required. The examination determines stability as there is dynamic physiologic loading of spine. They alter the management plan in up to 25% of cases in which they are performed.

Computed tomography (CT)
Helical CT will detect 99.3% of all spinal fractures and has the benefit of also detecting visceral and pelvic injuries. It is becoming the gold standard in the acute trauma setting. CT is employed to establish:
- The bony anatomy of the fracture.
- Fracture stability.
- Spinal canal compromise.

Reconstructions identify degree of deformity and severity of injury. If a patient undergoes CT head for a head injury then concurrent cervical spine CT should be considered. Similarly, if the chest, abdomen, and pelvis are being imaged then the clinician should request reformatted thoracolumbar films. CT is frequently used to visualize the occipitocervical and cervicothoracic junctions as X-rays of these areas are often difficult to interpret.

Magnetic resonance imaging (MRI)
MRI is the most sensitive method for detecting spinal injuries. It may allow prognostic assessment of final motor function (intraspinal haematoma). However, there may be significant logistical problems obtaining an MRI in the polytrauma or intubated patient. It is used to look for:
- Spinal cord injury.
- Haematoma.
- Intervertebral disc disruption.
- Soft tissue/ligamentous injury.

    Emergency MRI is indicated when there is:
- Worsening neurology.
- Unexplained neurological deficit.
- Discordant skeletal and neurological levels of injury.

In these cases it is used to evaluate spinal cord anatomy, identify cord compression, and rule out epidural haematoma.

Emergency interventions

Emergency indirect reduction of the spinal canal

Following appropriate investigation, closed reduction of traumatic cervical spine deformity may be indicated. Cervical traction can achieve indirect cord decompression by ligamentotaxis. This reduces bony canal encroachment and flattens the ligamentum flavum. The aim is to restore the spinal column to its premorbid alignment and re-establish the diameter of the bony spinal canal. Gardner Wells tongs or halo-ring devices are applied and then traction added. It is contra-indicated in distraction injuries, craniocervical dislocations, skull fractures, and injuries associated with ankylosing spondylitis. It is most commonly seen in the treatment of cervical facet dislocations and in the presence of deteriorating neurology—it may have to be performed in the emergency department.

Application of Gardner Wells tongs

The skin is shaved, washed with sterile prep and local anaesthetic applied. The pins are sited 1 cm above the upper earlobe in vertical continuation with external auditory meatus and they are torqued to 6 inch pounds (0.6 J) (Fig. 11.14). Gardner Wells tongs are not appropriate for children.

Application of a halo-ring

This requires 2 people and is rarely performed by non trained staff. The ring size is first determined. The clinician should be able to place 1–2 fingers between the ring and scalp circumferentially. The skin is shaved, washed with sterile prep, and local anaesthetic applied. With the eyes closed 2 anterior pins are sited 1 cm above the lateral half of the eyebrows. The frontal sinus medially and supraorbital nerve laterally need to be avoided. Two posterior pins are placed diametrically opposite—typically in a vertical line above mastoids. Each pin is torqued to 6–8-inch pounds (0.6–0.8 J) (Fig. 11.14). They should be retighten after 24 h (and at subsequent follow-up if used for definitive treatment in a halo jacket).

Cervical traction

Once the tongs or halo are applied, IV analgesia, muscle relaxants, and oxygen should be administered. Anaesthetic cover should be available because of the risk of respiratory depression and arrest. Weights are applied—5lbs per vertebral level in the cervical spine starting with 5-10lbs (2–5 Kg). This is incrementally increased with check lateral X-rays. Traction should be discontinued in the presence of:
• Neurological deterioration.
• Distraction > 1 cm.
• Reduction.

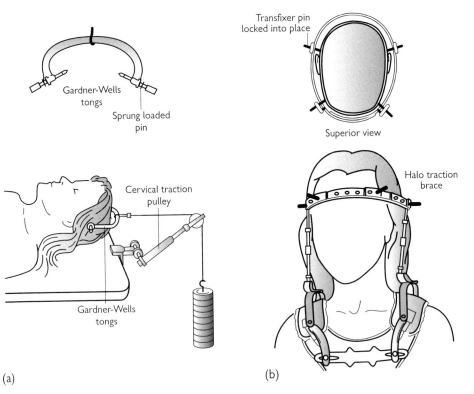

(a)   (b)

Fig. 11.14. Traction and stabilization (a) application of Gardner-Wells tongs; (b) halo immobilizer. (Reproduced from *Oxford Textbook of Orthopaedics and Trauma* with permission of Oxford University Press.)

Emergency surgery

Emergency surgery is indicated when there is:
- *Deteriorating neurology*: traumatic disc herniation, expanding epidural haematoma, irreducible facet dislocation.
- Unusual distraction injuries where traction or collar are contra-indicated or insufficient.
- Penetrating trauma and vertebral artery ligation is required.

The role of steroids

The British Association of Spinal Cord Injuries Specialists have concluded that the use of high dose steroids in the management of acute spinal cord injury should NOT be recommended or supported on the current evidence (*BOA Guidelines*, January 2006).

Definitive treatment options

In general, bony injuries heal well and ligamentous injuries will heal, but stability may be compromised. SCI alone is not an indication for surgery, but associated mechanical instability may be. Non-operative treatment modalities include bed rest, orthoses, halo, and traction.

Bed rest

Many spinal injury centres advocate bed rest in all patients with SCI for the first 6 weeks to allow autonomic recovery and prevent further damage due to loss of postural regulation of blood pressure. It is not without its complications (pressure sores, chest and urine infections, and deep vein thrombosis). It does not carry some of the high risks associated with surgery, but subsequent surgery following conservative treatment on bed rest may be required for symptomatic instability or potentially reversible neurological compromise.

Spinal orthoses

Cervical orthosis (CvO)

A collar is not a rigid form of immobilization, but it does increase the level of stability. They also act to unload the weight of the head from the cervical spine onto the shoulders. Types:
- Soft collar: foam rubber covered with stockinet used mainly for 'psychological' support it reminds the patient not to flex their neck.
- Hard collar: padded polyethylene it provides more effective control of flexion and extension.
- Bivalved hard collars: with reinforced anterior and posterior components.

Cervical-thoracic orthosis (CTO)

The sterno-occipital mandibular immobilizer (SOMI) provides better control than a hard collar, but it is less comfortable.

Cervico-thoracolumbosacral orthosis (CTLSO) and thoracolumbosacral orthosis (TLSO)

CTLSOs are mainly used in the treatment of scoliosis, but can be used in fracture management. Both the CTLSO and TLSO are made with polypropylene and operate on the principle of three-point fixation and prevent sway of the vertebral column. They can help to hold the spine in hyper-extension and reduce gross trunk motion.

Lumbosacral orthosis (LSO)

These are corsets made of fabric reinforced with polypropylene. They have adjustable velcro fasteners to allow the user to control the degree of tension for proper support and comfort. They reduce the pressure on the lumbosacral region by increasing the intra-abdominal pressure. They also act as a reminder to the patient to maintain correct posture.

Skull callipers and halo traction/vest

Callipers and halo traction are usually used for acute unstable cervical fractures (as discussed above). A halo vest permits mobility. Complications include:
- Pin site infection or loosening.
- Scars.
- Dural penetration.
- Nerve injury (supraorbital/supratrochlear).

Surgery

Indications for surgery fall broadly under neurological and biomechanical criteria:
- Neurological:
  - clearance of canal compromise;
  - improvement of neurological deficit;
  - progressive myelopathy;
  - worsening radicular symptoms.
- Biomechanical:
  - correction of deformity;
  - prevention of progressive deformity;
  - stabilization of instability.

Specifically, surgery may be indicated when there is:
- Progressive neurological deficit with persistent dislocation or neurocompression not corrected by closed traction.
- Persistence of incomplete spinal cord injury with continued impingement on neural elements.
- Unstable dislocations that have been reduced.
- Complete spinal cord injury with unstable fractures to enable early rehabilitation and aid nursing care.
- Late instability or deformity with continued cord percussion and neurological deficit or chronic pain.
- In the polytrauma setting to aid nursing and medical care.
- Prevent the development of, or to correct post-traumatic kyphotic spinal deformity.
- Unstable fractures.

Surgery can be performed anteriorly, posteriorly or both. Anterior surgery should be considered if there is
- Incomplete neurological deficit.
- Significant canal compromise.
- Excessive vertebral body damage.

Posterior surgery should be considered if there is:
- Damage to the posterior tension band.
- Significant translation deformity, which needs to be reduced.

There is no evidence that surgery improves neurological outcome. Complete cord injury or neurologically intact patients are likely to remain unchanged. Incomplete injuries tend to improve regardless of whether surgery or non-operative methods are employed. However, animal studies have consistently shown that neurological recovery is enhanced by early decompression. It is generally felt that timing to reduction does influence the degree and recovery of SCI in bilateral cervical facet dislocation. Urgent or acute decompressive surgery is recommended in bilateral locked facet dislocation in the incomplete tetraplegic or SCI patient with deteriorating neurology.

Canal compromise by bony fragments tends to remodel spontaneously and within 12 months there is up to 50% improvement in canal dimension. Exposure of the dura during surgery can result in further neuronal injury and complications such as cerebrospinal fluid leak.

Clearing the cervical spine

The treatment of life threatening injuries takes precedence over clearing the spine. There is no universally agreed protocol for intoxicated, multiply-injured, or head-injured patients.

In such patients a CT of the cervical spine is normally included in a standard head to hip protocol. In the unconscious patient when both X-ray and CT are negative a significant injury to cervical spine is unlikely (<1%). Further assessment may include waiting for the patient to wake to comply with clinical assessment, or MRI scanning. The clinician must weigh up the risks of continued immobilization of a normal spine versus the potential risk of mobilizing a spine with ligamentous instability.

In the patient with more minor injury, there are several clinical decision rules that may enable clinical clearance of the cervical spine without need to perform any radiological investigation. Examples of these include the NEXUS criteria and Canadian C-Spine Rule (Fig. 11.15a). Another suggested algorithm was published in *Injury* in 2005 (Licinia and Nowitzke, 2005) (Fig. 11.15b)

NEXUS criteria (all must apply to allow clinical clearance):

- No posterior midline tenderness.
- No evidence of intoxication.
- Normal level of alertness.
- No focal neurological deficit.
- No distracting injury.

If X-rays are taken and are normal, but there is a neurological deficit attributable to the trauma then continued immobilization and an MRI scan are indicated.

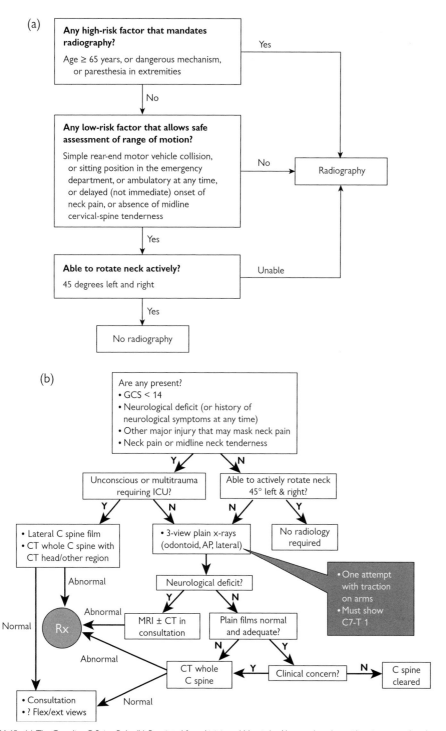

Fig. 11.15. (a) The Canadian C-Spine Rule. (b) Reprinted from Licinia and Nowitzke, 'Approach and considerations regarding the patient with spinal injury'. *Injury* 2005; **36:** S2–12, with permission from Elsevier; and Stiell *et al.* 'The Canadian C spine rule' *N Engl J Med* 2003, ©Massacheusetts Medical Society, all rights reserved.

Transfer of patients with spinal injuries

Before transferring a patient with spinal injuries some form of checklist should be used to ensure that nothing is missed. The *BOA Guidelines* (January 2006) recommend that:

- Immobilization of the spine is adequate and secure.
- Long bone fractures are immobilized.
- The airway is clear and can be maintained during transfer.
- Supplemental oxygen administered and ventilation is adequate (spontaneous or assisted).
- Voluntary vital capacity > 15 mL/kg.
- Chest drainage is performed if indicated.
- IV line is patent and infusing at desired rate.
- NG tube *in situ* is draining freely and connected to low suction.
- Urinary catheter *in situ* and draining freely.
- The skin is protected from injury.
- Level of SCI is documented.
- Records and images are sent with the patient.
- Other injuries documented and stabilized.
- Head injury documented and monitored.
- The time of departure is noted.

Classification of vertebral fractures

Classification systems can be used to aid communication, decide on treatment options, predict outcome, and for research purposes. None of the classification systems for vertebral fractures fulfil all of these criteria. In the axial cervical spine there are several systems used reflecting the unique anatomy (discussed below). In the subaxial cervical spine there are three main systems—the Allen and Ferguson classification, and the Denis and AO/ASIF modification of the thoracolumbar classifications (Arbeitsgemeinshchaft fur Osteosynthesefrage or Association for the Study of Internal Fixation). The Allen and Ferguson system is mechanistic and injuries fall into six groups (Fig. 11.16).

Several classification systems are used in the thoracolumbar spine. The two most commonly used are the Denis and AO/ASIF classifications. The Denis classification is based on a three-column theory and the AO/ASIF on two columns (Figs 11.17). The integrity of the middle column was felt to be the most important factor in determining stability. However, recent evidence suggests that this may not be the case. The Denis classification is descriptive and has 4 major categories of injury - compression, burst, flexion-distraction and fracture-dislocation. The AO/ASIF classification is mechanistic but also hierarchical (Fig. 11.18). There are three major categories of injury—A, axial compression; B, bending distraction; and C, circumferential/shear.

Sacral fractures are classified by a different system described by Denis et al. (discussed below).

More recently, two new systems, the Cervical Injury Severity Score (C-ISS) and the Thoracolumbar Injury Severity Score (TL-ISS) have been developed. They are based on the mechanism of injury, morphology of the fracture (in particular the integrity of the posterior ligamentous complex) and the neurological status of the patient.

Compression fractures demonstrate failure of the anterior half of the vertebral body without disruption of the posterior body cortex or retropulsion into the spinal canal. Burst fractures show compressive failure of the vertebral body with extension into the posterior body cortex and some degree of bony retropulsion into the spinal canal.

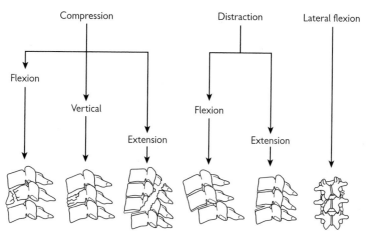

Fig. 11.16. The Allen and Ferguson Classification of Subaxial Cervical Spine Fractures. (Reprinted from Licinia and Nowitzke, 'Approach and considerations regarding the patient with spinal injury'. *Injury* 2005; **36:** S2–12.)

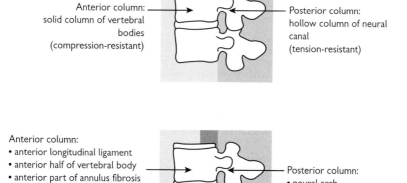

Anterior column:
solid column of vertebral
bodies
(compression-resistant)

Posterior column:
hollow column of neural
canal
(tension-resistant)

Anterior column:
• anterior longitudinal ligament
• anterior half of vertebral body
• anterior part of annulus fibrosis

Middle column:
• posterior longitudinal ligament
• posterior half of vertebral body
• posterior part of annulus fibrosis

Posterior column:
• neural arch
• ligamentum flavum
• facet joint capsules
• interspinous ligament

Fig. 11.17. The anatomy of the two- and three-column models.

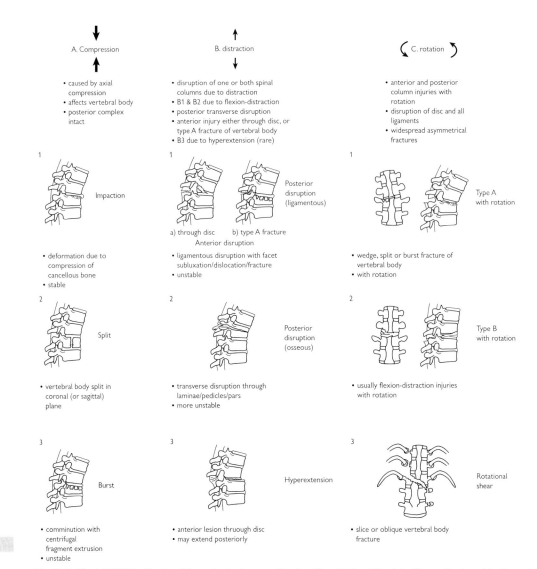

Fig. 11.18. The AO/ASIF Classification of Thoracolumbar Fractures. (Reprinted from Licinia and Nowitzke, 'Approach and considerations regarding the patient with spinal injury'. *Injury* 2005; **36**: S2–12.)

Specific spinal injuries by region

Cervical spine injuries

All cervical spine fractures should be considered unstable until proven otherwise because of the risk of devastating neurological injury. 10% of unconscious patients will have a cervical spine injury.

Axial fractures C0–2

The commonest cause of death from spinal injury occurs in this group and is usually immediate (at the time of injury).

Occipital condyle fractures

Occipital condyle fractures occur due to rapid deceleration or a direct blow to the head (axial compression). They are difficult to identify on plain X-ray and are usually picked up on CT. Associated injuries result in a mortality rate of around 10%, and 30% have associated cervical spine fractures. They are associated with cranial nerve palsies and chronic suboccipital pain. They are classified according to the Anderson and Montesano classification (Fig. 11.19):

- *Type 1 (3%):*
  - impaction;
  - stable;
  - treat with hard collar.
- *Type 2 (22%):*
  - associated base of skull fracture;
  - stable;
  - treat with hard collar.
- *Type 3 (75%):*
  - alar ligament avulsion with condyle;
  - *unstable*: 50% associated with occipito-atlanto instability;
  - may require halo immobilization or surgery.

Atlanto-occipital/occipitocervical dislocation

These are rare, but often fatal. They are associated with significant facial and chest injuries. They occur with deceleration and up to 20% may have normal neurology on presentation. Cervical traction must be avoided. They are generally treated with surgery (posterior occipitocervical fusion). Classification is based on the position of the dislocation (Fig. 11.20):

- *Type 1:* anterior.
- *Type 2:* longitudinal.
- *Type 3:* posterior.

Atlas fractures

Atlas fractures comprise 7–10% of all cervical spine fractures. They occur secondary to axial compression with or without flexion or lateral flexion. They are rarely associated with SCI (there is a large space for the cord). They are commonly associated with dens and non-contiguous spinal fractures (50%). Incomplete formation of the posterior arch of the atlas is not uncommon. They are classified according to Levine and Edwards, and Jarrett and Whitesides classifications (in which there are five types) (Figure 11.21). In summary:

- Posterior arch or non-displaced fractures are likely to be stable and can be treated in a cervical orthosis.
- Asymmetric lateral mass fractures or Jefferson 'burst' type fractures are unstable and often require halo immobilization.
- Transverse ligament rupture without a bony avulsion requires fusion as they are unlikely to heal.

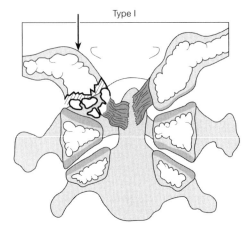

Type I

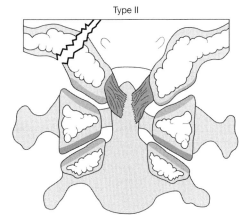

Type II

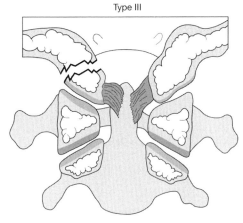

Type III

Fig. 11.19. Anderson and Montesano Classification of Occipital Condyle Fractures. (Reproduced from *Oxford Textbook of Orthopaedics and Trauma*, with permission from Oxford University Press.)

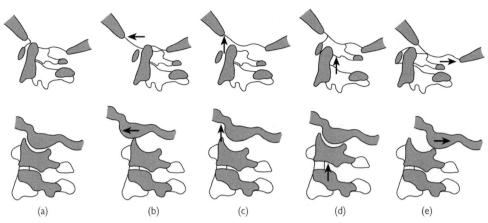

Fig. 11.20. Classification of atlanto-occipital/occipitocervical dislocation. (Reproduced from *Oxford Textbook of Orthopaedics and Trauma*, with permission from Oxford University Press.)

Atlantoaxial subluxation

Injury to the transverse ligament can occur in isolation or associated with a C1 fracture (above). They occur in flexion or with anterior translation. On the lateral cervical X-ray an increase in the ADI is seen (Fig. 11.22). Conservative management should only be contemplated if there is a large undisplaced bony avulsion fracture (this has healing potential). The majority require posterior fusion.

Odontoid peg fractures

Peg fractures comprise 10–20% of all cervical spine fractures and 60% of C2 fractures. As with atlas fractures, there is a low incidence of SCI. A bimodal age distribution is seen—young patients with high energy injuries at one end and elderly patients with low energy injuries (simple household falls) at the other. They are difficult to diagnose on plain films when they are minimally displaced or in the presence of degenerative change. They are classified according to Anderson and D'Alonzo (Fig. 11. 23):
- *Type 1 (<5%):*
  - rare, oblique avulsion fracture above the transverse ligament;
  - rule out atlanto-occipital dislocation;
  - treat with collar.
- *Type 2 (~65%):*
  - prone to non-union (35–85%—small surface area with little cancellous bone);
  - non-union associated with increasing age, displacement, and angulation;
  - treat with reduction followed by cervical orthosis, halo immobilization, anterior screw fixation versus posterior C1–2 instrumentation +/– fusion.
- *Type 3 (~30%):*
  - fracture extends into body of C2;

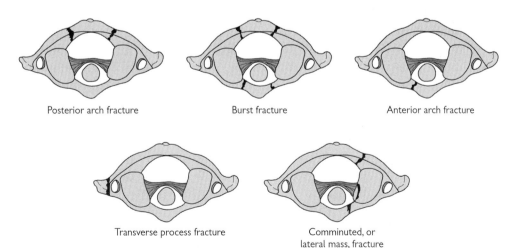

Posterior arch fracture   Burst fracture   Anterior arch fracture

Transverse process fracture   Comminuted, or lateral mass, fracture

Fig. 11.21. Classification of Atlas fractures. (Reproduced from *Oxford Textbook of Orthopaedics and Trauma*, with permission from Oxford University Press.)

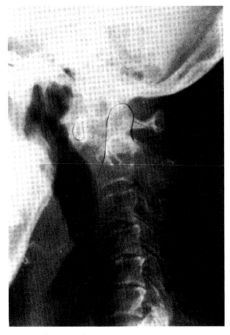

Fig. 11.22. Atlantoaxial subluxation.

- treat with reduction followed by cervical orthosis or halo immobilization (surgery may be required);
- large surface area of cancellous bone very unlikely to progress to non-union.

The majority heal in 10–12 weeks in an orthosis or halo. If fibrous non-union is suspected then supervised flexion extension views (or CT scan) are indicated.

Axis fractures

Traumatic spondylolisthesis (Hangmans fracture) is the 2nd most common fracture of C2. The term refers to bilateral pars fractures and they comprise 5–10% all cervical spine fractures. They often occur with high energy and are associated with other spinal fractures in 30%. They occur in hyperextension and compression, and additional flexion results in a very unstable pattern of injury. Neurological involvement is rare and the lateral cervical spine film will show the injury in 95% of cases. The Levine Edwards modification of the Effendi classification describes four main types of injury (Fig. 11.24):

- *Type 1:*
  - most common (70%);
  - minimally displaced bilateral pars fractures;
  - treat in collar.
- *Type 2:*
  - type 1 plus >3 mm displacement, disc and partial ligament injury present;
  - 2nd most common;
  - ensure the disc is intact on an MRI;

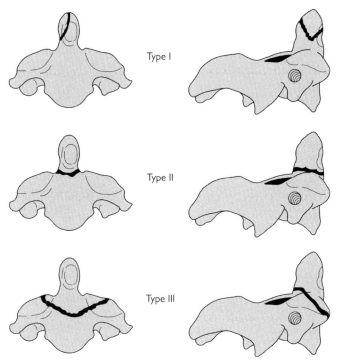

Type I

Type II

Type III

Fig. 11.23. Classification of odontoid peg fractures. (Reproduced from *Oxford Textbook of Orthopaedics and Trauma*, with permission from Oxford University Press.)

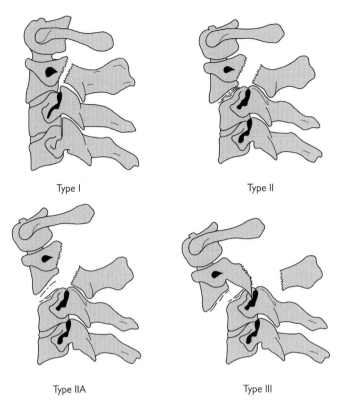

Type I   Type II

Type IIA   Type III

Fig. 11.24. Classification of Hangman's fractures. (Reproduced from *Oxford Textbook of Orthopaedics and Trauma,* with permission from Oxford University Press.)

- treat with reduction followed by immobilization (halo);
- malunion common.
- *Type 2A:*
  - minimal translation, but significant angulation (flexion component);
  - definite disc injury and possible anterior longitudinal ligament injury;
  - avoid traction;
  - treat in halo. Surgery is often required.
- *Type 3:*
  - associated facet dislocation;
  - often requires surgery.
- *Atypical:* the fracture crosses the pars and enters the body of C2.

Combination C1–2 fractures
It is relatively common to see C1–2 fractures occurring together in combination. They do, however, have a higher morbidity and mortality than the sum of the individual injuries and are more likely to require surgery.

Subaxial Fractures C3–7
Compression and burst fractures
In the absence of neurology, deformity, or instability, conservative treatment in a collar can be considered for compression fractures in the cervical spine. They often require CT to define the fracture and determine stability. Injury to the posterior ligaments must be ruled out as this indicates instability and can result in neurological injury, or progressive kyphotic deformity and pain. Burst fractures show a higher rate of instability and neuronal damage and often require surgery. Small anterior vertebral body avulsion fractures must be distinguished from the more sinister teardrop fractures. Teardrop fractures are unstable coronal fractures through the vertebral body. They indicate disruption of the disc, ligaments and facets. Small avulsion fractures show no malalignment, no prevertebral soft tissue swelling and no loss of vertebral body height or disc space. CT may be required to distinguish the two.

Facet dislocations
Facet dislocations are associated with a high rate of SCI. The possibility of herniated nucleus pulposus must be ruled out prior to reduction in the neurologically intact patient. This is because subsequent compression of the spinal cord could occur. It is thought the risk of herniation is between 1.5 and 35%, being twice as common in bilateral facet dislocations as unilateral ones. Some advocate emergency relocation of facet dislocations, whereas others advocate MRI first—the evidence for this is inconclusive. However, it is generally agreed that in the presence of deteriorating neurology, relocation of a dislocated cervical spine should not be delayed.

Bilateral facet dislocations typically show 25–50% vertebral body displacement on the lateral film and are associated with a high incidence of SCI. All of the ligaments except the anterior longitudinal ligament are disrupted and vertebral artery injury is increased with increasing vertebral body translation.

Unilateral facet dislocations are the most frequently missed significant cervical spine injury. They occur with flexion and rotation of the cervical spine. They typically show <25% vertebral body displacement on the lateral cervical spine film. Nerve root injury is more common than SCI and radiculopathy often improves with traction. They are most frequently treated by closed reduction with a halo.

25% of all facet dislocations will fail closed reduction. In all cases, the posterior ligaments are disrupted and most patients will require surgery to achieve stability. 40% of patients treated conservatively in a halo will remain unstable at 3 months. Subsequent kyphotic deformity, subluxation or radiculopathy may require surgery.

Spinous process fractures
Clay Shoveller's fractures require symptomatic treatment only. More sinister injury (especially posterior ligamentous injuries) should be considered and excluded.

Thoracolumbar spine injuries

The incidence of thoracolumbar fractures is:
- *T1–10:* 16–18%.
- *T11–L2:* 50–54%.
- *L3–5:* 28–34%.

The vertebral bodies in the thoracic spine are smaller anteriorly and it is most stable in flexion. The stability is increased by the ribs and sternum. The central thoracic spine has a relatively sparse blood supply and the canal is small compared with size of cord. Fractures are often the result of high energy trauma and they are associated with injuries to the thoracic aorta.

The thoracolumbar junction is an area of transition from a relatively rigid thoracic spine to a mobile lumbar spine and the majority of fractures occur here. The spine also changes from kyphosis to lordosis and the facet alignment

from coronal to sagittal. In the lumbar spine, burst fractures are common because the load bearing axis lies more posterior.

Criteria for a stable thoracolumbar fracture are:
- No transient or persistent neurological injury.
- Acceptable alignment.
- At least 1 column intact (2 column model).
- No significant ligamentous disruption.

Stable injuries can be managed in orthoses (with follow-up advised). Surgery in the thoracolumbar spine is indicated for:
- Progressive neurological deficit.
- Unstable fracture in the multiply injured patient.
- Complete spinal dislocation with partial cord injury.

Caution should be exercised in the presence of a thoracic fracture combined with a sternal fracture, as there is a significant risk of instability.

Compression fractures

These are the commonest type of thoracolumbar spine fracture. The majority occur between T11 and L2 and by definition the fracture does not extend into the posterior vertebral body wall. Compression fractures rarely require surgery—the majority are stable (Fig. 11.25). A hyperextension thoracolumbar orthosis and radiographic follow-up will suffice. Fractures with >50% loss of vertebral body height or >30° of kyphosis can be treated conservatively, but require follow-up (risk of progressive kyphotic deformity). They should have a CT to assess the bony anatomy and stability prior to mobilization. Any neurological deficit indicates instability. Fractures above T6 require a cervical extension on the orthosis to improve control.

Burst fractures

These fractures should be considered unstable and by definition the fracture extends into the posterior vertebral body wall. They can be treated with a period of bed rest (hyperextension) followed by mobilization in an orthosis. Alternatively, surgery can be performed. In both cases, radiographic follow-up is essential. In patients with complete cord injury the fracture can be stabilized posteriorly

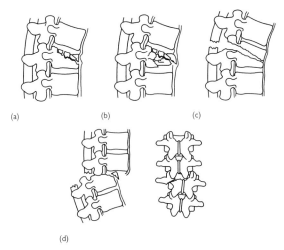

(a)   (b)   (c)

(d)

Fig. 11.25. Simple diagram of (a) compression, (b) burst, (c) chance, and (d) # dislocation.

to facilitate rehabilitation, and prevent deformity. Canal remodelling of retropulsed fragments occurs and up to 50% of the canal space can be restored. Burst fractures are commonest in the lower lumbar spine because the load-bearing axis is more posterior (Fig. 11.25). Occasionally, acute cauda equina syndrome due to retropulsed fragments will need to be decompressed and fixation at the time of surgery should be performed.

Flexion-distraction injuries (chance fractures)

These so called 'seatbelt' injuries are highly unstable (all columns are disrupted). They are commoner in children and up to 30% present with neurological injury. They are associated with life-threatening intra-abdominal injuries and up to 50% may have associated bowel perforation. The sentinel sign is transverse abdominal wall bruising from the lap portion of the seatbelt. Pancreatic and duodenal injury in particular should be excluded. The fracture can affect multiple spinal segments and the patient may not be able to wear a brace or orthosis due to their abdominal injuries. The majority require surgery. Pure ligamentous injuries can occur and the clinician should look specifically for widened dorsal processes on the AP and lateral X-rays.

Fracture-dislocations

These are high energy injuries and have the highest rate of SCI of all spinal fractures (90%). They should be suspected in polytrauma patients with sternal fracture, rib cage disruption, cardiac, or pulmonary injuries. Thoracic fracture dislocations carry the worst prognosis as there is very little space available for the cord. They are highly unstable injuries with multiplanar deformity and little residual stability. They frequently require surgical intervention. T1–2 fracture dislocations rarely reduce with skull traction.

Minor fractures

More serious injuries must be excluded. The following are generally stable injuries:
- Fractures of articular process (facet).
- Spinous process fractures (need to exclude chance fracture).
- Transverse process fractures (need to exclude renal tract injury).

Sacral injuries

The sacrum is the mechanical nucleus of axial skeleton—it is the base of spinal column and the keystone of pelvic ring. The sacral nerve roots exit anteriorly with the thecal sac terminating at the S1–2 level. Delay in diagnosis of these injuries occurs in 30% of cases. CT is the investigation of choice. They rarely occur in isolation and the clinician should think about associated pelvic and acetabular injuries and injuries at the lumbosacral junction. Surgery can be considered for stabilization and neural decompression but overall neurological improvement is seen in 80% regardless of treatment. Sacral fractures are classified according to Denis (Fig. 11.26):

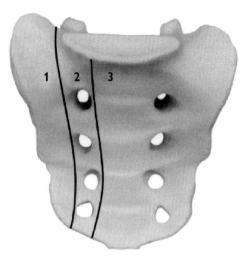

Fig. 11.26. Zonal classification of sacral fractures.

Zone 1
- Sacral alar fracture.
- Neurological injury rare (6%).
- Observe.

Zone 2
- Sacral foramina fracture.
- 28% neural injury commonly unilateral.
- Consider iliosacral fixation.

Zone 3
- Fracture medial to foramina.
- >50% neural injury.
- Mostly bilateral with bowel, bladder, and sexual dysfunction.
- Unstable, therefore, consider fixation.

Coccygeal fractures
These most commonly occur due to a direct blow following a fall. During assessment a rectal examination should be performed. Imaging is of little help unless there is suspicion of tumour or infection (in which case a CT or MRI may be appropriate). Analgesia and gentle mobilization is the mainstay of treatment.

Treatment options are summarized in Table 11.2.

Table 11.2. Summary of treatment options

		Observe	Collar	Halo Vest	Surgery
Cervical spine					
Occipital condyle fracture	Type 1		X		
	Type 2		X	X	
	Type 3		X	X	X
Atlanto-occipital dislocation				A	X
Atlas fracture	Stable		X	X	
	Unstable		X	X	
Axis—peg fracture	Type 1	X	X		
	Type 2		X	X	X
	Type 3		X	X	
Axis—Hangmans fracture	Type 1		X	X	
	Type 2		X	X	
	Type 2A		X	A X	X
	Type 3			X	X
Unilateral facet dislocation					X
Bilateral facet dislocation					X
Subaxial compression fracture			X	X	
Subaxial burst fracture			X	X	X
Unilateral facet fracture			X	X	X
Spinous process fracture	Stable	X	X		
Whiplash injury	Stable	X			

		Observe	Orthosis	Surgery	Bed Rest
Thoracolumbar spine					
Isolated transverse/dorsal process		X			
Compression fracture (intact PLC)		X	X		
Multiple Compression Fractures			X	X	X
Burst fracture (intact PLC)		(X)	X	X	X
Burst fracture (PLC disrupted)			X	X	X
Fracture dislocation				X	X
Flexion distraction (chance)			(X)	X	(X)
Osteoporotic fractures		X	X	(X)	

PLC – posterior ligamentous complex, A – avoid traction

Paediatric spinal injuries

Paediatric spinal injuries are uncommon. They account for 1–2% of all fractures in children and most occur in the cervical spine. Only 2–3% of all spinal injuries involve children and they represent only 0.1–0.2% of the total number of SCI per year. SCI is less common in children because of their increased musculoskeletal flexibility. Complete SCI in children shows little prospect of recovery, but of those with partial SCI 74% show significant improvement and 59% show complete recovery.

The definition of instability is less clear in children. They should be assessed in the same way as adults, however clinical and neurological assessment can be more challenging. The paediatric (growing) spine has several features that differ from the adult (mature) spine.

- *Aged 0–2 years:*
  - mobile and elastic spine;
  - underdeveloped neck musculature;
  - incomplete calcification of bones;
  - wedge-shaped vertebrae;
  - shallow horizontal cervical facet joints;
  - large head to torso ratio increases the likelihood of injury (especially at C0–1 junction);
- *Juvenile 2–10 years:*
  - muscle and ligament strengthening;
  - bone growth and calcification with mature shape;
  - head to torso ratio reduction (focus of injury becomes C5–6);
  - maturation of upper spine at 10 years, lower spine at 14 years.

There are several key radiological features seen during the development of the spine which are important in the interpretation of X-rays:

- *< 6 months:* C1 invisible, synchondroses open, vertebral bodies wedged anteriorly, no lordosis/kyphosis seen.
- *1 year:* body of C1 visible.
- *3 years:* spinous process synchondroses fuse, the dens ossifies.
- *3–6 years:* neurocentral body and C2-odontoid synchondroses fuse, anterior wedging of vertebral bodies resolves.
- *8 years:* pseudosubluxation and predental widening resolve, normal lordosis becomes evident
- *12–14 years:* secondary ossification centres of spinous process tips seen, summit ossification of odontoid fuses, superior and inferior epiphyseal rings seen on vertebral bodies.
- *25 years:* secondary ossification centres on tips spinous processes fuse, superior and inferior epiphyseal rings fuse

There can be marked variation in this development and there are several normal radiological points to bear in mind during the interpretation of X-rays (not to be confused with fractures):

- The presence of an apical ossification centre.
- Synchondrosis seen at the base of the peg.
- Rounded vertebral bodies.
- Secondary ossification centres at spinous process tips.
- Posterior peg angulation is seen in up to 5%.
- C2–3 pseudosubluxation is common (see below).

- Ossification centre in the anterior arch C1 is absent in the first year.
- The atlanto dens interval (ADI) can be up to 4.5 mm
- A prevertebral pseudomass is often seen—the pharyngeal wall is close to spine in inspiration which can give rise to increased soft tissue shadow in forced expiration (for example if crying).
- The facet joints are horizontal.
- In hyperextension the arch of C1 may appear to be in the foramen magnum (age < 2 years).
- Overriding of the atlas on odontoid on extension films is common.

As with adult trauma, the lateral X-ray of the cervical spine yields the greatest information. The ABC approach to interpretation is recommended. In particular, one should look for:

- Alignment.
- Atlanto dens interval and space available for the cord.
- Increased distance between adjacent spinous processes.
- Disruption of McGregors, Chamberlains, McRaes, or Wackenheims lines (indicating basilar invagination—movement towards the foramen magnum). These are often more important in assessing congenital anomalies (Fig. 11.27)
- Avulsion fracture of the endplate.
- Fracture of the spinous process.
- Widened disc spaces indicating apophyseal separation.

Paediatric cervical spine injuries

70% of all paediatric cervical spine injuries occur at C3 and above (85% in the under 8s). Up to 24% of cervical spine injuries occur at multiple levels and 50% of patients have significant associated injuries. There are several features which predispose the immature spine to cervical injury:

- Large head in proportion to body.
- Physiological ligamentous laxity.
- Weak cervical musculature.

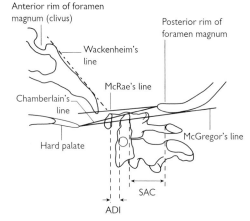

Fig. 11.27. Radiological measurements used to assess the C0–2 region.

- Orientation of facets less resistant to translation (more horizontal).
- Incompletely ossified wedged vertebrae with open growth plates.

Odontoid fractures are one of the more common paediatric cervical spine injuries. They are usually seen on the lateral X-ray and are commonly a Salter Harris 1 type fracture through the dentocentral synchondrosis. Neurological injury is rare. Wedge compression fractures are the most common subaxial injury. C3–7 physeal injuries are frequently missed. They are usually managed conservatively and tend to heal rapidly.

Os Odontoidum

This is thought to result from an unrecognized fracture of the base of the peg. A rounded ossicle is seen on the lateral X-ray separated from the axis by a transverse gap. A CT scan is often performed to look for congenital anomalies and surgery is generally required.

Atlantoaxial rotatory subluxation

This is a rare condition which presents typically with a tilted head or torticollis. A CT is required to confirm the diagnosis. It is classified according to Fielding and Hawkins (Figure 11.28)
- *Type 1:* unilateral facet subluxation.
- *Type 2:* unilateral facet subluxation with 3–5 mm anterior displacement.
- *Type 3:* bilateral anterior facet dislocation of > 5 mm.
- *Type 4:* posterior displacement of the atlas.

Treatment depends on the severity and duration ranging from halter traction to posterior arthrodesis.

Pseudosubluxation

This is a normal phenomenon seen in the immature cervical spine. There is an apparent anterior vertebral body slip of C2 on C3. It is seen in 25% of children <8 years old. At the C3–4 level it is seen in 14%. The posterior interlaminar line is undisplaced. Swischuk's line is used to assess whether the phenomenon is pathological. This is a line joining the spinolaminar arcs of C1 and C3, and it should pass within 2 mm of C2 (the C2 line should lie 1 mm anterior or posterior to Swischuk's line). This should not change with flexion or extension.

Paediatric thoracolumbar injuries

Thoracolumbar fractures tend to affect multiple levels and compression fractures are the most common type. They tend to occur in the thoracic region and most can be managed conservatively. Surgery should be considered if there is >50% compression or lateral compression >15°. The amount of wedging that will remodel is limited to less than 30 degrees. End plate damage can lead to a rapid increase in deformity during adolescent growth spurt and, therefore, follow-up is advised. Burst fractures are generally managed as for adults. Flexion distraction (Chance) fractures are more common in the paediatric population and they have a better prognosis in children. Surgery should be considered if there is kyphosis >20 degrees or a pure ligamentous injury.

The limbus fracture is an injury to the apophyseal ring (growth plate injury). It occurs most commonly at L4 in teenage boys, and presents like a herniated disc. The patient presents having lifted a heavy object, fallen, or twisted their back. They often describe a pop and then symptoms of radiculopathy. Delayed diagnosis is common, but non-operative management is rarely successful. MRI or

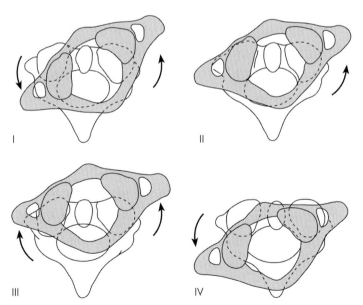

Fig. 11.28. Classification of atlanto-axial rotatory subluxation. (Reproduced from *Oxford Textbook of Orthopaedics and Trauma*, with permission from Oxford University Press.)

CT is required to identify the nature of lesion which can then be excised.

Acute spondylolytic spondylolisthesis is an acute fracture of the pars interarticularis, which occurs with high energy trauma. It usually occurs at L5 and early surgery is recommended. It should be distinguished from spondylolysis, which is seen in up to 5% of the general population. This is a defect in the pars thought to occur through both congenital and developmental mechanisms. It presents with low back pain, postural deformity, or gait abnormality. It is commonly precipitated by hyperextension of the lumbar spine. A bone scan or CT may be required to make the diagnosis if plain films are normal and it is usually managed conservatively.

SCIWORA

This is an acronym for *spinal cord injury without radiographic abnormality*. It is used when patients have clinical evidence of SCI, but the X-rays and CT are normal. It is becoming a misnomer because our diagnostic ability to detect the abnormality is improving—MRI can show cord oedema or haemorrhage, soft tissue, or ligamentous injury, apophyseal end plate, or disc disruption. However, MRI will be normal in 25% of cases. It is the cause of paralysis in 20–30% of children with SCI, 70% of which are complete SCI. It is commonest in the <8-year-old group. It can occur in the thoracolumbar spine, but >80% of cases are cervical. Up to 50% of cases have a delayed onset of neurological symptoms or a late deterioration after a less severe degree of injury. Ligamentous laxity, hypermobility, and immature spinal vasculature are thought to be contributory factors. Experiments have shown that the spinal column can stretch 2 inches without injury, but the cord ruptures after only 0.25 inches. The prognosis is related to MRI findings. Patients <10 years old are more likely to have been involved in a higher energy injury and are more likely to have permanent paralysis. Most cases can be treated in a collar with surgery occasionally required for unstable ligamentous injuries.

Complications of paediatric spinal injury

In addition to the complications seen in the adult spine (above) there are some of note specific to the paediatric spine. There is a high incidence of scoliosis following infantile paralysis—90% with quadriplegia and 50% with paraplegia—so follow-up is required. Late spinal deformity is related to age, severity of injury, and level of injury. It is recommended that a brace should be used in complete SCI until skeletal growth is complete. Growth arrest is rare and long-term back pain is uncommon in children after fracture.

Rehabilitation of spinal cord injury and complications

The following factors need to be considered in the reha-
bilitation of patients with acute traumatic SCI:
- Past and family history.
- Medications.
- Smoking, alcohol, drug abuse.
- *Neurology*: level, ASIA grade, brain and peripheral nerve
  function.
- *Spine*: deformity, stability.
- *Respiratory*: vital capacity, cough.
- *Cardiovascular*: hypotension, DVT, autonomic dysreflexia.
- *Bladder*: upper and lower renal tracts.
- *Bowels*: height, weight, nutrition, teeth, abdomen—stress
  ulceration, obstruction, function.
- *Sexual*: fertility, intercourse, sexuality.
- *Skin*: mattress, bed, cushion, pressure sores, foot care.
- *Joints*: heterotopic ossification, arthritis, joint, injury, long
  bones.
- Spasms and spasticity.
- *Pain*: nociceptive, neurogenic.
- *Mobility*: wheelchair, car modifications, orthoses, recrea-
  tional ability.
- *Transfers*: hoist, monkey pole, transfer board.
- *Activities of daily living*: aids, environmental controls.
- *Family*: partner, parents, children.
- Home.
- *Recreation*: holidays.
- Employment.
- *Care*: domestic, personal, therapy (occupational therapy,
  physiotherapy, hydrotherapy).
- *Psychology*: risk of suicide, depression.

Pneumonia
The commonest cause of death following SCI is pneumo-
nia. It accounts for nearly 20% of deaths in the first year
after injury. Chest infections occur secondary to bed rest
or respiratory dysfunction (in cervical injuries). It is impor-
tant to identify and manage secretions, atelectasis, and
hypoventilation. The following techniques may be
employed to prevent chest infections:
- Frequent position changes.
- Chest physiotherapy.
- Incentive spirometry.
- Assisted cough methods.
- Deep pulmonary suction.
- Abdominal binders.
- Mechanical insufflation-exsufflation.
- Positive pressure ventilation.
- Phrenic pacemakers.

Postural hypotension
Upper thoracic and cervical lesions can result in loss of
sympathetic outflow. This can put cord perfusion at risk
and cause secondary or ongoing neurological damage.
Some spinal injury centres advocate 6 weeks of flat bed
rest following SCI to prevent this complication. The
head is gradually raised and the bed tilted. The use of
abdominal binders, TEDS, mineralocorticoids, and ephe-
drine may be employed to prevent sudden falls in blood
pressure.

Deep venous thrombosis (DVT)
Patients with SCI are at very high risk of DVT and prophylaxis at the earliest safe opportunity is mandatory. The incidence of DVT lies somewhere between 15 and 80% within
the first 2 weeks of SCI. Chemoprophylaxis is recommended for the first 8 weeks, but in the presence of contraindications, an inferior vena cava filter should be
considered.

Autonomic dysreflexia
This is seen to some extent in up to 85% of patients with
SCI above T6, and is due to reflex sympathetic over-
activity by various triggering stimuli. Causes include:
- Bladder/bowel distension.
- Cholecystitis.
- Anal fissure.
- Pressure sores.
- In-growing toenails.
- Childbirth.
- Instrumentation/operation.

Hence, a general anaesthetic is still required if a patient is
undergoing an operation even if they have no apparent
sensation. The symptoms and signs include:
- Headache.
- Sweating.
- Chest tightness.
- Hypertension.
- Bradycardia.
- Cardiac dysrhythmia.

  Above the spinal lesion there is:
- Pallor then flushing.
- Sweating around lesion.
- Pupillary dilatation.

  Below the spinal lesion:
- Cold peripheries.
- Pilo erection.
- Contraction of bladder and large bowel.
- Penile erection and seminal fluid emission.

The treatment is guided towards the cause. It is important
to note that the hypertension can result in intracranial
haemorrhage. The bed should be tilted head up. Nifedipine
or GTN should be administered. Aspirin and NSAIDs
should be avoided.

Renal failure
Shock and reduced end organ perfusion can cause renal
failure. The bladder tends to be flaccid during spinal shock
and over distension damage must be avoided. Hence, a urinary catheter should be placed and left on free drainage (in
the presence of priapism a suprapubic catheter is recommended). Patients with SCI are at risk of urinary tract infections, sepsis, and renal tract calculi (secondary to in-dwelling
catheters or urinary stasis). Renal function should be monitored because of the risk of long-term renal damage.

Ileus and large bowel pseudo-obstruction
Paralytic ileus (small bowel) and large bowel pseudo-
obstruction are common in patients with spinal trauma.
They occur mostly in the first 72 h and is secondary to
neurological injury, immobility, and spinal and pelvic
fractures. They usually present with abdominal distension,

pain, and vomiting. The treatment is usually conservative. The patient is kept starved, a large bore NG tube is sited on free drainage and occasionally a flatus tube is inserted. Surgical decompression is rarely needed, but bowel perforation can occur if distension is not relieved.

Sexual function

In male patients with SCI normal spontaneous intercourse with ejaculation and orgasm are commonly lost (although medications and stimulation methods can be used). Infertility due to oligoaesthenospermia can occur.

In female patients sexual intercourse becomes passive although clitoral and uterine orgasm may occur depending on sacral and thoracolumbar innervation (long tracts).

Skin

The risk of pressure sores is very high. At least 80% of patients with SCI will have a pressure sore at some point and 30% will have more than one. The commonest sites are the heels, sacrum, and buttocks. Prevention is by regular turning (every 2 h), and the use of pressure mattresses and pillows (to prevent heel sores). It is important to check the skin behind braces and collars.

Psychological aspects

Most patients adapt to their disability although it can take up to 5 years. Counselling can be helpful, but most patients decline it. There is an increased risk of depression and suicide and family relationships are often understandably strained.

Outcome following spinal injury

Outcome is directly associated with age and the severity of disability. It is improved in patients who are transferred to a spinal injuries unit within 24 h. Experimental evidence has shown that the severity of SCI is dependent on:

- Force of compression.
- Duration of compression.
- Displacement/canal narrowing.

Persistent compression is a potentially reversible cause of secondary injury, but there is no clinical evidence that surgical decompression of the spinal cord or delay in surgical decompression influences the outcome of SCI (although experimental evidence does support early decompression). Recovery of motor function has been documented >2 years following injury. Improved recovery is associated with vertebral displacement <30% and age <30 years. Most recovery occurs in the first 6 months and is greatest during the first 3. An MRI finding of cord haemorrhage carries the worst prognosis, followed by contusion then oedema, with a normal MRI carrying the best prognosis.

Some facts:

- A 25-year-old tetraplegic has >60% of normal life expectancy (level below C5).
- A 25-year-old paraplegic has >80% of normal life expectancy.
- A 25-year-old partial paraplegic with mobility has >85% of normal life expectancy.
- 90% of patients with complete tetraplegia will recover some level of function in the muscles below the neurologic level of injury
- Patients with MRC 1–2/5 strength at 30 days will have a 97% chance of progressing to 3/5 at 1 year.

- In patients with MRC 0/5 at 1 month only 57% will recover to 1/5 and 27% to 3/5 at 1 year.
- 76% of patients with complete paraplegia do not change from 1 month to 1 year.
- 80% of patients with incomplete paraplegia recover to grade 3/5 in their hip flexors and knee extensors at 1 year (enough to stand with aids).

Treatment strategies that may improve outcome following SCI include:

- *Primary injury* nerve regeneration strategies:
  - stem cell transplants;
  - gene therapy;
  - electrical stimulation.
- *Secondary injury* neuroprotection strategies:
  - oxygenation and cord perfusion;
  - GM 1 ganglioside;
  - Minocycline;
  - Cethrin;
  - Activated macrophage implantation;
  - Thyrotropin releasing hormone;
  - Nimodipine;
  - Gacyclidine;
  - Riluzole;
  - Erythropoietin;
  - Fusogen polyethylene glycol;
  - Mild hypothermia.

Further reading

Surgery in Spinal Trauma. *Injury* 2005; **36** Supplement 1.

Aebi M, Thalgott JS, Webb JK (eds). *AO/ASIF Principles in Spine Surgery.* New York: Springer-Verlag, 1998.

American College of Surgeons Committee on Trauma. *Advanced Trauma Life Support for Doctors,* 8th edn. Chicago: ACS, 2008.

American Spinal Injury Association. Available at: www.asia-spinalinjury.org

Anderson LD, D'Alonzo RT. Fractures of the odontoid process of the axis. *J Bone Jt Surg* 1974; **56A**: 1663–74.

Anderson PA, Montesano PX. Morphology and treatment of occipital condyle fractures. *Spine* 1988; **13**: 731–6.

Beaty JH (ed.). Rockwood and Wilkin's Fractures in Children, 6th edn. Philadelphia: Lippincott Williams and Wilkins, 2005.

British Orthopaedic Association. *The Initial Care And Transfer Of Patients With Spinal Cord Injuries.* London: British Orthopaedic Association, 2006.

Bucholz RW (ed.). *Rockwood and Green's Fractures in Adults,* 6th edn. Philadelphia: Lippincott Williams and Wilkins, 2005.

Bulstrode C, Buckwalter JA, Carr A, Marsh L, Fairbank J, Wilson-Macdonald J,et al. (eds) *Oxford Textbook of Orthopaedics and Trauma.* Oxford: Oxford University Press, 2005.

Canale ST. *Campbell's Operative Orthopaedics,* 10th edn. Philadelphioa:Mosby 2002.

Corbett S. Introduction. *Spine Surgery AO Spine.* New York: Thieme, 2006.

Denis F, Davis S, Comfort T. Sacral fractures: an important problem. Retrospective analysis of 236 cases. *Clin Orthopaed Related Res* 1988; **227**: 67–81.

Denis F. The three column spine and its significance in the classification of acute thoracolumbar spinal injuries. *Spine* 1983; **8**: 817–31.

DeVivo MJ. Causes and costs of spinal cord injury in the United States. *Spinal Cord* 1997; **35**: 809–813.

Devlin VJ (ed.). *Spine Secrets.* Philadelphia: Hanley and Belfus, Inc., 2003.

Dormans JP. Evaluation of children with suspected cervical spine injury. *J Bone Jt Surg* 2002; **84A**: 124–32.

Effendi B, Roy D, Cornish B, Dussault RG, Laurin CA. Fractures of the ring of the axis. A classification based on the analysis of 131 cases. *J Bone Jt Surg* 1981; **63B**: 319–27.

Ferguson RL, Allen BL. A mechanistic classification of thoracolumbar spine fractures. *Clin Orthopaed Related Res* 1984; **189**: 77–88.

Fielding JW, Hawkins RJ. Atlanto-axial rotatory fixation. *J Bone Jt Surg* 1977; **59A**: 37–44.

Hendey GW, Wolfson AB, Mower WR, Hoffman JR, National Emergency X-Radiography Utilization Study Group. Spinal cord injury without radiographic abnormality: results of the National Emergency X-Radiography Utilization Study in blunt cervical trauma. *J Trauma* 2002; **53**: 1–4.

Hoffman JR, Wolfson AB, Todd K, Mower WR. Selective cervical spine radiography in blunt trauma: methodology of the National Emergency X-Radiography Utilization Study (NEXUS). *Annl Emerg Med* 1998; **32**: 461-9.

Jarrett DJ, Whitesides TE. Injuries to the cervicocranium. In Browner B, Jupiter AM, Levine AM, Trafton PG (eds). Skeletal Trauma. Philadelphia: WB Saunders, 1992, pp. 669–73.

Levine AM, Edwards CC. Fractures of the Atlas. *J Bone Jt Surg* 1991; **73A**: 680–91.

Levine AM, Edwards CC. The management of traumatic spondylolisthesis of the axis. *J Bone Jt Surg* 1985; **67A**: 217–26.

Magerl F, Aebi M, Gertzbein SD, Harms J, Nazarian S. A comprehensive classification of thoracic and lumbar injuries. *Eur Spine J* 1994; **3**: 184–201.

Mini-Symposium: Spinal Trauma. *Curr Orthopaed* 2004; **18**: 1–32.

National Spinal Cord Injury Statistical Centre. Available at: www.nscisc.uab.edu.

Orthopaedic Trauma Association. Available at: www.ota.org.

Rothman S. In: Herkowitz HH, Garfin SR, Eismont FJ, Bell GR, Balderston RA (eds), The Spine, 5th edn. Philadelphia: Saunders Elsevier, 2006.

Rubino LJ, Miller MD. Whats new in sports medicine. *J Bone Jt Surg* 2006; **88A**: 457–68.

Spine Trauma Focus Edition. *Spine* 2006; **31**(No. 11 Supplement).

Stiell IG, Clement CM, McKnight RD, Brison R, Schull MJ, Rowe BH, et al. The Canadian C-Spine Rule versus the NEXUS low-risk criteria in patients with trauma. New England Journal of Medicine 2003; **349**: 2512.

Vaccaro AR, Kim DH, Brodke DS, Harris M, Chapman J, Schildhauer T, et al. Diagnosis and management of thoracolumbar spine injuries. *J Bone Jt Surg* 2003; **85A**: 2456–70.

Vaccaro AR, Kim DH, Brodke DS, Harris M, Chapman J, Schildhauer T, et al. Diagnosis and management of sacral spine injuries. *J Bone Jt Surg* 2004; **86A**: 166–75.

Vaccaro ARE. *Orthopaedic Knowledge Update,* Vol. 8. Rosemont: American Academy of Orthopaedic Surgeons, 2005.

White AA, Panjabi MM. *Clinical Biomechanics of the Spine,* 2nd edn. Philadelphia: Lippincott, 1990.

Abdominal trauma

Abdominal trauma

Anatomy

The abdominal cavity extends from the inguinal ligaments below, to the costal margins above, with the domes of the diaphragm rising to the level of the 4th or 5th intercostal space in full expiration—the anterior axillary lines represent its lateral extremes. The flanks lie between the anterior and posterior axillary lines on both sides, and the back between the two posterior axillary lines. The abdominal viscera are distributed between the intraperitoneal and retroperitoneal compartments, both of which extend into the pelvis.

Intraperitoneal compartment

This contains the stomach, liver, spleen, 1st part of duodenum, the small bowel from jejunum downwards, the transverse and sigmoid colon, as well as the gynaecological organs in the female pelvis. The upper viscera lie under the protection of the lower rib cage but are susceptible to injury to the lower thoracic cage—the 'intrathoracic abdomen'.

Retroperitoneal compartment

Lying posterior to the intraperitoneal cavity, the retroperitoneum is bounded behind by the thick musculature of the back and flanks; it is usually subdivided into four regions. The central zone contains the aorta, vena cava, pancreas and 2nd, 3rd and 4th parts of the duodenum. The kidneys with the adrenals and ureters, ascending and descending colon lie in the respective left or right lateral zones, and the pelvic retroperitoneum contains the rectum, bladder and iliac vessels.

Mechanisms of injury

Abdominal trauma may result from either blunt or penetrating injury. The majority of abdominal trauma in the UK is a result of blunt injury, most commonly from motor vehicle collisions (MVCs); the penetrating trauma that does occur is largely from stab wounds, with gunshot wounds remaining uncommon in British hospitals. In urban America and South Africa, up to 35% of trauma admissions are from penetrating injury, with more gunshot wounds than stabbings. Penetrating injury may also result from MVCs, domestic and industrial accidents. Blast injury represents a special mechanism of injury for both blunt and penetrating abdominal injury and is considered in detail in Chapter 24.

Injuries to both solid and hollow abdominal viscera may be graded, the most commonly used system being the one devised by the American Association for the Surgery of Trauma (AAST). This largely relies on the radiological appearances of the injury, with grade increasing with size of laceration, subcapsular haematoma, or involvement of the vascular pedicle in solid organ injury and degree of tissue loss in hollow organ damage.

Pathophysiology of blunt trauma

There are four mechanism of blunt traumatic injury.

Compression

Direct compression by a lateral or antero-posterior force will crush immobile viscera against the unyielding restraints of the abdominal cavity. Those organs with strong peritoneal attachments, such as the liver and spleen, as well as the duodenojejunal (DJ) flexure, are prone to this form of injury as are the retroperitoneal viscera. Direct rupture can occur with associated massive haemorrhage.

Shearing

Rotational or deceleration forces applied to the abdomen result in differential movement of its viscera, with areas of relative fixity becoming the points of force concentration. The insertion points of blood vessels into viscera typically act as stress risers and these are commonly avulsed, leading to significant haemorrhage, as well as potential devitalization of distal parenchyma.

Bursting

Acute compression of the abdominal cavity generates a sudden rise in intra-abdominal pressure and pressure within the lumen of hollow organs, which if sufficient will cause bursting. The oesophagogastric junction is particularly prone to this mechanism of injury, and most diaphragmatic ruptures occur in this manner as the increased abdominal pressure decompresses into the thorax.

Penetration

Blunt injury to the bony pelvis, lumbosacral spine, or ribs may generate bone spicules that penetrate both hollow and solid organs—the pelvic organs are particularly vulnerable.

Pathophysiology of penetrating injury

The pathophysiology of penetrating injury is dependant on the degree of energy transfer. Stab wounds create injury confined to the wound track, unless the stab severs neurovascular structures causing downstream ischaemic damage. The peritoneum is violated in only about half of abdominal stab wounds and only about one-half of these injure abdominal viscera. The mechanisms of ballistic injury are described in detail in Chapter 24, but in brief are caused by an energized projectile passing through tissue and being retarded by the drag exerted by the tissues. This transfers energy from the missile to the tissues and this energy performs work. There is a high pressure region in front of the missile which creates a permanent track analogous to that created by a knife wound; in addition, as the energy transfer increases, so does the degree of radial dissipation of energy in the form of a low pressure shear wave which pushes the tissue away from the permanent track in a temporary cavity, which may achieve a diameter of 30 times that of the missile. The temporary cavity is at subatmospheric pressure and sucks debris and contamination into the cavity, which is dissipated through the tissues as the cavity collapses.

Penetrating abdominal trauma may exist in the absence of external abdominal injury as the cavity may be breached transdiaphragmatically from the thorax, or from below through the buttocks, perineum, and groins.

Solid organ injury

The solid organs most frequently injured in blunt abdominal trauma are the spleen, liver, kidneys, and pancreas; the liver is more susceptible than the spleen to penetrating injury.

Diaphragm

Diaphragmatic injury in blunt trauma is usually due to bursting as the abdominal pressure rises acutely and decompresses into the thorax; the left side is affected three times more frequently than the right, as the pressure is absorbed to some degree by the liver. Abdominal viscera may follow as a diaphragmatic hernia either immediately or many years later (Fig. 12.1).

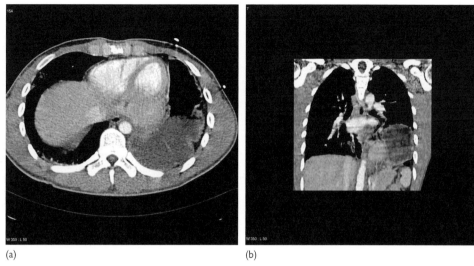

(a)   (b)

Fig. 12.1. Axial (A) and sagittal reconstruction (B) CT scan of the chest following blunt trauma in an MVC. The stomach and left lobe of the liver are present in the left hemithorax.

The incidence of traumatic diaphragmatic injury is approximately 0.63%, two-thirds of which are in penetrating injury. In stab wounds the direction of the wound track may suggest a potential diaphragmatic injury, but such prediction is impossible after a gunshot wound. The diaphragmatic injury may occur in the opposite direction with the penetrating agent traversing from thorax *into* abdomen. Diaphragmatic injuries generally occur in association with other injuries in both blunt and penetrating trauma, and are a marker of increased injury severity. Nearly half of all diaphragmatic injuries, irrespective of mechanism, are associated with liver injuries and haemopneumothoraces.

Liver

The liver remains the most commonly injured organ in abdominal trauma, even though it is shielded by the lower right rib cage. In blunt trauma, compression and shearing are the predominant mechanisms of injury. The liver is covered in a fibrous capsule and attached to the abdominal wall by the triangular, coronary and falciform ligaments. When compressed, commonly against the lower ribcage, the liver cannot easily move out of the way and the parenchyma is lacerated.

If the overlying fibrous capsule remains intact then haemorrhage is contained as a subcapsular haematoma, with the possibility of subsequent capsular rupture and profuse haemorrhage. More significant degrees of energy transfer may rupture the liver capsule and parenchyma resulting in free intraperitoneal bleeding. The greater the level of energy transfer the deeper the liver is injured with severe injuries crushing the central segments and caudate lobe. In shear injuries, which may also be caused by compression, as the liver attempts to move out of the way of the compressive force, the attachment of the supporting ligaments to the capsule are disrupted, tearing the parenchyma attached beneath. In severe injury the entire porta hepatis may be avulsed.

Stab wounds cause injury only along the path of the implement and unless a large vessel or biliary radical is transected, usually have low clinical impact. Ballistic wounding of the liver, however, has the potential for massive disruption. Low energy transfer ballistic wounds are largely akin to stab wounds in that the damage caused is largely confined to the direct tissue track. As energy transfer increases, so does the degree of temporary cavitation; the liver parenchyma is relatively non-elastic and accepts the stretch of cavitation poorly, hence, hepatic tissue tends to disrupt, rather than stretch. In addition, the fibrous capsule resists elastic expansion of the cavity compounding the tissue disruption—high energy transfer gunshot injury to the liver results in significant tissue damage.

Injuries to the portal triad are rare, but more common after penetrating trauma. Injuries to the extrahepatic biliary tree are extremely rare; approximately one-third are from blunt injury. The mortality rate is approximately 50%, largely due to vascular injury and this increases to 99% if both portal vein and hepatic artery are injured.

Spleen

In terms of trauma, the spleen bears many resemblances to the liver. It resides high in the abdominal cavity underneath the overlying ribcage, is surrounded by a capsule, and is anchored to the abdominal wall by a serious of fascial condensations referred to as the splenic ligaments. It is thus susceptible to injury from similar mechanisms. However, the capsule is more friable and tears more easily (Fig. 12.2).

Despite its relatively protected position inside the rib cage, the spleen is commonly injured in blunt abdominal trauma, most frequently from MVCs, although sporting injuries, iatrogenic damage, and spontaneous rupture are well recognized. The vascular pedicle of the spleen is closely related to the tail of the pancreas and injuries involving the pedicle invariably involve the distal pancreas as well. Blunt splenic injury may generate parenchymal lacerations or subcapsular haematomas (Fig. 12.3); injury with capsular disruption leads to profuse free intraperitoneal haemorrhage. Penetrating splenic injury is less common

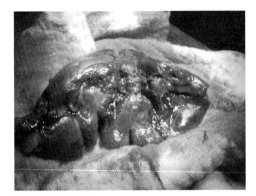

Fig. 12.2. Spleen removed after blunt abdominal trauma demonstrating multiple capsular lacerations.

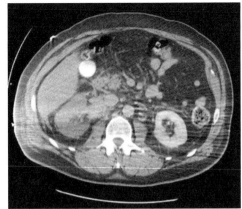

Fig. 12.4. Axial CT scan of right renal subcapsular haematoma following blunt MVC trauma.

than for the liver as the target is smaller and relatively more mobile but the pathological effects are similar.

Kidneys

Relatively protected in the retroperitoneum with the renal pedicle as the only point of fixation, the kidneys are normally only damaged in severe trauma (renal injury occurs in approximately 10% of all cases of abdominal trauma) (Fig. 12.4). Compression injuries require great force because of the protection offered by the posterior abdominal wall musculature, but the kidneys are susceptible to shearing of the pedicle in deceleration injuries.

The closed space of the retroperitoneum may tamponade the haemorrhage from significant renal injury. Blunt mechanisms predominate, even in gunshot-rich countries such as the USA. Injury rates are increased if the kidneys are abnormal, such as with cystic kidney disease, renal malignancy, and horseshoe kidneys.

Pancreas

The pancreas traverses the posterior abdominal wall from the duodenum to the spleen and, in contrast to the other abdominal solid viscera, is not encapsulated. Blunt pancreatic injuries are usually compression injuries as unrestrained

vehicle drivers strike their torsos against the steering wheel, crushing the pancreas, in the region of its neck, against the vertebral column (Fig. 12.5). In children, up to 75% of pancreatic injuries result from bicycle handlebars compressing the epigastrium; the duodenum is also often injured in this manner.

Blunt pancreatic injury requires a significant degree of force and there will usually be associated visceral injury. Parenchymal disruption by compression may also injure the pancreatic duct, which markedly increases morbidity and mortality, as the cycle of pancreatic enzyme activation and autodigestion accompanied by a systemic inflammatory response is unlikely to abate spontaneously. Pancreatic injury in isolation occurs in less than 10% of cases with a mean of four associated injuries. Pancreatic trauma, whether blunt or penetrating, has a high mortality. Large institutional series describe death rates of 3–32% in penetrating injury with that from shotguns and gunshots far outweighing stab-related deaths. Blunt injury has a mortality rate of 17–21%. Most deaths occur within 48 h of injury from haemorrhage or associated injuries.

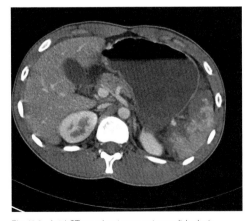

Fig. 12.3. Axial CT scan showing extensive medial splenic subcapsular haematoma.

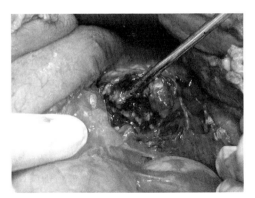

Fig. 12.5. Transected pancreas at laparotomy following blunt trauma.

Hollow viscus injury

The gastrointestinal and urinary tracts comprise the abdominal hollow viscera. The majority of the gut is protected from injury by its mobility, which suggests that it is vulnerable at points of fixed attachment such as the DJ flexure, ileocaecal junction, and the retroperitoneal segments. The gut, when injured, suffers either from direct trauma, particularly shearing at the fixed points, or injury to the mesentery and disruption of the blood supply giving rise to segmental ischaemia (Fig. 12.6).

Stomach

Gastric injury is relatively uncommon with direct penetrating injury commoner than blunt trauma. Blunt injury is often of the bursting type from acutely raised intra-abdominal pressure when the stomach is full, or shearing at the gastro-oesophageal junction. Penetrating injury to only one gastric wall is uncommon and surgery must inspect both anterior and posterior walls of the stomach. Blunt gastric perforations usually require significant force, are associated with multiple injuries, and have an increased mortality when compared with other gastrointestinal perforations.

Duodenum

Isolated duodenal injury is uncommon due to its proximity to other organs and the abdominal vessels. Epigastric compression (e.g. from handlebar injury) classically compresses the 2nd and 3rd parts of the duodenum against the vertebral column. If direct rupture does not occur, a mural haematoma may ensue, which increases in size over time and typically may present as epigastric pain and vomiting 2 or 3 days after injury as the haematoma obstructs the duodenal lumen. Shear injuries at the DJ flexure are common.

Small intestine and mesentery

The small intestine is injured by shear at the DJ and ileocaecal junctions and, occasionally, at other points fixed by congenital bands or adhesions. Direct injury may generate a mural haematoma, which if large will perforate immediately, but smaller lesions may gradually necrose the intestinal wall perforating up to 2 weeks after initial injury. Small bowel injury also occurs as a result of interruption of its blood supply because of mesenteric injury from either compression, shearing, or penetrating injury. If the ensuing ischaemia is not sufficient to cause acute perforation, segmental stenosis and later obstruction may occur. Mesenteric haematomas can extrinsically compress structures including the blood supply to their segments of gut. Free intraperitoneal bleeds from mesenteric vessels are often profuse as there is little ability for tamponade to limit the bleeding.

Colon

Blunt colonic trauma accounts for only about 5% of colon injuries. Deceleration causes shearing at the junctions of the intra- and retroperitoneal portions; the whole colon is susceptible to compression, and burst injuries and mural contusions follow the same pattern as in the small bowel. Colonic perforation may also occasionally occur as a result of extraperitoneal passage of energized missiles by virtue of the shear wave generated by temporary cavitation. Damage to the colonic blood supply is less common, but again may cause ischaemic perforation or delayed ischaemic stricturing. Colonic injuries are present in over one-third of patients with penetrating abdominal trauma with the transverse colon being most commonly affected; multiple colonic penetration occurs in a quarter of cases. Stab wounds tend to produce through-and-through wounds rather than injuring only one wall of the colon. Iatrogenic colonic injury during endoscopic examination occurs in approximately 0.1% of colonoscopies.

Rectum

The rectum is protected by the bony pelvis, which limits its susceptibility to compression and shear injuries. Blunt rectal injury is rare. It is prone to penetrating injury by bone fragments generated by pelvic crush injury and by any pelvic or gluteal gunshot. It may also be injured by anal insertion of foreign bodies (Fig. 12.7a&b).

Ureters

Both ureters are well protected in the retroperitoneum. Blunt trauma accounts for only 10% of ureteric injuries (and ureteric injury accounts for only 3% of all urinary tract trauma aside from iatrogenic surgical damage), but such injuries should be considered in children who have suffered spinal hyper-extension trauma, as this may avulse the ureters at the pelvi-ureteric junction. Pelvic injuries involving the ureters are usually associated with concurrent iliac vessel injury and a high mortality rate. The ureters are at risk more from anterior than posterior stab wounds as the paravertebral muscles protect from behind, and injury in gunshot wounds is again associated with multi-organ injury (Fig. 12.8).

Bladder

The bladder is an extraperitoneal organ and may be injured by blunt or penetrating injury. Blunt trauma, usually from MVCs, can shear the bladder at its attachments to the pelvis or pelvic compressive trauma will generate penetrating bone spicules, typically causing extraperitoneal injuries. Direct trauma to the dome of a full bladder, typically a kick to the lower abdomen in a drunken brawl, may cause the bladder to rupture intraperitoneally and generate a chemical peritonitis.

External genitalia

In the male, the external genitalia is susceptible to blunt and penetrating trauma. The commonest blunt injury is a penile fracture after forced bending of the erect penis during sexual intercourse. Blunt scrotal trauma has a high rate of testicular rupture. Penetrating penile or scrotal injury is associated with a high incidence of related injuries such as rectal penetration and femoral nerve and vessel injury.

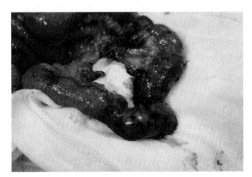

Fig. 12.6. Devitalized small bowel segment after blunt abdominal injury to the mesentery.

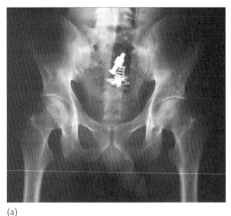

(a)

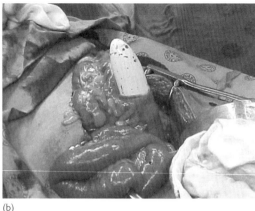

(b)

Fig. 12.7. (a) Plain pelvic radiograph showing rectal foreign body (a large dildo), which has perforated the sigmoid colon (shown at laparotomy, b).

Vascular injury

The abdominal vasculature is considered in five separate, but contiguous regions. Zone 1 is the midline retroperitoneal structures, which are further subdivided into those above the transverse mesocolon [suprarenal aorta, coeliac axis, superior mesenteric vein (SMV), and artery (SMA) and proximal renal arteries] and those below (infrarenal aorta and infrahepatic vena cava); zone 2 is the upper lateral retroperitoneum containing the renal vessels; and zone 3 (pelvic retroperitoneum) contains the iliac vessels. The retrohepatic vena cava, hepatic artery and portal vein constitute the final area.

Abdominal vascular injury occurs predominantly from penetrating mechanisms as all the major vessels are relatively

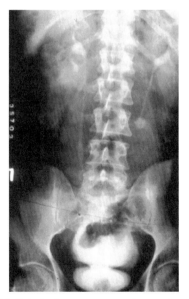

Fig. 12.8. Single shot Intravenous urogram demonstrating disruption of the left ureter by a penetrating fragment injury

well protected from blunt mechanisms throughout their abdominal course. Rapid deceleration during an MVC generates shearing forces on the origins of small vessels and may avulse them—typically either proximal or distal intestinal branches of the SMA. Direct trauma will either cause rupture, which may be intra- or retroperitoneal, with mortality being much higher for free intraperitoneal bleeds or intimal injury giving rise to later thrombotic occlusion. A well-recognized injury is the *seatbelt aortic injury*, where direct abdominal crush raises an intimal flap in large vessels, such as the infrarenal aorta or superior mesenteric artery. Ninety-five per cent of abdominal vascular trauma has a penetrating aetiology and vascular injury can account for nearly one-third of all abdominal trauma in a civilian context although this figure is much lower (approximately 5%) in military conflicts. This difference is a combination of the widespread use of personal ballistic protection of the torso in the military (body armour) and the tendency for military wounds to be of much higher energy transfer. Such wounds within the abdomen result in significant cavitation and extensive damage and, if accompanied by a major vascular injury, are unlikely to survive to definitive hospital care. Abdominal vessel injury is rarely an isolated phenomenon and associated small bowel injuries are common.

Injury complexes

Each organ and mechanism of injury have been described in isolation, but it is clear that many injuries occur as part of well recognized injury complexes, often with a specific aetiology.

Seat belt sign

Bruising of the anterior abdominal wall in the pattern and distribution of a restraining seatbelt is well recognized as a marker of potential underlying internal injury. This is true for three-point, shoulder and solitary lap belts, although the risk is greatest from a lap belt alone. There is a three fold increase in the risk of small bowel perforation if a seatbelt is worn (6 versus 2.2%) and a similar increased risk but substantially higher incidence (64 versus 21%) if a seatbelt sign was present or not. The commonest sites of injury are the proximal jejunum (deceleration injury), terminal ileum (shearing or crushing) and blowouts from sudden rises in intraluminal pressure.

Chance fracture

The Chance fracture is a purely bony injury of the spinal column as a result of forced forward flexion—typically as a motor vehicle occupant is thrown forward against a lap belt in an MVC. This flexion-distraction injury typically occurs at the level of the thoracolumbar junction or first 2 lumbar vertebrae; in children the injury may be lower due a lower centre of gravity. This fracture pattern is associated with a high rate of intra-abdominal injuries, most commonly small bowel perforation—rates of up to 60% have been reported, but a recent multicentre study of 79 patients reported a 33% incidence intra-abdominal injury, most of which were small bowel perforations. The incidence is usually reported as being slightly higher in paediatric Chance fractures. Approximately three-quarters of children with seatbelt bruising and a Chance fracture will require therapeutic laparotomy.

Pelvic fractures

Blunt pelvic fractures may be classified by the net direction of the applied force and the degree of haemorrhage is related to this. Lateral compression injuries of the pelvis are typically associated with significant injuries elsewhere (classically from an MVC side impact), but as they act to shorten the pelvic vasculature, haemorrhage is relatively modest. A similar effect is seen with vertical compression injuries, such as those suffered when jumping from a height. Anteroposterior (AP) compression, however, widens the pelvis and the hypogastric plexuses are frequently injured. High grades of AP compression may also disrupt the iliac vessels.

Pancreaticoduodenal injury

Figure 12.9 offers clues as to the likely concomitant injuries after pancreaticoduodenal trauma. The profusion of major vessels means that significant vascular damage is usually associated with injuries to the pancreas and duodenum, and this contributes to the significant morbidity and mortality previously described. There is a 40% chance of major vessel injury after pancreatic injury and 22% rate of aortocaval injury with duodenal wounds.

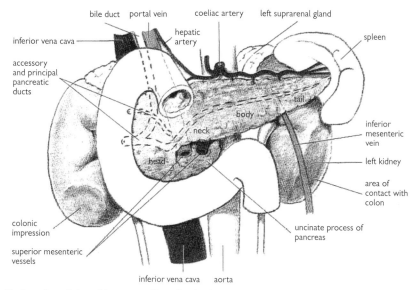

Fig. 12.9. The immediate relations of the pancreas. (Reproduced with permission from the *Oxford Textbook of Functional Anatomy*).

Initial assessment

Presentation

The presentation of abdominal trauma varies widely between haemodynamic stability and complete cardiovascular collapse with abdominal signs across the spectrum from normality to frank peritonism. Thus, assessment must be concise and timely, and should be repeated as often as necessary to ensure that nothing is missed.

Injury to the solid organs, blunt or penetrating, usually presents with hypotension from haemorrhage. Blood can be surprisingly non-irritant and so peritoneal signs may be absent initially, but tenderness in the respective upper quadrant is common. Lower rib fractures raise the suspicion of hepatic or splenic injury in blunt trauma. If the visceral injury is contained within the fibrous capsule then a subcapsular haematoma develops. Upper quadrant tenderness is present, but widespread peritoneal signs are generally absent as free rupture has not (yet) occurred. Significant intraperitoneal haemorrhage also occurs from damage to the mesenteric vessels and can be life-threatening, as there is nothing to tamponade the bleeding, especially if partial transection has occurred. Complete transection of any vessel normally results in retraction and contraction of the injured vessel with arrest of haemorrhage.

Different patterns of pain can offer clues as to the site of injury. Peri-umbilical pain arises embryologically from the mid-gut, which extends from the 2nd part of duodenum to distal transverse colon, while low abdominal pain arises from the hindgut. Pain between the shoulder blades is typical of diaphragmatic peritoneal irritation, although in cases of deceleration injury thoracic aortic transection can give similar pain. Epigastric pain boring through to the back is typical of pancreatic disease. Retroperitoneal injury requires a high degree of suspicion as the signs and symptoms may be subtle. Fullness, bruising, and tenderness in the flank raise the possibility of renal tract injury—haematuria offers confirmation, but not anatomical localization.

Assessment

Abdominal trauma, particularly blunt injury, is rarely an isolated occurrence and a systematic approach to the whole patient is required. The traditional approach of primary and secondary survey places the abdominal assessment into the secondary survey, but abdominal injury may be the contributing aetiology of a persistent hypotension that must be addressed in the circulatory section of the primary survey or junctional vascular injury leading to catastrophic cardiovascular collapse, which necessitates intervention even before management of the airway.

History

This may be obtained from the patient, friends and relatives, bystanders, or the police and ambulance crews. Information about the mechanism of injury gives useful clues to the potential for intra-abdominal injuries, but should be viewed in the context of the clinical presentation. In blunt trauma, details of the mechanism of injury allow an estimation of the level of energy transfer—in MVCs this includes the speed of impact, and the use of seatbelts and airbags. Other features such as collapse of the steering column, distortion of the steering wheel or ejection from the vehicle suggest an increased degree of energy transfer. In penetrating trauma, knowledge of the weapon is useful, in particular the length and type of knife blade used, the number of potential stab wounds, and the angle from which the wounds were inflicted. In gunshot wounds, the type of weapon offers a guide to the *potential* energy transfer, but this should not detract from a thorough clinical assessment. The adage *treat the wound not the weapon* remains apposite. The number of shots and distance between gun and victim is useful, the latter particularly relevant in shotgun wounds where the available energy diminishes rapidly at ranges above 5 m—the majority of shotgun pellets do not penetrate skin at a range of greater than 12 m. An AMPLET history should be taken.

Examination

A single abdominal examination is unreliable in detecting intraperitoneal injury (sensitivity of approximately 50%), whereas serial examination by the same observer is much better at detecting the onset of subtle signs and changes. The examination must include inspection of the back and posterior torso, as it is an area where penetrating wounds are notoriously well hidden. The presence or absence of bowel sounds correlates poorly with the presence of intra-abdominal injury. Digital rectal and vaginal examination and inspection of the external genitalia are mandatory. It should be noted that, in certain circumstances, resuscitative laparotomy, or thoracotomy in the case of multi-cavity injury, may form part of the circulation section of the primary survey. Assessment of the abdomen should also include notice of other specific injuries known to be associated with intraperitoneal injury, such as seatbelt bruising and lumbar spine fractures.

Clinically evident peritonitis may be absent or difficult to distinguish from abdominal wall injury, or overlooked because of the distraction of other injuries. Assessment must include the haemodynamic status and response to fluid resuscitation, as this will guide the choice of further investigations.

Gastrointestinal injury is notoriously difficult to diagnose. Traditionally, small bowel perforation was diagnosed at laparotomy for visceral haemorrhage—an opportunity denied to the modern surgeon in the era of non-operative management of up to 90% of hepatosplenic injuries. In the absence of free intraperitoneal air, CT may only show a small amount of free fluid and is insensitive for the direct demonstration of small bowel injury. Delays in diagnosis of small bowel perforation are associated with increased mortality and morbidity. The remaining retroperitoneal gut gives rise to diffuse signs initially (non-specific anterior abdominal pain, and vague flank and back pain) and it may be the onset of sepsis that prompts consideration of retroperitoneal gastrointestinal injury. The overall impact of abdominal trauma is significant as it contributes to 20% of all trauma deaths by way of haemorrhage and sepsis.

Haemodynamic monitoring

In most instances of abdominal trauma it is the degree of haemodynamic instability and response to resuscitation that informs the decision making process as to the need and urgency of laparotomy and choice of investigation. Thus the abdominal assessment should pay attention to those parameters and adjuncts that may have been instigated in other parts of the primary and secondary surveys. Pulse and blood pressure are easily measured parameters and the level of haemorrhagic shock has been equated with the volume of blood loss. It should be remembered that such estimates may prove wildly inaccurate in the young and the old. Young fit adults may tolerate significant blood loss without a rise in pulse rate or fall in systolic blood pressure; similarly, the elderly may have little physiological reserve and cardiovascular collapse may ensue very early in the injury process. Urine output is a sensitive indicator of end-organ perfusion and a urinary catheter should be inserted early in the resuscitation. The urethral route should be used unless there is a contraindication suggestive of urethral injury. Markers of potential urethral injury are:

• Blood at the external urethral meatus.
• High riding prostate on digital rectal examination.
• Scrotal or perineal haematoma.
• Significant pelvic fracture.

In the adult, resuscitation should aim for a minimum urine output of 0.5 mL/kg/h (1–2 mL/kg/h in children). Arterial blood gas analysis may give evidence of worsening acidosis, falling oxygenation, or rising CO_2 levels.

Resuscitative laparotomy

Where there is catastrophic cardiovascular collapse in the context of abdominal trauma—usually taken to mean imminent cardiorespiratory arrest from hypovolaemia—then immediate laparotomy to control haemorrhage is indicated. This should ideally be undertaken in the operating theatre. In such instances, it is important to remember to complete the remainder of the primary and secondary surveys as soon as is practicable so that other injuries are not overlooked.

Resuscitation room investigations

Blood should be sent for laboratory analysis. The serum amylase is normal in nearly half of all cases of pancreatic injury on presentation but resampling every 6 h for the first 24 h may demonstrate a rising titre suggestive of pancreatic damage.

The abdominal assessment of a trauma victim seeks to answer three basic questions:

- Has the abdomen been injured?
- Does the patient need a laparotomy?
- How quickly is that laparotomy needed?

Any investigations performed in the resuscitation room should add to the clinician's ability to answer those questions. More recently, a fourth question—does the patient require damage control surgery (DCS)?-has been added, the answer to which is based more on physiological data than investigations *per se*. Investigations that may be undertaken in the resuscitation room are to some degree dictated by the facilities and expertise available.

Plain radiographs

Antero-posterior chest and pelvic radiographs form part of the initial trauma assessment and should be performed in all patients with significant trauma. Aside from disclosing thoracic pathology, an erect or semi-erect chest X-ray may show free sub-diaphragmatic air indicative of intra-abdominal visceral perforation (Fig. 12.10); however, this is rarely possible in the trauma situation due to the necessity for spinal protection.

Fracture of the lower ribs increases the likelihood of injury to the spleen and liver, and gastric or small bowel shadows within the thorax—typically the left—suggest diaphragmatic rupture. Pelvic fractures on plain radiography should raise the suspicion of associated visceral injury. This can include avulsion of the prostatic urethra in males, extraperitoneal bladder rupture, or penetration of bladder or rectum by spicules of pelvic bone.

In ballistic penetrating trauma, plain abdominal X-ray may show radio-opaque foreign bodies and wounds should be marked on the surface (paperclips are ideal for this purpose). Free gas may be identified on an abdominal X-ray: clear delineation of both sides of the bowel wall by extraluminal air (Rigglers sign), linear gas streaks in the upper abdomen (falciform ligament sign), or loss of density overlying the liver (hepatic lucency), or odd-shaped air pockets may be evident on close inspection (Fig. 12.11).

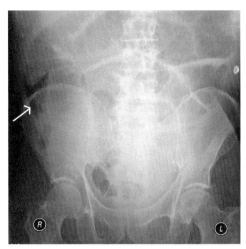

Fig. 12.11. Plain abdominal radiograph showing the peculiar shaped shadow of free intra-abdominal air (arrowed) following hollow viscus perforation.

Contrast radiographs

If there is suspicion of urethral injury the integrity of the urethra can be easily checked in the resuscitation room by a retrograde urethrogram. The technique is described in Box 12.1. In the past, when renal injury was suspected, a one shot intravenous urogram (IVU) may have been performed, but this has largely been superseded by contrast enhanced CT.

Wound exploration

When undertaken in the resuscitation room under local anaesthesia this is an imprecise technique with up to an 88% false positive rate. It is not recommended except when it can be performed in the operating theatre with the patient prepared and consented for proceeding to laparotomy as necessary.

Diagnostic peritoneal lavage (DPL)

DPL remained the gold standard investigation of blunt abdominal trauma for 30 years until the advent of readily-available CT and FAST scanning. Its role continues to be widely debated and whilst certainly no longer a first line

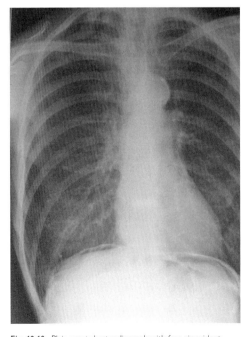

Fig. 12.10. Plain erect chest radiograph with free air evident beneath both hemidiaphragms.

Box 12.1. Technique of retrograde urethrography

- Aseptic preparation of the external urethral meatus
- Insert a conventional 16F Foley catheter so that the balloon sits in the fossa navicularis of the penile urethra and inflate the retention balloon with 1ml of sterile saline.
- The penis is placed laterally over the proximal thigh with moderate traction.
- 20 mL of iodinated contrast material is injected under fluoroscopy to fill the anterior urethra.
- In an intact urethra, contrast should flow freely into the bladder; if injured contrast will extravasate into surrounding issues. Extravasation of contrast from the bladder *may* be seen, but is unlikely with a low volume study.

investigation in most circumstances, it remains a useful, rapid, bedside investigation that can offer valuable information to the decision making process after abdominal injury, particularly if ultrasound and CT are unavailable.

The only definite contraindication to DPL is the presence of an indication for laparotomy, but DPL is relatively contraindicated in the uncooperative, the obese, children, pregnant women and those with previous multiple abdominal surgery. It may be performed by an open or Seldinger technique, which is quicker, but has a higher rate of complications. Insertion of both a nasogastric (or orogastric) tube and urinary catheter are mandatory before DPL. The main complications of DPL are gut injury, haemorrhage and intraperitoneal infection. The technique is described in Box 12.2.

A macroscopically positive result is seen when:

Box 12.2. Technique for open diagnostic peritoneal lavage

- Aseptic preparation of the infraumbilical midline and infiltration of local anaesthetic if not intubated and ventilated. In cases of pregnancy or pelvic fracture the DPL may be performed through a left or right upper quadrant entry.
- Sharp dissection through skin, subcutaneous fat, anterior fascia (posterior fascia if above the umbilicus) onto peritoneum.
- Open the peritoneum between two curved artery forceps and insert the end of a sterile giving set connected to 1 L of warmed crystalloid.
- Infuse 1 L of fluid (20 mL/kg in children), directing the giving set toward the pelvis.
- After infusion, place the fluid bag below the level of the patient (or the patient head up) and collect the lavage return (Fig. 12.12).
- If not obviously positive, send samples urgently to the laboratory for microscopy, Gram stain, amylase, and Red and White Cell counts.

The Seldinger technique is identical except entry to the abdomen is made by needle insertion and the giving set is inserted over a guide wire.

- >10 mL of frank blood is drained; *or*
- Gastric contents are aspirated; *or*
- Urine is aspirated; *or*
- The lavage return contains bile or vegetable material.

If the result is not macroscopically positive then the results are determined by laboratory analysis. This is often a lengthy process and one of DPL's greatest attributes (immediacy) is lost.

A microscopic positive result is seen when:
- RBC >100,000/mm^3; or
- WCC >500/mm^3; *or*
- Amylase >200 U/L.

Using these criteria, DPL after blunt trauma has a sensitivity and specificity of 94.4 and 99%, respectively, with an overall accuracy of 98.1%. When applied to penetrating trauma, these lavage counts yield an unacceptably low sensitivity, and the threshold for a positive result may have to be lowered to as low as RBC >1000/mm^3 to achieve satisfactory results.

A positive DPL has traditionally mandated laparotomy and in circumstances where no further imaging is available this should still hold true. The non-therapeutic laparotomy rate after positive DPL was historically given as approximately 15%, but in an era where selective non-operative management of abdominal injury is increasingly commonplace, this would now undoubtedly be higher. Mandatory laparotomy after a positive DPL precludes the concept of non-operative management of abdominal injury and now represents one of the biggest drawbacks of the technique. In a stable patient, a positive DPL may be augmented by a CT scan to quantify the level of solid organ injury

Focused abdominal sonography in trauma (FAST)

Ultrasound is an excellent non-ionizing radiation modality for identifying solid organ injuries and intra-abdominal free fluid. However, its utility in the management of trauma patients is limited partly by the lack of high quality mobile machines, but more usually by the lack of availability of a trained sonographer. This is particularly noticeable outside normal working hours.

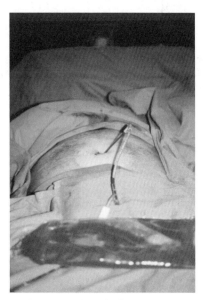

Fig. 12.12. Positive result from DPL. (Reproduced from *Trauma* 2007; **9:** 47–71, with permission from Sage Publications, London).

To overcome this difficulty, FAST has been developed as an easily applicable technique for non-radiologists using readily available portable equipment. It uses an ultrasound scanner, usually a 3.5–5.0 MHz convex transducer, in four defined positions on the abdomen to identify fluid in the hepatorenal and splenorenal pouches, and the pelvis (Figs 12.13 and 12.14). The fourth FAST position scans the lower mediastinum for evidence of pericardial effusion.

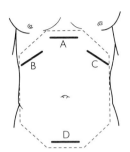

Fig. 12.13. The four FAST positions.

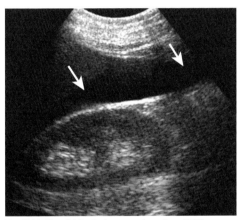

Fig. 12.14. Free fluid in the hepatorenal pouch on FAST (arrowed).

The technique is specifically designed to look for the presence of fluid in these four positions, and it is a rapid, easily repeatable bedside investigation that does not necessitate the patient being moved from the resuscitation room. It is not designed to identify solid organ injury. It is operator dependent and the view quality may be degraded by patient obesity and overlying bowel gas artefact. A small amount of pelvic free fluid in women of reproductive age is normal.

Studies have shown radiologists and non-radiologists who have been appropriately trained to be equally good at detecting free fluid. Volumes below 100 mL are unlikely to be identified by FAST, with only 10% of scanners able to detect 400 mL with a mean threshold volume for detection of 619 mL. For the assessment of blunt abdominal trauma in experienced hands FAST is reported to have sensitivity and specificity of 73–88% and 98–100%. In penetrating trauma, the evidence base is smaller, but the specificity remains extremely high, although the sensitivity falls to between 46–67%.

A positive FAST is a strong predictor of intra-abdominal injury, and when combined with haemodynamic instability necessitates laparotomy. In the stable patient, further imaging may be appropriate and consideration of conservative management. The problems arise when considering what to do with a negative FAST. There is currently insufficient evidence to safely allow discharge after a single negative FAST in abdominal trauma. If the patient is stable then they should undergo alternative imaging, ideally CT. An alternative is a repeated FAST scan—this may be performed after 30 min in the resuscitation room or after 6 h when admitted to a ward and this has been shown to increase the pick-up rate of occult injuries.

Investigations outside the resuscitation room

If abdominal assessment has not been completed in the resuscitation room then consideration can be made of continued investigation outside of the resuscitation room. This is usually in the form of computed tomography (CT) scanning. CT utility in managing both blunt and penetrating trauma has increased in line with the technological advantages in CT scanners, culminating in multi-slice CT scanning, which enables the entire abdomen to be scanned in a single breath hold, utilizing thinner slices, and reducing artefact.

CT scanning

CT scanning is indicated in abdominal trauma patients in whom suspicion of intra-abdominal injury remains after initial assessment, and who are haemodynamically stable. It is important to recognize the difference between haemodynamic stability and normality at this juncture. It is not necessary for a patient to exhibit normal vital signs to proceed to scanning, but they must have parameters that need minimal fluid infusion to maintain them. In addition, scanning of the abdomen should be considered when there are obvious injuries above and below the abdomen, a pattern which is highly suggestive of abdominal injury in between, and in the obtunded or unconscious patient in whom abdominal assessment is difficult or unreliable.

CT is the best modality for imaging the solid organs and retroperitoneum and gives useful information about bony injury, especially the pelvis where 60% of significant fractures are associated with visceral injury. It has to date been used predominantly in blunt trauma, as penetrating abdominal injury has traditionally been treated by mandatory laparotomy. With the advent of a more conservative approach in some centres, CT has been used to address the issue of peritoneal penetration, especially by tangential gunshot wounds (Fig. 12.15).

A non-contrast scan gives little information about the vascularity of organs or bleeding, but will identify free air within the peritoneum. Intravenous contrast and scanning

in the portal venous phase will identify haematomas within solid organs and a delayed scan 3–5 min later will identify ongoing extravasation of blood. The addition of oral (or nasogastric) contrast may increase the detection rate of gastrointestinal injury, although the evidence is conflicting; it also risks aspiration and delaying the scan at least 30 min to allow contrast to pass through the small bowel is often not possible. It is perhaps of most use to delineate suspected duodenal injury, as contrast passes quickly and scans are not delayed. If there is a suspicion of lower gastrointestinal tract injury, especially the rectum and left colon, then rectal contrast may also prove useful (the so called triple-contrast scan).

In penetrating abdominal injury, the sensitivity and specificity of predicting the need for laparotomy are both over 96% in most studies and approach 100% in some. The greatest contribution of CT scanning to modern abdominal trauma management has been its ability to reliably define the degree of solid organ injury, enabling the concept of selective non-operative management (SNOM) of abdominal injury. The American Association for the Surgery of Trauma (AAST) has produced specific organ injury scales for all abdominal and thoracic organs, which in most instances depend on CT evaluation of the organ. The scale for liver injury is shown in Table 12.1.

Features of injury on CT scanning

Pneumoperitoneum If not evident on the trauma series chest radiograph, a CT scan will clearly demonstrate extraluminal air as a black shadow (Fig. 12.16). If doubt still

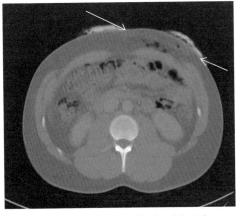

Fig. 12.15. CT scan of patient who suffered an abdominal gunshot wound. The wound track (between the arrows) can clearly be seen to be extraperitoneal throughout its course, sparing the patient a laparotomy. Reproduced from Whitfield & Garner (2007) with permission from Sage Publications, London.

Table 12.1. The AAST liver injury scaling system

Grade	Injury type	Description
I	Haematoma	Subcapsular <10% surface area
	Laceration	Capsular tear <1 cm parenchymal depth
II	Haematoma	Subcapsular 10–50% surface area; intraparenchymal <10 cm in diameter
	Laceration	Capsular tear 1-3 cm parenchymal depth, <10 cm in length
III	Haematoma	Subcapsular >50% surface area or ruptured subcapsular/parenchymal haematoma; intraparenchymal haematoma >10 cm or expanding
	Laceration	3 cm parenchymal depth
IV	Laceration	Parenchymal disruption involving 25–75% hepatic lobe or 1–3 Couinaud's segments within a single lobe
V	Laceration	Parenchymal disruption involving >75% of hepatic lobe or >3 Couinaud's segments within a single lobe
	Vascular	Juxtahepatic venous injuries such as to retrohepatic vena cava/central major hepatic veins
VI	Vascular	Hepatic avulsion

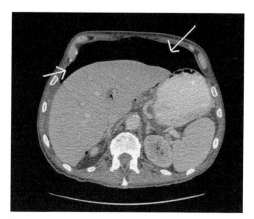

Fig. 12.16. Abdominal CT scan with abundant extraluminal intra-abdominal free air (arrowed).

exists, viewing the scan using lung windows will highlight extraluminal air more clearly.

Solid organ injury. Lacerations appear as linear hypodense areas, usually extending from one surface of the organ. Haematomas are often either centrally placed (Fig. 12.17A) or lie beneath the capsule (Fig. 12.17B) and are usually oval or round.

Bleeding. This may be evidenced by free fluid in the abdomen (blood has a CT density of 40 Hounsfield units) or by active leak of intravenous contrast which is best seen in the arterial phase of the scan.

Bladder injury. This is best demonstrated by a dedicated CT cystogram performed before intravenous contrast is given. 100 mL of dilute iodinated contrast is instilled via the urethral catheter and if no leakage of contrast is seen, further contrast is instilled. If a dedicated cystogram is not performed then bladder injury may be identified from the presence of intra-peritoneal free fluid, blood clots within the bladder or a deformation of the bladder shape.

Bowel injury. Identification of bowel injury is notoriously the weak point of CT scanning and many signs of bowel injury are indirect. The presence of free fluid without solid organ injury should raise the suspicion of gut perforation. Bowel wall thickening, mesenteric fat streaking and mesenteric haematoma are all predictors of bowel injury.

Magnetic resonance imaging

MRI scanning is rarely utilized in the acute management of abdominal trauma. It is often not available out of hours, and requires experienced MRI radiologists to interpret the images. The caveats that apply to transfer of a trauma patient to the CT scanner with regard to haemodynamic instability are equally if not more applicable to the acute use of MRI. Metal objects are not allowed within the scanner room and, thus, ventilation of a critically ill patient in the MRI suite requires specialist equipment not commonly available. MRI scanning may have a role to play in the investigation of the stable trauma victim in specific circumstances, such as pregnancy or renal failure where either high dose radiation or intravenous contrast media are contraindicated. MRI is also useful to delineate complex anatomy prior to reconstructive surgery, especially following hepatopancreaticobiliary injury.

Laparoscopy

Diagnostic laparoscopy in trauma is uncommon, but can be useful in certain circumstances. It is poor at visualizing the retroperitoneum and assessing the whole small bowel can be technically demanding and time-consuming. It is, however, excellent at assessing peritoneal penetration in stabbings or tangential gunshot wounds and at visualizing the diaphragms. If used to assess peritoneal violation any entry wounds should not be used as port sites due to the risk of restarting bleeding. Laparoscopy risks precipitating a tension pneumothorax or venous gas embolism if there has been significant vascular injury. Laparoscopy normally requires a general anaesthetic and should be performed in the operating theatre, although at least one study has used laparoscopy in the Emergency Department (ED) under

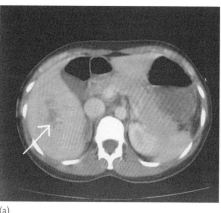

(a)

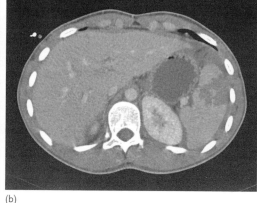

(b)

Fig. 12.17. Abdominal CT scan showing (A) a small centrally placed liver haematoma after blunt injury and (B) a subcapsular splenic haematoma.

local anaesthetic and sedation, to evaluate peritoneal breach after penetrating injury, facilitating discharge of 10 out of 16 patients from the ED. Therapeutic trauma laparoscopy is still in its infancy although laparoscopic splenectomy or splenic salvage surgery in isolated injury has been reported.

Laparotomy

Laparotomy remains an important investigation in abdominal trauma and the surgeon should have little compunction in opting for surgical exploration of a patient who remains persistently haemodynamically unstable after adequate resuscitation.

The trauma laparotomy and damage control

Trauma laparotomy

Trauma laparotomy is a demanding undertaking, and requires the input of experienced surgeons who must possess a wide range of surgical skills outwith those in routine practice. The basic technique is described in Box 12.3.

Box 12.3. The basic technique of trauma laparotomy

- *Preparation:* ensure a warm patient in a warm operating theatre with warm fluids being infused. The abdomen thorax and thighs are prepared aseptically and draped to expose this entire area, allowing for extension of the abdominal incision into other body cavities and junctional areas if necessary. Antibiotic prophylaxis including a second generation cephalosporin or co-amoxiclav is given; gentamicin should be avoided because of its adverse renal profile.
- *Incision:* a long midline from xiphisternum to pubis skirting the umbilicus to the left.
- *Procedure:* scoop out clots and free blood, and eviscerate the small bowel. Rapidly identify the source of massive bleeding and control by direct pressure or aortic clamping.
- *Packing:* use large abdominal packs. Start in the left upper quadrant under the left hemi-diaphragm and then the left paracolic gutter, the pelvis right paracolic gutter, and then above below and lateral to the liver. If bleeding is controlled allow the anaesthetist to resuscitate the patient further and place invasive monitoring at this stage.
- *Pack removal:* starting in the area thought least likely to be the main source of haemorrhage. Splenic bleeding can be dealt with by either splenectomy or splenic salvage techniques. As the right upper quadrant packs are removed, dissect free the free edge of the lesser omentum and compress the portal triad. Cessation of bleeding indicates portal venous or hepatic arterial bleeding. Continued bleeding suggests a hepatic venous or retrohepatic caval injury.
- *Visceral mobilization:* most of the duodenum is retroperitoneal and must be mobilized fully for assessment. Kocher's manoeuvre starts laterally and divides the peritoneal attachments, allowing it to be rotated upwards and medially. This allows inspection for the duodenum, head of pancreas, right kidney, and inferior vena cava. Incision of the peritoneal attachments of the small bowel from right lower quadrant to ligament of Treitz allows the small bowel, right colon, and caecum to be rotated medially to the left upper quadrant (Cattell–Braasch manoeuvre) exposing the IVC, aorta, 3rd and 4th parts of duodenum and inferior border of pancreas. Bile staining of the periduodenal tissues is strongly suggestive of duodenal injury. Incision of the left-sided peritoneal reflection and division of the splenic ligaments allows the left-sided viscera to be rotated medially exposing the aorta, and the origin of its midline branches and the left kidney (Mattox manoeuvre). Pelvic haematomas should not be disturbed.

Specific details of the many techniques required to deal definitively with many of the injuries mentioned are beyond the scope of this chapter (see Chapter 19 and further reading). The need to convert to a damage control approach should always be borne in mind when embarking on a trauma laparotomy.

Damage control surgery

Background

Mortality and morbidity from definitive surgery in the abdominal trauma victim has historically been high. The early surgical literature contained passing references to a concept of not operating in some types of severe injury, and packing of hepatic injuries (with a reasonable degree of success) was reported by Pringle in 1908 and Halsted in 1913, but fell from favour during the Second World War, due to further bleeding on pack removal and problems with sepsis attributed to the packs. Thereafter, sporadic successes from hepatic packing were reported, but it was the work of Rotondo and colleagues in 1993 that most clearly demonstrated the potential advantage of a damage control approach in the most critically ill trauma victims. Although he reported no overall significant difference between the two groups who had definitive or damage control laparotomy, when the subset of the most severely injured was analysed, DC had a significantly improved survival rate (10/13 = 77%) compared with (1/9 = 11%; p = 0.02) with traditional definitive laparotomy.

The basis of damage control surgery (DCS) is that it is the deranged physiology of the trauma victim that is responsible for the poor outcome and this is exacerbated by stress of embarking on lengthy definitive surgery.

Pathophysiology of DCS

- *Coagulopathy:* the coagulopathy of trauma has a dual aetiology. Exsanguinating haemorrhage depletes the reserve of clotting factors, which is further diluted by large volume fluid resuscitation. This, in turn, causes platelet and coagulation factor dysfunction and activation of the fibrinolytic system leading to a hypocoagulable state. Ongoing blood loss diminishes cellular perfusion and contributes to acidosis and hypothermia.
- *Acidosis:* prolonged haemorrhagic shock leads to cellular hypoperfusion, anaerobic cellular metabolism, and lactic acid production. This produces a profound metabolic acidosis, which reduces the efficiency of the clotting cascade, and promotes coagulopathy and blood loss.
- *Hypothermia:* hypothermia is a consequence of severe exsanguinating injury and subsequent resuscitative efforts, as well as climatic effects before arrival in hospital. Severe haemorrhage leads to decreased tissue perfusion and diminished oxygen delivery, a result of which is reduced heat generation.

These three physiological derangements are synergistic and have been termed the 'bloody vicious triad' of trauma (Fig. 12.18).

In short, the concept of DCS begins with an abbreviated laparotomy aimed at minimizing the metabolic insult, rather than restoration of anatomic integrity by temporary cessation of haemorrhage and limitation of gastrointestinal contamination, followed by admission to the Intensive Care Unit for restitution of physiology followed 24–72 h later by a return to theatre and completion of definitive surgical repair of the injuries.

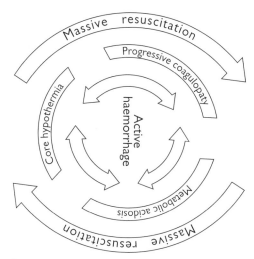

Fig. 12.18. The three interacting components of the bloody vicious triad of trauma.

Indications for damage control laparotomy
The decision for DCS should ideally be taken before laparotomy is started, by recognition of the poor physiological state of the patient during the resuscitation phase, when the need for laparotomy is first identified, or identification of injury complexes that would adversely affect the patient's physiology if definitive treatment were undertaken.

Surgical triggers for DCS are:
• Inability to achieve haemostasis.
• Combined vascular, hollow, and solid organ injury.
• Inaccessible vascular injury.
• Lengthy operative procedures.
• Need for surgical treatment of other injuries, e.g. craniotomy for intra-cranial haematoma.
• Need for non-surgical control of other injuries, e.g. angio-embolization of pelvic haemorrhage.
• Inability to close the abdomen or surgical reason for re-look laparotomy.

Physiological triggers for DCS are:
• pH < 7.2.
• Core temperature < 34°C.
• Coagulopathy (prothrombin time >16 s or activated partial thromboplastin time >60 s).
• Serum lactate >5 mmol/L.
• Probable operation time >60 min.
• 10 unit blood transfusion.
• Systolic BP < 90 mmHg for more than 1 h.

Technique of damage control laparotomy
The patient should be fully prepared and draped from the nipples to the knees to allow exposure and extension into the junctional areas and chest if necessary. The three main principles of the laparotomy are to arrest haemorrhage, limit contamination and temporarily close the abdomen.

Arrest bleeding: intra-abdominal free blood and clots are rapidly evacuated and four quadrant packing performed, or if haemorrhage is torrential a supra-hepatic aortic clamp may be applied. Packs are then removed,

starting in the quadrant thought least likely to harbour significant bleeding. Haemorrhage is temporarily controlled when found as definitive treatment may waste time on what may not be the major source of haemorrhage.

Liver bleeding can be reduced by bimanual compression or Pringles manoeuvre. These are unlikely to stop liver bleeding definitively and the commonest DCS manoeuvre is firm liver packing after mobilization of the liver by division of its supporting ligaments. If a single penetrating liver track is bleeding balloon tamponade by a Foley catheter can be used (Fig. 12.19).

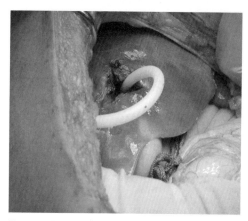

Fig. 12.19. Foley catheter balloon tamponade of hepatic bleeding.

If the spleen is bleeding a swift splenectomy is appropriate rather than wasting time on temporary haemorrhage control. Retroperitoneal haemorrhage not controlled by its own tamponade requires visceral mobilization for access (Cattell–Braasch or Mattox manoeuvres). Major vessel injury can be temporarily shunted.

Limit contamination: gastrointestinal contamination is limited by temporary exclusion of damaged segments of bowel. This can be rapidly achieved by soft bowel clamps, nylon tapes or linear stapler cutters. Biliary and pancreatic leakage can be managed emergently by drainage in the first instance either by sump drains or a biliary T-tube if easily placed.

Temporary abdominal closure: temporary abdominal closure (TAC) is a sensible technique because DCS mandates re-look laparotomy, and definitive closure is time consuming and markedly increases the risk of abdominal compartment syndrome (ACS). It may be achieved by suture of the skin alone or more commonly by application of a Bogota Bag (Fig. 12.20a, b) or Opsite sandwich closure.

Abdominal compartment syndrome
An acute rise in intra-abdominal pressure leads to a series of well defined physiological consequences, which have been termed the abdominal compartment syndrome (ACS). The aggressive fluid resuscitation of trauma is a well-recognized contributing factor to the development of ACS. Increased intra-abdominal pressure reduces venous return and decreases cardiac output; decreased perfusion pressure and direct compression of abdominal vessels reduces splanchnic and renal perfusion, which manifests as

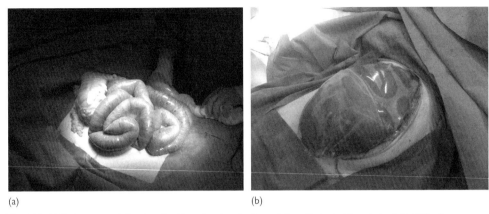

(a)   (b)

Fig. 12.20. (a) Oedematous and dilated small and large bowel protruding well above the level of the anterior abdominal wall.
(b) Protruding bowel enclosed in an opened intravenous fluid bag sutured to the anterior abdominal fascia as a Bogota bag closure.

gut acidosis and oliguria. Splinting of the diaphragms increases intra-thoracic pressure and requires increased ventilatory pressures to maintain oxygenation.

Treatment is by reduction in intra-abdominal pressure; whilst some medical measures, such as decompression of the intestinal contents by enemas or nasogastric aspiration, complete muscle relaxation, and the use of osmotic agents to offload abdominal oedema may help, the mainstay of management is surgical decompression of the abdomen. This may then be left open as a laparostomy (with or without temporary coverage from a Bogota bag or Opsite dressing) or closed temporarily with a mesh sutured to the abdominal fascia. It should be noted that ACS may recur even after TAC.

Resuscitation in intensive care

On completion of the damage control laparotomy the patient is transferred to ICU for restitution of normal physiology. Rewarming by electric blankets and warm intra-venous fluids can be augmented by warmed bladder or thoraco-abdominal cavity irrigation in severe hypothermia. Optimization of cellular perfusion is achieved by restoration of circulating volume with crystalloid and blood products coupled with supplemental oxygenation and inotropes as required. Aggressive replacement of clotting factors by infusion of platelets, fresh frozen plasma and cryoprecipitate is used to correct coagulopathy. The timing of re-laparotomy depends upon the speed with which normal physiological parameters can be restored, but is

normally scheduled for 24–48 h after initial surgery. If there is evidence of ongoing haemorrhage, contamination or development of ACS (which may occur even in the presence of TAC) then the return to theatre may be brought forward for further damage control.

Second look laparotomy

When the patient is normothermic with neither coagulopathy nor acidosis then they can be returned to theatre for definitive repair of injury. Packs are removed and any re-bleeding attended to; vascular shunts are replaced by definitive interposition grafts. Gastrointestinal injury can be resected and continuity restored or stoma created. Hepatopancreaticobiliary injury may be best served by surgery from a specialist as reconstructive surgery can be complex—this may necessitate transfer to a specialist centre prior to re-look laparotomy. In the absence of specialist skills T-tube drainage of the biliary tree is safe, as is the placement of large sump drains adjacent to an injured pancreas. In the face of pancreatic duct injury, definitive control of the duct is required otherwise a persistent systemic inflammatory response ensues, adding significantly to the mortality and morbidity. A complete inspection of the abdomen is repeated to detect missed injuries. It is often impossible to definitively close the abdomen at this stage and a variety of temporary abdominal closure techniques including vacuum systems, meshes and Velcro patches are available.

Selective non-operative management

Several decades ago haemodynamic instability after blunt abdominal trauma or any penetrating mechanism of abdominal injury was a mandate for laparotomy. Historically, this has led to a negative and non-therapeutic laparotomy rate of approximately 25%. It was thus realized that not all abdominal injuries injure the contents of the abdomen and that not all injuries within the abdomen require surgical intervention. This revelation coupled with the high complication rate (up to 41% following non-thera-peutic trauma laparotomy) and attendant financial costs, are the underlying rationale for the advent of selective non-operative management (SNOM). It was initially applied to blunt injuries only, and it is only recently that non-operative management of stab wounds to the abdomen has been adopted. The incidence of intra-abdominal injury after gunshot wounding is about 98% in most studies, and so non-operative management of gunshot wounds remains a controversial technique although high volume trauma centres such as the LA County trauma room report successful non-operative management in up to 30% of abdominal gunshot injuries.

Selective non-operative management of abdominal injuries now has fairly standard requirements as patients managed in this way have an enormous capacity for rapid, catastrophic deterioration. The following general criteria should be met before consideration of SNOM:

- Appropriate injuries (Grade I–III solid organ injuries on CT).
- No suspicion of hollow viscus injury.
- Cardiovascular stability (and an acute transfusion requirement of <2 units).
- Minimal physical signs.
- Availability of high dependency or critical care facilities for observation.
- Patient available for repeated frequent reassessment (preferably by the same senior clinician) to detect subtle changes in condition. Thus, patients requiring urgent surgery for non-abdominal injuries such as fracture fixation will not be available for repeated evaluation and must be excluded from non-operative management strategies.

Individual organ injuries generate their own criteria for SNOM and should be considered, as well as these general criteria. The investigation that underpins selection for SNOM is CT scanning, and thus by definition patients must be stable enough to undergo CT; this automatically precludes the haemodynamically unstable, which are usually the high grade injuries. Certain CT features, such as contrast 'blush' or active extravasation suggest that SNOM without intervention is unlikely to succeed.

SNOM may be achieved without any intervention, but the advent of more readily available interventional radiology has revolutionized non-operative management.

Basic technique of interventional angiography in trauma

Angiography requires a degree of haemodynamic stability as ongoing resuscitation is difficult in a radiographic screening room. Critical care facilities should be available in the angiography suite. Arterial access is usually gained by the femoral or brachial routes.

If active extravasation is demonstrated then embolization can be achieved by instillation of coils, gelfoam particles or a combination of both. The more selective

(and, therefore, distal) the embolization, the smaller the territory of ischaemia that is induced. If superselective embolization is not possible, for instance in the pelvis, then more proximal control of the internal iliac arteries may be indicated to obtain haemodynamic control, accepting the increased risks of collateral ischaemic injury.

Pelvic fractures

Significant bony pelvic injury is associated with a high risk of massive bleeding, usually contained within the loose tissues of the retroperitoneum, and this may be arterial or venous. Interventional radiology is now the mainstay of treatment. If CT scanning shows evidence of ongoing pelvic bleeding, such as contrast extravasation, bladder compression from haematoma or continuing transfusion requirement in the absence of other causes, then therapeutic angiography is required. If free intra-abdominal bleeding occurs, or temporizing measures, such as fracture stabilization by pelvic wrapping or external fixation fail to achieve haemodynamic stability then the patient may require immediate DCS with extraperitoneal pelvic packing to establish stability before diagnostic angiography +/– arterial embolization.

Spleen

Indications for angiography in blunt splenic injury include contrast extravasation (extrasplenic) or blush (intrasplenic), falling haemoglobin with known splenic injury and pseudoaneurysm formation. Superselective embolization of the distal vessels limits the area of ischaemic injury and maximizes the volume of functional splenic tissue. In cases where superselective embolization is not possible embolization of the splenic artery will significantly reduce the arterial pressure within the spleen, which may be sufficient to allow spontaneous arrest of haemorrhage, whilst maintaining perfusion from collateral vessels. Such a reduction of the perfusion pressure may also allow an operative splenic preservation technique to be achieved if embolization is insufficient and the patient ultimately requires surgery.

The increasing success of SNOM for splenic injury is reflected in the literature. A large retrospective review of nearly 1500 patients with blunt splenic injury identified attempted SNOM in 55% of cases with an 11% failure rate; increasing grade of splenic injury, increasing degree of haemoperitoneum and an Injury Severity Score >15 were all identified as predictors of failure of SNOM in blunt splenic injury. Interestingly, of those who failed SNOM, two-thirds did so within the first 24 h and only 10% went on to have splenic conservation surgery. Many reports suggest that the incidence of splenic salvage after SNOM is as high as 90% but these reports, as the EAST report does, count only those *considered* for SNOM—overall the rate of organ preservation is between 45 and 60%. The overall rate is much higher in children (~85–90%), potentially because the splenic capsule is relatively thicker in children, tears tend to lie parallel to the distribution of the blood vessels, thereby limiting haemorrhage, and children have a greater physiological reserve and no pre-morbid conditions to limit SNOM.

Liver

The indications for angiography in blunt hepatic trauma are similar to those for splenic injury and the same caveats apply. Most blunt liver injuries are low pressure venous injuries and will stop bleeding spontaneously, but contrast blush on CT suggests hepatic arterial injury and is likely be suitable for embolization using techniques similar to those for the spleen, aiming to place coils as peripherally as possible. A high grade hepatic injury is not a contraindication to potential SNOM, but it must be realized that the chances of failure are greater. Low grade injuries have a failure rate of 3–7.5% compared with 14% for grade IV and 22.6% for grade V injuries. Arterial embolization may be employed *after* liver packing at DCS.

Complications of SNOM of liver injury

- *Bile leaks:* occur in up to 20% of liver injuries, but can be managed without recourse to surgery. The majority can be treated by a combination of percutaneous drainage and endoscopic management of the biliary ducts.
- *Hepatic abscess:* these are a relatively rare complication and, again, are usually managed by percutaneous drainage. Persistent or recurrent infected collections will require laparotomy.
- *Delayed haemorrhage:* the advent of interventional radiology early in the management pathway has reduced the previously high rate of delayed bleeding from rupture of subcapsular haematoma; such delayed bleeds can be equally well treated by delayed embolization.
- *Ischaemia:* may occur as a result of the injury itself or embolization may disrupt vascular supply to hepatic segments giving rise to rising liver enzyme levels, abdominal pain and sepsis—resection of the dead segments is indicated.

Abdominal SNOM and head injury

Attempted non-operative management is not contraindicated by a concomitant head injury. The presence of neurotrauma increases the likelihood of disseminated intravascular coagulopathy which may exacerbate any intra-abdominal bleeding, so coagulopathy should be aggressively treated in these circumstances. Head injury increases the likelihood of SNOM failure but should not deter the attempt.

Critical decision making in abdominal trauma

Surgical decision-making in abdominal trauma can be complex, and should be performed by the most senior and experienced surgeon available. It is also true to say that decisions are not final and should be re-evaluated in light of each new piece of information or change in the patient's clinical condition.

Choice and timing of investigation

Which investigation to choose, and when, is largely based on individual operator experience, local availability of resources and, most importantly, the haemodynamic stability of the patient. The following rules are widely applicable and should encompass all clinical scenarios.

- *Catastrophic haemodynamic collapse with abdominal signs:* the patient is moribund and delay may prove fatal. The primary survey should be cut short for immediate resuscitative laparotomy. If the abdomen is negative then thoracotomy should be considered with cross-clamping of the descending aorta to achieve haemodynamic stability.
- *Gross haemodynamic instability with abdominal signs:* investigation is contraindicated and immediate laparotomy is required.
- *Gross haemodynamic instability without abdominal signs:* if a likely alternative source of haemorrhage is clear, such as obvious thoracic injury or multiple long bone fractures, then rapid resuscitation room abdominal assessment by FAST (or DPL) is appropriate. If this is negative, treatment priorities lie elsewhere. If positive, or no other likely cause of the ongoing haemodynamic compromise is evident then laparotomy should follow.

- *Haemodynamic instability with temporary response to fluid resuscitation (transient fluid responders):* if they are too unstable to move from the resuscitation room to the CT scanner then FAST (or DPL) is required. If positive and the patient remains unstable then laparotomy is indicated. If haemodynamic stability is achieved after a positive test then further imaging by CT will allow accurate grading of solid organ injury. If FAST is negative and haemodynamic stability is achieved, then the patient should be admitted and observed. In the face of haemodynamic compromise and a negative test then the decision lies between further imaging such as CT if stability allows, a period of further resuscitation with close monitoring and repeat test, or if haemodynamic parameters are worsening then laparotomy is permissible despite normal tests.
- *Stable patient with signs of abdominal injury* OR *an equivocal abdominal examination in the face of minor injuries:* these patients should undergo CT evaluation and the decision on observation, SNOM or laparotomy made on the basis of the findings.

Figure 12.21a–c summarize investigation algorithms for haemodynamically stable, labile, and unstable trauma patients.

Who needs laparotomy?

The indications for laparotomy have changed over the years and now depend on the degree of experience of the managing clinicians with abdominal trauma, as some experienced trauma physicians will now manage many cases of penetrating trauma conservatively.

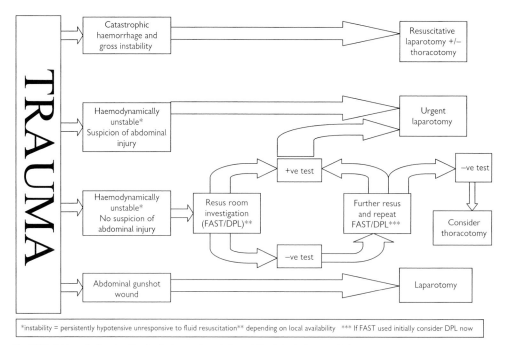

*instability = persistently hypotensive unresponsive to fluid resuscitation** depending on local availability   *** If FAST used initially consider DPL now

Fig. 12.21. (a) Investigation algorithm for the haemodynamically unstable abdominal trauma victim.

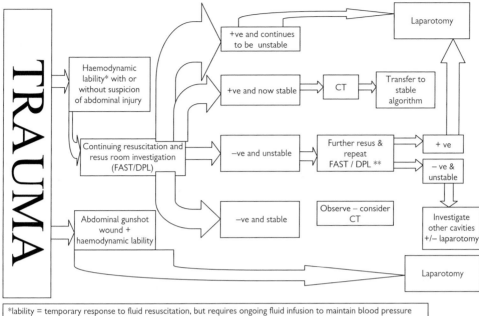

*lability = temporary response to fluid resuscitation, but requires ongoing fluid infusion to maintain blood pressure
**consider using DPL if FAST used initially

Fig. 12.21. (b) Investigation algorithm for the haemodynamically labile abdominal trauma victim.

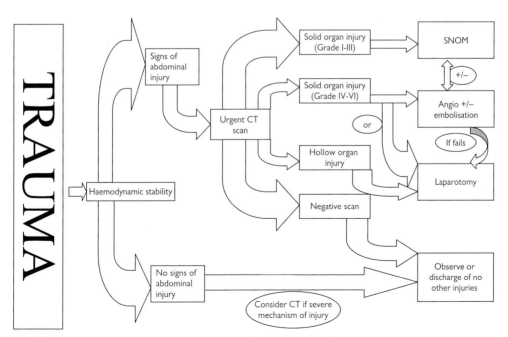

Fig. 12.21. (c) Investigation algorithm for the haemodynamically stable abdominal trauma victim.

In the UK the following remain recognized indications for laparotomy:

- All abdominal gunshot wounds (excluding those where the patient is stable and CT convincingly demonstrates an extraperitoneal wound track).
- Unstable patients after resuscitation with abdominal signs of trauma
- Unstable patients after resuscitation with a positive FAST (or DPL).
- Positive CT findings unsuitable for conservative management.
- Intra-abdominal haemorrhage uncontrolled by interventional radiology.
- Abdominal stab wounds with evidence of peritoneal penetration.
- Evisceration of abdominal contents or retained foreign body, as removal without visualization risks incurring further injury or instigating further bleeding (Fig. 12.22a,b).

Thoracotomy or laparotomy first?

In cases where there is actual or potential thoraco-abdominal injury the decision must be made as to which cavity is attended to first. A large study from USA has indicated that penetrating thoraco-abdominal trauma is associated with a high mortality (31%) and this is almost doubled (59%) if there is a need to explore both cavities. The authors assessed how many cavity procedures had to be interrupted to access another cavity (an indication of incorrect sequencing), which occurred in 36% of cases where thoracotomy was the first procedure compared with 53% of laparotomy first procedures. The commonest reason for inappropriate initial thoracotomy was a high thoracostomy output derived from abdominal injuries draining via a diaphragmatic rent.

Duration of observation period?

Whilst the indications and techniques for SNOM of solid organ injury are now well established, what is less clear is how long patients should be observed in hospital, and for how long they should be advised to refrain from strenuous activity, especially contact sports. CT evidence of organ healing appears to be related to the grade of injury with the more severe grades of injury taking longer to heal. The recommendations of the American Paediatric Surgical Association are that grades I, II, III, and IV liver and spleen injuries should be observed in hospital for 2, 3, 4, and 5 days, and refrain from strenuous activity for 3, 4, 5, and 6 weeks, respectively. No such guidance exists for adult patients. Routine re-imaging is not indicated for either adult or paediatric patients managed conservatively after blunt trauma; all imaging is directed by changes in haemodynamic status.

Haemodynamic instability with a pelvic fracture

As pelvic fractures have the potential for both intra- and retro-peritoneal haemorrhage it is important to ascertain the likely cause of instability urgently. Vertical and lateral compression injuries are usually associated with a lower degree of blood loss, which is commonly extraperitoneal. Instability in the face of these fracture patterns should prompt a search for other injuries. In both stable and unstable pelvic fracture patients pelvic stabilization should be promptly instigated; a pelvic binder or sheet is probably the easiest and quickest technique if the fracture pattern is suitable for this approach. In stable patients CT is the investigation of choice; in the unstable, a resuscitation room evaluation of the abdomen is necessary by FAST (or DPL). Peritoneal lavage in the face of a pelvic fracture should be performed by an open technique and in a supra-umbilical site to reduce the incidence of false positive tests—a negative DPL rules out the abdominal cavity as the source of haemodynamic instability. A positive FAST or DPL, plus instability merits laparotomy and if there is a large pelvic haematoma, extraperitoneal packing is used to achieve stability. At whatever stage haemodynamic stability is achieved, or the FAST is negative, pelvic angiography should be used to identify and embolize the source of haemorrhage. When definitive haemorrhage control has been achieved and physiology normalized, attention is then turned to more formal stabilization of the pelvic fracture.

Combined abdominal and head trauma

This combination of injuries is relatively uncommon, with large series suggesting an incidence of 5.7–13.4% of severe

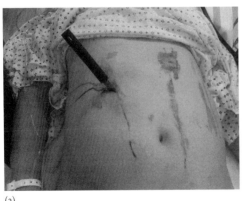

(a)

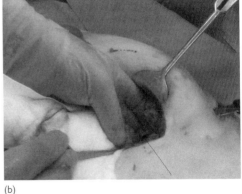

(b)

Fig. 12.22. (a) Self-inflicted stab wound to the abdomen. CT scanning suggested no intra-abdominal injury, but the knife was removed at laparotomy (b), which allowed control of omental bleeding. The tip of the knife is arrowed.

blunt head injury (GCS<8) and abdominal injuries on CT scanning. When present in combination, there are difficulties in both assessment and management. Neurological impairment will reduce the sensitivity of abdominal examination, and the permissive hypotension often used in the non-operative management of solid organ abdominal injury will aggravate secondary brain injury.

In the unstable patient, laparotomy takes precedence irrespective of neurological status, but consideration must be given to intra-operative intracranial pressure monitoring or burr holes if the GCS <9 or there were lateralizing signs before anaesthesia. Injuries to the abdomen and head are unlikely to have spared the intervening torso and the assessing clinician should be aware of the possibilities of thoracic injury as well.

Further reading

American College of Surgeon Committee on Trauma. *Advanced Trauma Life Support* (ATLS®) Chicago: ACS, 2007. Available at: www.trauma.org

Amin SN, Rowlands BJ. Colorectal trauma. *Trauma* 2000; **2**: 211–21.

Boffard KD (ed.). *Manual of Definitive Surgical Trauma Care*, 2nd edn. London: Hodder Arnold, 2007.

Bowley DMG, Barker P, Boffard KD. Damage control—concepts and practice. *J Roy Army Med Corps* 2000; **146**: 172–82.

Feliciano DV, Mattox KL, Moore EE. *Trauma*, 6th edn. New York: McGraw-Hill, 2008.

Herr BW, Gagliano RA. Historical perspective and current management of colonic and intraperitoneal rectal trauma. *Curr Surg* 2005; **62**(2): 187–92.

Nahum AM, Melvin J. *Accidental Injury: Biomechanics and Prevention*. Berlin: Springer, 2001.

Pietzman AB, Heil B, Rivera, et al. Blunt splenic injury in adults: multi-institutional study of the Eastern Association for the Surgery of Trauma. *J Trauma* 2000; **49**: 177–89.

Rotondo M, Schwab CW, McGonigal MD, et al. Damage control: an approach for improved survival in exsanguinationing penetrating abdominal injury. *J Trauma* 1993; **35**(3): 375–82.

Paterson Brown S. *A Companion to Specialist Surgical Practice: Core Topics in General and Emergency Surgery*, 3rd edn. London: Elsevier Sanders, 2008.

Stylianos S, and the APSA Trauma Committee. Evidence based guidelines for resource utilization in children with isolated spleen or liver injury. *J Paediat Surg* 2000; **35**: 164–9.

Whitfield C, Garner JP. The early management of gunshot wounds part II: the abdomen, extremities and special situations. *Trauma* 2007; **9**: 47–71.

Whitfield C, Garner JP. The early management of gunshot wounds part II: the abdomen, extremities and special situations. *Trauma* 2007; **9**: 47–71.

Whitfield CG, Garner JP. Beyond splenectomy—options for the management of splenic trauma. *Trauma* 2008; **10**: 247–59.

Pelvic injuries

Pelvic injuries

Anatomy

Pelvis means 'basin-like'. True to its name, the pelvis is a basin formed by a strong bony ring whose stability depends on ligamentous integrity. Disruption of the ring can fill the basin with blood from adjacent vascular structures. Damage to urogenital, gastrointestinal, and neurological structures must also be considered in the presence of pelvic injury.

Bones and ligaments

The pelvis consists of the union of the sacrum and the two innominate bones. The latter are derived from the fusion of three ossification centres, of the ilium, pubis, and ischium through the triradiate cartilage at the acetabulum. Rotational deformation of the pelvis by external or internal rotation, and vertical deformation are resisted by horizontally and vertically orientated ligaments, respectively.

Horizontal stability

Horizontal stability is provided by:
- The symphysis pubis, which unites the two innominate bones anteriorly.
- Sacrospinous ligaments that run horizontally from the sacrum and coccyx inserting onto the ischial spine.
- Sacro-iliac ligaments (anterior and short posterior) that bind the sacrum and innominate bones.
- Ilio-lumbar ligaments that originate from the lumbar 4th and 5th vertebrae and insert on the posterior iliac crest.

Vertical stability

Vertical stability is provided by:
- Sacrotuberous ligaments running vertically from the sacrum and coccyx inserting on the ischial tuberosity.
- Sacro-iliac ligaments (long posterior) binding the sacrum and innominate bones posteriorly.
- Lumbosacral ligaments originating from the transverse process of L5 and inserting onto the sacral ala.

Vascular structures

The common iliac artery divides into the internal and external iliac arteries anterior to the sacroiliac joint. The external iliac artery descends along the psoas muscle, giving off the inferior epigastric and deep circumflex iliac arteries, before passing under the inguinal ligament to leave the pelvis.

The internal iliac artery descends into the pelvis dividing into anterior and posterior divisions at the greater sciatic foramen. These vessels give rise to various named branches.

Venous anatomy is named according to the arterial anatomy. In addition there is also a venous plexus anterior to the sacrum, which is at risk of traumatic injury.

Urogenital anatomy

The bladder lies immediately posterior to the pubis, with the urethra arising from its inferior aspect. In men the urethra descends through the prostate and urogenital diaphragm to enter the penis.

In women the urethra is only about 4.5 cm long and courses directly through the urogenital diaphragm. The uterus is suspended by 2 round ligaments, and sits between the bladder and rectum.

Gastrointestinal anatomy

The sigmoid colon terminates anterior to the 3rd sacral vertebral body where it becomes the rectum. From here the rectum descends anterior to the sacrum and coccyx.

Neurological anatomy

Neurological supply is from the anterior rami of the 4th and 5th lumbar nerves form the lumbosacral trunk. This joins the anterior sacral rami to form the sacral plexus on the piriformis muscle.

Classification of injury

Various classifications have been proposed. A widely used system is the Young and Burgess modification of the Pennal classification. The system is based on mechanism of injury and radiographic evidence of instability.

The system divides injuries into four mechanisms:
- Lateral compression (LC)
- Anterior-posterior compression (APC).
- Vertical shear.
- Combination.

APC and LC are defined according to the anterior pelvic injury. Both are subdivided into 3 subsets according to the degree of posterior disruption of the pelvis.

Lateral compression

A lateral compression force is applied either directly to the innominate bone or indirectly via the iliac crest and proximal femur. All of the three subsets involve transverse fracture of the pubic rami; this may be ipsilateral or contralateral to the posterior injury (Figs 13.1–13.3). The subsets are classified according to the posterior injury as outlined in Box 13.1.

> 2.5 cm symphyseal diastasis implies rupture of sacrospinous liogament.

Avulsion fractures of lateral sacrum and ischial spine indicate rotational instability (Fig. 13.1).

Whilst compression fractures of the sacrum are generally stable, a sacral fracture with a gap may imply vertical instability.

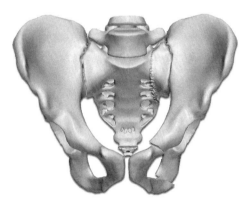

Fig. 13.1. Lateral compression I fracture. Highlights transverse fracture of the ipsilateral pubic ramus. There will often be a compression fracture of the sacrum as the hemipelvis is driven into the sacrum.

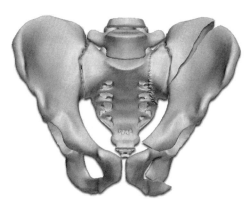

Fig 13.2. Lateral compression II fracture. Highlights transverse fracture of the ipsilateral pubic ramus. Additionally, there is a fracture through the iliac wing, with medial rotation of the separated segment.

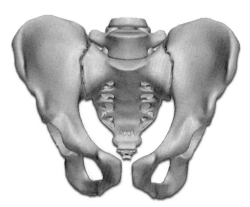

Fig. 13.4. AP compression fracture showing mild diastasis of the pelvic ring.

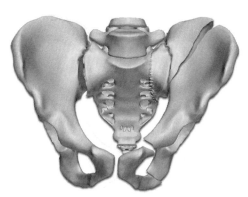

Fig. 13.3. Lateral compression III fracture. Highlights transverse fracture of the ipsilateral pubic ramus. Additionally, there is a fracture through the iliac wing. Furthermore, there is SI disruption of the contralateral hemipelvis and external rotation of the segment. An 'open book' appearance may be seen on the contralateral side.

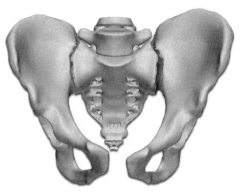

Fig. 13.5. AP compression II fracture. Showing diastasis of the pubic symphysis and anterior disruption of the left SI joint; the posterior ligaments keep the left hemipelvis attached to the ring, causing the 'open-book' appearance.

AP compression

An anterior-posterior force results in a pubic symphyseal diastasis or vertical fracture of the pubic rami (Figs 13.4–13.6). This injury is differentiated from the vertical shear category by the absence of cranial displacement of the hemi-pelvis.

Vertical shear

This results from vertically applied forces, such as when a patient has fallen from a significant height. Such forces result in a symphyseal injury or vertical rami fractures anteriorly and vertical displacement of the hemi-pelvis. These injuries are horizontally and vertically unstable (Fig. 13.7).

Combination patterns

Injuries to the pelvis may result from a combination of the injury mechanisms described. These injuries vary in their instability.

Mechanism of injury

The types of incidents in which the pelvis is typically at risk of fracture are:
• Frontal impact MVC.

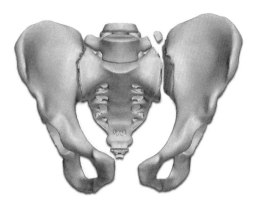

Fig. 13.6. AP compression III fracture. There is complete separation of the left hemipelvis from the ring. This is caused by total SI disruption, which is associated with high energy transfer and serious associated injury.

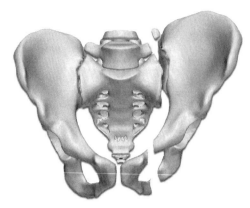

Fig. 13.7. Vertical shear injury. Showing complete anterior ring disruption on the left (which could also be symphyseal diastasis) and complete left-sided SI disruption with the left hemipelvis moving in a cephalad direction.

- Lateral impact MVC.
- Motorcycle collision.
- Significant fall from height.
- Crush injury.

Thus, patients presenting with these mechanisms should be assumed to have a pelvic fracture until ruled out by appropriate radiography.

Management of pelvic ring fractures

Patients with suspected pelvic trauma require assessment along established trauma guidelines. Approximately 5% of all polytrauma patients will have a pelvic injury. Bony disruption and concomitant vascular injury can lead to significant circulatory compromise or, indeed, fatal haemorrhage into the pelvis. For this reason, the pelvis should be considered during the primary survey and initial resuscitation. The pelvic girdle is a strong structure and a significant amount of energy is required to disrupt the ring. The force resulting in bony injury will have been transmitted to the pelvic viscera, and also to other organ systems, resulting in associated injuries in the majority of cases. Fewer than 30% of pelvic injuries will be isolated to the bony pelvis. Therefore, the pelvic injury should be sought, but associated injuries are often as life-threatening:
- Head injuries   40%
- Chest injuries   30%
- Limb injuries   35%
- Abdominal injuries   15%

Pelvic fractures may present in one of several ways:
- Reported from pre-hospital team.
- Binding in place from pre-hospital team.
- Mechanism of injury.
- Complaining of pain in lower back/groin/hips.
- Limb deformity.
- Bleeding from urethra, vagina or rectum.
- X-ray findings.
- Unexplained hypotension.

Pre-hospital care

Pre-hospital teams are increasingly aware of the need for early identification and management of serious pelvic injuries. Initial assessment and management follows established trauma guidelines. Pre-hospital teams need to assess the scene, and useful information can be gleaned by reading the wreckage. Injury patterns can be predicted to an extent, but the patient still requires full assessment and appreciation of the likely forces involved. Any concern regarding the potential for pelvic fracture should result in a cautious approach using immobilization until injury is excluded. The reliability of clinical examination in this environment is poor. Additional movement of the pelvis during clinical examination may provoke clot disruption and further bleeding. Thus, the pelvis should be splinted, and patients will be packaged and presented to the emergency department with immobilization devices in situ. Fluid therapy should be given judiciously—250 mL boluses of crystalloid titrated to the presence of a radial pulse. When moving and handling the patient, movement should be kept to a minimum. Different pre-hospital systems have different packaging protocols, but the following system is advocated in pelvic injury. The clothing should normally be removed, and the patient should be log rolled to approximately 15 degrees each side to facilitate placement of binding devices and immobilization on a scoop stretcher within a vacuum mattress.

Emergency department

On arrival in the emergency department, the patient should be moved and handled with great care to avoid clot disruption. Log rolling should be to approximately 15 degrees to facilitate clinical examination, removal of debris, and transfer. Pelvic binding devices should be left in situ. No attempt should be made to remove them, as inadvertent movement of bony fragments may worsen bleeding and cause circulatory collapse. During the primary survey, initial radiographs should include a pelvic film. Pelvic splinting devices allow penetration of X-rays and should therefore be left in place. Following radiographic confirmation of fracture, significant bleeding should be assumed to be present if there is:
- Unexplained tachycardia.
- Narrowing of pulse pressure.
- Hypotension unresponsive to judicious fluid challenge.

A patient who does not respond to initial attempts at fluid replacement and who has a pelvic fracture should be considered to be bleeding from the pelvis until proven otherwise.

The primary treatment of the bleeding is not fluids; it is to stop the bleeding.

Pelvic injuries bleed extensively. The pelvic girdle is large enough to contain all the circulating volume and more. Haemorrhage can be from four sources:
- Arterial haemorrhage.
- Venous plexus bleeding.
- Soft tissue capillary bleeding.
- Bone end bleeding.

Reduction in mortality from these injuries relies on stopping haemorrhage by appropriate splinting, early recognition of severity of injury and early involvement of appropriate specialities.

Definitive options include angiography, external fixation, laparotomy, and pelvic packing. The resuscitation team should take all steps necessary to preserve clotting function, whilst the definitive treatment is organized. This includes early involvement of laboratory services, and a massive transfusion protocol should be invoked at an early stage, facilitating release of red blood cells and appropriate blood products. Early involvement of senior team members is vital in these patients.

The decision regarding the definitive treatment strategy depends to a degree on the resources available. A sample protocol is given in Fig. 13.8. Once the decision has been made, it should be communicated effectively to all respective team members, stating clearly that the patient has pelvic fracture with haemodynamic compromise.

External fixation has a limited role and offers little benefit over simple binding techniques. Its use in the resuscitation phase is questionable. Angiographic embolization works well for arterial haemorrhage, but does not control venous or bone-end bleeding. It has the disadvantage of being a specialized procedure requiring access to interventional radiologists and appropriate equipment. Additionally, the clinical state of the patient and associated injuries may require intubation and ventilation. The radiology suite is often a remote area of the hospital and arrangements should be made before, during, and after transfer to this area to optimize patient safety. Laboratory and portering staff should be informed of exactly where the patient is going. On-going massive transfusion and critical care are often required during angiography.

Radiography

Several radiological techniques may be required in the diagnosis and early stabilization of pelvic fractures and associated injuries, including plain radiographs, ultrasound (FAST), CT scanning, and angiography.

The first plain AP radiograph should be performed during the primary survey. Box 13.1 highlights the radiographic features relevant to pelvic fractures. Posterior injury may not be appreciated on standard AP radiographs. Subsequent imaging, such as inlet/outlet views, or more commonly CT evaluation, is required for definitive classification. Note that pelvic binding may reduce the fracture to such an extent that it is difficult to see on plain radiography, so careful haemodynamic monitoring is required once pelvic binding is released, and in cases where there is high suspicion, further imaging should be performed to exclude significant injury.

Box. 13.1. Radiographic signs of pelvic fracture seen on pelvic radiography

Anterior features
- Diastasis of symphysis.
- Public rami fractures.

Posterior features
- SI joint disruption.
- Sacral fracture.
- Iliac fracture.

During the immediate resuscitation period, focused sonography (FAST) may identify free intraperitoneal fluid. In the context of haemodynamic instability this points to intra-peritoneal haemorrhage. The patient with both abdominal and pelvic injury will require multi-speciality intra-operative management. Early consultation and liaison between orthopaedic and general surgical specialities is key to a successful outcome.

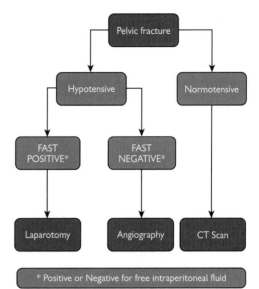

Fig. 13.8. Example of a guideline for the immediate management of pelvic fractures.

Pelvic stabilization

Reduction and stabilization of the pelvic ring is the key to arresting haemorrhage. This acts via a variety of mechanisms:

- Tamponade effect; reduction in pelvic volume (this will not stop active arterial haemorrhage).
- Increasing apposition of bone fragments, reducing bony haemorrhage.
- Stabilization of fragments thus reducing clot disruption.

Non-invasive external fixation

Displaced pelvic fractures can be successfully reduced and temporarily stabilized with the use of a bed sheet pulled tightly round the pelvis and fixed with forceps. Commercially-designed devices are also available, such as the SAM Splint™. This is applied as shown is Figures 13.9–13.11. Many trauma organizations recommend early application of such devices to provide external compression in any unstable pelvic fracture. other non-invasive methods of immobilizing pelvic fractures are:

- Kendrick extrication device (inverted).
- Broad bandages.
- Bed sheet.
- Feet tied together.
- Vacuum mattress.

When placing pelvic binding devices it is essential to avoid covering up the femoral vessels. These may be needed during subsequent management for central venous access or for femoral arterial access for angiography.

Invasive external fixation

This may be sub-classified into anterior and posterior fixation.

Anterior external fixation requires 2–3 pins to be driven down from the iliac wing centrally towards the thinner portion of the ilium. The pins are connected via a modular device, thus restoring anterior stability. They require significant skill and fluoroscopy to apply, often needing 30–40 min in theatre for their application. Such devices cannot provide posterior stability in vertically unstable fractures.

A posteriorly placed C-clamp was developed by Ganz to provide posterior stability in the resuscitation phase. Large percutaneous pins are placed 3–4 fingers breath anterolateral to the PSIS. These are joined by a C-shaped clamp with threaded bolts to close the posterior diastasis and provide stability.

Invasive internal fixation

In general, external fixation is applied as a damage control measure whilst internal fixation is the definitive treatment, only to be carried out once the patient has been physiologically optimized. Internal fixation may require anterior, or a combination of anterior and posterior stabilization.

In cases of pubic symphyseal diastasis anterior fixation is usually achieved with the use of open reduction via a pfannenstiel incision and fixation with a plate. Superior pubic rami fractures may be managed in a similar manner or with percutaneous screw fixation.

Posterior fixation may be achieved via open or percutaneous techniques.

Open reduction involves an anterior approach that parallels the iliac wing or a posterior approach parallel and adjacent to the posterior iliac spine.

Crescent fractures of the ilium and sacroiliac joint disruptions may be fixed with a closed manipulation and percutaneous screw fixation. Alternatively, open reduction via anterior or posterior approach and fixation with plate or screws may be employed.

Sacral fractures may be fixed via an open posterior approach with plating, or with closed manipulation and percutaneous screws.

Angiography techniques

Invasive angiographic techniques have unquestionably improved the mortality of this difficult patient group. Those who require open surgery to control bleeding points have a high mortality. Angiography and associated embolization techniques can successfully stop arterial bleeding and obviate the need for open surgery. It is limited by a lack of availability and expertise in all centres. The technique involves placement of arterial cannulae, often on the contralateral side to the injury. Once cannulated, fluoroscopic guidance allows advancement of smaller catheters into distal arteries, such as the superior gluteal artery. Fluoroscopic angiography confirms distal bleeding points and allows the practitioner to decide on the site for embolization. There are a variety of methods available including placement of foams, coils, and beads. The exact method used will be operator-, site-, and patient-dependent. Of note, some methods provide only temporary occlusion, dissolving over the subsequent weeks. Physiological clotting should occur at the distal site before native repair of the blood vessel. When the foam dissolves, normal flow should be restored to distal tributaries. This has the theoretical advantage of reducing long-term ischaemic complications. Coils remain *in situ* and should provide long-term haemostasis.

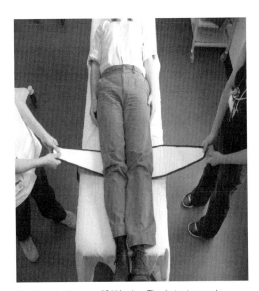

Fig. 13.9. Application of SAM splint. The device is passed underneath the patient's legs.

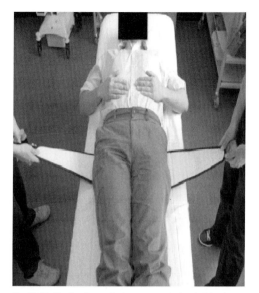

Fig. 13.10. The band is worked up to sit at the level of the greater trochanters.

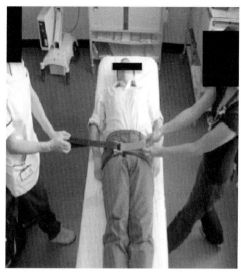

Fig. 13.11. The belt is passed through the buckle and traction applied bilaterally until a click is heard. Finally, the strap is attached to the velcro strip.

Other pelvic injuries

Avulsion fractures
Avulsion fractures may occur at any of the insertion points of the powerful muscles that support the function of the pelvis and lower limbs. These may include the anterior superior iliac spine, anterior inferior iliac spine, posterior spine, iliac crest, and ischial tuberosity. In general, these are treated symptomatically. An exception is a displaced avulsed ischial tuberosity. Open reduction and internal fixation is sometimes considered as they have a tendency towards non-union and chronic pain.

Stable ring fractures
Pubic ramus fractures are common, especially in the elderly. Typically, they are an isolated superior or inferior pubic ramus fracture, sustained following a fall. Alternatively, both rami on the same side may be fractured. If the contra-lateral side of the ring and posterior elements are intact, all of these injuries may be treated with conservative management, with analgesia and mobilization as comfort allows.

Acetabular fractures
These injuries are usually a result of high energy trauma. The nature of the fracture is dependent on femoral head position, bone stock, and direction and magnitude of applied force.

The acetabulum is commonly described as two columns, forming an inverted Y-shape. The anterior column is formed from the ilium and symphysis pubis; the posterior column runs from the superior gluteal notch to the ischial tuberosity.

An AP pelvic view may be supplemented by a CT scan, or an iliac oblique and obturator oblique radiographs, which provide additional information on the posterior and anterior columns respectively.

Initial management consists of reduction of any hip dislocation and use of traction to maintain the position. Definitive management should be carried out following appropriate resuscitation, imaging, and planning. Non-operative or operative treatment may be indicated depending on fracture configuration and patient factors.

Hip dislocations
Dislocation of the native hip joint is an orthopaedic emergency as delay in reduction increases the risk of avascular necrosis of the femoral head. This results from occlusion of the ascending branch of the medial circumflex femoral artery, which supplies the majority of blood to the weight-bearing femoral head.

Hip dislocations may be posterior (the majority) or anterior. The direction of dislocation and presence, or absence of associated acetabular or femoral head fractures depends on the position of the femur at the time of impact and the direction of applied force.

Hip dislocations are high-energy injuries and, therefore, warrant a full assessment and exclusion of associated injuries. Neurovascular status should be assessed. The sciatic and femoral nerves may be damaged in posterior and anterior dislocations respectively. Leg position warrants careful assessment. Posterior dislocation results in internal rotation and adduction of the limb. Anterior dislocation results in external rotation and abduction.

Hip dislocations should be managed with an urgent reduction under sedation or general anaesthesia. If fluoroscopic imaging is not used, a postoperative radiograph to confirm reduction is mandatory.

Posterior reductions are commonly relocated using the Allis method.

Anterior dislocations are relocated with the use of in line traction. If closed reduction fails an open reduction should be untaken.

Dislocation of a hip prosthesis may occur following minimal trauma. Indeed, sometimes moving around in bed can be the precipitant. These should be reduced in the emergency department under sedation, or if this is not possible under general anaesthesia in the operating theatre.

Femoral head fractures
These are usually associated with hip dislocations. The femoral head is crushed or sheared upon dislocation. The initial assessment should be as described above for hip dislocations. The Pipkin classification describes femoral head fractures:

- *Type 1:* inferior to fovea.
- *Type 2:* superior to fovea.
- *Type 3:* (1 or 2) + associated femoral neck fracture.
- *Type 4:* (1 or 2) + associated acetabular fracture.

Following emergency reduction of the dislocated hip, subsequent management depends on the classification and patient factors. A CT is usually required to guide definitive management.

Fractured neck of femur
The vast majority of femoral neck fractures occur as a result of low velocity trauma in the osteoporotic elderly population following a fall. Radiographic classification of the fracture and patient factors dictate further management.

Long-term sequelae
Following an unstable pelvic injury many patients are left with disability. Chronic pain is a common problem in those sustaining serious injury. Sexual dysfunction in male and females has been reported as 12 and 2%, respectively. Furthermore, pelvic fractures in women can affect delivery method in future pregnancy. Women who have sustained previous pelvic injury are at risk of difficulties during delivery and should be considered for specialist obstetric management. Of those working at the time of injury, approximately 75% return to work within a year.

A retrospective review of patients sustaining open pelvic fractures showed a survival rate of 75%. Their acute care was characterized by substantial blood transfusions, frequent need for a colostomy and extended hospitalization. In the long-term most were able to care for themselves, but had residual pain and ongoing unemployment.

Further reading

Brenneman FD, Deepak K, Boulanger BR, Tile M, Redelmeier DA. Long term outcomes in open pelvic fractures. *J Trauma* 1997; **42**(5): 773–7.

British Orthopaedic Association Standards for Trauma (BOAST). *Pelvic and Acetabular Fracture Management*, December 2008. Available at: http://www.boa.ac.uk/site/showpublications. aspx?ID=59 (accessed 1 September 2009).

Burgess AR, Eastridge BJ, Young JWR, Ellison TS, Ellison PS, Poka A, et al. Pelvic ring disruptions: effective classification system and treatment protocols. *J Trauma* 1990; **30**(7): 848–56.

Canale T, et al. *Campbell's Operative Orthopaedics*, 11th edn. New York: St Luis: WC Campbell, 2008.

Faringer PD, Mullins RJ, Feliciano PD. Selective Faecal Diversion in complex open pelvic fractures from blunt trauma. *Arch Surg* 1994; **129**: 958.

Geeraerts, T. et al. Clinical review: Initial management of blunt pelvic trauma patients with haemodynamic instability. *Crit Care* 2007; **11**(1): 204.

Gruen GS, Leit ME, Gruen RJ, Garrison JD, Auble TE, Peitzman AB. Functional outcome of patients with unstable pelvic ring fractures stabilised with open reduction and internal fixation. *J Trauma* 1995; **39**(5): 838–45.

Joint Royal Colleges Ambulance Liaison Committee. (JRCALC) *Pelvic Trauma*, April 2009. Available at: http://www2.warwick. ac.uk/fac/med/research/hsri/emergencycare/prehospitalcare/ jrcalcstakeholderwebsite/clinicalpracticeupdates/pelvic_ trauma__final_published_version_issued_21apr2009.pdf (accessed 1 September 2009).

Koval KJ, Zuckerman. *Handbook of Fractures*, 3rd edn. Philadelphia: Lippincott Williams and Wilkins, 2006.

Lee C, Porter K. The prehospital management of pelvic fractures. *Emerg Med J* 2007; **24**: 130–3.

Miller PR, Moore PS, Mansell E, Meredith JW, Chang MC. External fixation or arteriogram in bleeding pelvic fracture: initial therapy guided by markers of arterial hemorrhage. *J Trauma* 2003; **54**: 437–43.

Miranda M, Riemer, B. Butterfield, S. Burke, Charles. Pelvic ring injuries: a long term functional outcome study. *Clin Orthopaed Related Res* 1996; **329**: 152–9.

East Practice Management Guidelines Work Group. *Practice Management Guidelines for Hemorrhage in Pelvic Fracture*. Allentown: Eastern Association for the Surgery of Trauma 2001.

Limb injuries

Limb injuries

The first consideration in managing orthopaedic trauma is to *treat the patient, not only the fracture*. The initial assessment of a patient with polytrauma should follow a standard trauma protocol and include the identification and treatment of life-threatening injuries.

In general, the orthopaedic injuries will not be considered until the secondary survey, but major haemorrhage from pelvic or multiple fractures, particularly open femoral fractures, may have to be considered under the circulation element of the primary survey.

Once the patient has been adequately resuscitated, a systematic secondary survey should be conducted. Depending upon the clinical condition of the patient, this may only occur several days after the incident.

History

The mechanism of injury can provide useful information on both the severity and pattern of injury likely to be encountered. The pattern of fracture can often be related to the mechanism of injury. A direct blow will break the bone at the point of impact and usually causes a transverse fracture. A significant crush injury may cause a comminuted fracture with extensive soft-tissue injury. A twisting mechanism causes a spiral fracture, whereas compression causes a short oblique fracture. Bending forces result in fractures with a triangular butterfly fragment. If the fracture pattern seen is not consistent with the mechanism of injury, then the possibility of non-accidental injury (NAI) should be considered in the differential diagnosis. NAI is not seen exclusively in children and should be a consideration when also assessing vulnerable adults.

Any associated events surrounding the injury should also be elicited. For example, a fall resulting in a fractured neck of femur in the elderly may be caused by a cardiac or neurological event. The fracture can therefore distract from the true life-threatening condition.

A full medical and surgical history should be taken and a record of previous injuries noted. Medications such as chronic steroid use can inhibit fracture healing. Additionally, heavy smoking has been shown to inhibit healing.

Examination

When examining any limb, Apley's method of LOOK, FEEL, and MOVE provides a systematic approach.

Look

The limb is examined for open wounds or previous operation scars. Limb deformity or signs of a crush injury should be noted. Wounds associated with open fractures should be photographed in the emergency department before covering it with a sterile dressing.

Feel

The limb should be felt for tenderness or crepitus in an unconscious patient. In particular, it is important to feel for tenderness at the site of commonly missed injuries, the clavicle, isolated fibula, or single forearm bones, and hand and feet injuries.

It is also vital to feel for pulses, and in a co-operative patient sensation can be assessed at this stage.

Move

The patient should be asked to move the limb if possible. A patient who can comfortably lift their leg off the bed and bend the knee to 90 degrees is unlikely to have significant leg injuries, but see the missed injuries above. If the patient can't move the limb, it will be necessary to assess whether this is due to pain or neuromuscular injury and attempt gentle passive movement. As well as assessing movement, stability of the joints can be assessed.

X-rays

When ordering radiographs in limb trauma, it is important to remember the *rule of twos*:

- *Two views*: a fracture or dislocation may not be seen on a single X-ray film, and at least two views must be taken.
- *Two joints*: in the forearm or leg, angulation of one bone cannot occur without the other being broken or the joint dislocated. The joints above and below the fracture must be included on the X-ray film.
- *Two injuries*: severe force often causes injuries at more than one level (e.g. with fractures of the calcaneum or femur it is important to exclude pelvic or spinal injury).
- *Two occasions*: some fractures (e.g. scaphoid) are notoriously difficult to detect soon after injury, but repeat films 1–2 weeks later may show a lesion. Similarly, post-reduction X-rays should be taken to confirm adequacy of the fracture alignment.

There are a number of methods to describe a fracture, but they all invariably include the following information:

- *Anatomy* (e.g. proximal tibia).
- *Articular surface involved* (e.g. intra- versus extra-articular).
- *Angulation* (usually describes the orientation of the distal fragment).
- *Apposition* (described as a percentage of total contact).
- *Rotation*
- *Length* (e.g. shortening from bone overlap or lengthening from fracture distraction).

Associated vascular injuries

The artery may be cut, torn, compressed, or contused, either by the initial injury or by the jagged bone fragments. Even if the outward appearance of the vessel is normal, intimal damage may have occurred or a segment of artery may be in spasm. Common sites of injury include the knee (popliteal), elbow (brachial), and the shaft of the femur (femoral).

Clinically, the patient may complain of paraesthesia or numbness in the affected extremity. The limb may be cold, pale, or cyanosed, and the distal pulse maybe weak or absent; however, the majority of arterial injuries are associated with 'hard signs' of an absent pulse, pulsatile bleeding, or an expanding haematoma.

If a vascular injury is suspected, early discussion with a vascular surgeon is recommended. Any compressive dressings or splints should be removed. If the fracture is grossly displaced, then this should be reduced. If there is no return of pulse, then exploration of the vessel is indicated with or without an on-table angiogram. Fracture stabilization should be performed if vascular repair is contemplated.

Associated nerve injury

Nerves can also be damaged in trauma and, for this reason, a full neurological assessment should be undertaken and documented in the medical notes at initial and subsequent assessments. This is particularly important following reduction and fixation of a fracture. As in vascular injury, if a nerve injury is found, then the fracture should be reduced as soon as possible to prevent further damage.

Damage to the peripheral nerves can be classified into three major groups: *neuropraxia*, *axonotmesis*, and *neurotmesis*.

- *Neuropraxia* is characterized by local myelin damage, usually secondary to compression. Axon continuity is preserved, and the nerve does not undergo distal degeneration.
- *Axonotmesis* is defined as a loss of continuity of axons, with variable preservation of the connective tissue elements of the nerve.
- *Neurotmesis* is the most severe injury, equivalent to physiological disruption of the nerve; it may or may not include actual nerve transection.

After injury, function fails sequentially in the following order: motor, proprioception, touch, temperature, pain, and sympathetic innervation. Recovery occurs sequentially in the reverse order. Neuropraxia has the best prognosis and complete recovery can be expected within weeks. In axonotmesis a full recovery can be expected, but may take weeks to months. Neurotmesis, being the most severe injury, may require surgical repair or grafting, and full recovery cannot be guaranteed.

Nerves commonly at risk include the anterior interosseous nerve in supracondylar fractures of the humerus, axillary nerve in shoulder dislocation, radial nerve in humeral shaft fractures, sciatic nerve in hip dislocation, and peroneal nerve in knee dislocations. The incidence of acute median nerve compression following distal radius fracture has been reported as 4%.

In closed injuries, the nerve is rarely severed, so recovery can be expected. However, if recovery has not occurred by the expected time and if nerve conduction studies fail to show evidence of recovery, then the nerve should be explored. Nerves can become entrapped within the fracture site (e.g. radial nerve in humeral shaft fractures), and will not recover without surgical exploration.

Acute nerve compression can occur after surgery, with cases of acute carpal syndrome reported after volar buttress plating of distal radius fractures. If the symptoms do not settle after elevation of the limb, then surgical decompression is indicated.

Compartment syndrome

Compartment syndrome is a limb-threatening condition observed when perfusion pressure falls below tissue perfusion pressure in a closed anatomical space. Bleeding, oedema or inflammation may increase the pressure within one of the osteofascial compartments. This leads to reduced capillary flow, which results in ischaemia, oedema and further increase in the pressure of the compartment. A vicious cycle occurs that ultimately leads to the necrosis of the nerves and muscles in the compartment within about 12 h. Once infarcted, the muscles are replaced by inelastic fibrous tissue (Volkmann's ischaemic contracture).

Risk factors for compartment syndrome include high-energy injury, concomitant vascular injury, crush injuries, and burns. The presence of an open fracture does not preclude compartment syndrome, as not all compartments may be fully decompressed.

The classical diagnostic features of compartment syndrome are the 5P's; pain, paraesthesia, pallor, poikilothermia, and pulselessness. However, these are mostly late signs and are not apparent in ventilated or paralysed patients. One of the most important symptoms is pain out of proportion with the injury. Increasing pain or analgesic requirements despite adequate splintage are warning signs that compartment syndrome is present. This can be confirmed with pain on passive stretching of the muscles in the suspected compartment. Clinically, the compartment will feel tense. The use of compartment pressure testing may be useful in ventilated patients and can also be useful in monitoring trends of compartment pressures. Delta-p is a measure of perfusion pressure (diastolic pressure—intracompartment pressure). McQueen found a correlation between a Delta-p less than 30 mmHg and the development of compartment syndrome.

The management of compartment syndrome is dependent on early diagnosis. Full compartment fasciotomies of the affected limb segment is required and if performed within 6 h of onset then almost full recovery of limb function can be expected.

Fat embolus syndrome

Fat embolus syndrome (FES) usually occurs 24–48 h after trauma and occurs in 2–5% of patients with long bone fractures. The embolization of fat from fractures is extremely common and has been reported as high as 95% in femoral fractures. The classical triad involves pulmonary changes, cerebral dysfunction, and a petechial rash. There are no reliable radiological or laboratory tests to confirm the diagnosis, so clinical diagnosis remains key. Schonfeld proposed a fat embolism index that gives points for different diagnostic criteria (Table 14.1). A score of 5 or more is diagnostic of fat embolus syndrome.

The pathophysiology of FES is still uncertain, although there are two theories. Gauss established the mechanical theory in which injury to adipose tissue and rupture of veins within the zone of injury causes the passage of free fat into the circulation. Lehman proposed the biochemical theory where plasma mediators mobilize fat from body stores and cause it to form large droplets. Once fat has been mobilized it can occlude the pulmonary, cerebral, retinal, and skin microcirculatory beds.

The management of FES is supportive with positive pressure ventilation. Early fracture fixation may be critical in reducing recurrent liberation of fat into the circulation as a result of fracture movement. Fluid resuscitation remains key in shocked patients and human serum albumin may be a useful adjunct as it has several binding sites for free fatty acids.

Table 14.1. Diagnostic criteria for fat embolus syndrome.

Points	
Diffuse petechiae	5
Alveolar infiltrates	4
Hypoxemia (<70 mmHg)	3
Confusion	1
Temp >38°C	1
Heart rate > 120/min	1
Respiratory rate > 30/min	1

The mangled extremity

The treatment of severe, leg-threatening injuries often necessitates an immediate or early decision between limb reconstruction and amputation. This initial decision requires a prediction of treatment outcomes on the basis of patient and injury characteristics. Factors that may tend towards amputation include;

- Irreparable vascular injury, warm ischaemia greater than 8 h, or severe crush with minimal remaining viable tissue.
- The severely damaged limb may constitute a threat to the patient's life.
- Even after revascularization, the limb remains so severely damaged that function will be less satisfactory than that afforded by a prosthesis.

A number of scoring systems have been developed to aid the surgeon in making the difficult decision to amputate. The most commonly used is the MESS (Mangled Extremity Severity Score) proposed by Johansen in 1990 (Table 14.2). A score of greater than 7 predicts amputation. However, it should be noted that the sensitivity of these scoring systems was 63%.

The decision to amputate should be made by the most senior surgeon available and ideally should be made by two surgeons and documented clearly in the medical notes. It has previously been thought that the presence of an insensate foot at the time of injury was an indication for amputation. However, evidence from the LEAP study has shown that plantar sensation can return and therefore should not be used as a determining factor for amputation. The huge psychological cost of such injuries cannot be underestimated and often patients are unwilling to under-go primary amputation following injury. In these cases, where the patient's physiological state is favourable, initial salvage may be attempted, with amputation occurring at a later stage.

Table 14.2. MESS scoring system.

		Points
A. Skeletal/soft-tissue injury		
1	Low energy (stab, simple fracture, low velocity gunshot wound).	1
2	Medium energy (open/multiple fractures)	2
3	High energy (close range shotgun, high velocity gunshot, crush)	3
4	Very high energy (above plus gross contamination)	4
B. Limb ischaemia (double score if >6 h)		
1	Pulse reduced or absent, perfusion normal	1
2	Pulseless, paraesthesia, diminished cap refill	2
3	Cool, paralysed, insensate, numb	3
C. Shock		
1	Systolic BP > 90 mmHg	0
2	Hypotensive transiently	1
3	Persistent hypotension	2
D. Age (years)		
1	<30	0
2	30–50	1
3	>50	2

Open fractures

An open fracture refers to osseous disruption in which a break in the skin and underlying soft tissue communicates directly with the fracture and its haematoma. The term is also applied when a fracture is in communication within a body cavity. In the UK, the annual incidence of open long bone fractures is 11.5 per 100,000 with 40% occurring in the lower limb. Any wound occurring on the same limb segment as a fracture must be suspected to be a consequence of an open fracture until proven otherwise.

Soft tissue injuries related to an open fracture have these important consequences:
- Contamination of the fracture site by exposure to the external environment.
- Crushing, stripping, and devascularization resulting in soft tissue compromise and increased susceptibility to infection.
- Destruction of the soft tissue envelope affects the options for fracture fixation. There is also a loss of function from damage to muscle, tendon, nerve, vascular, or ligamentous structures.

The extent of the associated soft tissue injury is one of the major determinants of the infection risk after a civilian open fracture. Gustilo and Anderson (1976) have reported a grading of wounds, which remains a universally accepted classification of the wound associated with an open fracture:
- Type I: an open fracture with a wound less than 1 cm long and clean.
- Type II: An open fracture with a laceration more than 1 cm long without extensive soft tissue damage, flaps, or avulsions.
- Type III: Either an open segmental fracture, an open fracture with extensive soft tissue damage, or a traumatic amputation.

For Gustilo type I fractures an infection rate of 1% or less can be expected, and for type II fractures a rate of approximately 3% has been reported. A modification to this grading was made by Gustilo et al. in 1984, when the type III fractures were subdivided:
- Type IIIA: adequate soft tissue cover of the bone despite extensive laceration.
- Type IIIB: extensive soft tissue loss, with periosteal stripping, and exposed bone. Usually associated with massive contamination.
- Type IIIC: open fracture with vascular injury that needs repair.

For type IIIA fractures an infection rate of 17% has been reported, and for type IIIB 26%. Type IIIC fractures have a variable infection rate, depending on the soft tissue injury and delays in revascularization.

Management in the emergency department
One-third of patients with open fractures have multiple injuries. Patients should be assessed using standardized trauma protocols with appropriate management of life-threatening conditions. Clinical evaluation of the limb should include:
- Addressing wound haemorrhage with direct pressure using a sterile dressing.
- A full neurovascular assessment of the injured limb. If necessary, Doppler ultrasound can be used to assess distal pulses. The location of the pulse should be marked for future examination. Consideration of early referral to a vascular surgeon, if vascular injury is suspected.
- Assessment of skin and soft tissue damage. If possible, photograph the wound, and then cover the wound with a sterile dressing.
- Following adequate analgesia, reduction of the fracture if possible and splintage. If the fracture is manipulated in the emergency department, the neurovascular status must be rechecked and documented in the medical notes.
- Senior help must be sought early.

It is essential not to:
- Irrigate, debride, or probe the wound in the emergency department, if immediate operative intervention is planned. Doing so may further contaminate the tissues.

Antibiotic prophylaxis
In 1974, Patzakis et al. established the role of antibiotics in the treatment of open fractures in a prospective, randomized, controlled trial. After treatment, the subsequent infection rate was 13.9% in the placebo group and 2.3% in the cephalosporin group. Antibiotics should be commenced promptly as delays >3 h increases the risk of infection.

Recommended treatment regimen
For Type I and II open fractures Staphylococcus aureus, streptococci, and aerobic Gram-negative bacilli are the most common infecting organisms, and these can be covered with a 1st or 2nd generation cephalosporin or alternatively with a quinolone (e.g. ciprofloxacin).

Type III open fractures These should be managed with better coverage for Gram-negative organisms, and the addition of an aminoglycoside to the cephalosporin is recommended.

For severe injuries with soil contamination and tissue damage with areas of ischaemia, a penicillin should be added to provide coverage against anaerobes, particularly Clostridia species.

A 3-day course of antibiotics is sufficient for Type I and II fractures, whereas Type III fractures will require a longer 5-day course.

Tetanus prophylaxis
If the patient has not been vaccinated in the last 10 years, then they will require 0.5 mL im tetanus toxoid. Consider giving tetanus immunoglobulin in all patients with grossly contaminated open fractures.

Principles of management
The aim of fracture management is to produce a united fracture with intact soft tissues and normal function. The essential features of management are:
- Antibiotic prophylaxis.
- Wound debridement.
- Early stabilization of the fracture.
- Early wound cover.

In fractures with significant soft tissue damage, this will require a multi-disciplinary approach, and early communication with a plastic surgical unit is advised. The traditional dictum is that the original debridement should occur within 6 h of injury. However, Webb et al. (in 2007) demonstrated that delays up to 24 h did not increase infection rates.

Debridement

The aim of debridement is to render the wound devoid of foreign material and of non-viable tissue, in order to leave a clean healthy bed for soft tissue reconstruction. As open fractures are frequently high-energy injuries with severe tissue damage, the most experienced surgeon available should perform the debridement. The principles of debridement are:

- *Wound excision:* skin is generally very resistant to trauma and has a good capacity to heal. Therefore, the wound edges should be excised with care.
- *Wound extension:* the zone of soft tissue injury will often extend far beyond the wound. Therefore, the wound will need to be extended proximally and distally to enable full examination of the injured tissue.
- *Removal of non-viable tissue:* devitalized tissue, especially muscle, will provide a focus for infection and needs to be excised. When assessing damaged tissue, the key is to look for the 4 C's:
- *Colour*—dead muscle is often dark and discoloured;
- *Consistency*—non-viable tissue has a mushy consistency;
- *Contractility*—dead muscle will not contract when crushed with forceps or touched with a diathermy probe;
- *Capillary bleeding*—non-viable bone fragments should be removed.
- *Wound toilet:* an essential feature of wound debridement is copious wound irrigation. A minimum of 6 L of saline is recommended.
- *Nerves and tendons:* damaged nerves and tendons can often be left and repaired at the time of wound closure once the wound is free of infection.

Fracture stabilization

Early fracture stability is required to prevent further soft tissue damage and reduce the risk of infection. Traditionally, the external fixator has been the method of choice as it allows management of the fracture without placing metalwork within the zone of injury and it does not require further exposure of the damaged soft tissue. However, pin site infection is a problem with infection rates of 25% in Type IIIA and 50% in Type IIIB reported.

In low energy Type I fractures and selected Type IIIB fractures, an intramedullary nail can be placed with no significant increase in infection. A meta-analysis of fixation methods in open tibial fractures showed that use of an intramedullary nail significantly reduced the incidence of superficial infection and reoperation rate compared with external fixation. There was no difference in deep infection or non-union rates.

Wound coverage

Small uncontaminated Type I wounds may be primarily sutured after the initial debridement, or just left to heal. However, in general, it is advisable to dress the wound with sterile gauze and consider wound closure at 48 h. A number of reconstructive options are available and form the 'reconstructive ladder', which ranges from delayed primary closure to application of a free flap. 70% of all Gustilo type IIIB open tibial diaphyseal fractures require flap cover. Whichever option is used, soft tissue coverage within 3–5 days of injury has been reported to reduce the risk of osteomyelitis and deep infection.

BOA/BAPS guidelines for timing of surgery

The British Orthopaedic Association/British Association of Plastic Surgeons working group has developed guidelines for the management of open tibial fractures. They recommend that the first orthopaedic procedure should be undertaken within the first 6 h of injury. At the initial operation, details of the injury should be passed onto the plastic surgeons. In the first procedure, the wound should be adequately debrided and the fracture stabilized to permit subsequent plastic surgery. This includes fasciotomies for suspected compartment syndrome. The patient may require further wound inspection or debridement at 48 h. Soft tissue coverage should be performed within the first 5 days of injury (BOA/BAPS working group, 1997).

Fracture healing

Fracture healing is a complex physiological process of repair in which bone heals for the purpose of transferring mechanical loads. Unlike other tissues that heal by the formation of connective scar tissue of poor quality, bone is regenerated, and the pre-fracture properties are mostly restored.

Fractures can heal by:
- Primary (direct) bone healing.
- Secondary (callus formation) bone healing.

The vast majority of fractures heal by secondary bone healing. Secondary bone healing proceeds in five distinct stages:
- *Stage 1*: tissue destruction and haematoma formation.
- *Stage 2*: inflammation and cellular proliferation.
- *Stage 3*: callus formation.
- *Stage 4*: consolidation.
- *Stage 5*: remodelling.

Tissue destruction and haematoma formation
Bleeding occurs from the medullary cavity, the periosteum, as well as adjacent soft tissue and muscle. This results in the formation of a haematoma within and around the fracture site. The disruption of the Haversian systems leads to death of the osteocytes at the fracture surface.

Inflammation and cellular proliferation
Without an inflammatory process, bone will not heal. Within the first 8 h, the fibrin mesh within the haematoma forms a framework for the influx of various cells (e.g. platelets, neutrophils, lymphocytes, monocytes, macrophages, and mast cells).

The haematoma organizes over the next week into granulation tissue. The inflammatory cells and platelets release a variety of cytokines (see Table 14.3). These activate cell migration, proliferation, and differentiation of mesenchymal stem cells (MSCs). Angiogenesis occurs as the haematoma organizes and osteoclasts resorb the dead bone ends. Inflammatory mediators increase vascular permeability, causing an exudate of plasma and promoting phagocytosis of necrotic material.

Callus formation
Callus is a physiological reaction to inter-fragmentary movement, and requires the existence of residual cell vitality and adequate blood flow. The initial haematoma matures into granulation tissue at the fracture gap. Soft callus or cartilage then forms and, finally, the soft callus is replaced by endochondral ossification to become hard callus or woven bone. The chondrocytes become hypertrophic, calcify, and die. Angiogenesis occurs and osteoblasts lay down bone matrix on the collagen scaffold left by the chondrocytes.

The composition of the callus is not only dependent upon the growth factors released during the inflammatory phase but is also highly dependent on the biomechanical strains at the fracture site. *Strain* is defined as the change in length of a material when a given force is applied. Osteoblasts are very sensitive to strain and cannot tolerate strains of >1% and chondrocytes proliferate when the strain is <10%. In the initial stage after fracture, the area between the bone ends has a strain of >100%. This environment is not conducive to bone formation. The

Table 14.3. Inflammatory mediators in fracture healing

Mediator	Cell line	Action
Interleukins (IL-1, IL-6)	Inflammatory cells	Regulate osteoclastogenesis and early differentiation of osteoblasts
Transforming growth factor β (TGFβ)	Platelets Extracellular matrix	Stimulation of MSCs
Fibroblast growth factor (FGF)	Macrophages, MSCs, osteoblasts and chondrocytes	Mitogenic for MSCs, chondrocytes, and osteoblasts
Insulin-like growth factor (IGF)	Bone matrix, osteoblasts, and chondrocytes	Proliferation of osteoprogenitor cells
Platelet derived growth factor (PDGF)	Platelets and osteoblasts	Mitogenic for MSCs and osteoblasts and promotes macrophage chemotaxis.
Bone morphogenic proteins (BMP)	osteoprogenitor cells, osteoblasts	Promote differentiation of progenitor cells into osteoblasts

increasing size and stiffness of the callus reduces movements and strain at the fracture site. Cyclical micromovement stimulates the growth of cartilage and then bone.

Osteoblasts beneath the periosteum (cambium level) deposit a subperiosteal layer of woven bone at the fracture site. This woven bone forms the framework of the bridging external callus. External callus forms on the outside of the fractured bone to bridge the gap. Internal callus forms more slowly from the medullary canal. Finally, the cortical continuity is restored.

Consolidation
Consolidation is the conversion of woven bone into lamellar bone. Woven bone can be considered as 'temporary' callus. The collagen fibres that run through the osseous matrix are arranged in an irregular network. Lamellar bone, on the other hand, is the permanent bone of the mature trabeculae and the shafts of long bone. Lamellar bone is laid down in orderly layers and the osteocytes are distributed evenly between the layers. The fibres in each layer run in parallel, but at a different angle to adjacent layers. This configuration increases the bone's strength.

Lamellar bone cannot be deposited in fibrous tissue and cannot therefore bridge a moving gap spanned only by fibrous tissue. The solid framework on which lamellar bone is normally deposited, is the woven bone of callus which has formed a temporary scaffold. The woven bone is finally removed by osteoclasts when the lamellar bone has acquired an adequate thickness.

Remodelling
Remodelling can continue long after the fracture has clinically healed; eventually the temporary woven bone is replaced by lamellar bone and there is reconstitution of the medullary canal and restoration of the bone shape.

Excessive callus is formed initially to reduce strain at the fracture site in order to produce a favourable biomechanical environment for osteoblastic activity. In non-aligned fractures the callus is preferentially distributed on the concave surface of the fracture.

In remodelling, osteoclastic and osteoblastic activity occurs in synergy to regain the shape of the bone based on the stresses to which the bone is exposed. Wolff's law states that bone is laid down in areas of excess stress and removed from areas where there is little.

In children, the remodelling is so effective that even completely displaced fractures may heal and remodel without trace. Axial rotation deformity should not be accepted as it will persist.

In adults there is very little correction of angulation or axial rotation. Therefore, both should be corrected before the fracture heals.

Primary bone healing

If the fracture is anatomically reduced, at a micrometric level, osteonal healing occurs. Osteoclasts can tunnel across the fracture line, and establish a 'cutting cone' across the fracture. Osteoblasts follow and lay down bone matrix and re-establish continuity between Haversian systems. Vessel in-growth is absent and the bone filling the interfragmentary gap appears without the intermediate formation of cartilage or granulation tissue.

For primary bone healing to occur, interfragmentary strain must be minimal and the fracture gap between the bone ends should be <200 μm. This requires anatomical reduction with intra-fragmentary compression to prevent motion. Primary bone healing is essentially the same biological process as occurs in normal bone turnover and late remodelling. This can, therefore, be a slow process and any internal fixation device implanted must be maintained until this healing process is complete.

Implications for fracture fixation

The principles of fracture management should take into consideration the mechanisms of fracture healing. In fractures of long bones, accurate reduction of axes, and rotation are important. Whenever possible, the blood supply at the fracture site should not be compromised.

If secondary fracture healing is the goal, movement of the fracture along the axes is beneficial for the formation of soft callus. However the movement should be small (ideally amplitude 0.2–1.0 mm and fracture gap <2 mm). Higher strain amplitudes may inhibit osteoblastic activity and delay fracture healing. In the later stages, the formation of hard callus is compromised by vigorous mechanical stimulation. Therefore, motion should be limited in the final phase of consolidation. Ideally, this increase in fracture site stiffness is a biological response from formation of hard callus.

If fracture fragments are rigidly fixed but the fracture gap is greater than 200 μm, then neither secondary bone healing or primary (direct) healing can occur and the fracture is at risk of developing into non-union and ultimately the implant failing.

With intra-articular fractures, where absolute stability and accurate reduction is required, primary fracture healing is desirable and can be achieved with lag screw fixation.

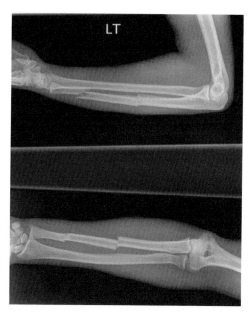

Fig. 14.1. A segmental fracture of the ulna.

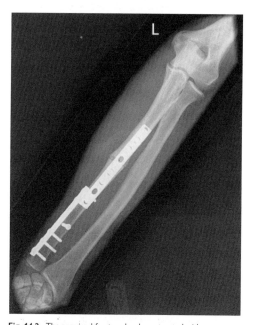

Fig. 14.2. The proximal fracture has been treated with a compression plate. The fracture has healed by secondary healing with callus visible. The distal fracture has been treated by a compression lag screw with a neutralization plate. The fracture has healed by primary (direct) healing. Note there is no callus formation and the fracture is no longer visible.

Methods of reduction

The goal of early fracture management is to control haemorrhage, provide pain relief, and remove potential sources of infection (necrotic tissue or foreign material). The overall aim in managing fractures is to ensure that the limb, when healed has returned to its maximal possible function. This is accomplished by obtaining and subsequently maintaining a reduction of the fracture with an immobilization technique that allows the fracture to heal, and at the same time, provides the patient with functional aftercare. Reduction should aim for adequate apposition and normal alignment of the bone fragments. This can be achieved with operative (open) or non-operative (closed) measures.

Non-operative methods (closed reduction)

Closed reduction should be performed initially for any fracture that is displaced, shortened, or angulated. Even if the fracture is inherently unstable, closed reduction of grossly displaced fractures in the emergency department can help to reduce further soft tissue damage prior to internal fixation.

The principles of closed reduction are:
- The distal part of the limb is pulled in the line of the bone.
- As the fragments disengage, they are repositioned by reversing the original direction of force.
- Alignment is adjusted in each plane. This is most effective when the periosteum and muscles on one side of the fracture remain intact; the soft-tissue strap prevents over-reduction and stabilizes the fracture after it has been reduced.

Closed reduction is not required if the fracture is undisplaced or if the displacement is not clinically significant. Close methods are likely to be unsuccessful in the following scenarios:
- If reduction is impossible (e.g. severely communited fractures, soft tissue interposition between the fracture fragments, or haematoma formation that creates tension in the soft tissues).
- If the reduction, when achieved, cannot be maintained.
- If the fracture has been produced by traction forces (e.g. displaced patellar fracture).

If the fracture has been reduced then it can be held by casting, splintage or traction.

Casting

Cast splintage is commonly used in distal limb fractures. It can be made from fibreglass or plaster of Paris. After the fracture has been reduced, a layer of wool is applied. It protects the bony prominences and the elastic pressure of the wool actually enhances the fixation of the limb by compensating for slight shrinkage in the tissues after application of the cast. Once the plaster is applied, the plaster is moulded with three-point pressure to keep the intact periosteal hinge under tension and, thereby, maintain reduction. If the fracture is recent, further swelling is likely

and it is therefore prudent to split the cast to prevent compartment syndrome.

Complications

Pressure sores can develop when a cast presses upon the skin over a bony prominence. Thermal burns may also occur during plaster hardening. If a cast is applied badly, then fracture reduction may not be maintained and further manipulation maybe required. Similarly, once the swelling has subsided the cast may no longer hold the fracture securely. If it is loose, the cast should be replaced.

Prolonged cast immobilization can result in circulatory disturbances, inflammation, and bone disease, which results in fracture disease. This manifests as osteoporosis, chronic oedema, soft-tissue atrophy, and joint stiffness. These problems can be avoided by early elevation of the fracture to reduce oedema and early mobilization.

Traction

Traction has been used for the management of fractures for hundreds of years. Traction is applied to the limb distal to the fracture, so that continuous pull is applied along the long axis of the bone with counterforce in the opposite direction. If the soft tissues around the fracture are intact, then traction should align the bony fragments. Traction can be applied:
- By gravity.
- By skin traction.
- By skeletal traction.

Gravitational traction is only relevant in upper limb fractures. A hanging cast utilizes the weight of the arm to apply traction to a humeral shaft fracture.

Skin traction is applied by using Elastoplast stuck to shaved skin and held on with a bandage. Skin traction can only be used as a temporary measure, as most of the forces created by skin traction are lost and dissipated in the soft-tissue structures. Skin traction will usually allow up to 10lb of weight. At weights greater than 10lb, superficial skin layers are disrupted and irritated.

Skeletal traction is most commonly used in femur fractures. It is applied by placing a pin (e.g. Steinmann or Denham pin) through the bone distal to the fracture. Weights are applied to this pin, and the patient is placed in an apparatus to facilitate traction and nursing care (Fig. 14.3).

Complications

The complications from skeletal traction include the development of pressure ulcers, pulmonary, and urinary infections, permanent footdrop contractures (if the foot is positioned in equinus), peroneal nerve palsy, pin tract infection, and thromboembolic events. These complications are mainly related to patient immobility, whilst on traction. Traction requires a long in-patient stay that has both economic and psychological effects on the patient. The introduction of intramedullary nailing has meant that traction is now rarely used in developed countries.

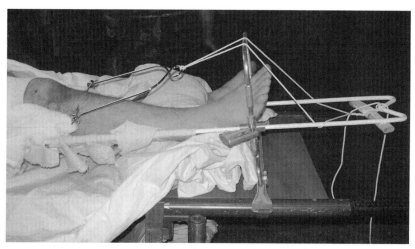

Fig. 14.3. An open femoral fracture temporarily treated with skeletal traction and a Thomas splint.

Internal fixation

In 1958, the Association for the Study of Internal Fixation (ASIF) created 4 treatment goals for surgical fracture management.
- *Anatomical reduction of the fracture fragments.* For the diaphysis, anatomic alignment ensuring that length, angulation, and rotation are corrected as required, whereas intra-articular fractures demand an anatomic reduction of all fragments.
- *Stable internal fixation to fulfil biomechanical demands.*
- *Preservation of blood supply to the injured area of the extremity.*
- *Active, pain-free mobilization of adjacent muscles and joints to prevent the development of fracture disease.*

There are a number of indications for internal fixation that include:
- Fractures that cannot be reduced except by operation.
- Fractures that normally unite poorly and present with nursing difficulties (e.g. fractures of the femoral neck).
- Fractures that are inherently unstable and prone to redisplacement after reduction (e.g. mid-shaft forearm fractures).
- Pathological fractures where disease can prevent healing.
- Displaced intra-articular fractures.

Contraindications to internal fixation include
- Soft tissues that compromise the overlying fracture or the surgical approach due to soft-tissue injury or burns.
- Medical conditions that contraindicate surgery or anaesthesia (e.g. recent myocardial infarction).

The method of internal fixation is dependent upon the location and configuration of the fracture. A multitude of internal fixation implants are available and each have their advantages and complications. The types of internal fixation are:
- Wires.
- Interfragmentary screws.
- Plate fixation.
- Intramedullary nails.

Wire fixation

Kirschner wires (K-wires) are commonly used for temporary and definitive treatment of fractures. K-wires resist only changes in alignment, they do not resist rotation and they have poor resistance to torque and bending forces. Therefore, they have to be used in conjunction with casting or splinting. They can be placed percutaneously. K-wire fixation is useful for fractures in metaphyseal and epiphyseal regions, especially in fractures of the distal foot, wrist, hand, and in displaced metacarpal and phalangeal fractures after closed reduction (Figs 14.4. and 14.5).

Cerclage and tension band wires are loops of wire that pass around two bone fragments and then tightened to compress the fractures together. The tension band wire is placed such that the maximum compressive force is over the tensile surface, which is usually the convex side of the bone.

Interfragmentary screws

Interfragmentary screws provide compression when inserted across two fracture fragments. This is achieved by

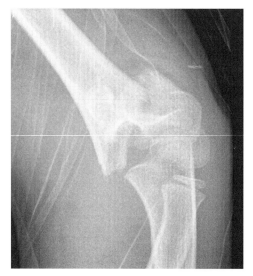

Fig. 14.4. A Gartland Type III supracondylar fracture of the humerus.

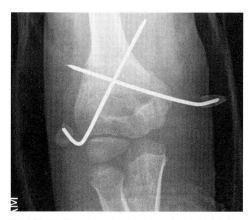

Fig. 14.5. The fracture is reduced and the reduction is held with crossed K-wires supplemented with cast immobilization.

using either a partially-threaded screw or by over-drilling the near cortex. This technique is useful for reducing single fragments onto the main shaft of a tubular bone or fitting together fragments of a metaphyseal fracture.

Plate fixation

Since the late 1950s, open reduction and internal fixation has been employed to overcome the limitations encountered with casting or skeletal traction. The aim of 'osteosynthesis' is to produce *absolute stability* to allow primary (direct) fracture healing. Early techniques emphasized the need for exact anatomic reduction and rigid fixation. This technique permitted early rehabilitation of the patient and has become the standard management for many types of fractures. Depending on the location and the application of the plate, they can perform many different functions:

- *Neutralization:* neutralization plates are used in combination with interfragmentary screw fixation. The interfragmentary compression screws provide compression at the fracture site. This plate function neutralizes bending, shear, and torsional forces on the lag screw fixation, as well as increases the stability of the construct. Protection plates are commonly used for fractures involving the fibula, radius, ulna, and humerus.

- *Compression:* compression plates counteract bending, shear, and torsional forces by providing compression across the fracture site via the eccentrically loaded holes in the plate. Compression plates are commonly used in the long bones, especially the fibula, radius, and ulna, and in non-union or malunion surgery. Compression plates provide a minimum strain environment to allow primary (direct) healing (Fig. 14.6).

- *Buttressing:* buttress plates counteract the compression and shear forces that commonly occur with fractures that involve the metaphysis and epiphysis. These plates are commonly used with interfragmentary screw fixation. The buttress plate is always fixed to the larger main fracture fragment, but does not necessarily require fixation through the smaller fragment, because the plate buttresses the small fragment into the larger fragment. To achieve this function requires appropriate plate contouring for adequate fixation and support (Fig. 14.7).

- *Tension-band:* a tension band plate technique converts tension forces into compressive forces, thereby providing absolute stability. An example of this technique is when a tension band plate is used for an oblique olecranon fracture.

- *Bridging:* bridging plates are used in multifragmented diaphyseal and metaphyseal fractures. Once the fracture

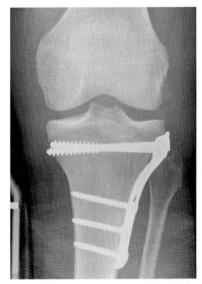

Fig. 14.7. A Schatzker Type II (split depression) fracture of the tibia treated with a buttress plate.

is adequately reduced the plate is applied across the fracture and the fracture is allowed to heal by secondary intention. This has the advantage of not disrupting the soft tissues around the fracture site (Figs 14.8 and 14.9).

Complications

- Conventional plating techniques often require extensive operative exposure to achieve an anatomic reduction. This results in devitalization of the bone and surrounding tissues, as well as evacuation of the fracture haematoma that has osteogenic potential. Surgical devitalization of the remaining vasculature in a displaced fracture has been clearly shown to inhibit healing. Additionally, plates cause necrosis to the periosteum, which disrupts the fracture environment beneath. Significant soft tissue dissection may be required to expose the fracture site. Further damage to already injured tissue may result in wound problems.

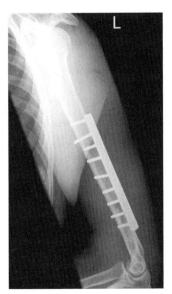

Fig. 14.6. A compression plate applied to treat a humeral shaft fracture. The low strain environment produced by the plate should allow the fracture to heal by primary (direct) healing.

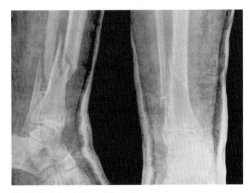

Fig. 14.8. A distal tibia and fibula fracture.

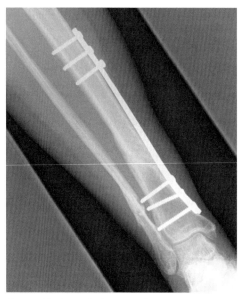

Fig. 14.9. The fracture has been treated with a percutaneous bridging plate. The fracture has healed by secondary healing with minimal disruption of the fracture site.

During the initial post-operative period, the plate has to counter the torsional and bending forces. In conventional plates, this load is borne at the screw-bone interface. In poor quality bone, toggling of the screw at the interface can lead to movement, and ultimately either screw loosening, breakage, or plate fracture.

If the bone ends are fixed rigidly with no compression at the fracture site, then neither primary (direct) or secondary (callus) bone healing can occur, and this may ultimately lead to delayed or non-union.

Locking plates

To overcome the disadvantages of conventional plating, more 'biological' fixation systems have been developed. These attempt to provide mechanical fracture stability without disturbing the fracture environment. As a result, the locking plate and percutaneous plating technique has become increasingly popular in orthopaedic practice. In cadaveric studies, Farouk (1997) showed that with percutaneous plating of the femur, no perforating or nutrient arteries were damaged compared to 80% in the conventional plating group.

Locking plates are fracture fixation devices with threaded screw holes, which allow screws to thread to the plate and function as a fixed-angle device. They follow a similar biomechanical principle of external fixators and in effect can be considered as 'internal fixators'. They have improved mechanical stability compared with external fixators in that the distance between the plate and bone is very short. Unlike conventional plates that require friction between the plate and bone to provide fracture stability, the mechanical stability is maintained at the angular-stable screw-plate interface. Therefore, there is little requirement for plate and bone contact, which helps to preserve the periosteal blood supply and bone perfusion. Also, as the screws are locked to the plate, it is difficult for one screw to pull out or fail unless adjacent screws fail.

Modern design of locking plates allows the use of unlocked and locked screws with the plate. Therefore, where absolute stability is required, an unlocked lag screw can be placed through the plate. The locking screws can then be inserted according to the neutralization principle to protect the lag screw in osteoporotic bone, with the increased pullout resistance of the locking screws. This combination technique is also indicated for fractures with a simple pattern (e.g. intra-articular split) at one level and comminution (e.g. metaphyseal-diaphyseal comminution) at a different level.

The classical use of the locking plate is as a bridging plate across a comminuted diaphyseal fracture. Indirect reduction is performed by ensuring adequate axial alignment, length, and rotation of the extremity, while the fracture fragments are not exposed or directly reduced. The bridging plate provides elastic fixation that leads to secondary fracture healing by callus formation.

The advantage of the minimally invasive percutaneous plate osteosynthesis (MIPPO) technique includes faster bone healing, reduced infection rate, decreased need for bone grafting, and better aesthetic results.

Although locking plates may be seen as the panacea for fracture fixation by combining the advantages of minimal exposure seen with intra-medullary nailing and the mechanical stability of conventional plating, it is not without its complications. As the fracture site is not exposed, non-direct methods of reduction are required and the surgeon must ensure that limb alignment is correct before attempting plating. Once a locking screw has been placed through the plate into a bone segment, this segment can no longer be manipulated by insertion of additional screws or by using compression devices. Therefore, the sequence of screw placement is crucial to avoid mal-reduction. Locking plates will not improve fracture reduction and if poorly reduced fractures are then fixed with the stiff construct of locking plate and screws, then this is a recipe for mal or non-union.

Intramedullary nails

The development of intramedullary nailing, introduced in 1939 by Küntscher, has revolutionized the treatment of fractures of the long bones. It has now become the standard management of many long-bone diaphyseal fractures that require surgical stabilization.

Intramedullary nails have undergone significant design changes from Küntscher's solid cloverleaf nail, which provided fracture stabilization by close contact and friction between the implant and the inner cortex. Since then, the development of intramedullary reaming and interlocking screws has widened its indication for use. The use of very distal, multiplanar interlocking screws has allowed the use of nails in complex metaphyseal fractures and intra-articular fractures, where the distal screws can provide compression of the fracture fragments. Cephalomedullary nails have become increasingly popular and are routinely used for subtrochanteric proximal femoral fractures. In addition, elastic nails have been increasingly used in the surgical management of paediatric diaphyseal fractures.

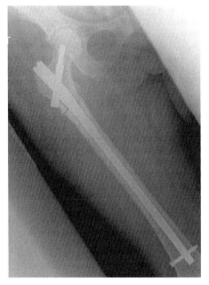

Fig. 14.10. A subtrochanteric fracture treated with a cephalomedullary intramedullary nail.

Biomechanics of intramedullary nails

Intramedullary implants are introduced into the bone remote to the fracture site. They act as internal splints and have load-sharing characteristics. The amount of load borne depends on the stability of the fracture/implant construct. In the initial phases, the intramedullary nail bears most of the load, and then gradually transfers it to the bone as the fracture heals.

Three types of loads act on a nail:
- Torsion.
- Compression.
- Tension.

Physiological loading is a combination of all three. With reaming of the canal and the use of locking screws, physiological loads are transmitted to the proximal and distal ends of the nail through the screws. During axial loading a bending moment is produced that creates compressive forces on the concave side of the nail and tension forces on the convex side. When cortical contact across the fracture is achieved, most of the compressive loads are transferred to the bone. In the absence of cortical contact, compressive loads are transferred to the interlocking screws, which result in screw bending and eventual screw failure.

The rigidity of the nail is dependent upon its diameter. In a solid circular nail, the bending rigidity is proportional to the nail diameter to the third power, and the torsional rigidity is proportional to the fourth power.

Interlocking screws placed proximally and distal to the fracture site restrict translation and rotation at the fracture site. This is important in oblique and multifragmentary fractures that rely on the screws for stability. Therefore the largest possible screw diameter should be used to increase its stability. As a rule the diameter of the screw should not exceed 50% of the nail diameter. The closer the fracture is to the distal locking screw, the less cortical contact the nail has, which leads to increased stress on the screw. Similarly, the further the distal screw is from the fracture site, the more rotationally stable the fracture becomes because of friction of the nail within the medullary canal.

Biomechanics and biological effects of reaming.

The clinical merits of reaming have been studied in a number of studies. In a meta-analysis comparing reamed and unreamed nailing of femoral shaft fractures, Forster et al. (2005) found significantly longer time to union, higher non-union rate, higher delayed union rate and higher revision rate in the unreamed group. Its use in open fractures has been the cause of considerable debate. It has been postulated that because reaming damages the endosteal blood supply it may theoretically increase the incidence of non-union and deep infection. However, Keating et al. (1997) found no increase in complications comparing unreamed and reamed nails in the management of open tibial fractures.

Biomechanics

Intramedullary reaming can act to increase the contact area between the nail and cortical bone by smoothing internal ridges. When the nail is the same size as the reamer, 1 mm of reaming can increase the contact area by 38%. Increased reaming allows insertion of a larger-diameter nail, which provides more rigidity in bending and torsion.

However there are also disadvantages to reaming. Depending on the outer diameter of the bone and amount of bone removed, reaming the canal diminishes the cortical wall thickness and can weaken the bone. This effect can be mitigated by the load sharing characteristics of the nail.

Biological effects

Reaming can cause both local and systemic effects. Locally reaming can cause significant disruption to the osseous blood supply. The vascular supply to bone is comprised of medullary arteries that supply the inner two-thirds of the cortex and of periosteal arterioles that penetrate the cortex at fascial attachments and supply the outer one-third.

The haversian system acts as a conduit between the endosteal and periosteal flow circulation, with flow occurring in a centrifugal manner.

Reaming destroys the medullary canal and the endosteal blood supply and has a negative effect on cortical blood flow. However, in animal studies, this effect is reversed within 12 weeks. In spite of the damage on the endosteal circulation, reaming also significantly increases the vascular perfusion of surrounding muscles and deep soft tissues.

One local effect of reaming is the deposition of autologous medullary contents and osteo-inductive factors at the fracture site. Experiments in sheep have shown 24% of reaming debris is deposited at the fracture site. Reamings have been found to have higher levels of growth factors such as insulin growth factor (IGF-1) and TGF-b1 than iliac bone graft.

The heat generated from reaming has been thought to cause thermal necrosis and alterations to the endosteal architecture. The critical temperature for thermal injury of bone is considered to be 56°C, the level at which denaturation of alkaline phosphatase occurs. Although the complication of thermal necrosis as a result of intramedullary reaming is commonly quoted, clinical evidence of this is rare and fewer than 10 cases have been reported in the medical literature. Similarly, the use of tourniquets with reaming has been discouraged due to the perceived risks of thermal damage, but studies have shown that the application of a tourniquet and reaming to 1.5 mm above the required diameter of the nail appear to be safe clinical practice.

The systemic effects of reaming include the embolization of marrow contents into the circulation. Reaming causes transient rises pulmonary artery pressure and pulmonary vascular resistance. This may be related to the release of pro-inflammatory mediators such as IL-6.

Elastic nails

In paediatric diaphyseal fractures of the forearm, femur, and tibia, elastic nails can be inserted percutaneously to stabilize the fracture. These flexible nails are made of either titanium or steel, and are placed in the metaphysis of the bone away from the epiphyseal plate. If these cases, are treated conservatively they often require a considerable period of cast immobilization that interferes with schooling. With flexible nailing, in-patient hospital stay is reduced and time to weight bearing is also reduced. The nails are usually removed 6–9 months after insertion.

Complications

A number of complications have been reported with intramedullary nailing;
- *Infection*: the rate of deep infection following intramedullary nailing has been reported between 1.8% for closed tibial fractures up to 9.5% for Type III open tibial fractures.
- *Compartment syndrome*: the incidence of compartment syndrome following intramedullary nailing of the tibia has been reported as high as 7%. This maybe related to prolonged longitudinal traction during nailing. Although compartmental pressures increase significantly during reaming, these pressures return to normal soon after surgery.
- *Anterior knee pain and shoulder dysfunction*: anterior knee pain (AKP) is commonly reported following intramedullary nailing of both the femur and tibia. Meta-analysis has revealed the mean incidence of AKP following tibial nailing was 47%, 25.6% for retrograde femoral nailing, and 18.6% for antegrade femoral nailing. The cause of AKP is multi-factorial and may be related to malposition of the nail, damage to the patella, irritation of the infrapatellar fat pad, and damage to the infrapatellar branches of the saphenous nerve. Removal of the nail may alleviate symptoms when the nail is protruding, but in many cases AKP remains problematic despite removal.

Shoulder dysfunction and pain has been reported following antegrade intramedullary nailing of the humerus. A meta-analysis comparing intramedullary nailing and plating of humeral shaft fractures found a higher incidence of shoulder pain and reoperations in the intramedullary nail group.
- *Implant failure*: intramedullary nails are load-sharing devices. Over-enthusiastic weight-bearing in the early post-operative stage, before fracture callus has formed places considerable strain on the nail, which may then subsequently fail. As with all metallic implants, there is a relative race between bone healing and implant failure. An implant may break when fracture healing is delayed or when a non-union occurs. Unlocked nails typically fail either at the fracture site, or through screw hole or slot. Locked nails fail by screw breakage or fracturing of the nail at locking hole sites, most commonly at the proximal hole of the distal interlocks.
- *Mal-union and non-union*: if the fracture is distracted following IM nailing then this may result in non-union. Compression of the fracture site once the distal locking screws are inserted may reduce the risk of distraction. In cases of non-union, dynamization of the construct by removing the proximal screws or exchange nailing are possible treatment options. Mal-union can arise if the limb is not properly aligned during nailing. Careful attention should be paid to the limb orientation to prevent malalignment.
- *Fat embolus syndrome*: the leakage of fat from lower limb fractures has been estimated to be about 20–50 mL. Reaming may cause an increase in fat release. This may, in turn, result in a higher degree of inflammatory response after reamed nailing. In combination with pre-existing pulmonary trauma, the effects may be accentuated and may have more clinical significance. Therefore, the use of an unreamed nail may be more appropriate in the presence of chest trauma.

External fixation

The external fixator has been utilized in orthopaedics for over 100 years. The first attempts at external fixation were reported by Malgaigne in 1843 and consisted of a claw-like device designed for patella fractures. By 1960, Vidal and Hoffmann had popularized the use of the external fixator to treat open fractures and infected pseudoarthroses.

External fixation provides fracture stabilization at a distance from the fracture site, reducing further damage to the soft tissues near the fracture.

Components of external fixators

There are a number of different external fixator systems available, as well as specialist configurations such as Ilizarov frames and Taylor Spatial Frames (Smith and Nephew, Tennessee, USA). However, in essence they all consist of the same component parts (Fig. 14.11:
- *Bone fixation elements*: these are either half pins (Schantz pins) or thick wire.
- *External supporting elements*: these connect wires or pins from a fixation segment. They can be either blocks, rings or arches.
- *Connecting elements*: these are rods or hinges that connect the external supporting elements together and can be manipulated to alter the position between the supporting elements.

Indications for use

External fixators can be applied as either a damage control orthopaedic procedure or as a definitive fracture stabilization device. The indications for their use include:

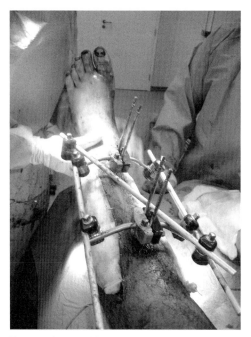

Fig. 14.11. An external fixator applied as a damage control procedure. The patient also had compartment syndrome and full fasciotomies have been performed. Courtesy of Surg Cdr M Brinsden, RN.

- As a damage control procedure in critically ill or multiply-injured patients.
- Open fractures with severe soft tissue damage.
- Infected fractures, where internal fixation is not suitable.
- Severely comminuted femoral shaft fractures in children.
- In cases of non-union or mal-union, where deformity or limb length correction is required.

Damage control orthopaedics requires the adequate stabilization of the major orthopaedic injury until the patient's condition has been optimized, at which point definitive fracture stabilization is undertaken, usually with internal fixation methods. External fixators provide an excellent option for damage control procedures as they can be applied at a distance from the fracture site without causing significant soft tissue damage and can generally be applied faster than internal fixation devices.

Biomechanics of external fixators

The external fixator is an ideal device with which to obtain healing because it is one of the few devices which provides a stable construct in which the mechanical parameters (rigidity and alignment) can be modulated as needed throughout treatment. Based on the biology of fracture healing, a stable construct is required to reduce strain to the fresh fracture environment. This stimulates the mesenchymal cells to differentiate towards chondrogenesis and subsequently endochondral ossification. Once there is evidence of biological activity (early fracture callus), the fixator can be made more flexible to allow micromotion to help stimulate healing of the fracture. This is achieved quite easily by removing bars,

The stiffness of the external fixator construct is based on a number of factors:
- *The number of pins in each fixation segment*: each fixation segment should have a stable configuration of pins or wires. 2 half pins are sufficient for diaphyseal fragments, although more are required in metaphyseal fragments. More pins can potentially increase the probability of infection. However, if a pin does become infected, then it can be removed without reducing the stiffness of the construct.
- *The diameter of pins*: the stiffness of the pin is proportional to the diameter of the pin. Therefore, the greater the diameter of pin, the stiffer the construct.
- *The number and position of bars*: the number of interconnecting bars or rods can increase the stiffness of the fixator. In addition, the closer the bar is to the fracture, the stiffer the construct. The position of the bar is often dictated by the intervening soft tissues and patient comfort.
- *Multiplanar fixation*: bars placed perpendicular to each other provide greater stability than monolateral frames.
- *Pin configuration*: pins placed further away from the fracture site provide greater protection from torsional forces. Pins placed closer to the fracture site allow greater compression at the fracture site, and help to reduce strain. Therefore, the ideal pin placement is a 'near-far' configuration with pins placed both closer and further away from the fracture site to counter the physiologic loads at the fracture.

Ilizarov frames

The Ilizarov apparatus was developed by Professor Gavril Ilizarov in the Kurgan region of Siberia in the 1950s. It is a specialized circular fixator in construction. It is commonly used to correct deformity and to treat bone defects by bone transportation techniques. It is also used to treat complex or open fractures and infected non-unions.

Deformity correction is produced by callostasis. A low energy osteotomy (corticotomy) is produced. The fracture callus is then formed during the initial latency period. At this stage there should be minimal displacement of the fracture fragments. Following the formation of the fracture callus, the distraction period begins. Lengthening or deformity correction occurs at a rate of 1 mm a day. Once the correction has been made, the limb remains in the fixator until adequate consolidation of the new bone has occurred. Typically, the consolidation period is approximately twice the distraction period. The advantage of the Ilizarov system is that the patient does not have to remain immobilized during the process and is able to mobilize on crutches from the early post-operative period.

The surgeon must be aware of the multiple complications that can arise from the Ilizarov technique. This is related not only to the procedure, but is also significantly affected by patient factors. This technique is usually seen as a final salvage procedure and is frequently used in the presence of infection. Therefore, complications are more likely to be encountered.

Neurovascular damage can occur from direct injury during transfixion. Injury can also occur secondarily during lengthening because of excessive distraction or impingement of nerves or vessels against wires or half-pins. An incomplete corticotomy may result in tension developing at all wire-bone interfaces leading to limb pain. Early X-rays show bending of the fixation elements without distraction of the osteotomy site. Premature consolidation can occur if the rate of distraction is inadequate to maintain continued fragment separation or if the patient is non-compliant with the distraction prescription.

Joint subluxation is a serious complication that can permanently jeopardize the function of the affected limb. Subluxation may occur when the lengthening exceeds soft-tissue tolerance or when lengthening continues despite the development of contractures. The response of muscle to lengthening is the stretching and increase in the number of sarcomeres. However, this only occurs in the initial stages and the threshold of soft tissue lengthening is often limited to 15–20% of the original limb segment length. Articular cartilage reacts negatively to lengthening procedures, and this may be related to joint compression during lengthening.

Taylor Spatial Frames

Taylor Spatial Frames (TSFs) were designed 10 years ago and based on the Stewart–Gough Platform. The Stewart–Gough Platform consists of two orthogonal platforms connected by six struts. By manipulating the length of the struts it is possible to change the orientation of one platform in relation to the other with 6 degrees of freedom (x, y, z, pitch, roll, and yaw). In order to correctly orientate the two platforms, inverse kinematics equations are used to calculate the appropriate length of each connecting strut.

Clinically, a ring is placed orthogonal to the proximal and distal fracture fragments. The two rings are connected by six adjustable struts. The software accompanying the frame produces a prescription of strut adjustments to allow correction of a limb deformity, by realigning the rings to the mechanical axis of the limb segment.

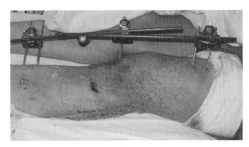

Fig. 14.12. A monolateral external fixator spanning the knee joint. Note the pin tract infection of the proximal pin sites, which would complicate future internal fixation.

Complications

Pin site infection

Pin site infection following external fixation has been commonly reported, and can result in deep infection and subsequent fixation failure (Fig. 14.12). Pin site infection normally starts as cellulitis with organisms such as Staph. aureus predominating. Pins closest to joints are most frequently affected as they are subject to the greatest movement. The contributory effect on the development of infection with the accumulation of fluid at the interface of the pin has also been described.

Deep infection from pins may require removal of the pin and the onset of osteomyelitis may require the removal of the fixator and can be extremely difficult to treat. Pin site infection can also interfere with future surgical management. Animal studies have shown that infected pin sites lead to contamination of the medullary canal within 2 weeks. Nowartarski found that early closed intramedullary nailing (less than 7 days) after external fixator application resulted in an infection rate 1.7% in femoral fractures of multiply injured patients. If intramedullary nailing is considered after prolonged external fixation, most authors recommend a delay between the external fixator removal and intramedullary nailing to allow the pin sites to dry.

A number of different regimes have been proposed for the management of pin sites. The aim of any regime is to reduce the number of superficial and deep infections related to the pins. In a prospective study by Davies et al. (2005), they showed a significantly lower proportion of pin site infections and increased time to first infection, utilizing a protocol from the Russian Ilizarov Scientific Centre for Restorative Traumatology and Orthopaedics. This protocol includes:

- Non-touch handling of wires and pins.
- Pulsed drilling with irrigation.
- Bone swarf removal.
- Immediate pin-site dressings in alcoholic solution of chlorhexidine with pressure to reduce haematoma formation.
- Pin sites cleaned daily for the 1st 3 days with 70% alcohol solution.
- Pressure occlusive dressing after day 3; pin sites then cleaned as above every 7–10 days.

Other complications include neurovascular damage from pin insertion and patient difficulties with the frame. External fixators require active management with regular outpatient visits and careful clinical and radiographic monitoring.

Late complications of fractures

A number of late complications can arise following limb injury and can develop even if the fracture is appropriately managed. They include:
- Delayed, non-, and mal-union.
- Avascular necrosis.
- Myositis ossificans/heterotrophic ossification.
- Tendon ruptures.
- Nerve compression.
- Muscle contracture.
- Complex Regional Pain Syndrome.
- Osteoarthritis.

Non-union of fractures

Definition
Non-union of a fracture is defined as a fracture that occurred a minimum of 9 months previously and has not shown radiographic signs of progression toward healing for three consecutive months (US Food and Drug Administration definition).

Delayed union is an ununited fracture that continues to show progress toward healing or that has not been present for long enough to satisfy the definition of a non-union.

Mal-union is a fracture that has healed, but in a non-anatomic position.

Prevalence
The prevalence varies for different bones, but as an example in a meta-analysis of 5517 tibial fractures, the combined prevalence of non-union was 2.7% and the prevalence of delayed union was 4.4%.

Classification of non-union
Non-unions can be classified according to their radiographic appearance (LaVelle, 1998).
- *Hypertrophic non-unions:* they have abundant callus. This indicates an adequate blood supply, but insufficient mechanical stability for completion of fracture healing.
- *Oligotrophic non-unions:* they have little callus, but still have an adequate blood supply. They are typically due to inadequate reduction with little or no contact between the fracture surfaces.
- *Atrophic non-unions:* they have no or little callus and have resorption of bone. This is due to a deficient biologic process.

Causes of non-union
Non-union of fractures is a multifactorial phenomenon. It can be the result of systemic conditions and local factors.

Malnutrition and vitamin deficiency
Patients with long bone fractures are frequently catabolic. Protein malnutrition affects callus composition and has a negative effect on early proliferation and differentiation of those cells required for repair.

Vitamin B6 deficiency causes changes in the coupling between osteoblasts and osteoclasts, as a result of decreased glucose-6-phophate (G6PD) activity in the periosteal region. This significantly delays the maturation of the callus and union.

Diabetes
Diabetes has been implicated in non-union in numerous elective orthopaedic procedures with non-union rates of 28% reported in diabetic patients undergoing ankle fusion.

This is due to the combination of vascular compromise and peripheral neuropathy. At a cellular level, diabetics are prone to deficiencies in the production of growth factors, angiogenic response, and macrophage function, which results in impairment of fracture healing. Sensory neuropathy is an independent risk factor in non-union and should be checked for at the time of injury.

Cigarette smoking
Smoking can significantly impair fracture healing by a number of mechanisms. It has been shown to decrease collagen deposition by 30–50%. Nicotine inhibits alkaline phophatase and collagen production, and stimulates deoxyribosenucleic acid synthesis. It also decreases bone blood flow. Clinically, this has been reported by Schmitz et al. (1999), who showed a 69% delay in the radiological union of tibial fractures in patients who smoke.

Non-steroidal anti-inflammatory drugs
There is a correlation between the use of non-steroidal anti-inflammatory drugs (NSAIDs) and non-union, especially when NSAIDs are used for more than 4 weeks. NSAIDs inhibit osteogenic activity, although the pathogenesis is not fully understood. Animal studies have shown decreased prostaglandin E2 levels with NSAIDs. The effects are likely to be reversible with prostaglandin levels being restored after short-term treatment. The newer generation of cyclo-oxygenase-2 (COX-2) inhibitors have been shown to inhibit fracture healing more than less specific NSAIDs. The avoidance of NSAIDs in the post-operative and post-injury period may prevent non-unions.

Infection
Infection can contribute to non-union through the creation of gaps by osteolytic granulation tissue, and motion from loosening of prosthetic implants. The inflammatory response to bacteria at the site of the fracture disrupts callus, increases the gaps between fragments and increases motion between fragments.

Inadequate vascularity
Insufficient vascularity is one of the potential causes of non-union, and particularly decreased vascularity in the first 3 weeks after fracture may prevent fracture union. Animal studies have shown that ischaemia at the fracture site decreased the amount of bone formation and significantly fewer blood vessels are seen in atrophic non-unions compared with normal fracture healing.

Biomechanical instability
The stability of the fracture directly affects the differentiation of mesenchymal cells towards either an osteoblast or chondrogenic cell line. Poor stability leads to the formation of more chondroblasts and fibroblasts in the fracture gap. This can eventually lead to hypertrophic non-union. Conversely, over-rigid fixation without compression of the fracture fragments can prevent both primary and secondary bone healing and lead to non-union.

Iatrogenic factors
Excessive stripping of the periosteum and damage to the bone and soft tissue blood supply during fracture fixation can decrease vascularity at the fracture site and contribute to non-union.

Diagnosis

Non-union or delayed union can often be painless, but tenderness over the fracture site or pain on movement can indicate problems. The presence of a draining sinus or infected soft tissue may be a result of osteomyeltis. The neurovascular status of the distal limb can indicate a sensory neuropathy or potential vascular problems, which can promote non-union. The mainstay of diagnosis is good quality X-rays which can be augmented by CT and MRI.

Treatment options

Correction of biological factors

- *Malnutrition:* albumin levels of <34 g/L and lymphocyte counts of <1.5 x 10^9/L are an indication of inadequate nutritional status and should be checked in the outpatient department.
- *Smoking:* patients should be advised on the effects of smoking and given smoking cessation support.
- *NSAIDs:* if the patient is on a prolonged course of NSAIDs, this should be discontinued.

Operative options

Infection, soft-tissue defects, and malalignment substantially alter the options of treatment. A closed, uninfected non-union with acceptable alignment requires intervention only to achieve union. In infected cases, thorough debridement and soft-tissue coverage in addition to bone stabilization and bone-grafting are required. A number of operative strategies are available:

- Intramedullary nailing.
- Compression plates.
- External fixation.
- Ilizarov technique.

Intramedullary nailing

Intramedullary nailing is the most commonly used form of stabilization in the management of unstable acute tibial fractures. Consequently, they may already be *in situ* when a non-union is diagnosed. If the fracture union does not occur relatively early, considerable stress is placed on the implant and it may consequently fail. In cases of un-infected non-unions, the fracture can be dynamized by removing one of the locking screws from one end of the nail. This maybe appropriate when the fracture ends have been distracted by the nail. Another option is exchange nailing, whereby the existing nail is removed and is replaced with a nail that is at least 1 mm larger. The advantages of exchange nailing are the osteo-inductive effects from the reamings, and better fixation between the larger diameter nail and the medullary canal. Intramedullary nailing also allows early full weight bearing.

Compression plates

Compression plates have been used with considerable success in the treatment of closed uninfected non-unions. They can be used on hypertrophic non-unions, but will require supplementary bone grafting in atrophic non-unions. As load-bearing devices, they do not tolerate weight-bearing until healing has occurred. There is an associated increased risk of infection compared with bone-grafting and they should not be used in the presence of previously infected fractures.

External fixation

External fixation may be indicated in patients with a previous infection. It allows free wound access, stabilization of bone fragments at a distance from the lesion, permits motion of adjacent joints, and encourages patient mobility.

Ilizarov technique

This technique is useful in the treatment of angulated malunions and non-unions associated with malalignment. The technique is also useful in cases of segmental bone defects where the techniques of corticotomy and bone transport need to be employed and in managing infected cases, where intramedullary nailing and compression plating are not possible. This method is usually only available in selected centres and requires good ancillary medical support.

Biologic adjuncts

Autologous bone graft aids bone formation by a process of *osteogenesis, osteo-induction and osteoconduction*. Osteogenesis refers to the synthesis of new bone at the recipient site by the cellular elements of the graft that survive the transplantation. Osteo-induction is the process by which host mesenchymal stem cells from the surrounding tissue are differentiated into osteoblasts as a result of chemotactic factors within the graft. Osteoconduction is the process by which the graft acts as a scaffold for new bone formation. Iliac bone graft remains the gold standard for autologous bone graft, although patients should be warned of potential pain, infection, and bleeding from the donor site.

Approximately one-third of bone grafts used are allografts. Allografts are either frozen, or sterilized with gamma radiation or ethylene oxide sterilization. Freeze-drying destroys all osteogenic capability, but the host immune response is less robust than the response to fresh allograft. Gamma radiation appears to affect the mechanical properties of allografts, whereas ethylene oxide affects the osteo-inductive properties. Large strut allografts have been used successfully in limb salvage following tumour resection. In trauma, Haddad et al. (2002) reported on a case series of 40 patients in whom a femoral fracture around a well-fixed prosthetic femoral stem was treated with strut allograft. Thirty-nine of the 40 fractures united.

Demineralized bone matrix is produced by acid extraction of allograft. It contains type-1 collagen, non-collagenous proteins, and osteo-inductive factors. Although osteo-inductive effects have been seen in animals, its effect in humans is less certain. It may have potential use as a bone graft extender used in conjunction with autologous bone graft.

Calcium phosphate synthetic substitutes are osteoconductive. They increase bone formation by providing an osteoconductive matrix for host osteogenic cells to create bone under the influence of host osteo-inductive factors. Pore size and porosity are important characteristics of bone graft substitutes. No osseous in-growth occurs with pore sizes of 15–40 µm. Osteoid formation requires pores sizes of 300–500 µm to be ideal for osseous in-growth. Interconnecting pores prevent the formation of blind alleys, which are associated with low oxygen tension; low oxygen tension prevents osteoprogenitor cells from differentiating into osteoblasts. Calcium phosphate comes in many forms and can be manufactured as a cement. It is resorbed in 26–86 weeks. In a prospective randomized study of 40 closed tibial plateau fractures with metaphyseal defects conducted by Bucholz, patients were randomized to have the defect filled with either autogenous bone or porous calcium phosphate. At 15 months follow-up, no significant radiographic or clinical differences were seen between the two groups.

Bone morphogenic proteins (BMP) are members of the transforming growth factor ß (TGF-ß) group of proteins that have strong osteo-inductive properties. BMP-7 has been shown to be as effective as autologous bone graft in non-union of the tibia. Although relatively expensive, their use may prevent the need for further procedures and, therefore, may be cost-effective overall.

Non-biological adjuncts
Direct electrical stimulation has been used in the management of non-unions, with some success reported in a few small-scale studies. However, no prospective randomized trials are available for review. Ultrasound has been proven to enhance the healing of fresh closed tibial fractures.

Avascular necrosis
Definition
Avascular necrosis (AVN) is defined as cellular death of bone components due to interruption of the blood supply; the bone structures then collapse, resulting in bone destruction, pain, and loss of function. Certain areas are more prone to develop AVN:
- The head of the femur.
- Proximal pole of the scaphoid.
- Lunate.
- Body of the talus.

These sub-articular regions lie at the most distant parts of the bone's vascular territory, and they are mostly enclosed by cartilage, giving restricted access to local blood vessels. The subchondral trabeculae are further compromised in that they are sustained largely by a system of endarterioles with limited collateral connections.

Pathophysiology
The medullary cavity is effectively a closed compartment containing myeloid tissue, marrow fat and capillary blood vessels. Therefore, swelling in one component can only occur at the expense of the other components within the compartment. In trauma, damage to the blood supply or haemorrhage leads to a vicious cycle of ischaemia, reactive oedema, marrow swelling, increased intra-osseous pressure, and further ischaemia.

Causes
There are a number of conditions that are associated with AVN. They are:
- Post-trauma.
- *Infection:* osteomyelitis, septic arthritis.
- *Haemoglobinopathy:* sickle cell disease.
- *Storage disorders:* Gaucher's disease.
- *Dysbaric osteonecrosis:* Caisson disease in deep sea divers.
- *Coagulation disorders:* familial thrombophilia, hypolipo-proteinaemia, thrombocytopaenic purpura.
- *Others:* SLE, steroid administration, alcohol abuse, Perthe's disease, ionizing radiation.

Diagnosis
In the initial stages, AVN is often asymptomatic. Pain and loss of movement are the most common complaints. Some patients complain of a 'click', which maybe due to catching a loose articular fragment.

Early signs of AVN cannot usually be detected by plain X-ray. When they appear (seldom before 3 months), the characteristic 'crescent' line of subchondral sclerosis is caused by osteoblastic proliferation at the interface between ischaemic and live bone. Other features include the loss of trabeculae in the necrotic region. MRI is a more useful modality in the early stages and the necrotic segment is defined as a hypodense band on the T1 weighted images.

In the late stages there is distortion of the articular surface and more intense sclerosis.

Treatment
The management of AVN is specific to the region affected, but the basic principles are as follows:
- *Early AVN*: when the bone contour is intact there is the possibility that structural failure may be prevented. Some lesions heal spontaneously or do not progress to bony collapse. In non-weight-bearing surfaces, a waiting policy may be warranted. Lesions in weight-bearing areas often progress to collapse and in these cases medullary decompression and bone grafting, or an osteotomy may be helpful. Medullary decompression is thought to decrease vascular engorgement and inflammation and to relieve the increased intramedullary pressure.
- *Intermediate AVN*: when there is distortion of the articular surface, conservative management will not suffice. However, the joint may still be salvageable and a realignment osteotomy may have a role.
- *Late AVN*: destruction of the articular surface may give rise to severe pain and loss of function. In these cases, treatment falls into three categories: non-operative management with analgesia, lifestyle modification and splintage; athrodesis of the joint (e.g. wrist or ankle), partial or total joint arthroplasty.

Myositis ossificans/heterotrophic ossification
Myositis ossificans is the presence of calcified tissue following an injury to muscle. This is due to the differentiation into osteoblasts of mesenchymal cells. It is more common following head and spinal injuries, suggesting there may be some neural control. Common sites are around the hip, following surgery for acetabular fractures, and also round the elbow. The patient presents with local swelling and soft tissue tenderness. Initial X-rays are usually normal, but by 2–3 weeks a fluffy calcification is seen in the soft tissues. By 8 weeks the bony mass is easily palpable and is clearly defined on X-ray. Initial treatment involves gentle physiotherapy to maintain ROM. Surgical excision should only occur once the condition has been stable for several months. Bone scan can help to determine this as can the appearances on CT. Indomethacin or local radiotherapy can help prevent a recurrence.

Tendon ruptures
Rupture of the extensor pollicis longus (EPL) tendon may occur 6–12 weeks after a fracture of the distal radius. The site of rupture is usually at the Lister tubercle. The rupture is far more common in association with undisplaced fractures, and it has been reported in patients who had a wrist injury without a fracture. The pathogenesis of the rupture appears to involve both mechanical and vascular factors. Displaced fracture fragments or healing callus can mechanically impale the EPL tendon or narrow the third dorsal compartment and contribute to rupture. A 5-mm length of the tendon adjacent to the tubercle is relatively avascular. A fracture of the distal part of the radius can compromise the extrinsic synovial nutrition to the EPL tendon by oedema or haematoma. This further limits the precarious blood supply of the EPL tendon and can lead to ischaemic rupture.

It presents as an inability to fully extend the distal phalanx of the thumb. Direct suture is rarely possible and is treated by transfer of the extensor indicis proprius tendon to the distal stump of the ruptured thumb tendon.

Another tendon at risk is the long head of biceps following a fractured neck of humerus. Tendinopathy of the tibialis posterior tendon can occur following medial malleolus fractures.

Nerve injury

Bone or joint deformity may result in local nerve entrapment. Typical features are numbness, paraesthesia, loss of power, and muscle wasting in the distribution of the affected nerve. Common sites are:
- Radial nerve injury complicating 10% of humeral shaft fractures.
- Median nerve following wrist injury.
- Posterior tibial nerve following ankle fractures.
- Common peroneal nerve following fractures of proximal fibula or tight cast application.

The diagnosis is made clinically but can be confirmed with neurophysiological studies. Treatment involves early decompression with or without transposition of the nerve.

Muscle contracture and joint stiffness

Following arterial injury or a compartment syndrome, the patient may develop ischaemic contractures of the affected muscle (Volkmann's ischaemic contractures). Nerves injured by ischaemia can sometimes recover, so patients present with deformity and stiffness, but numbness is inconstant. Treatment involves splintage, release of contractures, soft tissue reconstruction, and tendon transfer procedures.

Joint contractures can be caused by scarring of the capsule. Fixed flexion deformities can occur in prolonged immobilization of elbow injuries. If physiotherapy fails to resolve the problem, an anterior capsulectomy may be required. Shoulder stiffness and loss of flexion of the knee can also be seen following injury and may require surgical treatment if medical management fails.

Complex Regional Pain Syndrome
Definition
Complex Regional Pain Syndrome (CRPS) is a chronic condition characterized by burning pain and abnormalities in the sensory, motor and autonomic nervous systems. The syndrome typically appears after an acute injury to a joint or limb, although it may occur with no obvious precipitating event. In most cases, regardless of the site of injury, the symptoms begin and remain most intense in the most distal extremity.

Epidemiology
CRPS is thought to be present in 5–10% of patients with a peripheral nerve injury. In the UK, there are thought to be 11,500 patients suffering from the condition. 60–80% of cases are in females. It can occur in any age group, although paediatric cases often have a better outcome.

Pathophysiology
The pathophysiology of the condition is still uncertain, although some authors have proposed that sympathetic pain results from tonic activity in myelinated mechanoreceptor afferents. This, in turn, causes tonic firing in neurons that are part of the nociceptive pathway.

Classification
The International Association of the Study of Pain (IASP) classifies CRPS as Type I and Type II. Type II occurs in the presence of a documented nerve injury. The diagnostic criteria for CRPS are:
- The presence of an initiating noxious event or a cause of immobilization.
- Continuing pain, allodynia (perception of pain from a non-painful stimulus), or hyperalgesia disproportionate to the inciting event.
- Evidence at some time of oedema, changes in skin blood flow, or abnormal sudomotor activity in the area of pain.
- The diagnosis is excluded by the existence of any condition that would otherwise account for the degree of pain and dysfunction.

Disease progression
Stage I Pain is more severe than would be expected from the injury, and it has a burning or aching quality. It may be increased by dependency of the limb, physical contact, or emotional upset. The affected area becomes oedematous, may be hyperthermic or hypothermic, and shows increased nail and hair growth. Radiographs may show early bony changes. Duration is usually 3 months from onset of symptoms.

Stage II Oedematous tissue becomes indurated. Skin becomes cool and hyperhydrotic with cyanosis. Hair may be lost, and nails become ridged, cracked, and brittle. Hand dryness becomes prominent, and atrophy of skin and subcutaneous tissues becomes noticeable. Pain remains the dominant feature. It usually is constant and is increased by any stimulus to the affected area. Stiffness develops at this stage. Radiographs may show diffuse osteoporosis. The 3-phase bone scan is usually positive. Duration is 3–12 months from onset.

Stage III Pain spreads proximally. Although it may diminish in intensity, pain remains a prominent feature. Flare-ups may occur spontaneously. Irreversible tissue damage occurs. Skin is thin, shiny, and oedema is absent. Contractures may occur. Radiographs indicate marked demineralization.

Treatment
CRPS is a very difficult condition to treat requiring a multidisciplinary approach and, in most cases, early physiotherapy can help symptoms. Breaking the pain cycle early is important in relieving symptoms, using several drugs in combination. Tricyclic antidepressants have been used with mixed success using sub-therapeutic doses e.g. amitryptiline 10–25 mg nocte as opposed to the antidepressant dose of 75–150 mg. Anticonvulsant drugs, such as gabapentin and pregabalin, also have a role in management. Selective neural blockade and regional intravenous administration of local anaesthetic and clonidine have been successful in some patients.

Post-traumatic osteoarthritis
Post-traumatic arthritis is common in intra-articular fractures, particularly in intra-articular fractures that are not anatomically reduced. It can also occur following malunited fractures. Malalignment of the tibia can affect the biomechanics of the ankle joint by decreasing the total area of contact pressure, which results in regions of increased pressure where the residual contact occurs. This increased pressure may cause increased shear stresses on

the articular cartilage in the areas of high stress, and the shear stresses may result in premature osteoarthritis of the joint. Management of post-traumatic arthritis depends on the joint involved and can include arthroscopic debridement (e.g. radio-capitellar degeneration of the elbow), osteotomy (e.g. high tibial osteotomy for unicompartmental degeneration of the knee), excision arthroplasty, or arthrodesis (e.g. ankle fusion).

Joint injuries

Injuries to the joints are commonly seen in the emergency department. They range in severity from minor sprains to significant intra-articular fractures. Clinically, they present with pain, swelling, and reduced ROM. Joint laxity suggests possible ligamentous damage. This should be compared with the contralateral limb, as patients may have generalized joint laxity. The presence of an acute haemarthrosis of the knee following an injury is indicative of ligamentous injury or intra-articular pathology, and a lipohaemarthrosis suggests an intra-articular fracture. X-rays can rule out fractures and dislocations. The presence of an avulsed fragment may suggest a detached ligament.

Intra-articular fractures

The AO principles of fracture care include the anatomic reduction of the fracture fragments and early joint range of movement exercises. These principles are particularly pertinent in intra-articular fractures where anatomical reduction is necessary to prevent post-traumatic osteoarthritis and early movement prevents joint stiffness and fracture disease (see Figs 14.13 and 14.14). To allow early weight bearing, rigid fixation of the articular fragments is required. This traditionally meant the use of lag screw compression, but the same effect can now be achieved with very distal locking screws of intramedullary nails and with external fixator frames.

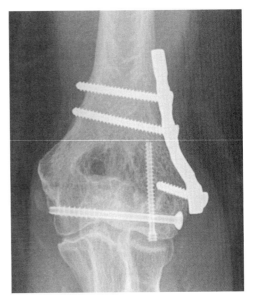

Fig. 14.14. The articular fragment has been anatomically reduced and fixed with two compression screws. The fixation has been protected with a buttress plate. This fixation allows early mobilization of the joint and thereby reduce the risk of joint stiffness.

On examination the shape of the joint is abnormal and bony landmarks may be displaced. A full neurovascular examination should be performed to exclude an associated vascular or nerve injury. The vessels frequently affected are listed in Table 14.4.

X-rays are diagnostic and will also show whether there is a related bony injury.

Treatment

The dislocation should be reduced as soon as possible. Reduction of a dislocated hip within 12 h of injury has been shown to reduce the incidence of complications. Reduction should be performed using closed methods. However, if there is soft tissue imposition or a fracture dislocation then open reduction may necessary. Whichever method is used, it is imperative that a pre- and post-reduction neurovascular examination be documented in the notes to exclude an

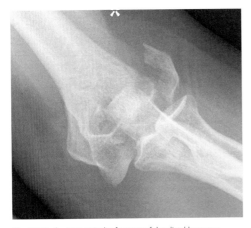

Fig. 14.13. An intra-articular fracture of the distal humerus.

Dislocation and subluxation

Dislocation occurs when the joint surfaces are completely displaced and are no longer in contact. Subluxation describes a lesser degree of displacement and the articular surfaces are still partly apposed.

Clinical findings

Following a dislocation the joint is painful and the patient is very reluctant to move it. There is usually a history of trauma, but in the case of recurrent dislocations, this may be very minor.

Table 14.4. Associated neurovascular injuries with dislocation

Joint dislocation	Vascular injury	Nerve injury
Shoulder	Axillary A	Axillary N
Elbow	Brachial A	
Hip	Superior gluteal A	Sciatic N
Knee	Popliteal A	Peroneal N

iatrogenic injury. Post-reduction radiographs are necessary to confirm joint reduction. Once the joint has been reduced, it is normally immobilized until soft tissue healing occurs.

Complications

Complications following an acute dislocation are similar to the general complications with fractures and include neurovascular damage, stiffness, avascular necrosis (hip dislocation), and secondary osteoarthritis. In addition, recurrent dislocation can also occur. In a 25-year follow-up study, 53% of patients suffered a recurrent dislocation of the shoulder. This figure is much higher in patients who played contact sports. Primary arthroscopic stabilization following first time anterior dislocation of the shoulder has been shown to reduce the risk of further dislocation by 76% and were more likely to return to sport at 2 years.

Further reading

Aderinto J, Keating JF. Intramedullary nailing of fractures of the tibia in diabetics. *J Bone Jt Surg Br* 2008; **90-B**: 638–42.

Bachiller FG, Caballer AP, Portal LF. Avascular necrosis of the femoral head after femoral neck fracture. *Clin Orthop Relat Res* 2002; **399**: 87-109.

Bar-On E, Sagiv S, Porat A. External fixation or flexible intramedullary nailing for meoral shaft fratures in children. A prospective, randomized study. *J Bone Jt Surg Br* 1997; **79-B**: 975–8.

Bhandari M, Guyatt GH, Swiontkowski MF, Schemitsch EH. Treatment of open fractures of the shaft of the tibia: A systematic review and meta-analysis. *J Bone Jt Surg Br* 2001; **83**: 62–8.

Bosse MJ, McCarthy ML, Jones AL, Webb LX, Sims SH, Sanders RW, et al. The insensate foot following severe lower extremity trauma: An indication for amputation? *J Bone Jt Surg Am* 2005. **87-A**: 2601–8.

Boyce T, Edwards J, Scarborough N. Allograft bone. The influence of processing on safety and performance. *Orthop Clin N Am* 1999; **30**: 571–81.

Cammisa FP Jr, Lowery G, Garfin SR, Geisler FH, Klara PM, McGuire RA, et al. Two-year fusion rate equivalency between Grafton DBM gel and autograft in posterolateral spine fusion: a prospective controlled trial employing side-by-side comparison in the same patient. *Spine* 2004; **29**: 660–6.

Canale ST. *Campbell's Operative Orthopaedics*. 10th edn. St Louis: Mosby-Year Book, 2003.

Charnley J. *The closed treatment of common fractures*, Golden Jubilee edn. Cambridge: Cambridge University Press, 1950.

Claes LE, Heigele CA, Neidlinger-Wilke C, Kaspar D, Seidl W, Margevicius KJ, et al. Effects of mechanical factors on the fracture healing process. *Clin Orthop Relat Res* 1998; **335**(Suppl): S132–47.

Clasper JC, Cannon LB, Stapley SA, Taylor VM, Watkins PE. Fluid accumulation and the rapid spread of bacteria in the pathogenesis of external fixator pin track infection. *Injury* 2001; **32**: 377-81.

Clasper JC, Parker SJ, Simpson AH, Watkins PE. Contamination of the medullary canal following pin-tract infection. *J Orthop Res* 1999; **17**(6): 947–52.

Davies R, Holt N, Nayagam S. The care of pin sites with external fixation. *J Bone Jt Surg Br* 2005; **87-B**: 716–19.

Dickson KF, Munz JW. Locked plating: biomechanics and biology and clinical indications, part II. *Techn Orthopaed* 2007; **22**(4): E1–6.

Egol KA, Kubiak, EN, Fulkerson E, Kummer FJ, Koval KJ. Biomechanics of locked plates and screws. *J Orthop Trauma* 2004; **18**: 488–93.

Einhorn TA. The cell and molecular biology of fracture healing. *Clin Orthop* 1998; **355**(Suppl): 7–21.

Farouk O, Krettek C, Miclau T, Schandelmaier P, Guy P, Tscherne H. Minimally invasive plate osteosynthesis and vascularity: Preliminary results of a cadaver injection study. *Injury* 1997; **28**(Suppl 1): S7–12.

Feitelson JB, Rowell PP, Roberts CS, Fleming JT. 2 week nicotine treatment selectively increases bone vascular constriction in response to norepinephrine. *J Orthop Res* 2003; **21**(3): 497–502.

Forster MC, Aster AS, Ahmed S. Reaming during antegrade femoral nailing; Is it worth it? *Injury* 2005; **36**: 445–9.

Fransen M, Neal B. Non-steroidal anti-inflammatory drugs for preventing heterotopic bone formation after hip arthroplasty. *Cochrane Database Syst Rev.* 2004;**3** CD001160.

Friedlaender GE, Perry CR, Cole JD, Cook SD, Cierny G, Muschler GF,et al. Osteogenic protein-1 in the treatment of tibial non-unions. *J Bone J Surg Am* 2001; **83**(Suppl 1): S151–8.

Gerstenfeld LC, Al-Ghawas M, Alkhiary YM, Cullinane DM, Krall EA, Fitch JL, et al. Selective and nonselective cyclooxygenase-2 inhibitors and experimental fracture-healing. Reversibility of effects are short-term treatment. *J Bone Jt Surg Am* 2007; **89**(1): 114–25.

Giannoudis P, Snowden S, Matthews SJ, Smye SW, Smith RM. Friction burns within the tibia during reaming: are they affected by the use of a tourniquet? *J Bone Jt Surg Br* 2002; **84-B**: 492–6.

Glover P, Worthley L. Fat Embolism. *Crit Care and Resusc* 1999; **1**: 276–84.

Gustilo RB, Anderson JT. Prevention of infection in the treatment of one thousand and twenty- five open fractures of long bones: retrospective and prospective analyses. J Bone Jt Surg Am 1976; **58**(4): 453–8.

Gustilo RB, Mendoza RM, Williams DN. Problems in the management of type III (severe) open fractures: a new classification of type III open fractures. *J Trauma* 1984; **24**(8): 742–6.

Haddad FS, Duncan CP, Berry DJ, Lewallen DG, Gross AE, Chandler HP. Periprosthetic femoral fractures around well-fixed implants: use of cortical onlay allografts with or without a plate. *J Bone Jt Surg Am* 2002; **84**: 945–50.

Hente R, Füchtmeier B, Schlegel U, Ernstberger A, Perren SM. The influence of cyclic compression and distraction on the healing of experimental tibial fractures. *J Orthop Res* 2004; **22**(4): 709–15.

Holton PD. Antibiotics prophylaxis: current recommendations. *J Am Acad Orthopaed Surg*, 2006; **14**(10): S98–100.

Hovelius L, Olofsson A, Sandström B, Augustini BG, Krantz L, Fredin H, Tet al. Nonoperative treatment of primary anterior shoulder dislocation in patients forty years of age or younger. *J Bone Jt Surg Am* 2008; **90**: 945–52.

Jagodzinski M, Krettek C. Effect of mechanical stability on fracture healing – an update. *Injury* 2007; **38S1**: S3–10.

Johansen K, Daines M, Howey T, Helfet D, Hansen ST Jr. Objective criteria accurately predict amputation following lower extremity trauma. *J Trauma*. 1990; **30**: 568–73.

Keating JF, O'Brien Pj, Meek RN, Broekhuyse HM. Interlocking intramedullary nailing with and without reaming for the treatment of closed fractures of the tibial shaft: a prospective, randomized study. *J Bone Jt Surg Am* 1997; **79**: 640–6.

Kozin SH, Wood MB. Early soft-tissue complications after fractures of the distal part of the radius. *J Bone Jt Surg Am* 1993; **75-A**: 144–53.

LaVelle DG. Delayed union and nonunion of fractures. In: Canale TS (ed.). Campbell's Operative Orthopaedics. 9th edn. St. Louis: Mosby, 1998, pp. 2579–629.

Maffulli N, Binfield PM, King JB, Good CJ. Acute haemarthrosis of the knee in athletes. A prospective study. *J Bone Jt Surg Br* 1993; **75**(6): 945–9.

McQueen MM, Gaston P, Court-Brown CM. Acute compartment syndrome. Who is at risk? *J Bone Jt Surg Br* 2000; **82**(2): 200–3.

Metaizeau J-P. Stable elastic intramedullary nailing for fractures of the femur in children. *J Bone Jt Surg Br* 2004; **86B**: 954–7.

No authors listed. The early management of severe tibial fractures: the need for combined orthopaedic and plastic management. *Br J Plast Surg* 1997; **50**: 570–83.

Nowotarski PJ, Turen CH, Brumback RJ, Scarboro JM. Conversion of external fixation to intrameduallry nailing for fractures of the shaft of the femur in multiply injured patients. *J Bone Jt Surg Am* 2000; **82-A**: 781–8.

Phillips AM. Overview of the fracture healing cascade. *Injury* 2005; **36**: S5-7.

Robinson CM, Jenkins PJ, White TO, Ker A, Will E. Primary arthroscopic stabilization for a first time anterior dislocation of the shoulder. a randomized, double-blind trial. *J Bone Jt Surg Am* 2008; **90**: 708–21.

Ruedi TP, Buckley R, Moran C, (eds.) AO *Principles of Fracture Management*. 2nd edn. New York: Thieme Medical Publishers, Inc; 2007.

Schmitz MA, Finnegan M, Natarajan R, Champine J. Effect of smoking on tibial shaft fracture healing. *Clin Orthop Rel Res* 1999; **365**: 184–200.

Smith WR, Ziran BH, Anglen JO, Stahel PF. Locking plates: tips and tricks. *J Bone Jt Surg Am* 2007; **89-A**: 2298–307.

Solomon L, Warwick DJ, Nayagam S. *Apley's system of orthopaedics and fractures*, 8th edn. London: Arnold Publishers.

Templeman DC, Gulli B, Tsukayama DT, Gustilo RB. Update on the management of open fractures of the tibial shaft. *Clin Orthop Relat Res* 1998; **350**: 18–25.

Watson JT. Current concepts review: treatment of unstable fractures of the shaft of the tibia. *J Bone Jt Surg Am* 1994; **76**: 1575–84.

Webb LX, Bosse MJ, Castillo RC, MacKenzie EJ. Analysis of surgeon-controlled variables in the treatment of limb-threatening Type III open tibial diaphyseal fractures. *J Bone Jt Surg Am* 2007; **89-A**: 923–8.

Williams J, Gibbons M, Trundle H, Murray D, Worlock P: Complications of nailing in closed tibial fractures. *J Orthopaed Trauma* 1995; **6**: 476–81.

Wolff J. *Das gesetz der transformation der knochen*. Berlin: Verlag von August Hirschwald, 1892.

Crush injury

Crush injury

Definitions

A consensus meeting on crush injury and crush syndrome held in 2001 agreed the following definitions, although many others exist:

A crush injury is a direct injury resulting from crush. Crush syndrome is the systemic manifestation of muscle cell damage resulting from pressure or crushing.

These systemic manifestations include acute respiratory distress syndrome, disseminated intravascular coagulation, electrolyte disturbances, and acute renal failure.

History and epidemiology

Crush injury first appeared in the English language literature in 1941 during the London Blitz. Bywaters described two patients who, having been extricated from several hours of burial under building debris, were initially thought to be unharmed, but rapidly deteriorated and subsequently died.

However, substantial reference had already been made to this condition in the German literature. It was described in 1909 in victims of the Messina earthquake and, subsequently, in 1916 in (German) First World War injuries. As far back as the early 1800s Larrey, the Napoleonic surgeon, reported skin and muscle necrosis in the pressure areas of comatose patients. Little was published on crush injuries in the years following the Second World War until the 1976 Tangshan earthquake, where it was thought that up to 5% of deaths were complicated by crush syndrome.

Following his initial discovery, Bywaters continued to study the effects of crush injury and established some principles for its management that are still accepted today, albeit modified as a result of technological advancement.

Aetiology

Crush injury and crush syndrome are most commonly reported during mass casualty events, such as earthquakes, explosions, mine accidents, and other such catastrophes. However, they have also been described in smaller scale trauma and in non-traumatic situations.

For a crush injury to occur there must be continuous prolonged pressure on tissue. There are three variables, namely pressure, area of affected tissue, and duration of crush.

Pressure

In a disaster situation where a casualty has to be extricated from debris the fact that pressure has been applied is obvious. However, at the other extreme crush injury can occur as a result of the patients own body weight if they are comatose for long enough, for example, after a narcotic overdose or a cerebrovascular event.

Affected region

Treatable crush injury tends to occur in limbs. If the pressure required to cause a significant crush injury was applied to the torso the injury would be non-survivable. The scale of the injury may not be immediately obvious as there may be minimal external evidence of injury.

Duration

The longer the period of crush the more likely a significant crush injury is to occur. Hence, a massive force applied for a short time, or a minimal force applied over several hours can both cause crush injury.

Incidence and mortality

Its incidence is difficult to estimate, but crush injury is one of the leading causes of death after earthquakes. Following the terrorist attack in New York on 11 September 2001 only one case of crush injury-induced renal failure was reported, but this was thought to be due to the low number of survivors.

Around the world many densely populated regions lie in areas where seismic activity is not unusual, for example, California and Turkey. This fact, together with the current trend in international terrorism, lead to the potential for crush injuries to become more common.

Pathophysiology

The sarcolemma is the cell membrane of an individual skeletal muscle cell which maintains cell integrity. It houses various energy-dependent pump mechanisms used to control homeostasis (for example, the Na^+/K^+ ATP-ase pump). Sodium is largely an extracellular ion, and potassium and calcium are largely intracellular ions. Without the pump mechanisms, the basic principles of diffusion would apply and the concentration of each ion would be similar on either side of the cell membrane.

Myoglobin is an oxygen-carrying protein contained within muscle cells. It has a greater affinity for oxygen than haemoglobin and so oxygen diffuses from blood into muscle. Because of its action as an oxygen store, myoglobin is present in greater concentration in the postural muscles of the lower limbs, and accounts for their dark red or brown colour. When present in the urine it causes rusty discolouration (typical in crush syndrome).

The cellular damage inflicted by crush injury can be separated into the ischaemic injury and the reperfusion injury, although these are related.

The ischaemic injury

External pressure from crush causes a decrease in arterial blood supply leading to hypoperfusion, resulting in anaerobic metabolism and the accumulation of lactic acid. This situation is viable for a short period of time, but if the ischaemia continues the muscle damage will become irreversible.

The external pressure also causes a pressure-stretch myopathy, which involves an influx of sodium, chloride, and water from the interstitium into the muscle cells. Initially, the cellular pump mechanisms will actively remove these materials from the cytosol, but they soon become overwhelmed and the cells become swollen. This interferes further with normal cellular respiration.

The pressure may result in damage to the muscle sarcolemma, causing substances that are normally maintained inside the cells to leak into the interstitial fluid. This is exacerbated by cell death.

The reperfusion injury

In crush injury, the following substances are released from muscle cells:
- Myoglobin.
- Potassium.
- Phosphorus.
- Calcium.

These remain local to the injury while the external compressive force is still in place, but when released the affected area will re-perfuse, becoming bathed in oxygen.

Those substances normally isolated inside cells are introduced into the circulation. The re-perfusion injury has two elements, namely the reperfusion of damaged and hypoxic muscle, and the introduction of intracellular material into the circulation.

Recent work has shown that the damage on a microvascular level which is responsible for reperfusion injury is largely governed by oxygen free radicals (also termed 'reactive oxygen species'). A free radical is an atom with an unpaired electron in the outer shell. Many substances are implicated in the generation of these, the most important of which is xanthine oxidase. Mitochondria, activated leucocytes, prostaglandin synthase, and catecholamine oxidation also have a role.

Xanthine oxidase is normally present in the liver and is integral to the uric acid cycle. The presence of xanthine oxidase in a crush injured muscle leads to cellular oedema and ultimately cell death.

Muscle cells do not normally contain xanthine oxidase, but they contain xanthine dehydrogenase, which can cleave to form xanthine oxidase in the presence of calcium and oxygen. In crush injury, the amount of calcium in the cytosol is increased (because of the pressure-stretch myopathy) and xanthine oxidase is produced during the reperfusion phase when oxygen is present.

Xanthine oxidase is an 'electron acceptor', taking an electron from the (stable) outer shell of the O_2 molecule to create an (unstable) superoxide anion (O_2^-) and hydrogen peroxide (H_2O_2). This free radical (O_2^-) is unstable and will in turn 'steal' an electron from other molecules, often from the electron transport chain of damaged mitochondria.

In addition, there is an influx of activated neutrophils to the affected region, which produce reactive oxygen species causing further damage to the endothelium and microvasculature.

It is this microvascular damage that causes muscle and tissue oedema in crush injury. The reperfusing muscle is oedematous and hypoxic, and the subsequent deranged cellular respiration further exacerbates this by the production of reactive oxygen species. The oedema can be substantial, with volumes in the region of 10 L lost from the intravascular compartment in a 24-h period.

Acute renal failure

The aetiology of renal failure in crush syndrome has several aspects, but is incompletely understood. The biggest cause is thought to be the hypovolaemia resulting from fluid sequestration, which also activates various constrictor mechanisms, such as the renin-angiotensin system. Myoglobin also has a direct toxic effect on the renal parenchyma, as it is a large protein, which obstructs the distal convoluted tubules causing an obstructive nephropathy.

Once reperfusion occurs the damaged or necrotic muscle cells will leach their contents into the circulation and the renal tubules will have to process a large potassium load.

Systemic acidaemia occurs because of several mechanisms including:

- Intracellular production of lactic acid as a result of anaerobic metabolism, which subsequently leaks into the circulation.

- Production of uric acid by the xanthine oxidase pathway.

- Amino acids are produced as a result of muscle necrosis, and also lead to acidaemia.

Principles of management

As with all medical conditions, the main aim of treatment is to prevent deterioration and further complications.

Pre-hospital care

Attention should be paid to scene assessment and rescuer safety prior to individual patient assessment. This is particularly important in situations where building debris may not have settled and there is potential for further injury. There may also be fire, electrical, or explosive risks.

The priority in each patient, in common with any trauma situation, is the primary survey:

Control of exsanguinating external haemorrhage

Any critical external haemorrhage must be controlled before the airway is assessed. Minor bleeding wounds can be treated at a later stage.

Airway with cervical spine control

The airway should be assessed and patency ensured. All patients should receive high flow oxygen. The possibility of burns or smoke inhalation should be considered. Patients who are trapped after the collapse of a building have a high risk of having incurred a spinal injury so full precautions should be initiated and maintained.

Breathing with ventilation

The chest wall should be assessed for signs of trauma and associated conditions. Ventilation should be supported as necessary.

Circulation with haemorrhage control

Shock should be identified and potential sources assessed, remembering that crush injury causes third space losses in addition to the possible other sources of blood loss from associated injuries. Peripheral venous access should be obtained.

Disability

The conscious level should be assessed and the pupils examined.

Exposure

Whilst it is important for the entire body to be examined to detect injury, hypothermia should be avoided. The limbs should be examined; inspection of the skin may reveal breaches, bruising, blistering, or a shiny appearance suggesting raised internal pressure. Distal pulses should be assessed along with distal motor and sensory function.

If the patient has been trapped for a period of time greater than 4 h, or if it is estimated that extrication will take that period of time, then treatment for crush syndrome should be initiated. The essential principle is safety, and it may be necessary for the patient to be extricated promptly.

Removal of the crushing force is a potentially painful experience, notwithstanding the pain from the original insult. Proportional use of analgesia should be considered, which can be delivered in several forms:
- Inhaled nitrous oxide/oxygen mixture (Entonox™).
- Intravenous morphine sulphate, titrated to effect. Use of the intramuscular route is discouraged.
- Intravenous ketamine, if appropriately trained personnel are present.

The key is to begin fluid resuscitation as soon as is possible. The incidence of renal failure in crush-injured patients increases with delay in treatment.

There continues to be debate about the fluid of choice for resuscitation. The crush-injured patient is already prone to hyperkalaemia from muscle breakdown, and infusing exogenous potassium (contained in Hartmann's Solution) could exacerbate an already deranged biochemical picture. It is therefore recommended that initial resuscitation should be with 0.9% sodium chloride (normal saline), warmed to body temperature when possible.

This should be given initially as a 2-L bolus followed by an infusion of 1–1.5 L/h. As soon as the compressing force is removed the damaged muscle will begin to re-perfuse and toxic substances will enter the circulation. It is therefore vital that the release is co-ordinated with the attending medical team.

The Consensus Statement discusses the use of a venous tourniquet proximal to the injury that, in theory, would prevent the release of these metabolites. However, it concludes that there is no evidence supporting this and the use of tourniquets should be restricted to the treatment of life-threatening, non-compressible limb haemorrhage. Once extricated, the affected limb should be splinted at heart level, to prevent oedema and assist perfusion.

The use of sodium bicarbonate during trauma and other resuscitation is controversial, but there is a definite role in the management of crush injury. Whilst controversy surrounds the efficacy of bicarbonate in reversing intracellular acidaemia, its use in crush injury is to alkalinize urine and prevent renal failure. The initial dose is 1 mmol/kg, which equates to 1 mL/kg of 8.4% sodium bicarbonate, the concentration available in most emergency drug packs.

Once the treatment regime is in progress, evacuation of the patient to an appropriate facility should occur. The circumstances of the incident will dictate whether this is by road or air. Patients should be taken to a facility with
- Surgical support.
- Critical care support.
- Renal support—haemodialysis or haemofiltration.
- Facilities relevant to the associated injuries.

The receiving facility should be alerted by radio or telephone so they can be prepared for the arrival of the patient and have appropriate personnel present.

Emergency Department care

On arrival in the Emergency Department the patient should be met by an appropriately experienced team and a MIST handover given.

The primary survey should be performed, and cardiac monitoring and pulse oximetry should be applied at an early stage.

Sufficient venous access should be obtained (usually multiple large-bore cannulae). A bedside capillary blood glucose test should be performed. Blood should be sent for full blood count, cross-match if indicated, electrolyte profile, creatine kinase, and liver function. If available a serum myoglobin may be performed.

Arterial blood gas analysis will provide information on acid-base status and may also provide key biochemical measurements.

As long as there was no requirement to proceed to urgent operation a full secondary survey should be performed, including a log-roll. At this stage, a urinary catheter should be inserted if there is no contraindication. Examination of the urine specimen begins with inspection, as the presence of myoglobin will cause a dark red or brown colour. A bedside urine dipstick will show large amounts of protein and blood if myoglobinuria is present, as standard urinalysis sticks cannot differentiate between haemoglobin and myoglobin. The absence of blood can only be confirmed by direct microscopy, which should be requested. The presence of red blood cells on microscopy suggests renal tract trauma and is not indicative of crush injury, and alternative diagnoses should be considered.

Urgent biochemical analysis is important as life-threatening abnormalities may be present, the most important of which is hyperkalaemia. Untreated, this may cause arrhythmia and lead to cardiac arrest.

If hyperkalaemia is present the following actions should be considered

- 10 mL of 10% calcium chloride or gluconate IV. This helps to stabilize the myocardial membrane, but will not in itself lower the potassium level. It should be available in the emergency drug pack. It can be repeated every 10–20 min until the ECG normalizes.
- *Insulin*: this should be given in the soluble, rapid-acting form, e.g. Actrapid™ (Novo Nordisk). 10 units is the usual dose, and this will drive extra-cellular potassium into cells. It should be co-infused with 50% dextrose (50 mL) to prevent hypoglycaemia.
- *β₂-agonists*: e.g. salbutamol. Administered by nebulizer, this will also cause a transient movement of potassium into cells, which lasts for approximately 2 h. Over-use will precipitate a sinus tachycardia.

It should be considered that all of these methods are temporary and the injured muscle will continue to cause hyperkalaemia, therefore:

- Cardiac monitoring should be continuous.
- Regular capillary blood glucose measurements should be taken if insulin is being administered.
- Serum potassium should be re-checked regularly with an expected fall of 1 mmol/L/h.

Further management of hyperkalaemia may be necessary, with the most appropriate methods being haemodialysis or haemofiltration. Continuous infusions of frusemide are often used to increase urinary potassium loss—this should not be used in the crush-injured patient as it can counter attempts to alkalinize the urine. It can also precipitate myoglobin in the renal tubules.

Hypocalcaemia should not be treated as 'rebound' hypercalcaemia occurs later.

The key outcome in the following advanced aspects of management is the prevention of renal failure. If this develops then the mortality increases significantly.

Definitive care

Once the initial assessment and emergency treatments have been performed, the priorities for treatment should be established. In the case of multiple injuries, the patient may require urgent laparotomy or skeletal fixation. If this is not the case, then the patient should be transferred to a high dependency or intensive care unit where close observation is possible.

Monitoring and access

The treatment will involve infusion of large volumes of fluid and central venous access should therefore be obtained to help guide fluid status. Invasive cardiac output monitoring should be considered. As has previously been intimated, continuous cardiac monitoring should be in place and arterial pressure monitored invasively.

Urinary alkalinization

This involves infusing sodium bicarbonate to a level sufficient to maintain a urinary pH, in the case of crush syndrome, of greater than 6.5.

Its mechanism is to enhance the excretion of acid, as well as to prevent the deposition of myoglobin and uric acid in the renal tubules, which cause acute renal failure. Haem in its ferric form is directly nephrotoxic, whereas if this can be converted to its ferrous form (by alkalinization) it is much more benign.

There are various concentrations of sodium bicarbonate available. Possibly the easiest to infuse is 8.4%, 1 mL of which contains 1 mmol of sodium bicarbonate. This should be given in 50-mL aliquots and urinary pH monitored. Urinary pH can be measured using standard urinalysis strips. If excessive sodium bicarbonate is administered a metabolic alkalosis may result, which can be treated with a 500 mg intravenous bolus of acetazolomide.

Intravenous fluid

As has been discussed, patients with crush syndrome have hypovolaemic shock secondary to traumatic fluid loss and third space losses. Pre-hospital treatment involves resuscitation with 0.9% sodium chloride, but continued use of this fluid may cause a hypernatraemic hyperchloraemic metabolic acidosis. It is, therefore, recommended that treatment should alternate between 0.9% sodium chloride and 5% dextrose solutions in hospital.

The use of packed red cells and other blood products should be reserved for situations where there is confirmed blood loss. If transfusion is indicated then there should be close monitoring of serum potassium as the risk of hyperkalaemia is higher.

The quantity of fluid required is large and is guided by the urine output and cardiovascular status of the patient. It is recommended that the approximate rate is 500 mL/h, but this will vary between patients and the combination of fluids and mannitol should achieve a urine output of 300 mL/h.

Mannitol diuresis

This is the other major tenet in the prevention of renal failure. Mannitol is an osmotic diuretic and a mild acid, so is usually buffered with sodium bicarbonate. Its mode of action is renal, increasing sodium and free water excretion by its osmotic effect. Mannitol also has a role in neutralizing reactive oxygen species.

Its use is contraindicated in anuric renal failure. It should only be given if the urine output exceeds 20 mL/h (6). This is important as the urine output may fall as a result of developing renal failure and, if this is the case, the mannitol infusion should be stopped. It is usually administered as a 20% solution (20g mannitol per 100 mL, although other concentrations are available), and is given in two stages. The initial dose is 1-2 g/kg (1–2 mL/kg) and this should be continued for 4 h. After this the dose is dependent on response.

The aim is to have a urine output of 300 mL/h (or approximately 3 mL/kg/h), and this should be achieved by combined use of fluid and mannitol. It is suggested that patients will require about 12 L daily, alternate litre bags of which should contain 1 mmol/kg of sodium bicarbonate. This is a large amount of fluid and close invasive monitoring of the fluid status is essential. A daily positive balance in the region of 4 L is to be expected. If the patient is fluid replete (as judged by cardiac output monitoring or pulmonary capillary wedge pressure), but the urine output is insufficient, then a bolus of mannitol is indicated. A continuing fall in urine output indicates acute renal failure and the patient should be considered for haemofiltration or haemodialysis.

Along with cardiovascular monitoring, it is important to measure the serum electrolytes (especially sodium and potassium, but also magnesium, phosphate, and calcium) and osmolality twice daily to ensure that measured values are normalizing and that therapy remains appropriate.

Analgesia

In a high dependency setting either continuous or patient-controlled intravenous opioid infusion are appropriate. Regional nerve blocks are discouraged as they may mask the early symptoms of compartment syndrome.

Amputation

In theory this could be a prophylactic measure, which could prevent renal failure and other complications, but there is no supporting evidence at present, and it is not advocated unless there is a non-salvagable limb or one that has life-threatening septic complications.

Hyperbaric oxygen therapy

Although theoretically beneficial, hyperbaric oxygen is logistically difficult to provide. At present only eight centres in the UK are capable of managing critically ill patients. It would be reasonable to discuss a patient with an isolated crush injury with a regional hyperbaric oxygen centre, but it is not recommended that this forms part of first line treatment.

Complications

If crush syndrome is anticipated and appropriate treatment instigated at an early (i.e. pre-hospital) stage complications should be preventable. The treatment, however, requires advanced equipment and skills, and the potential for deterioration should not be under-estimated.

Renal failure

This is the most serious complication of crush injury. Rhabdomyolysis is implicated in 7% of all cases of acute renal failure. The causes of renal failure are traditionally divided into pre-renal, intrinsic-renal and post-renal factors. The first two are important in crush injury.

Pre-renal

Caused by hypovolaemia, hypotension, and shock.

Treating the pre-renal causes involves adequate and monitored fluid resuscitation as covered in the previous section. Sub-optimal fluid administration can result in renal hypoperfusion and subsequent ischaemia.

Intrinsic-renal

Acute tubular necrosis caused by:
• Ischaemia secondary to hypotension.
• Toxins (e.g. myoglobin).
• Septicaemia.
• Prolonged pre-renal oliguria.

There are several factors that have been shown to be predictive of the crush injured patient developing intrinsic renal failure (13):
• Hypovolaemia.
• Elevated creatinine phosphokinase (CPK).
• Hyperkalaemia.
• Hyperphosphataemia.
• Hypoalbuminaemia.
• Low venous bicarbonate (< 17 mmol/L).

The creatinine phosphokinase level relates to the amount of muscle damage incurred and very high values (>20,000 IU) are associated with increased mortality. A patient with a relatively low CPK may still progress to renal failure and therefore the figure should not be interpreted in isolation.

Indications for initiation of renal replacement therapy

If a patient has required emergency treatment for hyperkalaemia then, due to the nature of the insult, it is likely they will require some form of renal replacement therapy (RRT) until the muscle damage is arrested. The decision to begin RRT relates to the patient's biochemical and general medical condition: the following criteria were proposed by Bellomo et al. in 1998:
• Anuria or oliguria (urine output <200 mL/12 h).
• Hyperkalaemia (K$^+$ > 6.5 mmol/L).
• Severe acidaemia (pH < 7.1).
• Azotaemia (urea > 30 mmol/L).
• Clinically significant organ oedema (particularly lung).
• Uraemic encephalopathy.
• Uraemic pericarditis.
• Uraemic neuropathy or myopathy.
• Severe dysnatraemia (Na$^+$ > 160 or <115 mmol/L).
• Hyperthermia.
• Drug overdose with a dialysable toxin.

One criterion can be an indication for the initiation of RRT. Two or more criteria make RRT mandatory. Multiple criteria are a reason for early initiation of RRT. The first five criteria are particularly relevant to the crush injured patient.

Methods of renal replacement therapy

There are three options in the provision of RRT and the choice is dependent on local policy, technical support, and available resources. The available modalities are:
• Peritoneal dialysis.
• Intermittent haemodialysis or haemofiltration.
• Continuous haemodialysis or haemofiltration.

Continuous therapy is more suitable in a patient whose cardiovascular status is unstable as there is less of an acute insult. However, this restricts the use of a machine to one patient and will use more dialysis fluid than intermittent therapy. It also requires continuous anticoagulation, which may prove to be contra-indicated in a patient with multiple injuries. Intermittent therapy should be sufficient to prevent hyperkalaemia, the most important consequence of ARF in this situation.

Haemodialysis and haemofiltration require a dedicated vascular access device, which is usually a double-lumen polyurethane catheter inserted into the femoral, subclavian, or internal jugular vein. Use of the subclavian vein is discouraged as the patient may subsequently require a permanent arterio-venous fistula for long-term dialysis, and the risk of subclavian vein stenosis precludes the use of that side of the body.

Peritoneal dialysis is the least resource-intensive as it does not require fresh water or electricity. However, it requires high standards of sterility and may not be possible if the patient has also suffered abdominal or pelvic trauma. In addition, a gastrointestinal ileus (common in critically ill patients) will reduce the efficiency of this method.

There are no clear guidelines on when RRT can be safely stopped. Electrolytes should be closely monitored and cessation of RRT considered when they are normalizing and the urine output increases to the region of one litre daily.

Compartment syndrome

This can be defined as a limb-threatening condition observed when perfusion pressure falls below tissue perfusion pressure in a closed anatomical space. It has multiple causes, which can be divided into non-traumatic and traumatic. In the case of a crush-injured patient, compartment syndrome occurs when the previously crushed muscle reperfuses and becomes oedematous within the confines of its compartment. Compartmental pressure can be increased significantly by application of a plaster or relatively tight dressing over a limb. Care should be taken that any splint applied to a crush-injured limb is not so tightly attached as to cause or exacerbate a compartment syndrome.

Symptoms and signs

The patient will complain of severe pain in the affected limb, classically out of proportion to the pain expected from the original injury and will be reluctant to move the limb. There may also be some neurological symptoms (commonly paraesthesiae).

In the sedated patient, an unexpected rise in the heart rate and blood pressure can indicate pain. However, this is not specific and there should be a low threshold for affected compartmental pressure monitoring in patients unable to verbalize symptoms.

On examination the affected compartment may feel tense when compared with the other side. The classical sign of compartment syndrome is a sudden increase in pain in response to passive stretching of the affected muscle. It is possible that the limb distal to the insult feels cool with weaker or absent pulses, but a significant compartment syndrome can exist with normal temperature and pulsation. Compartment pressure in health is normally less than 12 mmHg, and this will need to rise significantly before arterial pulsation will be lost, by which stage considerable damage will already have occurred.

Compartment pressure monitoring
There are various methods employed to monitor the pressure inside particular compartments, but one of the simplest involves using a standard intra-arterial catheter connected to a pressurized intravenous giving set filled with 0.9% sodium chloride and a transducer. The use of an actual figure is controversial and there is no agreement on an acceptable compartment pressure. In general, a pressure of 30–40 mmHg will indicate hypoperfusion.

Treatment
All constraining bandages should be removed from the limb. The mainstay of treatment is fasciotomy—an opening of all compartments of the affected limb along their entire lengths. However, it is now accepted that, in the absence of neurovascular compromise, a bolus of mannitol may reduce the need for operative management. If symptoms persist despite this then immediate fasciotomy should be performed. This not only involves incising the compartments, but also removing necrotic muscle and several visits to the operating theatre may be required.

The fasciotomy incisions are left open out of necessity but also because of the bulging, oedematous muscle. The major complications of fasciotomy are bleeding and infection. These are much more common if fasciotomy is carried out when the injury was a pure crush injury, rather than compartment syndrome and, for this reason, the differentiation between the two conditions is important.

Volkmann's ischaemic contracture
If a compartment syndrome is not recognized, or treatment is delayed, the muscle in that compartment will become necrotic. If not debrided, or incompletely debrided, the necrotic muscle will undergo fibrosis and a contracture will result. This is a difficult condition to manage, and often requires tendon transfer surgery. It is preventable by careful assessment and timely use of mannitol or surgical intervention.

Other complications
Patients with crush syndrome are prone to other conditions including:
- Adult Respiratory Distress Syndrome.
- Sepsis/ventilator-associated pneumonia.
- Oxygen toxicity.
- Disseminated intravascular coagulation.
- Thromboembolic disease.

Outcome

The outcome of the crush-injured patient is dependent on the severity of other injuries, as well as co-morbidities. In an otherwise healthy patient who is appropriately managed, a favourable result of treatment is possible.

Good outcome relies on:

- Early suspicion, recognition, and diagnosis.
- Early intravenous fluids.
- Early alkaline diuresis.
- Prompt treatment of electrolyte disturbances.
- Recognition and treatment of complications.

Key points

- A high index of suspicion should be maintained if the history is compatible.
- Patients who have had prolonged immobilization should not be extricated without due consideration of crush injury.

- Treatment should ideally begin pre-extrication.
- Subsequent renal failure carries a high mortality and early management should be directed towards its prevention.
- Early intravenous fluids are vital.
- Early renal protection by induction of an alkaline diuresis helps prevent acute renal failure.
- Electrolyte disturbances should be anticipated and treated.
- Analgesia should be titrated to effect.

Further reading

American College of Surgeons. *Advanced Trauma Life Support for Doctors (ATLS) 7/e* (2004). American College of Surgeons, Chicago: ACS, 2004.

Bellomo R, Ronco C. Indications and criteria for initiating renal replacement therapy in the intensive care unit. *Kidney Int* 1998; **66**(Suppl): S106–9.

Better OS, Rubenstein I, Reis ND. Muscle crush compartment syndrome: fulminant local oedema with threatening systemic Effectseffects. *Kid Int* 2003; **63**: 1155-115–7.

Better OS. History of the Crush Syndrome: from the earthquake of Messina, Sicily 1909 to Spitak, Armenia 1988. *Am J Nephrol* 1997; **17**: 392-39–4.

Bywaters EGL. 50 years on: the Crush Syndrome. *Br Med J* 1990; **301**: 1412-14–15.

Bywaters EGL, Beall D. Crush injuries and renal function. *Br Med J* 1941; **I**: 427-4–32.

Goldfarb DS, Chung S. The absence of rhabdomyolysis-induced renal failure following the World Trade Centre Collapse. *Am J Med* 2002; **113**: 260.

Greaves I, Porter K, Smith JE. Consensus statement on the early management of crush injury and prevention of crush syndrome. *J R Army Med Corps* 2003; **149**: 255-25–9.

Krost WS, Mistovich JJ, Limmer DD. Beyond the basics: crush injuries and Compartment Syndrome. *Emerg Med Serv* 2008; **37**: 67-–71.

Major Incident Medical Management & Support (MIMMS). London: BMJ Publishing, London 2002

Michaelson M. Crush injury and Crush Syndrome. *World J Surg* 1992; **16**: 899-–903.

Odeh, M. The role of reperfusion-induced injury in the pathogenesis of the Crush Syndrome. *N Engl J Med* 1991; **324**: 1417, 14–22.

Reis ND, Better OS. Mechanical Muscle-Crush Injury and Acute Muscle-Crush Compartment Syndrome. *J Bone Joint Surg [Br]* 2005; **87-B**: 450-45–3.

Sever MS, Vanholder R, Lameire N. Medical progress: management of crush-related injuries after disasters. *N Engl J Med* 2006; **354**: 1052, 10–63.

Von Schroeder HP, Botte MJ. Crush Syndrome of the Upper Extremity. *Hand Clin* 1998; **14**: 451-45–6.

Ward MM. Factors predictive of acute renal failure in rhabdomyolysis. *Arch Intern Med* 1998; **148**: 1553-155–7.

Vascular trauma

Vascular trauma

Introduction

Vascular trauma is challenging for the vascular specialist and non-specialist alike. As might be expected, vascular injuries are frequently the cause of profound haemorrhage and physiological disturbance, are time-critical and require expeditious treatment. However, they are particularly intolerant of hasty, rushed, or sub-optimal technique. In these frequently critically-injured patients, the surgeon and the wider trauma team must at once balance the twin priorities of haemorrhage control and definitive repair with the imperative to address other life-threatening injuries, whilst minimizing operative time. Furthermore, when considering extremity injury, there is the need to set the costs of intervention against the likelihood of restoring adequate limb function, taking into consideration the totality of damage to integument, soft tissue envelope, and axial skeleton.

This chapter describes the injury pattern (aetiology and pathophysiology), diagnosis, and assessment (history, examination, and investigation) and treatment (damage control options, interventional radiology, and surgical repair) of vascular injuries.

Patterns of injury

In both military and civilian practice, the vascular trauma patient is likely to be a young male, average age 30 years, with penetrating injury. There are, however, noticeable differences in the mechanisms of injury. In contemporary military settings, around two-thirds of vascular injuries are caused by explosions, with a quarter caused by high velocity gunshots and the remainder from blunt trauma, such as motor vehicle collisions and crush injuries. The extremities bear the brunt of injury and extremity haemorrhage remains a significant cause of battlefield death.

The aetiology of injury observed in the civilian setting typically reflects the level of urban violence local to the reporting centre. Case series from inner city centres in the United States and South Africa report high levels of vascular trauma secondary to gun and knife violence. Reports from Europe, Asia, and Australasia tend to be dominated by blunt trauma, iatrogenic damage from cardiological or interventional radiology, industrial trauma, or infrequent stabbings. It is from civilian centres that most evidence has been gathered pertaining to the management of trauma to the great vessels of the torso. Such injuries are usually fatal in military circumstances due to the high energy nature of the munitions used and extended casualty evacuation (casevac) times.

In both civilian and military practice the most commonly injured arteries are the femoral, brachial and popliteal arteries. Worldwide, the most commonly injured vein is the superficial femoral vein, although venous injuries are probably under-reported and under-diagnosed as they are rarely limb-critical.

Mechanisms of vessel injury

Vessels may be penetrated by ballistic projectiles (a bullet fired from a rifled or non-rifled weapon, or shotgun pellet), explosively-borne fragments (shell casing, preformed fragments), secondary fragments (bone splinter), or by sharp, impaling objects, such as edged weapons (knives) or medical instrumentation (vascular access sheath). Projectiles possessing large amounts of kinetic energy (usually, but not always, fired from rifled weapons) can cause tissue damage beyond the track of their passage through the tissue by the propagation of shock waves and cavitation effect. This may result in disruption to the intima of the vessel without accompanying breach of the vessel wall.

Vessel wall breach may be limited to an isolated puncture, or may be more extensive. Partial vessel transection is classified mild (<25% diameter involved), moderate, severe (>50% involved) through to complete transection. Haemorrhage will result, and vessel spasm will accompany arterial injury, but the haemostatic effect of this is likely to be far more effective in complete transection (when cut vessel ends can retract). Where the magnitude of the injury is not great, and where the injury is constrained, closed, or compressed, such that exsanguination does not result, the natural history of penetrating vascular injury is for the surrounding haematoma to form an encasing pseudo-aneurysm. Such aneurysms may thrombose spontaneously, or grow over time to compress adjacent arterial or venous structures, or they may erode through overlying skin with devastating consequences. Disruption to adjacent artery and vein may result in direct communication between the vessels, as a traumatic arterio-venous fistula. Haemorrhage itself may be classified as compressible (extremity) or incompressible (torso cavity).

Non-penetrating or closed vascular injury can occur secondary to direct blunt trauma over a vulnerable vessel (such as a blow to the femoral artery in the groin), but is usually seen following a high energy limb injury (fall from height, motor vehicle collision) resulting in long bone fracture or joint dislocation. The same loading force that results in injury to the axial skeleton can shear, stretch, or compress adjacent vessels resulting in contusion and damage to the delicate intimal layer, without vessel wall breach or haemorrhage. In such circumstances vessel thrombosis occurs, with attendant risk of end-organ ischaemia, as the intima is dissected off the underlying muscular layer by antegrade blood flow. The clinical consequences of such dissections should never be optimistically attributed to vessel spasm (with the expectation that sequelae will spontaneously resolve). Positive proof that the vessel is patent and intact should be obtained, usually by operative exploration or radiological imaging. As with penetrating injury, the degree of end-organ ischaemia depends upon the degree of collateralization, extent of arterial disruption, tissue susceptibility to ischaemia (with nerve tissue being more sensitive than skeletal muscle) and the length of time to revascularization.

Diagnosis and assessment

The fundamental aims of assessing the trauma patient with a potential vascular injury are four-fold. First, to determine if there is a vascular injury present; secondly, to establish if the vascular injury is the cause of significant compromise in terms of haemorrhage or ischaemia; thirdly, to prioritize management of the vascular injury within the overall injury burden of the patient; and fourthly, to establish the best strategy for treatment of the injury (open versus endovascular, damage control surgery (DCS) versus definitive repair, immediate versus deferred treatment; see Table 16.1).

Table 16.1. Key questions in assessing vascular trauma.

Question	Subsidiary questions
Is there a vascular injury?	What is the patient history and mechanism of injury? What are the physical findings? • Hard signs & soft signs—see Table 16.2 • ABPI, hand-held Doppler. Are there any associated markers of vascular injury? What special investigations are available? • Angiography. • Angio suite. • On-table. • CT angiography. • Duplex Doppler ultrasound
Is there significant compromise of patient or limb?	What is the extent of haemorrhage, and is it on-going? • Physiology of patient, • Blood pressure, pulse, respiratory rate, mentation, urine output, • Base excess, lactate. • Physical evidence of bleeding. • Dressings, drains, distended abdomen. What is the extent of ischaemia, and is it getting worse? • Physical examination (the '6 P's'). • Duration. • Tissue affected.
How urgently does this vascular injury require treatment?	What is the injury burden? Are there other over-riding life-threatening injuries? Is the haemorrhage incompressible or compressible? Is there significant compromise?
What is the best management strategy?	Open versus endovascular? • Is the injury complex amenable to an *advantageous* endovascular solution? • What are the local facilities, resources and expertise, and how long will it take to muster these? DCS vs definitive repair? • What is the patient's physiology? • What is the injury burden? • Will the patient survive the repair? Immediate versus deferred treatment? • Is the end organ/limb threatened (likely to become non-viable without repair)? • Does patient instability preclude any attempt to address re-vascularization?

Clinical features

The presentation of a vascular injury depends on the pattern of the injury and the location of the vessel. In the absence of obvious external haemorrhage, the diagnosis of vascular injury can be difficult, especially in the shocked polytrauma patient. In evaluating such patients it is imperative to understand the injurious force that has been applied to the patient and determine the vascular structures at risk. Pre-hospital personnel must be interrogated to ensure that all relevant details (such as height of fall, speed of impact) are handed over. Details of weapon type, range of use, and type of knife are desirable in understanding the wound track and potential for damage. The time since injury is crucial in determining the potential warm ischaemic time. Elderly patients, although infrequent, are increasingly prevalent amongst the trauma population, and a proportion will have degenerative vascular disease that will need to be distinguished from acute injury.

By tradition, clinical signs of extremity vascular injury are classified as hard or soft (Table 16.2). Hard signs are considered sufficient evidence to be diagnostic of vascular injury, whereas soft signs are merely indicative and their presence or absence is not confirmatory—further investigation is required. A full survey of the injured limb, searching for lacerations, fragment, or bullet wounds, fractures, dislocations, neurological deficit, and distal ischaemia is mandatory. The traditional features of extremity ischaemia, the 6 P's, (painful, pale, pulseless, paraesthetic, paralysed, and perishingly cold) lose a good deal of their utility when dealing with the intubated, sedated, shocked, and hypothermic major trauma patient, but are a useful baseline. Fractures and joint dislocations are often associated with vascular injury, particularly so in the case of the popliteal artery, which is particularly vulnerable in dislocations of the knee. Certain patterns of injury should alert the clinician to potential vascular trauma (see Table 16.3). Compartment syndrome, with a tense, swollen extremity and severe pain on passive flexion, may occur with or without an underlying fracture (whether open or closed) in severe trauma. Reliance on the presence of pulses (which are rarely lost) and the measurement of intra-compartment pressure (a one-off result means little) should not override clinical suspicions and appropriate action in such circumstances.

Hand-held Doppler is an easily portable, cheap, and accurate tool in the diagnosis of extremity vascular trauma and should be utilized liberally (Box 16.1), although the limitations of hearing a Doppler signal should be understood (see Table 16.4). The gold standard is to measure the ankle-brachial pressure index, although this requires the careful placement of a pressure cuff around an injured, painful limb, and an accurate assessment of Doppler signal that may be difficult in the hectic circumstances of a trauma resuscitation, the pay off is that a normal ABPI is almost never associated with significant vascular injury.

Penetrating injuries to the great vessels of the torso, resulting in haemothorax or haemoperitoneum, will often present with profound shock as the haemorrhage is not constrained and is not amenable to external compression. Blunt disruptive injuries to these vessels (typically caused by rapid deceleration or acceleration forces) may not be associated with such profound shock as bleeding is constrained, at least initially, within the overlying peritoneal or pleural reflection.

Table 16.2. Clinical features of vascular injury

Hard signs	Soft signs
Pulseless cold pale limb	History of active bleeding
Expanding haematoma	Penetrating injury close to major vessel
Palpable thrill or audible bruit	Non-expanding haematoma
Active bleeding	Neurological deficit

Table 16.3. Patterns of skeletal trauma and associated vascular injury in blunt trauma.

Injury	At risk vascular structures
Cervical skin contusion (seat belt sign)	Carotid artery
Fracture of 1st/2nd ribs or sternum	Descending thoracic aorta
Supracondylar fracture of humerus	Brachial artery
Supracondylar fracture of femur	Popliteal artery
Posterior dislocation of knee	Popliteal artery
Open tibial fracture	Popliteal/crural arteries

Box 16.1. Hand-held Doppler in lower extremity trauma

- *Use:* apply manual sphygmomanometer cuff around lower calf.
- *Locate posterior tibial (PT) vessel* (halfway between prominence of medial malleolus and tip of heel): if PT not found, document and use dorsalis pedis (DP) instead (midpoint of dorsal surface of ankle, halfway between malleoli).
- Place tip of probe against vessel position, angling probe 60° incident to flow.
- Confirm Doppler signal.
- Inflate cuff until signal lost.
- Release cuff and observe pressure upon which signal regained.
- Repeat for other limb.
- Repeat for both arms.
- *Ankle Brachial Pressure Index (ABPI):* systolic pressure (leg)/systolic pressure (ipsilateral arm)

Penetrating injuries to the junctional zones of the torso (axilla, thoracic outlet, groin) may lead to the signs of unconstrained haemorrhage into an adjacent cavity (haemothorax, haemoperitoneum), to features of ischaemia in the adjacent extremity (6 P's, neurological change in carotid or vertebral trauma) or indeed both.

Investigation in the resuscitation room

Where the combination of clinical findings and hand-held Doppler assessment has indicated the likelihood of vascular injury, further investigations should only be ordered on the following basis. Firstly, where there is doubt about which segment of vessel is injured (such as shotgun injuries or multiple fractures along the axial course of a vessel); secondly, to investigate and triage other associated injuries (such as injuries to mediastinal structures); and, thirdly, where information garnered from the investigation will change the strategy of intervention (from open surgery to endovascular intervention if a vertebral artery injury is suspected).

Patients who have suffered blunt trauma should undergo the usual radiographs as part of the primary survey. The chest X-ray allows confirmation of associated pneumothorax or haemothorax. It is a non-specific indicator of disruption to the thoracic aorta, with signs including a widened

Table 16.4. Pitfalls in diagnosis of extremity vascular injury

Pitfall	Comment
No vascular injury as pulses present	Pulses often present below level of injury if good collaterals present
No vascular injury as good Doppler signal	Phasicity of hand-held Doppler is a poor marker of proximal vascular injury due to collateralisation
Lack of distal blood flow due to vessel spasm	Vessel spasm is a diagnosis of exclusion
Failure to appreciate patterns of injury	Knee dislocation→popliteal artery injury Supracondylar elbow fracture→brachial artery injury
Failure to follow-up suspicion of vascular injury with timely definitive investigation	Reluctance to mobilise diagnostic resources out-of-hours—investigate in the morning
Failure to institute neurovascular observations in patients being managed conservatively	Failure to appreciate evolutionary nature of vascular injury (dissection → flap → occlusion → thrombosis)

mediastinum, widened heart shadow or indistinct border, apical capping, odd-looking aortic arch, wide paraspinal lines, depressed left main bronchus, and deviated tracheal or nasogastric tube (the most reliable sign).

In penetrating trauma, particularly ballistic trauma, radio-opaque wound markers prior to plain radiography of the affected zone allow interpretation of trajectory. Bi-planar series of injured extremities are helpful in assessing the mangled extremity, although they may be deferred if the urgency of the situation warrants immediate vascular control or revascularization. An image intensifier in theatre will often be sufficient to allow temporizing skeletal fixation.

Catastrophic vascular injury requires location of the bleeding to cavity or limb and expeditious control of haemorrhage with or without revascularization. Focused assessment with sonography for trauma (FAST) is useful in blunt trauma (and to a lesser degree in penetrating trauma) in helping to triage the body cavities, but will not delineate the retroperitoneal structures. If doubt exists regarding the site of vascular injury in the torso or extremity, if the patient's condition allows it, and if the infrastructure is readily available, then the contemporary investigation of choice is contrast enhanced multi detector CT (MDCT) angiography, which has largely replaced the historical gold standard of contrast angiography.

Investigation beyond the resuscitation room
Computed tomography
Conventional CT takes several cardiac and respiratory cycles to acquire a full set of images. These scanners are less sensitive at detecting active haemorrhage due to difficulty in co-ordinating the timing of image acquisition with the bolus of intravenous contrast, and motion artefact. Multi-slice or multi-detector CT scanners (MDCT) use a two-dimensional array of detector elements and can

acquire multiple slices simultaneously, greatly increasing the speed of image acquisition. High resolution CT angiography (CTA) can reliably delineate the large and medium-sized vessels within the thorax, extremity, or neck with sufficient sensitivity to permit accurate delineation of the injury tract, to rule out vessel wall breach, active haemorrhage, occlusion, or thrombosis (see Figs 16.1 and 16.2). Views in any plane can be reconstructed from MDCT and these have further improved the detection of haemorrhage, although the time taken to process these images may offset their diagnostic utility in the emergency situation. Subtle flaps may be missed and angiography is still warranted in certain, infrequent circumstances (for instance, prior to aortic root replacement in proximal aortic injury, or for the investigation of subtle injuries in the carotid or vertebral arteries). Furthermore, CTA, whilst defining vascular injury well, is less good for detecting solid organ parenchymal injury. Consequently, CT is often performed during the portal venous phase of contrast enhancement to give the best compromise between arterial and solid organ diagnostic information. No matter how fast CT can be performed, grossly unstable patients should not be placed in the CT scanner, particularly when the purpose of the scan is to triage the body cavities for haemorrhage. All patients requiring CT should be accompanied by the trauma team and associated resuscitation equipment. Decompensation should be anticipated and a plan formulated should this eventuality occur.

Formal angiography

Angiography used to be performed for asymptomatic patients with penetrating wounds in close proximity to a major vessel. However, this tends to detect only minor injuries that do not require operative repair and this practice has now been abandoned.

Formal angiography can be utilized in a number of ways. Antegrade single-shot studies, administered in the resuscitation room, require percutaneous placement of a suitable cannula in the proximal artery, an X-ray cassette beneath the affected limb centred on the injury zone, injection of 20 mL of intravenous contrast material, and exposure. While useful in austere circumstances, such angiograms are rarely done in centres equipped with digital subtraction angiography (DSA), image intensification, and dedicated angiography suites. Such facilities, combined with the appropriate expertise, allow precise definition of injury extent and site with lower contrast and radiation loads than conventional angiography (Fig. 16.3), but DSA is challenged by the growing ubiquity of spiral MDCT. However, the ability to combine DSA with wire or catheter endovascular techniques to control arterial haemorrhage, via proximal intra-arterial balloon control, covered stents and embolization, is advantageous. It is especially useful in surgically challenging areas, such as the thoracic outlet and the pelvis, and allows single-room diagnosis and therapy (Fig. 16.4). Finally, intra-operative on-table angiography, either as a single-shot study or via mobile C-arm image intensification, is occasionally required in the polytrauma patient with extremity trauma. Circumstances where this may be necessary include follow-on in-theatre investigation of suspected vascular injury in patients who have completed their primary non-vascular surgery, or as a quality control measure post-vascular repair. It is prudent to ensure that, before commencing any operation in patients with suspected or confirmed vascular trauma, the operating table is X-ray compatible and that the appropriate radiological resources are notified that angiography may be required. It is worth noting that the images from DSA can be distorted by metallic and bony fragments, so shotgun wounds and comminuted fractures may be better evaluated by conventional angiography.

Duplex Doppler ultrasound

Duplex ultrasound combines real-time brightness modulation (B-mode) imaging with pulsed-Doppler flow detection, velocity sampling and depiction of flow wave-forms. Vessels can be imaged non-invasively and the velocity and direction of the flow interpreted according to colour representation. Although operator dependent, Duplex is very sensitive (95–100%) and specific (97–99%) in the diagnosis of vascular injury in the hands of accredited personnel. Unfortunately, it has limited utility in the diagnosis of acute vascular trauma, principally because Duplex services are usually not available out-of-hours. Nonetheless, Duplex is an excellent modality for assessing the late complications of vascular trauma, such as arterio-venous fistulae and false aneurysms, and for the surveillance of graft patency following vascular reconstruction.

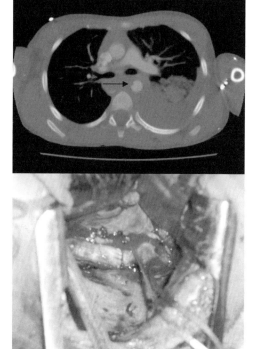

Fig. 16.1. (Top) Contrast CT of a 9-year-old child struck by fragments from a mortar round. Note luminal irregularity in aorta at the 9 o'clock position (black arrow) associated with mediastinal blood and left haemothorax. (Bottom) Aorta viewed through a left thoracotomy, following proximal and distal aortic clamping with debridement and direct suture repair of injury.

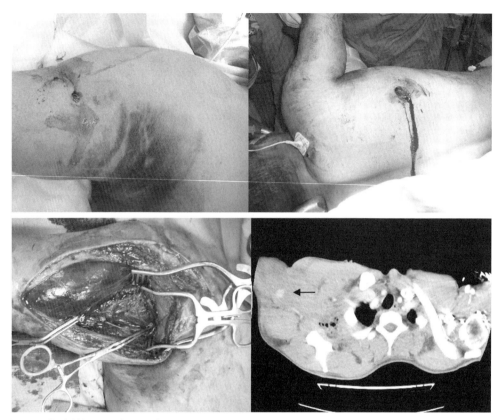

Fig. 16.2. (Top left) Entry gun shot wound in proximal right arm anterior surface (from AK 47 variant). (Top right) Exit wound on posterior right chest wall. (Bottom right) Contrast-enhanced angiogram revealing blush (arrow) from proximal right brachial artery (lower cuts revealed extra-pleural track of round). (Bottom left) Proximal and distal vascular clamps to lower axillary/upper brachial artery; damaged segment excised and vessel awaiting reversed saphenous vein interposition graft.

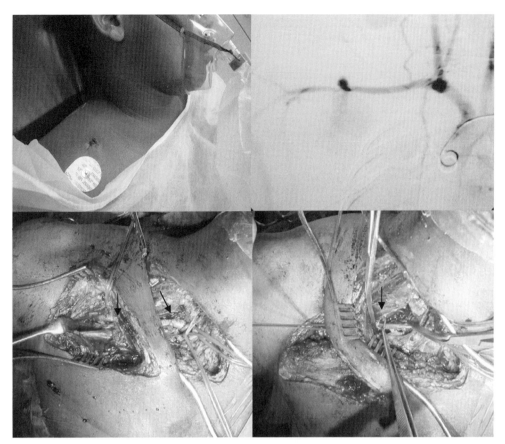

Fig. 16.3. (Top left) Stilleto-type stab wound to right supraclavicular area associated with 'normal' ipsilateral pulse. (Top right) Digital subtraction arch angiogram of the aorta revealing extravasation of contrast at junction of distal subclavian/proximal axillary artery. (Bottom right) Supraclavicular-infraclavicular counter incisions to expose and control vessels and reveal injury (arrow). (Bottom left) Interposition graft using ring-reinforced polytetrafluroethylene graft (arrows).

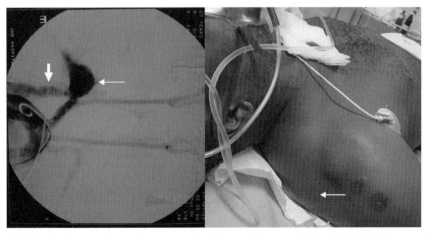

Fig. 16.4. (Top) Handgun-shot wound sustained to suprasternal notch, covered by gauze swab. Round palpable in subcutaneous tissues of left shoulder (arrow). Loud machinery murmur on chest ausculatation. (Bottom) Digital subtraction arch angiogram of the aorta, demonstrating false aneurysm between subclavian artery and vein (thin arrow), back-filling superior vena cava (thick arrow)—patient was treated with a covered subclavian stent.

Management of vascular trauma

Resuscitation
The initial management of all patients suffering with suspected vascular injury should follow a standard primary and secondary survey, with two important areas of emphasis. First, the compression of actively bleeding wounds by direct pressure is performed concurrently with assessment of the airway and cervical spine control (<C>ABCDE). Secondly, surgical control of incompressible haemorrhage is performed as part of the circulatory assessment and intervention stage, with rapid diversion to the interventional radiology suite or operating theatre when shock is present or decompensation likely. Blood and blood products should be administered as part of a damage control resuscitation (DCR) process, with near equivalent usage of plasma and packed cells. Such a strategy appears not to compromise graft patency.

Obtaining control of compressible haemorrhage in the resuscitation room, particularly with brisk bleeding, requires a co-ordinated sequence of manoeuvres (Box 16.2). The temptation to utilize haemostats in the emergency department environment and in the absence of proper lighting, suction, and trained assistance should be avoided as this risks further iatrogenic vessel damage. Poorly placed or ineffective dressings must be taken down and replaced prior to taking patients to other hospital areas. The insertion of a large bore Foley balloon catheter down deep, narrow tracks (with inflation of the balloon with saline and application of a haemostat across the drainage channel) may reduce external egress of blood, but may not reduce internal haemorrhage if the track communicates with an adjacent body cavity (see Fig 16.5). This technique has most often been described with respect to penetrating injuries to the root of the neck. Following insertion, inflation and traction, a second balloon may need to be inserted above the first to stop the bleeding.

Patients with suspected major torso vascular haemorrhage require urgent triage to theatre or angiography suite.

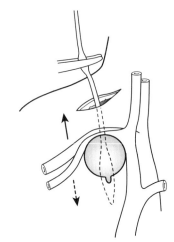

Fig. 16.5. Insertion of a deflated Foley catheter in to a bleeding supraclavicular wound track. The balloon is inflated and pulled upwards to exert traction on the adjacent subclavian artery with control of haemorrhage. A further Foley may be inserted on top of the first if required. The clip on the catheter is to prevent egress of blood down the catheter's lumen.

Emergency Department (ED) thoracotomy for in-extremis patients with infra-diaphragmatic exsanguination, for the purposes of cross-clamping of the thoracic aorta, has fallen from favour in the past decade due to very low salvage rates. Failure to recover a blood pressure after clamping is a good marker of futility of care.

Principles of surgery
Pre-surgical planning
The pre-operative surgical checklist prior to vascular repair is generic regardless of the vessel involved.

Position:
- Patient typically in cruciform position on an X-ray compatible table.
- Preparation of limb or body part plus adjacent junctional area and cavity.
- Preparation of uninjured groin and thigh (vein harvesting).

Equipment:
- Vascular set, including appropriate prosthetic grafts if required.
- Fogarty catheters.
- Heparinized saline.
- Magnification Loupes.
- Bair Hugger® and under-patient warming blanket.
- Properly positioned pneumatic tourniquet on proximal limb above injury.

Personnel:
- Vascular surgeon mobilized (if required).
- Interventional radiology and radiographer alerted (if required).
- Orthopaedic and plastics team consulted with regard to sequence of operating (if required).

Box 16.2. Dealing with active compressible haemorrhage

- Ensure personal protective equipment is adequate.
- Reassure patient and explain what needs to be done as it is being done.
- Rapidly remove any ineffective dressings.
- Surgeon applies robust wound compression:
  - force vector oriented to compress wound against the underlying axial skeleton;
  - small wounds can be managed with a single gauze swab and digital pressure;
  - larger cavities can be managed with internal gauze packing (kurlex) and palmar pressure;
  - it is always painful, so give iv opiate analgesia concurrently with any wound manipulation.
  - avoid application of haemostats to visible vessels;
  - transfer to theatre as soon as possible.
- In theatre: surgeon replaces digital compression of wound with sponge stick held by assistant who is prepped in to operative field.
- Proximal and distal vascular control obtained prior to release of sponge-stick control.

The key sequence in surgical management of injured vessels, whether in the extremity or the torso, is to make an incision that allows for axial extension, to obtain proximal and distal control of the injured vessel, then to explore the haematoma, and confirm the nature of vessel injury. Unlike conventional vascular surgery, systemic heparin is usually not given, due to the risk of bleeding in a patient who is often coagulopathic and has multiple other injuries. Thereafter, the vessel is debrided and carefully swept with a Fogarty catheter (a size 4Fr serves most above elbow or above knee injuries). In-flow and back-flow is confirmed prior to flushing the downstream and upstream segments with heparinized saline (5000 iU of heparin per 500 mL of normal saline). A decision should be made to either repair the injury definitively or to resort to a damage control manoeuvre. Distal, downstream injury should be ruled out before embarking upon revascularization, using on-table angiography if necessary. Following repair, the vessel and anastomosis must be covered by viable tissue to prevent break down, exsanguination or fistulation (exposed femoral vessels can be covered by dividing sartorius at its iliac insertion and rotating it across to cover the repair; omentum can be mobilized and interposed between bowel and vessel for intra-abdominal repairs). Common techniques for definitive repair, and their indications, are listed in Table 16.5. Monofilament, double ended prolene is the default suture for vascular repair (2-0/3-0 for aorta, 4-0 for iliac or subclavian, 5-0 for femoral or axillary, and 6-0 for popliteal and brachial injuries).

The importance of calm and effective communication between anaesthetist and surgeon cannot be over-emphasized, particularly with regard to major torso haemorrhage. It is vital for the anaesthetist to be regularly updated by the surgeon as to the state of vascular control and any anticipated blood loss. Equally, it is important to allow the anaesthetist a few moments to catch-up with any blood product administration as required, maintaining temporary control with firm pressure prior to continuing. The anaesthetist should also be forewarned of the restoration of perfusion to an extremity to allow mitigation of the effects of wash-through of the ischaemic tissues.

Fasciotomy

Compartment syndrome within an extremity occurs when intramuscular compartment pressure overcomes inflow pressure within the capillary bed. The driving mechanism appears to be reperfusion injury secondary to interruption in flow due to severe crush injury, prolonged hypotension or ischaemia, or combined arterial and venous injury. Muscle necrosis, rhabdomyolysis, and renal failure may result. Even if the limb is salvaged, fibrotic resolution frequently results in disabling contracture. Fasciotomies should be performed as a routine procedure given any of the above injury patterns, and performed prior to any arterial repair if there is prolonged limb ischaemia. Pressure measurements are no substitute for clinical suspicion.

In the lower limb, fasciotomies involve opening four muscular compartments with full length anterolateral and posteromedial incisions (Fig. 16.6). The anterolateral incision begins two finger-breadths below the lateral tibial crest, immediately below the level of the tibial tuberosity, and extends to the ankle. By dividing the fascia, the anterior compartment is opened. The intermuscular septum

Table 16.5. Techniques in definitive vascular repair

Technique	Comments
Primary closure	• Most appropriate with simple transverse lacerations with minimal tissue loss. • Continuous or interrupted sutures. • Sutures passed from out to in on upstream edge of laceration, inner surface to vessel exterior on downstream edge. • Risks compromising luminal diameter and vessel thrombosis if axial laceration closed primarily.
Vein-patch angioplasty	• Useful for complex vessel wall defects where vessel has not been transacted. • Excess tissue loss (>50% circumference) best served with resection/anastomosis. • Requires harvesting of vein patch (long saphenous vein, external jugular) or use of PTFE/Dacron®. • Continuous sutures, completing furthest side of patch first. • Common pitfall is narrowing of vessel at apices of patch. • Avoid by clock-facing sutures at patch apices.
Resection and primary anastomosis	• For cleanly transected vessels with minimal loss of vessel length after debridement. • Requires mobilisation of vessel ends and apposition without excess tension. • Avoid sacrificing side branches during mobilization. • Anastomose by triangulation/stay suture placement. • Continuous sutures, completing back wall first. • Spatulation of vessel ends reduces risk of luminal narrowing at suture line.

Interposition grafting	• Used when a primary repair will cause tension on the vessel.
	• Autologous vein grafts:
	  • long saphenous vein or external jugular vein are readily usable;
	  • internal jugular vein can be harvested from the neck assuming the contralateral side is patent;
	  • 'panel' grafts of composite vein can be constructed to create large diameter conduits if required (but are time-consuming).
	• Prosthetic grafts:
	  • quick to utilize; variety of calibers suited to large vessel repair;
	  • use in civilian arterial trauma is controversial and should not be used in military trauma except as short-term damage control option due to higher risk of infective complications.

Extra-anatomical bypass	• Infrequently indicated. • Used for injuries with gross soft tissue loss, contamination or loss of axial vascular length. • Must be routed away from zone of injury though viable tissue bed to minimize infective complications.

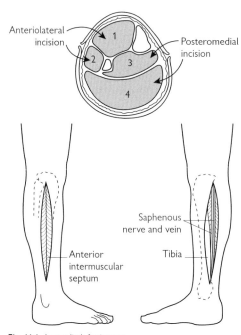

Fig. 16.6. Lower limb fasciotomy

state of the patient. Clearly, the cold, coagulopathic and acidotic patient will be further compromised by prolonged attempts at definitive reconstruction and the surgeon should perform a damage control procedure. This state should be anticipated before it develops, with early default to a damage control procedure in cases where multiple injuries compete for attention, or in combined arterial and venous trauma.

Shunting
Insertion of a temporary vascular shunt across a damaged section of vessel was first popularized in 1971 during the Israel–Egypt border war. Their use has become further established during the current conflicts in Iraq and Afghanistan. While commercial products such as the Javid, Brenner, or Sundt shunts are purpose-designed, appropriately-sized sterile intravenous tubing, nasogastric tubes, or feeding tubes are just as effective. The shunt is held in place with clamps or ligatures, umbilical tape, or Ramel tourniquets. A check of in-flow and back-flow, Fogarty sweep, and flush with heparinized saline must be accomplished prior to shunt deployment (Fig. 16.7 and Box 16.3).

Whilst the shunt is *in situ*, the saphenous vein can be harvested, the graft fashioned, the anastomoses constructed, any venous injury repaired and fractures stabilized. Patients with shunts *in situ* must have their distal perfusion monitored closely, by frequent clinical examination or continuous Doppler flow measurement proximal and distal to the shunt. Shunts are equally applicable in venous trauma and particularly advisable in combined venous and arterial injury.

Ligation
Ligation of bleeding vessels without attempting to reconstruct them is a valid damage control manoeuvre in certain circumstances. First, if limb or organ viability is not dependent

between the anterior and lateral compartments is then divided to release the lateral compartment, taking care to avoid the lateral peroneal nerve superiorly. The medial incision is made immediately posterior to the posterior border of the tibia, taking care to avoid the saphenous vein. By incising the fascia, the superficial posterior compartment is opened. The deep posterior compartment is reached by detaching soleus from the posterior aspect of the tibia.

In the forearm there are only two muscular compartments (flexor and extensor), and dorsal and volar incisions are made to decompress the upper limb. Each muscle within the forearm is contained within its own fascia and each of these must be opened to prevent ongoing compartment syndrome. The flexor retinaculum must be divided so the volar incision is continued into the wrist, taking care to avoid the median nerve and its superficial branch that runs medially.

Patients who have undergone fasciotomy should still be monitored closely with clinical examination, watching for myoglobinuria, and measuring creatine phosphokinase. Complications of fasciotomy wounds include infection and decreased efficacy of the calf muscle pump, although the procedure is generally well tolerated. Open wounds may be managed with delayed primary closure, split skin graft, gradual wound apposition using bootlace techniques, or topical negative pressure dressings.

Vascular damage control
Once control has been established, the haematoma has been opened and the injury defined, a decision must be made as to the ability of the patient to withstand a definitive surgical procedure. This requires clear communication between surgeon and anaesthetist regarding the physiological

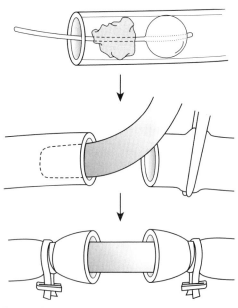

Fig. 16.7. Deployment of a temporary intra-luminal shunt.

Box 16.3. Use of vascular shunts

Use

- Ligation of juxta-injury tributaries/collaterals to prevent back-bleeding.
- Choose tube of appropriate diameter, cut to length and apply clip to mid-portion.
- Insert proximal end into upstream artery slung with 0 silk and tighten.
- Bleed through by releasing clamp.
- Reapply clamp and insert distal end in to downstream artery slung with 0 silk and tighten.
- Remove clamp and perfuse limb (forewarn anaesthetist).

Pitfalls

- Too much shunt outside vessel (looping)—shunt displacement if loop caught.
- Too much shunt length inside vessel—shunt ostia opposed against vessel side wall with occlusion.
- Damage to vessel luminal surface during shunt placement due to rough handling.

upon the vessel concerned (e.g. single calf or forearm vessel injuries, single visceral vessel injuries, internal iliac arteries, external carotid artery). Secondly, even if organ or limb loss may result, it may be necessary to resort to ligation *in extremis* (renal artery, external iliac artery, femoral artery, popliteal artery). The axillary or subclavian arteries can be ligated with little chance of limb loss due to collateralization. All limb veins and the infra-renal IVC can be ligated, but this may result in significant limb oedema. Ligation of the supra-renal IVC and portal vein is associated with poor outcome.

Amputation

Primary amputation is a legitimate damage control option for vascular injury when the limb is frankly unsalvageable or when the patient would not withstand an attempt at salvage in a potentially salvageable limb. The latter circumstance is heralded by the phenomena of ongoing haemodynamic instability, traumatic coagulopathy, acidosis, and hypothermia. While the decision to amputate should preferably be made by two consultants from different specialties, it is recognized that such council may not be possible *in-extremis*.

Endovascular therapy

The endovascular revolution has affected acute trauma care in three ways. First, proximal control of large bleeding vessels through remote placement of an endovascular balloon upstream of the injury zone, allowing for a more controlled surgical approach to the injury; secondly, sealing of vessel injury and restoration of vascular integrity by deployment of a covered stent across the injury zone; and thirdly, interruption of the blood flow to an injured vessel or organ by proximal embolization using thrombogenic material.

The place of endovascular therapies in the treatment of vascular injury has yet to be defined. Generically, such manoeuvres have found favour in vessels that are difficult to access conventionally (e.g. the vertebral artery or subclavian artery; see Fig. 16.8) or where the morbidity of

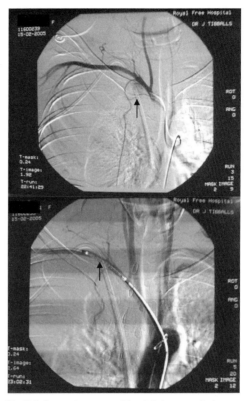

Fig. 16.8. Iatrogenic trauma to right subclavian artery distal to origin of vertebral artery. Patient was undergoing insertion of a subclavian line for chemotherapy and had a very depressed platelet count. (Top) Blush of contrast (arrow). (Bottom) Covered stent being pushed in to position (arrow).

open repair favours an endovascular solution (traumatic disruption of the aorta). The contraindications to stent and embolization therapy are detailed in Table 16.6. The main constraint to the use of such appealing technologies remains the 24/7 availability of staff and equipment.

The use of covered stents is becoming standard care in uncomplicated traumatic disruption of the aorta. Stent repair for injuries to the vertebral, subclavian, brachiocephalic, axillary, carotid, iliac, and lower extremity arteries have also been documented. Pseudo-aneurysms, arteriovenous fistulae, first-order branch avulsions, and intimal flaps may be managed with a suitable stent, although the presence of severe contamination, unsuitable proximal or distal landing zones, or injury across a mobile joint line (such as the third part of the axillary artery) favour conventional repair. The use of covered vascular stents in younger patients commits them to life-long follow-up and an ever-present risk of mechanical failure, stent dislodgement or embolization that does not accompany conventional repair.

Table 16.6. Contraindications to endovascular treatment (stent or embolisation)

Contraindication	Classification	Notes
Exposed vessel	Absolute	Vessel is accessible to open surgery. No advantage in minimally invasive approach
Acute surgical repair required of adjacent structures/organs	Absolute	Open approach required to manage invasive
Transected vessel	Relative	Difficult to bridge the guidewire across the two ends of the vessel unless dual access "top and bottom" snare approach employed
Patient instability	Relative	Depending upon institutional expertise

Specific vascular injuries

All patients with thoraco-abdominal injuries should be placed in a cruciform position with neck-to-knee preparation and draping in anticipation for both thoracotomy and laparotomy.

Thorax

In the exsanguinating patient there should be no hesitation in defaulting to clamshell thoracotomy if the injury pattern does not clearly direct the operator to one specific pleural cavity. This incision affords sufficient exposure to the great vessels and the arch of the aorta, but requires good traction on the upper rib cage. Median sternotomy gives good exposure to the heart and the great vessels, and can be extended across either clavicular area or in to the neck to allow for exposure of the vessels of the thoracic outlet. Postero-lateral thoracotomy gives good exposure to the aorta, oesophagus, lung, and posterior chest wall, but is seldom used in emergency trauma patients.

Thoracic aorta

Open surgical repair is the standard management for penetrating thoracic aortic injury. Injuries may be managed with 'clamp and sew' (with a paraplegia rate up to 20%), or formal cardiopulmonary bypass and interposition grafting depending on the extent of vessel damage. The majority of patients with blunt traumatic dissection of the thoracic aorta die at scene. Those who survive to hospital have contained leaks that are seldom the cause of ongoing shock. Open repair and interposition grafting has a mortality of between 5 and 28%, and a paraplegia rate of around 10%. Endovascular stenting is quicker and less invasive, with less blood loss, no single lung ventilation and no thoracotomy scar. Results show mortality rates of 0-4% and paraplegia rate of less than 1%, although the long-term durability of stent-grafts is not known.

Brachiocephalic artery

Contained injuries are repaired using a 'bypass and exclusion' technique. A segment of normal aortic arch is isolated via a side-biting clamp and a prosthetic graft sewn on to aorta with a distal anastomosis on to the distal brachiocephalic, carotid or subclavian vessel beyond the haematoma. The injury is then excluded by ligation of the brachiocephalic artery (Fig. 16.9).

Mediastinal venous injuries

Injuries to the superior vena cava are rare and should be repaired to prevent superior vena cava syndrome or cerebral oedema. Other injuries to the innominate or subclavian vein can be ligated in the unstable patient with few immediate complications.

Neck

Penetrating vascular injury is frequently associated with wounding to the aerodigestive tract and there is often need for emergency airway control. Unstable patients or patients with evidence of profuse bleeding, expanding haematoma, or neurological deficit should be triaged to the operating theatre immediately. Stable patients with injury that breaches the platysma should undergo CTA in order to determine the trajectory of the injury, proximity to vessel, presence of haematoma, or contrast extravasation, vessel patency, and integrity of aerodigestive structures. Classifying the wound in terms of its anatomical zone (Table 16.7) allows accurate description and assessment of surgical approach although the site of the skin laceration does not always match the level of vascular injury. In practice, CTA has become the triage tool of choice in managing penetrating neck trauma, permitting selection of patients for observation, intervention, or further investigation (formal selective angiography) as appropriate. Despite fears of converting an ischaemic cerebral insult into a haemorrhagic one, revascularization is always indicated unless the patient is profoundly comatose. Surgery is conducted with the aid of a beanbag beneath the shoulders to extend the neck with the head rotated away from the side of the injury. The field should always include the chest, in the event that proximal control from within the thoracic cavity is required.

Patients with a risk of blunt cervical vascular injury (blow to the neck, seatbelt restraint in motor vehicle collisions, suspension trauma) should also be investigated primarily with CTA, with follow-on angiographic documentation of the exact nature of the injury in positive scans.

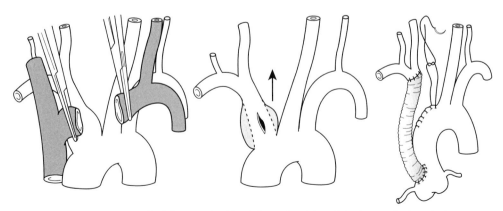

Fig. 16.9. Division of innominate vein (shaded) to access brachiocephalic vessel; exclusion of injury by suture ligation and prior extra-anatomic by-pass graft.

Table 16.7. Zones of the neck in penetrating injury

Zone	Description	Major vessels at risk	Implication	Approach to investigation†
1	From manubrium to cricoid cartilage (C6)	Subclavian, proximal carotid, mediastinal vessels	Median sternotomy/thoracotomy for proximal control	Mandatory CTA*
2	From cricoid cartilage to angle of jaw	Mid-carotid artery, carotid bifurcation, proximal internal and external carotid arteries, internal jugular vein	Proximal control probably achievable via standard surgical approach (anterior to SCM)	CTA* or selective surgery exploration
3	From angle of jaw to base of skull	Distal internal carotid	Distal control via extensive dissection/division of styloglossus/subluxation of mandible or endovascular stenting	Mandatory CTA*

*Or arch angiography where CTA equivocal or unavailable
†Assuming breach of platysma

Such injuries cause a range of neurological sequelae ranging from coma and death to lateralizing signs, which may be erroneously assigned to a concomitant head injury.

Carotid artery

Penetrating carotid artery injuries should be repaired using a patch or vein-graft for internal carotid artery (ICA) or narrow (<6 mm) common carotid vessels. Shunts should be used for ICA repairs in order to maintain pro-grade flow to the brain as 20% of patients lack a complete circle of Willis. There is no absolute requirement to shunt common carotid injuries in the presence of good backflow from the ipsilateral external carotid artery (ECA).

The standard approach involves a full length incision from mastoid process to jugular notch along the anterior border of sternocleidomastoid (SCM), developing the plane medial to the SCM and toward the carotid sheath and dividing the omohyoid muscle. The first structure to be encountered is the jugular vein, which can be mobilized laterally by dividing the facial vein to expose the carotid bifurcation.

The posteriorly sited vagus nerve, and the horizontally coursing hypoglossal nerve (crossing the proximal internal carotid) must be identified and spared. High internal carotid injuries require division of the overlying styloglossus and stylohyoid muscles, and subluxation of the jaw (seldom practical in the emergency situation). In circumstances where distal control cannot be achieved and ligation of the vessel is not possible, a Fogarty catheter should be passed in to the vessel upwards, inflated just beyond the injury, and left *in situ*, whilst further manoeuvres to expose the skull base are undertaken or additional expertise enrolled.

The use of stents is most valuable in high ICA injuries identified on CTA where the vessel is not transected and a guide wire can navigate the injury zone. Beyond this application or in cases where neck dissection will be difficult due to previous surgery or radiotherapy, the use of carotid stents in penetrating trauma remains an unconventional and controversial technique.

Internal jugular veins

Jugular veins can be repaired if the nature of the injury and the patient's physiology lend themselves to a quick and straightforward repair. If not, a single vein can be ligated with no consequence.

Vertebral artery

The vertebral artery can be controlled using a number of approaches, none of which are easy in the emergency patient. Proximally, it may be intercepted as it arises from the subclavian artery medial to the anterior scalene (see subclavian artery). In its middle territory the vessel can be found travelling upward in the foramen transversarium of each cervical vertebra between C6 and C2. Exploring the vessel here requires the standard approach to the carotid sheath, but with medial displacement of the sheath and lateral retraction of the anterior longitudinal ligament and anterior paraspinous muscles to expose the anterior arch of the transverse processes. An encircling suture around the vessel one level above and below the injury, or application of clips, may control the bleed without the need to remove the anterior arch but with risk to the adjacent cervical nerve roots. Direct repair is not usually feasible.

Endovascular embolization is the favoured management and rarely prejudices the posterior circulation.

Abdomen

The large vessels of the abdomen, and the origins of the major visceral vessels are located in the retroperitoneum. The site of haematomata and key techniques used to expose these vessels are detailed in Table 16.8.

Adequate exposure is the key to gaining rapid proximal and distal control of any vascular injury. A left medial visceral rotation, including the spleen, kidney, pancreas, and fundus of the stomach, can be used for complete exposure of the aorta and its branches (Fig. 16.10). The lateral peritoneal reflection attaching the sigmoid and left colon is divided and the left colon, spleen and kidney are swept medially. The left crus of the diaphragm can be divided or the laparotomy wound extended as a sternotomy to give better views of the proximal aorta. Injuries to structures on the right can be revealed by right medial visceral rotation, beginning with mobilization of the right colon along the line of Todt, bringing the mesentery of right colon and small bowel across the midline, and then liberally kocherizing the duodenum to allow full access to the IVC, right renal pedicle, bifurcation of the aorta and confluence of the iliac veins (Fig. 16.11).

Intra-abdominal aortic cross-clamping may be required to get proximal control of haemorrhage from the proximal zone of a visceral vessel. It can be performed at the supra-coeliac level by retracting the left lobe of the liver towards the right shoulder whilst having the body of the stomach retracted down and to the left. A window in the lesser omentum is made and the peritoneum overlying the left crus of the diaphragm incised longitudinally. The underlying muscular fibres are spread and parted to reveal the

Table 16.8. Injury pattern and key exposure techniques in abdominal vascular injury

Suspect injury to:	Haematoma position	Decision making	Expose vessel by:
Aorta or proximal visceral branches (celiac, SMA)	Central (to left of midline) and above/behind/beneath transverse mesocolon	Explore	Left medial visceral rotation
Portal triad vessels	Lesser omentum; central (to right of midline) and above transverse mesocolon	Explore	Clamping of portal triad above and below haematoma prior to opening haematoma
Retropancreatic vessels (SMV, splenic vein, proximal SMA)	Central, above/behind transverse mesocolon	Explore	Division of neck of pancreas (in extremis)
Renal vessels	Lateral to side of injury, retrocolic	Explore unless [blunt mechanism + non-expanding haematoma + patient stability]	Left or right medial visceral rotation
IVC	Central (to right of midline) above/behind/ beneath transverse mesocolon	Explore	Kocherization of duodenum, extended right medial visceral rotation
IVC (retrohepatic)	Behind liver (to right of midline)	Only explore if bleeding cannot be controlled by appropriate liver packing (vector of compression AP)	Kocherization of duodenum, extended right medial visceral rotation and control of supra-renal IVC; extension of laparotomy incision in to right thorax; complete mobilization of liver; intra-thoracic control of IVC

pearly white surface of the aorta lying to the left of the vertebral midline (Fig. 16.12). A space either side of the aorta should be developed such that the whole of the aorta can be engaged by an aortic clamp or else control will not be achieved. Clamp time should be minimized to less than 30 min. Digital pressure over the aorta, accessed through the lesser omentum, is a useful and rapid default when dissection is difficult (as it often is when the

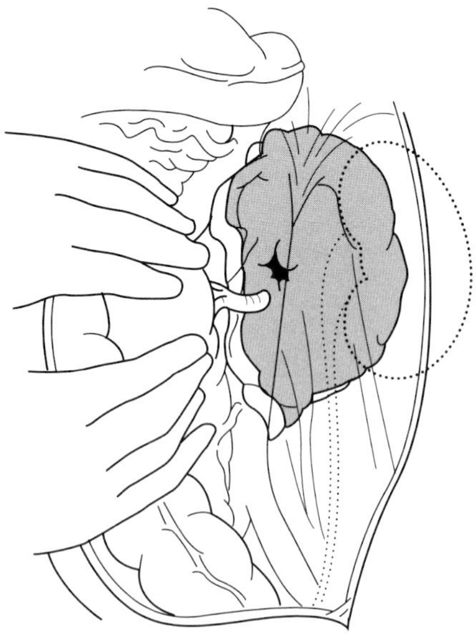

Fig. 16.10. Left medial visceral rotation.

aorta loses definition in the shocked patient) or when the operator is unfamiliar with the approach.

Abdominal aorta

Abdominal aortic injuries are rare. Disruption due to blunt and ballistic mechanisms is often associated with rapid exsanguination and death. For penetrating injuries, lateral repair usually suffices, and larger defects may be patched.

Inferior vena cava

Simple injuries are repaired primarily after right medial visceral rotation and sponge-stick control of the cava on either side of the injury, repairing through-and-through injuries to the posterior wall through the anterior laceration. Retrohepatic IVC injuries are highly lethal and should be managed using aggressive liver packing in the first instance. Failure of this commits the operator to extend the laparotomy incision in to the right chest to expose the supra-renal and intra-thoracic IVC, and full liver mobilization to facilitate adequate control and exposure. Formal hepatic isolation by using an atriocaval shunt is a salvage technique that rarely may result in success.

Coeliac axis and mesenteric vessels

Proximal penetrating injuries to these vessels are effectively side-holes in the aorta and present with profound haemorrhage and haemodynamic instability. Injuries to the proximal branches of the coeliac axis can usually be ligated without sequelae if the SMA remains patent. The inferior mesenteric artery can also be ligated in most cases due to collateral supply from the marginal artery of Drummond. The hepatic artery can be ligated provided that there are patent SMA collaterals and a patent portal vein.

The superior mesenteric artery should be repaired if possible, particularly if the injury lies proximally, as ligation is associated with a high risk of small bowel infarction. Proximal injuries are often lethally associated with

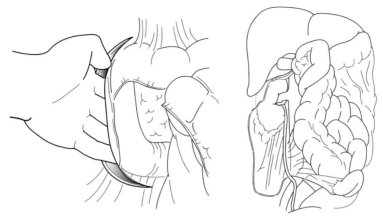

Fig. 16.11. Kocherization of the duodenum and medial visceral rotation from the right.

pancreaticoduodenal, right renal pedicle, and IVC injuries. The SMA can be repaired with a vein patch or alternatively the injury can be ligation-excluded and bowel perfusion assured by means of a retrograde aorta-to-SMA reversed saphenous vein graft, particularly if a concomitant pancreatic injury threatens a proximal repair.

Injury to the portal vein is challenging and often associated with proximity wounding to the hepatic artery and the common bile duct, both of which lie immediately adjacent and anterior. Repair should be attempted to maintain mid-gut viability, although ligation *in extremis* is acceptable, but associated with massive bowel oedema and fluid shift. The SMV can be ligated, but with similar consequences, plus the risk of venous gangrene of the bowel. Repair should be attempted if the patient's condition allows—splitting the pancreas if necessary to access the SMV injury near the confluence with the splenic and inferior mesenteric veins.

Renal vessels
Penetrating injuries to the renal artery can occasionally be repaired with lateral sutures, end-to-end anastomosis or interposition grafting, but associated injuries often preclude renal salvage. Blunt renal artery injury is usually confirmed on contrast-enhanced CT when one of the kidneys fails to opacify. An isolated dissection flap can be better delineated with formal angiography and then stented or repaired via open surgery. Injuries associated with major disruption to the renal parenchyma should be managed expectantly unless on-going haemorrhage mandates nephrectomy.

Lateral repair is the treatment of choice for injuries to the renal veins, although ligation on the left side is well tolerated if it is performed downsteam of the confluence with the left gonadal vein.

Upper limb junctional and extremity injury
Injury to the subclavian and axillary vessels is often associated with damage to elements of the brachial plexus. Vascular repair takes precedence over neurological repair, which may be safely deferred in the critically ill patient.

Subclavian vessels
Subclavian artery haemorrhage can result in both profound external and internal (pleural cavity) haemorrhage. Proximal siting of an intra-arterial occlusion balloon assists

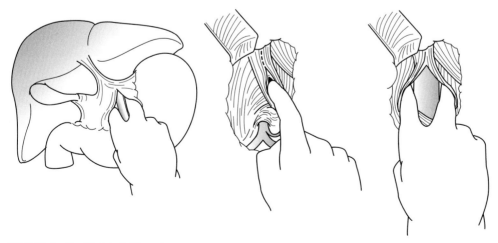

Fig. 16.12. Supracoeliac control of the aorta.

surgical exposure, and may be used to temporize while arrangements are made for endoluminal stenting, if facilities allow. Right-sided injuries are amenable to control via median sternotomy; dissection to the left subclavian takes longer as the vessel originates from the posterior aspect of the aortic arch. High (third space) left anterolateral thoracotomy is an alternative approach to the left subclavian, which is located behind the parietal pleura of the upper, medial apex of the left pleural cavity (Fig. 16.13). Limb loss after ligation is rare due to collaterals, although claudication and steal syndrome (if ligation is proximal to the vertebral artery take-off) may result.

Injuries to the distal subclavian may be controlled with supraclavicular and infraclavicular counter incisions, dissecting the second part of the subclavian and axillary artery, respectively. The supraclavicular approach involves division of the clavicular head of sternocleidomastoid to reveal the internal jugular vein (retracted medially) and the scalene fat pad (swept laterally) exposing the anterior scalene muscle (Fig. 16.14). The overlying phrenic nerve is protected and the muscle divided to reveal the second part of the artery. The clavicle can be divided to facilitate better exposure, but excision is unnecessary. Proximal control may be achieved by splitting the sternum and undertaking a dissection along the arch of the aorta if necessary, although this route is more difficult on the left than the right (Fig. 16.15).

Axillary vessels

These are accessed via an infraclavicular incision made from the mid-clavicle to the deltopectoral groove. Pectoralis major is split in the line of its fibres and the pectoralis minor divided to expose the clavipectoral fascia which is incised to reveal the neurovascular bundle (Fig. 16.16).

Brachial and forearm vessels

The proximal brachial artery is accessed via a medial upper arm incision between biceps and triceps, which can be easily extended distally (via an S-shaped incision across the antecubital fossa) or proximally (in to the deltopectoral groove) as required. Ligation of the brachial artery distal to the origin of the profunda brachii in the upper third of the

arm is well tolerated. A single intact radial or ulna vessel is sufficient to maintain perfusion of the hand.

Lower limb junctional and extremity injury

Fractures and dislocations should be reduced. Restoration of perfusion should be accomplished prior to bony fixation, if necessary using a temporary shunt prior to stabilization and then definitive repair. Extremity venous injuries should be repaired if possible, although the value of repair seems more established in military patients than in civilian ones, possibly because of the greater disruption to venous collaterals in battle injuries. Tibial level vein injuries may be safely ligated.

Iliac vessels

Penetrating iliac artery injury is controlled initially at laparotomy with digital pressure, whilst proximal control is gained at the level of the aortic bifurcation via a right medial visceral rotation. Clamps can be then 'walked' on to the vessel adjacent to the injury prior to repair. If necessary, the common iliac artery may be ligated and a femoro-femoral cross-over performed to maintain distal limb viability. When ligation alone is undertaken an amputation rate of 50% can be expected. There are usually no consequences to ligation of an internal iliac artery due to pelvic cross-flow.

Division of the overlying common iliac artery may be required to allow access to the injured common iliac vein (with follow-on repair of artery and interposition of omentum between artery and vein).

Ligation of iliac veins is accompanied by major limb swelling, which should be mitigated by compression stockings and limb elevation.

Femoral vessels

The femoral vessels are exposed via a mid-inguinal vertical incision halfway between anterior superior iliac spine and pubic symphysis. The inguinal ligament may be divided to gain control proximal to the haematoma (Fig. 16.17). Alternatively, an extra-peritoneal approach to the external iliac artery may be utilized via an oblique skin crease incision (Fig. 16.18) or by extending the axial vertical incision laterally toward the anterior superior iliac spine (inverted hockey stick approach). Simple injuries should be repaired with vein patch or suture repair. Complex injuries involving a long length of vessel should be repaired with interposition grafting. Repair of the profunda takes precedence over the superficial femoral artery in combined arterial injuries.

The superficial femoral artery is exposed by making a longitudinal incision over the anterior border of sartorius (retracting the muscle anteriorly in the upper and middle thigh and posteriorly in the middle and lower thigh). Opening the white fascia of Hunter's canal between adductor magnus and vastus medialis exposes the neurovascular bundle.

Popliteal and crural vessels

Popliteal artery injury carries the greatest risk of limb loss of any peripheral vascular injury (9% for penetrating injury, 18–30% for blunt injury). In-line flow should be restored whenever possible. Fasciotomies should be performed prior to either repair of the injured section or exclusion and vascular by-pass. The approach to the above-knee popliteal starts with a medial incision between vastus medialis and sartorius (Fig. 16.19). The posterior border of the femur is palpated and the deep fascia is incised revealing

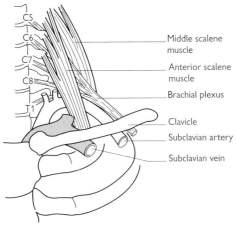

C5
C6
C7
C8
T1

Middle scalene muscle

Anterior scalene muscle

Brachial plexus

Clavicle

Subclavian artery

Subclavian vein

Fig. 16.13. Basic anatomy of thoracic outlet.

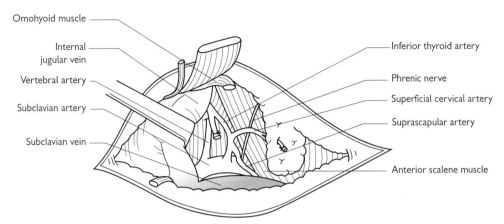

Fig. 16.14. Detailed anatomy of left supraclavicular approach to subclavian artery.

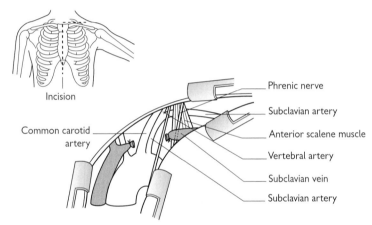

Fig. 16.15. Control of proximal left subclavian injury by median sternotomy and supraclavicular extension.

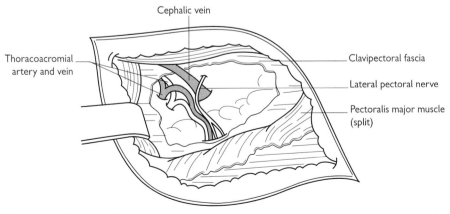

Fig. 16.16. Infraclavicular route to right axillary artery.

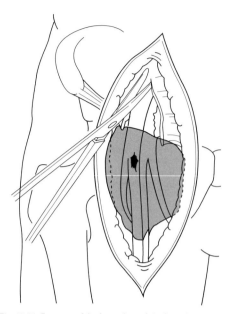

Fig. 16.17. Exposure of the femoral vessels in the groin.

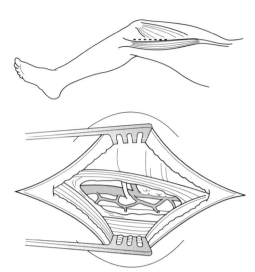

Fig. 16.19. Approach to the above-knee popliteal artery.

the popliteal fat. The popliteal vessels lie posterior to the femur. Distally, the popliteal artery is exposed through a separate incision 1 cm behind the posterior border of the tibia, beginning at the level of the medial femoral condyle (Fig. 16.18). Soleus is retracted posteriorly and the deep fascia opened to expose the fat of the popliteal fossa, in which lie the popliteal vessels behind the bone.

The tendons of semimembranosus, semitendinosus, sartorius, gracilis, and the medial head of gastrocnemius are divided for further exposure of the tibio-peroneal trunk and crural vessels (Fig. 16.20).

Calf and foot viability is usually assured if at least one of the three calf vessels (anterior tibial, posterior tibial, peroneal) is intact.

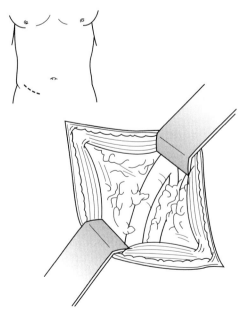

Fig. 16.18. Exposure of the external iliac vessels via an extra-peritoneal muscle splitting approach.

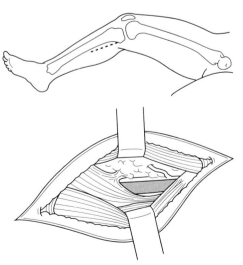

Fig. 16.20. Approach to the below-knee popliteal artery.

Conclusion

Even for the specialist vascular surgeon, the management of vascular trauma can be challenging. The key determinants of success remain early haemorrhage control and early default to damage control techniques, where appropriate. CTA and the development of endovascular therapies are exciting developments, but personal physical examination and attendance to the prime surgical directives of adequate control prior to vessel exposure are the foundations for good outcome. When faced with severe extremity injury the non-specialist must always attempt to muster expert help as efforts are directed to secure the patient's physiology, and only then should limb salvage be attempted.

Further reading

Bynoe RP, Miles WS, Bell RM, Greenwold DR, Sessions G, Haynes JL, et al. Noninvasive diagnosis of vascular trauma by duplex ultrasonography. *J Vasc Surg* 1991; **14**(3): 346–52.

Caps MT. The epidemiology of vascular trauma. *Semin Vasc Surg* 1998; **11**(4): 227–31.

Carrillo EH, Bergamini TM, Miller FB, Richardson JD. Abdominal vascular injuries. *J Trauma* 1997; **43**(1): 164–71.

Champion HR, Bellamy RF, Roberts CP, Leppaniemi, A. A profile of combat injury. *J Trauma* 2003; **54**(5 Suppl): S13–19.

Danetz JS, Cassano AD, Stoner MC, Ivatury RR, Levy MM. Feasibility of endovascular repair in penetrating axillosubclavian injuries: a retrospective review. *J Vasc Surg* 205; **41**(2): 246–54.

Demetriades D, Velmahos GC, Scalea TM, Jurkovich GJ, Karmy-Jones R, Teixeira PG,, ral. Operative repair or endovascular stent graft in blunt traumatic thoracic aortic injuries: results of an American Association for the Surgery of Trauma Multicenter Study. *J Trauma* 2008; **64**(3): 561–71.

Fox, CJ, Gillespie DL, Cox ED, Mehta SG, Kragh JF, Salinas J, et al. The effectiveness of a damage control resuscitation strategy for vascular injury in a combat support hospital: results of a case control study. *J Trauma* 2008; **64**(2 Suppl): S99–107.

Gupta R, Rao S, Sieunarine K. An epidemiological view of vascular trauma in Western Australia: a 5-year study. *Aust NZ J Surg* 2001; **7**(8): 461–6.

Holcomb JB, McMullin NR, Pearse L, Caruso J, Wade CE, Oetjen-Gerdes L, et al. Causes of death in U.S. Special Operations Forces in the Global War on Terrorism: 2001-2004. *Ann Surg* 2007; **245**(6): 986–91.

Lynch K, Johansen KA. Can Doppler pressure measurement replace 'exclusion' arteriography in the diagnosis of occult extremity arterial trauma? *Ann Surg* 1991; **214**(6): 737–42.

Menakuru SR, Behera A, Jindal R, Kaman L, Doley R, Venkatesan R. Extremity vascular trauma in civilian population: a seven-year review from North India. *Injury* 2005; **36**(3): 400–6.

Midgley PI, Mackenzie KS, Corriveau MM, Obrand DI, Abraham CZ, Fata P, et al. Blunt thoracic aortic injury: a single institution comparison of open and endovascular management. *J Vasc Surg* 2007; **46**(4): 662–8.

Mullenix PS, Steele SR, Andersen CA, Starnes BW, Salim A, Martin MJ. Limb salvage and outcomes among patients with traumatic popliteal vascular injury: an analysis of the National Trauma Data Bank. *J Vasc Surg* 2006; **44**(1): 94–100.

Peck MA, Clouse WD, Cox MW, Bowser AN, Eliason JL, Jenkins DH, et al. The complete management of extremity vascular injury in a local population: a wartime report from the 332nd Expeditionary Medical Group/Air Force Theater Hospital, Balad Air Base, Iraq. *J Vasc Surg* 2007; **45**(6): 1197–205.

Peck MA, Rasmussen TE. Management of blunt peripheral arterial injury. *Perspect Vasc Surg Endovasc Ther* 2006; **18**(2): 159–73.

Rasmussen, TE, Clouse WD, Jenkins DH, Peck MA, Eliason JL, Smith DL. The use of temporary vascular shunts as a damage control adjunct in the management of wartime vascular injury. *J Trauma* 2006; **61**(1): 8–15.

Starnes BW, Beekley AC, Sebesta JA, Andersen CA, Rush RM. Extremity vascular injuries on the battlefield: tips for surgeons deploying to war. *J Trauma* 2006; **60**(2): 432–42.

Tisherman SA, Bokhari F, Collier B, Cumming J, Ebert J, Holevar M, et al. P. *Clinical Practice Guidelines: Penetrating Neck Trauma.* Eastern Association for the Surgery of Trauma 2008. Available at: www.east.org.

Eye trauma

Eye trauma

Introduction

The eyes occupy only 0.1% of the total and 0.27% of the anterior body surface; however, injury to the eyes can have devastating consequences as vision is the most important sensory modality. Loss of vision is likely to lead to loss of career, major lifestyle changes and disfigurement. Eye injuries occur in economically active people, usually males (70%) with an average age of approximately 39 years. Eye and orbital injuries were responsible for approximately 3500 hospital consultant episodes in England in 2007, and are the commonest cause of extended hospitalization for ophthalmic patients. The home is now commonest place for a serious injury to occur (30.2%), followed by the workplace (19.6%), and sports or leisure facilities (15.8%). Tools or machinery are the most frequent cause of injury (25%), followed by assault (20%) and sports-related activities (12.5%). War-related eye injuries have become more common over the past few years and are often from high explosive devices associated with injuries from the blast wave itself or secondary to debris from the explosion. Eye injuries come at a high cost to society and are largely avoidable.

Birmingham Eye Trauma Terminology System

The Birmingham Eye Trauma Terminology System (BETTS) is the standardized system used to describe and share eye injury information (Fig. 17.1). The wall of the eye is composed of the sclera and cornea. For clinical and practical purposes ocular wounds are graded according to damage to the most external layer.

Assessment of the injured eye

The history

Meticulous note-keeping is essential as eye injuries will often require preparation of legal and insurance reports or police statements. Time and date of the injury, as well as the attendance in the eye emergency department (ED) should be recorded.

The mechanism of injury should be described in detail including the circumstances of the injury (e.g. hammering, metal, or machine tool use). Whether the patient was at work at the time of injury must also be recorded.

An accurate list of all injuries to the eye, its adnexae, and other injuries to the body should be made; this is especially important with multi-trauma cases. Any eye protection or eyewear used at the time of injury should be noted. This information is particularly important for medico-legal reasons.

The presence of foreign bodies should be sought and the patient asked about their composition or type. First aid treatment should be detailed.

Past ocular history should be recorded, as it may affect ophthalmic management and prognosis. Was the eye a seeing eye before the injury, is there a history of amblyopia in either eye? The general medical history may be important for patient management and the patient's tetanus status must be established. Known allergies are important as systemic antibiotics are often prescribed.

Examination

Ocular trauma patients are often particularly stressed as they are worried about losing their vision, and should be made as comfortable and relaxed as possible. It is, therefore, absolutely essential to assess whether both eyes are present and if they are grossly intact: this can be difficult to assess with extensive ocular adnexal swelling. Associated cranial trauma should be considered especially if there are associated facial injuries or penetrating orbital or ocular trauma.

Visual assessment

The best corrected visual acuity is measured for each eye separately using a Snellen chart and the patient's normal visual correction. The acuity is measured as a fraction of the distance from the chart (6 m) divided by the size of letter a normal observer should see at that distance. The fraction 6/6 represents what a normal person can see at 6 m; a vision of 6/12 is what the patient sees at 6 m and a normal patient sees at 12 m, half the acuity. A reduced chart using smaller letters at a closer distance can be used in the examination room. Spectacles are often lost or broken in ocular trauma; if the vision is measured while looking through a pin-hole the effects of uncorrected refractive error are counteracted. If no letters can be read, the ability to count fingers, to see hand movements, and to perceive light are recorded in that order as CF, HM, PL, and NPL (nil perception of light), respectively. If the vision is PL, whether the patient is able to detect from which quadrant the light is shining is recorded.

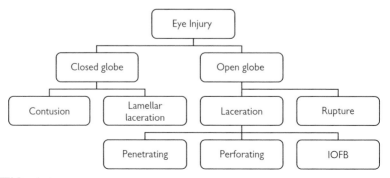

Fig. 17.1. BETTS flow chart.

Pupil examination

Pupil shape, symmetry, red reflex, and reactions are examined. A distorted pupil suggests anterior segment trauma, iris plugging of a penetrating injury or prolapse of vitreous or lens into the anterior segment (Figure 17.2a,b).

Transillumination defects of the iris may be due to iris root tears or the passage of an intra-ocular foreign body. Iris sphincter rupture causes notching of the pupil margin and indicates significant ocular trauma.

The pupillary red reflex is assessed using a direct ophthalmoscope at 50 cm. It is absent if there is opacity of the ocular media, such as cataract, vitreous haemorrhage, or total retinal detachment. Afferent pupillary reactions must be tested using the Marcus Gunn swinging flashlight test. A bright pen torch can be used even when one eye is closed. In an afferent pupillary defect there is a decreased direct response caused by decreased visual function in one eye due to optic nerve or retinal damage. In the swinging flashlight test a light is moved back and forth between the eyes every 2–3 s. The afferent pupillary defect becomes obvious when the flashlight is moved from the normal to the affected eye and the affected pupil dilates in response to light. Under normal conditions, the pupil remains constricted when the light is shone at it.

Facial injuries

Cheek swelling, flattening, or asymmetry from a malar fracture should be sought. Horizontal and vertical alignment of the pupils and canthi from the bridge of the nose should be measured with a ruler; an increase (telecanthus) indicates a mid-facial fracture. An inferiorly displaced lateral canthus indicates a zygomatic fracture.

Enophthalmos, where the eye is sunken, suggests a blow-out fracture, usually affecting the maxillary floor, whereas proptosis, a bulging eye, suggests an orbital haematoma. If combined with loss of vision and a tense orbit a retrobulbar haemorrhage should be diagnosed. This is an ocular emergency requiring immediate surgical decompression with a lateral canthotomy.

The orbital rim must be palpated for steps indicating a fracture or crepitus indicating a fracture in an air sinus. Infra-orbital hypoaesthesia indicates infra-orbital nerve involvement in an orbital floor fracture.

Eyelid examination

The lid contours must be examined; assymmetry may be from ruptured canthal tendons, which attach the ends of the lid to the orbit. A flattened upper lid may indicate a globe rupture. A lid notch or laceration may indicate an underlying penetrating ocular injury.

Lid foreign bodies should be sought by lid eversion. The conjunctiva can be anaesthetized with benoxinate hydrochloride 0.4% drops, then the upper lid everted by placing a cotton-wool bud stick over the lid crease, pinching the eyelashes, and folding the lid tarsal plate over the stick. If a foreign body is seen on the tarsal surface, it can be wiped off using the cotton wool bud. If a foreign body is suspected in the upper fornix (such as a lost contact lens) a Desmarres retractor can be used to double-evert the eyelid. If globe rupture is suspected the lid must not be everted.

Lid wound assessment includes the depth (partial or full-thickness), tissue loss (corneal exposure), lacrimal or canalicular involvement (epiphora), wound contamination and ptosis (levator damage).

Extra-ocular muscle testing

The cover/uncover test and alternate cover tests are performed with the eyes looking straight ahead and the eyes are tested for diplopia in all nine positions of gaze while following a pen torch (Fig. 17.3). The alternate cover test is performed to check the ocular balance in each position.

Globe examination

This includes pen torch examination of the anterior segment, pupil reactions, lids, and adnexae. An estimation of the anterior chamber depth can be made by holding the torch side on to the limbus. Direct ophthalmoscopy is a readily available and portable examination technique. The patient is asked to look straight ahead at a distant point. The same eye is used by the observer to look through the ophthalmoscope as is examined. Positive lenses are dialled to visualize the anterior segment and will

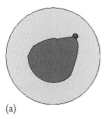

(a)

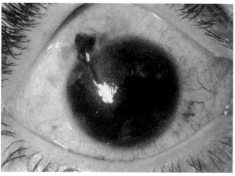

(b)

Fig. 17.2. (a,b) Distorted pupil due to iris extrusion through a corneal laceration. (Reproduced from Sundaram et al., Training in Opthalmology, 2009, with permission from Oxford University Press.)

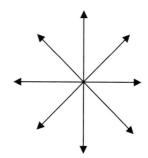

9 positions of gaze (includes straight ahead)

Fig. 17.3 Nine positions of gaze (includes straight ahead).

detect corneal lacerations, hyphaema, the red reflex, and pupil abnormalities.

The lens power is typically reduced to examine the posterior segment. The view is limited to the disc and macula; a more peripheral view is possible if the patient moves their eyes.

Slit lamp biomicroscopy is the best examination technique for the anterior segment and allows an excellent view of the posterior segment. Basic proficiency with the technique is recommended, even if just for anterior segment examination. Foreign bodies can be visualized and removed from the cornea and conjunctiva easily. Inflammation of the anterior segment can be assessed as the actual inflammatory cells and flare from aqueous protein can be seen.

Indirect ophthalmoscopy is used to diagnose retinal tears and detachments using a head mounted light and a hand-held lens, if combined with scleral indentation, a view of the retina up to the ora can be achieved.

If it is impossible to examine the injured eye, examination under anaesthetic (EUA) is indicated. An EUA is commonly performed if the patient is a child, unable to tolerate an examination, if there is too much swelling around the eye or if there is a suspected occult globe rupture.

Pupil dilation (mydriasis) is useful for posterior segment examination, but must only be performed after the pupil reactions have been assessed, an anterior penetrating injury or globe rupture has been excluded and the anterior chamber is judged not to be shallow. Topical tropicamide 1% (2–3 h dilation) or cyclopentolate 1% (12–24 h dilation) are used. Mydriatic drops paralyse the ciliary muscles (accommodation) and the sphincter pupillae muscle (dilation) by reversible muscarinic inhibition. The patient should be warned that their vision will be blurred, and driving is not advised while the drops are working.

Special investigations

A plain skull X-ray is performed to exclude cranial and facial fractures and to visualize radio-opaque foreign bodies. If an intra-ocular foreign body (IOFB) is suspected, the request should be for views in upward and downward gaze. An IOFB will move with the eye, and an orbital foreign body (FB) or artefact will remain still. CT scans are the investigation of choice for orbital and IOFB localization. Consultation with the CT technician is vital. Helical CT scanning has a high sensitivity for IOFB, but will also diagnose other unsuspected cranial and facial injuries.

Ultrasound is also useful for IOFB localization and can be used even if the globe is still open. It is capable of detecting some IOFB that are not radio-opaque or are very small and that will not be detected by X-ray or CT scan. Ultrasound can often localize orbital FB and help with surgical removal. Magnetic resonance imaging (MRI) is contraindicated for metallic IOFB as the magnetic flux may cause them to move within the eye and cause further intra-ocular damage

Microscopy and microbiological culture of aqueous or vitreous samples must be requested if endophthalmitis is suspected. Electrodiagnostic tests of optic nerve and retinal function can be useful in severe trauma to help decide if visual function has been lost. Electroretinography (ERG) is useful in the diagnosis of siderosis or chalchosis.

A visual field test is performed if optic nerve or tract damage is suspected. If an eye is lost a visual field test is performed of the good eye to confirm that it is normal.

Specific injuries

Corneal abrasions

Corneal abrasions are common, often from fingernail or tree branch scratches. They are intensely painful with a foreign body sensation in the eye. There is conjunctival injection with a swollen eyelid and, occasionally, mild anterior chamber inflammation. A history of eye trauma should be sought and also any details of contact lens use.

Diagnosis is made by slit lamp examination of the cornea with fluorescein staining, after anaesthetic drops have been instilled to allow examination of the eye. The abrasion stains, and can be measured and recorded. The underlying corneal stroma is clear in corneal abrasion.

The differential diagnosis of corneal abrasion is bacterial or fungal keratitis, where there is stromal infiltrate and often marked anterior chamber inflammation. In these cases, the patient is usually a soft contact lens wearer.

Corneal foreign bodies

Corneal FBs are intensely painful with a foreign body sensation in the eye. There is conjunctival injection with a swollen eyelid and occasionally mild anterior chamber inflammation (Fig. 17.4).

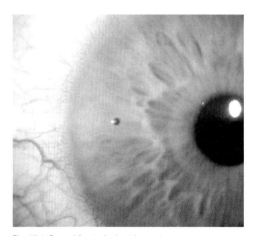

Fig. 17.4 Corneal foreign body with rust ring

A history of how the FB entered the eye is sought: if there is a chance of an IOFB then radiographic investigation is mandatory. Diagnosis is made by slit lamp examination of the cornea with fluorescein staining after an anaesthetic drop is instilled to allow examination of the eye. There is often a sterile infiltrate surrounding the FB, especially if it has been present for more than 24 h. There may be superficial punctuate staining of the cornea and mild anterior chamber inflammation. The eyelids must be everted to exclude the presence of multiple FB.

Conjunctival foreign bodies

Conjunctival FB usually causes a gritty foreign body sensation, but can be relatively painless. The history must exclude a scleral laceration or IOFB, and if there is a chance

of an IOFB then radiographic investigation is mandatory. Diagnosis is made by slit lamp examination with intra-ocular pressure measurement to exclude a penetrating injury. There may be a subconjunctival haemorrhage at the FB site. Eversion and double eversion of the eyelid should be performed if a subtarsal or forniceal FB is suspected (Fig. 17.5).

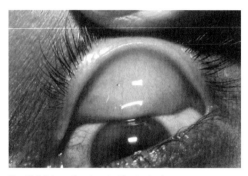

Fig. 17.5 Subtarsal conjunctival foreign body.

Ocular burns

Thermal burns often result from contact with hot liquids, hot gases, or molten metals. Tissue damage is usually limited to the superficial epithelium, but thermal necrosis and ocular penetration can occur.

Ultraviolet burns result from exposure to sources including sunlamps and welding arcs. Patients present with a superficial punctuate keratitis. Onset of pain may be delayed but is intense.

Chemical burns are blinding emergencies. Alkaline agents, such as lye or cement penetrate cell membranes and cause more damage than acidic agents. Acid burns are usually from battery acid explosions and acids precipitate when they react with ocular proteins.

Corneal epithelial defects in burns range from superficial epitheliopathy to total epithelial loss. Limbal ischaemia is a whitened area without blood flow. The whiter the eye, the worse the burn. Other signs include focal areas of conjunctival chemosis, hyperaemia, conjunctival haemorrhages, eyelid oedema, mild iritis, and periocular burns.

The Roper-Hall classification of ocular chemical burns relates the visual prognosis to the amount of corneal damage and limbal ischaemia (Table 17.1).

Intra-ocular foreign bodies

Intra-ocular foreign bodies (IOFB) cause approximately 15% of hospital admissions for eye injuries; 95% are males, with an average age of 37 years. They must be suspected if there is a history of high speed tool use or hammering. The final resting place of an IOFB, and the damage caused by it depend on the size, the shape, and the momentum of the object at the time of impact, and the site of ocular penetration. Over 90% IOFB are metallic; 5% are multiple. Appropriate eye protection would abolish virtually all IOFB injuries.

Table 17.1. Roper-Hall classification

Grade	Prognosis	Limbal ischaemia	Corneal involvement
I	Good	None	Epithelial damage
II	Good	Less than 1/3	Haze, but the iris details are visible
III	Guarded	1/3 to 1/2	Total epithelial loss, haze obscures iris details
IV	Poor	Greater than 1/2	Cornea opaque, iris and pupil obscured

Hammering metal is the cause of 70% of cases. Increasing IOFB mass is associated with posterior segment injury, retinal impact, and poor vision. The frequency of globe penetration by an IOFB is determined by its shape; blade-shaped > disc-shaped > cylindrical > spherical.

Secondary complications from IOFB occur in half of patients, including endophthalmitis, corneal scarring, elevated intra-ocular pressure, cataract, retinal detachment, and metallosis (e.g. chalcosis, siderosis). Siderosis occurs if a ferrous IOFB is left *in situ*, when iron dispersion throughout the globe causes retinal toxicity; IOFB removal is usually followed by visual and ERG recovery. Chalcosis occurs from IOFB, which contain more than 85% copper, which is highly retinotoxic and causes profound visual loss associated with a greenish hue to the affected cornea. The diagnosis is made by copper assay of an aqueous fluid sample.

Failure to diagnose an IOFB is a major cause of negligence claims.

Penetrating and perforating injuries

Penetrating eye injuries are sharp eye injuries that usually result in a single entrance wound (Fig. 17.2a). Perforating eye injuries have an entrance and exit wound; both wounds are caused by the same agent. The symptoms of these wounds include pain with decreased vision and a history of ocular trauma. The signs may be obvious with an entry or exit site and extrusion of ocular tissue, but if there is occult penetration there may be early ocular hypotony that recovers after a few hours; anterior segment disruption; vitreous haemorrhage and retinal breaks.

Vision can be lost if there is a suprachoroidal haemorrhage as the ocular contents are extruded through the wound.

Globe rupture

Globe rupture is a full-thickness wound of the eye wall from a blunt injury. The eye is filled with incompressible liquid and the impact causes sufficient pressure to rupture the eye at its weakest point. Rupture is commonly at the impact site, or an area of corneal or scleral weakness such as an old cataract wound.

The clinical signs of scleral rupture include periocular haemorrhage with haemorrhagic chemosis, a visual acuity of PL or less, afferent pupillary defect, ocular hypotony, an abnormally deep or shallow anterior chamber, and an irregular pupil. There is often extrusion of the ocular contents.

Globe rupture must be excluded by ultrasound scan in all cases of hyphaema or post-traumatic media opacity that prevents indirect ophthalmoscopy of the fundus.

Sympathetic ophthalmia

Sympathetic ophthalmia is a bilateral panuveitis that causes a painful red eye with visual loss in a patient with a history of eye injury. It occurs in approximately 1 in 500 cases of open globe injury. The injured eye is termed the exciting eye and the fellow eye is the sympathizing eye. Exposure of retinal specific proteins to the immune system during the injury of one eye causes an autoimmune reaction to both eyes at a later date. It can occur as early as 5 days and as late as 60 years after the injury, although 90% of cases occur within the first year. The typical appearance is of granulomatous panuveitis with mutton-fat keratoprecipitates, usually with multiple yellow Dalen-Fuchs subretinal nodules apparent on fundoscopy.

Lamellar lacerations

Non-penetrating lacerations of the cornea and sclera can be diagnosed by careful ophthalmoscopy. Siedel's sign indicates a penetrating injury of the anterior segment. Here, a drop of fluorescein dye is applied to the cornea and is observed with a slit lamp's cobalt blue light. Any fluid leaking out of the eye dilutes the yellow fluorescein and can be observed as a lighter green fluorescent wave.

Ocular contusion injuries

A blunt injury to the eye compresses the globe anteroposteriorly causing expansion around the equator. This stretches the intra-ocular tissues and can damage them. When the compressing object is larger than the orbit it pushes the globe posteriorly to suddenly increase the orbital pressure. The pressure is relieved by a blow-out fracture of the orbit, typically inferiorly into the maxillary sinus. This phenomenon often protects the globe from injury though there is up to a 30% incidence of ruptured globe reported in conjunction with orbital fracture.

Orbital blow-out fractures

Blow-out fractures are usually of the orbital floor with herniation of orbital contents into the maxillary sinus, or less commonly the medial wall with herniation into the ethmoidal sinus. The rectus muscles can be trapped as they herniate into the sinuses causing restriction of eye movement. Patients present after facial trauma with blurred vision, a sunken eye, diplopia, and restriction of eye movements, especially on up-gaze (Fig. 17.6).

Epistaxis and eyelid swelling following nose blowing occurs due to air being blown into the orbit through the maxillary sinus (surgical emphysema). Initially, there is

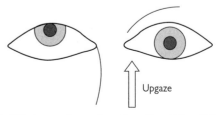

Fig. 17.6. Attempted upgaze in a patient with restriction of left inferior rectus muscle causing limitation of upward movement of the eye.

tender periorbital ecchymosis and oedema. Enophthalmos can be obscured by tissue swelling and the eye may be proptotic due to orbital haemorrhage. The swelling also may restrict extra-ocular muscle motility, mimicking entrapment. Palpation of the orbital rim may reveal a bony step and point tenderness due to a fracture.

Inferior periorbital hypoaesthesia indicates trauma (neuropraxia) to the infra-orbital nerve, which usually recovers over a few weeks.

Examination of the globe is essential to check ocular function and to exclude a rupture.

Ocular misalignment, hypotropia, or hypertropia, and limitation of eye movements indicate an orbital fracture. Forced duction tests differentiate entrapment or traumatic dysfunction of the rectus muscles.

Orbital X-ray and CT scanning will diagnose an orbital floor blow out fracture with characteristic herniation of orbital contents into the maxillary sinus and often a sinus haemorrhage (Fig. 17.7).

Retrobulbar haemorrhage

Retrobulbar haemorrhage is an ocular emergency where bleeding into the orbital space can result in compression of the optic nerve, leading to ischaemia and blindness. Rapid diagnosis and treatment may avoid permanent vision loss. It is particularly associated with infra-orbital, zygomatic and other facial fractures.

Retrobulbar haemorrhage is characterized by severe ocular **pain**, rapid tense **proptosis, pupil reactions** to light are lost, ocular **paralysis**, where ocular movements are lost and **visual loss**, where the vision is reduced like a falling curtain.

Anterior segment contusion

Hyphaema

Hyphaema is caused by bleeding in the anterior chamber which results in layering of red blood cells (RBCs) in the inferior anterior chamber. The height from the inferior limbus is measured to guide management and chart progress (Fig. 17.8).

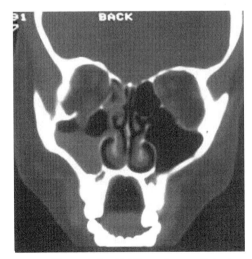

Fig. 17.7. CT scan of right orbital blowout fracture with herniation of orbital contents superiorly and a maxillary sinus haemorrhage inferiorly.

(a)

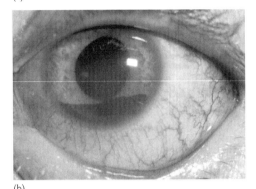

(b)

Fig. 17.8. a and b Hyphaema with a blood level in the anterior chamber.

Microhyphaema is a small hyphaema in which there are only suspended RBCs in the anterior chamber with no layered clot.

The main complications are raised intra-ocular pressure and re-bleeds. Approximately 10% of patients with traumatic hyphaema have associated retinal tears. Retinal detachment must be excluded by posterior segment examination or ultrasound if the view is obscured. Gonioscopy must be performed at some stage to exclude iridocorneal angle recession that may cause late secondary glaucoma.

Hyphaema can be graded according to the scale in Table 17.2.

Iris trauma

Traumatic iritis appears similar to uveitic iritis, but with a history of trauma. The condition presents with reduced vision, ocular pain, and photophobia. Examination shows perilimbal injection with cells and flare in the anterior chamber.

Corneal blood-staining may occur if there is prolonged hyphaema with a high intra-ocular pressure.

Iridocorneal angle recession is where the ciliary body is torn in a manner such that the longitudinal muscle remains attached to its insertion at the scleral spur, while

Table 17.2. Grade of hyphaema

Grade	Proportion of anterior chamber filled with blood
+	< 1/3
++	1/3 – 1/2
+++	> 1/2 but subtotal
++++	Total hyphaema '8 ball'

the circular muscle, with the pars plicata and the iris root, is displaced posteriorly. This damages the trabecular meshwork, impedes flow of aqueous from the eye and can cause a rise in the intra-ocular pressure with secondary glaucoma. It is common after blunt trauma and is diagnosed on slit lamp gonioscopy. In less than 20% of cases of angle recession, it progresses to glaucoma.

Cyclodialysis clefts result from traumatic separation of the ciliary body from the sclera, this allows aqueous to exit directly to the subchoroidal space and causes ocular hypotony (low intra-ocular pressure). The diagnosis is made by gonioscopy or an anterior segment ultrasound scan.

Iridodialysis is a detachment of the iris root from the ciliary body which can produce corectopia (displaced pupil) and pseudopolycoria (more than one pupil) (Fig. 17.9). Glare and diplopia are common symptoms as light enters the eye through two areas.

Lens trauma

Contusion rosette cataracts are classic consequences of blunt trauma and may not appear for years after the injury. Anterior and posterior subcapsular cataracts are also common after trauma. Cataracts cause glare and loss of vision.

Lens subluxation is a partially dislocated crystalline lens caused by incomplete zonular dehiscence from trauma. The lens equator is visible through the pupil and the lens (phakodonesis) and overlying iris (iridodonesis) (Fig. 17.10). If the zonular dehiscence is complete lens dislocation can occur into the anterior chamber or posterior segment. Lens dislocation and subluxation cause sudden loss of visual acuity depending on the position of the lens. If dislocation occurs after relatively minor trauma, Marfan's disease, homocystinuria, Weill–Marchesani syndrome, Ehlers–

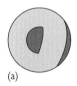

(a)

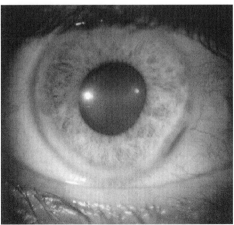

(b)

Fig. 17.9. (a and b) Traumatic iridodialysis with iris root disinsertion and 'D' shaped pupil.

Fig 17.10. Traumatic subluxation of lens inferiorly with abnormal red reflex and equator of the lens visible.

Danlos syndrome, and syphilis should be considered as underlying disorders.

Posterior segment injuries

Commotio retinae (Berlin's oedema) describes the transient grey-white opacification at the level of the deep sensory retina after blunt trauma. It settles over 4–6 weeks leaving retinal pigment epithelial disturbance, retinal atrophy, optic atrophy, and on occasion a traumatic macular hole. Visual loss may be transient or permanent according to the extent of macular involvement.

Choroidal ruptures are typically crescent-shaped and sited at the posterior pole. They occur when the eye is deformed by a blunt injury. They are associated with subretinal haemorrhages that clear to reveal the rupture. Visual recovery is the rule, but vision can be reduced if the rupture involves the fovea, if there is choroidal sub-retinal neovascularization, or massive intra-ocular scarring.

Sclopetaria, traumatic chorioretinal rupture is from a concussion injury where an object strikes the eye at high velocity, but does not penetrate the eye. The choroid and retina are locally disrupted by the shock wave (coup) and at the opposite side of the eye (contracoup) to give an acute traumatic degeneration of the choroid and retina. There are often dramatic retinal tears with associated shallow retinal detachment. These characteristically do not require active treatment as scarring from the surrounding tissue seals the retinal break.

Optic nerve avulsion typically when an object intrudes between the globe and orbital wall. There is sudden visual loss that is irreversible. Diagnosis is by ophthalmoscopy (where there is loss of the optic disc) and confirmed by ultrasound or CT scan. Traumatic optic neuropathy occurs when the concussive wave causes profound vasoconstriction of the pial vessels that supply the optic nerve. The ensuing neural deficit reduces the visual acuity, brightness sense, and colour vision. It is typically associated with a relative afferent pupillary defect.

Traumatic retinal tears and detachments

Retinal dialysis is a peripheral retinal disruption between the edge of the retina and the ora serrata from sudden expansion of the ocular equator from blunt injury. The condition is responsible for up to 84% of trauma-related retinal detachments. Myopic patients are more susceptible and the commonest areas for post-traumatic dialyses are the superonasal and inferotemporal retinal quadrants. The detachment evolves slowly, often years after the trauma, and diagnosis is made when vision is lost due to macular involvement or as an incidental finding during routine ophthalmic examination.

Irregular retinal breaks can form as a result of direct contusion. The retina is separated from the vitreous base and the retinal edge typically has a rolled edge. If the tear is greater than 3 clock hours it is termed a traumatic giant retinal tear. If left untreated, a retinal detachment occurs with a high chance of proliferative retinopathy (retinal scarring) and a poor visual prognosis, so early diagnosis and treatment are essential.

Traumatic macular holes form as a result of acute changes in vitreoretinal traction over the macular area from ocular contusion, they are typically 300–500 µ in diameter, but if there is an element of retinal necrosis they can be much larger. Only 1% progress to retinal detachment and there is a good visual prognosis with successful macular hole surgery.

Other retinal breaks can form as a result of an induced posterior vitreous detachment from the injury. If there is an area of increased vitreoretinal traction, typically over blood vessels a retinal tear forms often with a vitreous haemorrhage. The tears will often be associated with a retinal detachment.

Indirect ocular injury

Purtscher's retinopathy is a sudden-onset multifocal, vaso-occlusive event that is associated with head and chest trauma. It causes a sudden loss of vision that slowly recovers over weeks or months. The appearance is of multiple patches of superficial retinal whitening with retinal haemorrhages surrounding a hyperaemic optic nerve head. The phenomenon has also been described after acute pancreatitis, childbirth, amniotic embolism, connective tissue disorders, and retrobulbar anaesthetic injection.

Terson's syndrome is a vitreous haemorrhage that occurs after an intracranial haemorrhage. It is commonest (3–8%) after a subarachnoid haemorrhage and is often bilateral. It is thought to be related to an acute rise in intracranial pressure that is transmitted to the retina, and causes rupture of the papillary and retinal capillaries. The haemorrhage is thought to form initially between the retina and internal limiting membrane disperses into the vitreous haemorrhage. It is often diagnosed when a patient recovers from the subarachnoid haemorrhage on the intensive care unit and is found to be profoundly blind.

Shaken baby syndrome may be suspected in unexplained respiratory arrest, seizures, or coma in an infant, often with no external signs. Ocular findings include bilateral retinal and vitreous haemorrhages. These findings are extremely rare in isolated blunt head trauma or CPR, and should alert physicians to the possibility of child abuse. Careful documentation and if possible photography are important for medico-legal reasons.

Valsalva retinopathy is a sudden loss of vision from a pre-retinal haemorrhage that occurs when there is a sudden increase in intrathoracic pressure. It typically occurs after heavy lifting or straining at stool coughing or vomiting. Spontaneous recovery is the rule.

Fat embolism syndrome (FES) is a potentially fatal complication of long bone fractures that can affect the respiratory and central nervous systems. Visual involvement is found in 50% of FES cases and it will commonly cause reduced vision. The retinal appearance is similar to Purtscher's retinopathy with multiple patches of superficial retinal whitening and retinal haemorrhages surrounding a hyperaemic optic nerve head. Visual recovery is usually good, although permanent patchy visual field loss will occasionally occur.

Whiplash retinopathy is caused by an extreme flexion-extension of the head and neck without direct eye injury. It causes a mild reduction of visual acuity associated with subtle signs of central macular swelling and an abnormal central foveal pit. The vision will usually recover to a normal level although the foveal pit may remain. Careful documentation is advised as there is often a medico-legal case associated with these injuries.

Management and referral

Virtually all significant eye trauma should be referred to an ophthalmologist for assessment and treatment.

Eyelid trauma management

Simple cases do not require ophthalmic referral, but any full thickness lid laceration requires an ophthalmic opinion before a surgical repair is attempted. Eyelids have an excellent blood supply and healing potential so debridement of tissue should be avoided. Bleeding should be stopped using tacking sutures to hold the lids together if necessary. Pressure on the globe must be avoided in cases of rupture.

If there is lid avulsion a cartella shield should be used to protect the eye and lubricants to prevent corneal exposure. Superficial lacerations that do not involve the lid margins can be repaired with 6/0 vicryl sutures. Where the lid margins are involved, if the cannaliculi have been involved or the levator muscle has been damaged, referral to an ophthalmologist for an oculoplastic repair is recommended. Complex reconstruction of the lid with cannalicular repair as a first procedure can prevent future complications from inappropriate interventions. If there has been tissue loss normal plastic surgery repair may not be appropriate and referral to an oculoplastic surgeon is indicated so that tissue sparing techniques can be used to give the best possible cosmetic result.

The lids can be left for several days before repair as long as the cornea is protected from exposure.

Orbital fracture management

Orbital fractures are not urgent cases. They require referral to an ophthalmologist or maxillofacial surgeon for further investigation and management. The presence of an orbital foreign body should be excluded by radiography and CT scan. Prophylactic systemic antibiotics should be prescribed and the patient instructed not to blow their nose.

Management of orbital blow out fractures is conservative if there is no enophthalmos or rectus muscle tethering. Adult patients are observed for 1–2 weeks in case of spontaneous resolution; children are observed for a maximum of 1 week before definitive action is taken.

If there is more than 2 mm enophthalmos or significant restriction of eye movement, orbital floor reconstruction with an implant is performed.

Retrobulbar haemorrhage

Emergency referral to an ophthalmologist must be made and treatment started as soon as possible. Lateral canthotomy and inferior cantholysis should be performed immediately to decompress the orbit. Intravenous acetazolamide (500 mg) is given to lower the intra-ocular pressure. Intravenous mannitol (1 g/kg as 20% infusion) is an osmotic diuretic agent given to lower the intra-ocular pressure. It is contra-indicated in congestive heart failure and pulmonary disease.

Corneal abrasion

Non-contact lens wearers should be prescribed topical antibiotic ointment for 1 week to lubricate the eye surface and protect against infection. If the eye is painful, a topical cycloplegic (cyclopentolate 1% bd) should be prescribed. There is no evidence that application of an occlusive eye patch improves healing, comfort, or visual outcome.

The patient should be seen the next day to confirm healing of the defect and then a week later to confirm total healing. If the abrasion is persistent, a switch should be made to a non-preserved antibiotic along with topical ocular lubricants until healing occurs. More frequent follow-up in contact lens wearers is advised in case of corneal ulcer.

Recurrent erosions occasionally occur after an initial abrasion, these are particularly common against the background of a corneal epithelial dystrophy. They occur classically in the morning as the corneal epithelium sticks to the upper lid conjunctiva, while the lids are closed at night and is torn off on waking. Treatment is with frequent topical lubricant drops during the day and ointment at night.

Corneal foreign bodies

Corneal foreign bodies do not require ophthalmological referral. The foreign body is removed under topical anaesthesia at the slit lamp using the edge of a needle. Topical antibiotics should be prescribed and one follow-up visit to check healing at one week is usually sufficient. Occasionally a rust ring forms around a corneal foreign body that can be difficult to remove with a needle. These are removed with a rotating Alger brush.

Conjunctival foreign bodies

Once again ophthalmological referral is not necessary. Direct removal with a cotton wool bud under topical anaesthesia is performed. A pair of fine forceps is used to remove embedded foreign body. Multiple foreign bodies can generally be removed with saline irrigation and needle removal of the remainder. The ocular fornices may be swept using a cotton wool bud to remove any loose foreign bodies that may have been missed on examination. Topical antibiotics should be prescribed.

Thermal burns

Topical antibiotics are prescribed for epithelial defects and conjunctivitis. Initially, the lid swelling may protect the corneal surface, but sloughing and contracture can lead to corneal exposure. Topical ocular lubricants are used to prevent corneal exposure.

Ultraviolet radiation burns

Ultraviolet radiation burns do not require ophthalmological referral. Topical cycloplegics and antibiotic ointment are prescribed and an occlusive patch is applied to the eye for comfort.

Chemical burns

Immediate copious irrigation with Ringer's lactate solution for 30 min (normal saline or even tap water are alternatives) is essential. The pH should be measured after 5 min on ceasing irrigation and, if it is not neutral (pH7.0), then irrigation should be continued until the pH is neutral. The fornices must be swept to remove retained debris and break conjunctival adhesions. Topical antibiotic ointment and cycloplegic drops are prescribed along with oral ascorbic acid (vitamin C) up to 2 g qds to promote fibroblast activity. Oral analgesia will usually be required. Topical steroids are used cautiously within the first week as they may cause corneoscleral melting. Raised intra-ocular pressure is treated with topical or systemic ocular antihypertensives. Amniotic membrane grafts that promote corneal surface healing are especially useful in the management of severe burns.

IOFB

All suspected IOFB injuries must be referred to an ophthalmologist for potential emergency surgical management. Systemic and topical antibiotic therapy should be started prior to surgical intervention to prevent endophthalmitis. Topical corticosteroids are used to minimize inflammation and a tetanus booster may be appropriate.

Surgical removal of a posterior segment IOFB is by pars plana vitrectomy and is performed as an emergency if the risk of endophthalmitis is high. In most other cases, intervention can be deferred for a few days to reduce the risk of intra-operative haemorrhage as long as systemic antibiotics have been started. The posterior hyaloid is removed, and retinal impact sites are treated with prophylactic retinopexy.

Occasionally, an external electromagnet is used to remove IOFB, especially if it is buried in the ciliary body. Anterior chamber IOFB are not removed through the original wound, but through a paracentesis at 90–180° to it. Viscoelastics reduce the risk of iatrogenic damage to the lens and corneal endothelium. Intralenticular IOFB occasionally can be left *in situ* unless there is a risk of siderosis.

The prognosis from an IOFB injury is relatively good with over 50% of eyes achieving reading vision.

Penetrating and perforating injuries

The eye should be protected by a Cartella shield and the patient admitted for bed rest. Systemic antibiotics should be started, fluoroquinolone antibiotics, such as ciprofloxacin are recommended as they have an excellent spectrum of antibacterial action with good ocular penetration and can be administered orally. Tetanus toxoid is given if required. A CT scan should be performed to rule out an intra-orbital, intracranial, or intra-ocular foreign body or penetration, ultrasound can be used to localize a posterior rupture or exit site.

Management is by urgent primary surgical repair, which can be followed by a definitive secondary procedure at a later date depending on the experience of the surgeon. Associated retinal detachments and tears are managed by vitrectomy, retinopexy, and internal tamponade. Suxamethonium should be avoided during the anaesthetic as it may cause increased venous pressure and an intra-ocular haemorrhage.

Enucleation as a primary procedure should be avoided unless the patient has been properly counselled and consented. It is better to perform a primary repair and obtain consensus, before the eye is enucleated or eviscerated with an orbital implant as a secondary procedure.

Globe rupture

The eye should not be manipulated in case of extrusion of its contents. A protective Cartella eye shield is fitted to protect it until it can be surgically repaired. Surgical exploration and primary repair is performed if globe rupture is suspected. The conjunctiva is reflected back and the sclera is systematically examined with particular reference to the thinnest area of sclera that lies under the rectus muscles.

Secondary procedures for intra-ocular haemorrhage are delayed for up to 14 days to allow the blood clot to liquefy, when it can be surgically drained as part of a vitrectomy procedure.

Sympathetic ophthalmia

Prevention of sympathetic ophthalmia is by enucleation of blind traumatized eye within 7–14 days of the injury. If sympathetic ophthalmia occurs, enucleation may still be beneficial regardless of the time period after the injury. Treatment should be under the care of an ophthalmologist. Topical and systemic steroids are the mainstay of treatment with further immunosuppression, as required. Topical cycloplegia help relieve pain and discomfort.

Corneal lacerations

The treatment of corneal lacerations is usually by direct suturing using 10/0 nylon sutures under an operating microscope. Occasionally, corneal lacerations can be managed with a bandage contact lens. A contact lens will protect the eye until referral can be made to an ophthalmologist as it stops the flap from dislodging. Topical antibiotics must be given for 1–2 weeks after the laceration.

Conjunctival lacerations

The conjunctiva heals rapidly and rarely needs suturing. A 7/0 vicryl (absorbable) tacking suture is used if required. Topical antibiotic drops are given for 1 week.

Hyphaema

When hyphaema occurs, elective anticoagulants should be stopped and the patient rested in bed with 30° head elevation for 4 days to reduce episcleral venous pressure and promote cells settling. Only light activity is allowed for 2 weeks after this. Atropine 1% drops and topical steroids should be given for 2 weeks and sickle cell anaemia should be excluded in susceptible groups.

Raised intra-ocular pressure occurs in 30% of cases and is treated with oral or topical ocular anti-hypertensives. Acetazolamide is contraindicated in sickle cell disease. Re-bleeding occurs in 4–40% of cases, usually 2–5 days post-injury. Surgical wash-out of the anterior chamber is required for 5% of cases. Iridocorneal angle recession or iridodialysis occurs in 75%, but 5% develop secondary glaucoma.

Traumatic iritis

A topical cycloplegic agent is prescribed to relieve pain. Topical steroids are of limited value unless the iritis is prolonged. Retinal examination should be performed to exclude traumatic retinal tears.

Cyclodialysis cleft

Topical atropine 1% bd should be given for 6–8 weeks. Spontaneous resolution is usual. If persistent, transcleral diode laser is applied to the cleft. Direct surgical closure is required if medical treatments fail.

Iridodialysis

Patients require lifelong glaucoma monitoring as the iridocorneal angle damage predisposes to a raised intra-ocular pressure. If there is diplopia, a contact lens with an artificial iris can be considered. The best treatment is with direct surgical closure of the defect.

Cataract

Surgical removal of the cataract by phacoemulsification and lens implantation should be performed if there is a visually significant cataract.

Lens dislocation or subluxation

For anterior chamber dislocation, the lens should be repositioned after pupil dilation and supine positioning with corneal indentation with a gonioprism at a slit lamp.

Cases of posterior segment dislocation, if there is an intact lens capsule, can be managed conservatively. If there is a chance of capsular damage pars plana vitreolensectomy with intra-ocular lens implantation is performed. Leakage of lens protein in the vitreous causes severe inflammation and secondary glaucoma.

Traumatic optic neuropathy

Traumatic optic neuropathy management options include observation, high dose steroids (iv methylprednisolone) and surgical decompression of the optic canal. There is no evidence of superiority of medical and surgical treatment over observation and the interventional treatments carry a high risk of side-effects and complications. As a result, the available options should be discussed with the patient. Measurement of recovery is with visual acuity measurement, colour vision estimation, visual field analysis, and electrodiagnostic testing.

Retinal tears and detachments

These are managed surgically with retinopexy for retinal tears and vitrectomy and internal tamponade, or cryopexy and buckling procedures, for retinal detachment. If an intra-ocular gas is used, the patient cannot travel by air until it has resorbed in case of sudden gas expansion at altitude.

Retinal detachments associated with penetrating trauma are particularly susceptible to post-operative retinal scarring (proliferative vitreoretinopathy). This reduces the anatomical and visual outcomes of surgery and the patient should be warned of the guarded prognosis.

Important tips

The following tips may be helpful in the management of ophthalmological trauma cases:

- Anaesthetics should never be used except to examine a patient.
- It is vital to be extra vigilant with contact lens wearers.
- Fundoscopy should always be performed in cases where child abuse is suspected.
- Trauma prevention by the use of safety glasses should always be encouraged.

Further reading

Blanch RJ. Scott RA. Primary blast injury of the eye. *J Roy Army Med Corps* 2008; **154**: 76.

Chalioulias K, Sim KT, Scott RA. Retinal sequelae of primary ocular blast injuries. *J Roy Army Med Corps* 2007; **153**: 124–5.

Colyer MH, Weber ED, Weichel ED, Dick JS, Bower KS, Ward TP, et al. Delayed intra-ocular foreign body removal without endophthalmitis during Operations Iraqi Freedom and Enduring Freedom. *Ophthalmology* 2007; **114**: 1439–47.

Desai P, MacEwen CJ, Baines P, Minassian DC. Epidemiology and implications of ocular trauma admitted to hospital in Scotland. *J Epidemiol Comm Health* 1996; **50**: 436–41.

Kanski JJ. *Clinical Ophthalmology—A Systematic Approach*, 6th edn. Oxford: Butterworth-Heinemann.

Kuhn F, Pieramici DJ. *Ocular Trauma Principles and Practice*, 1st edn. New York: Thieme, 2002.

Kuhn F, Maisiak R, Mann L Morris R, Witherspoon CD. The Ocular Trauma Score (OTS). *Ophthalmol Clin N Am* 2002; **5**: 163–5.

Kuhn F, Morris R, Witherspoon CD Heimann K, Jeffers JB, Treister G. A standardized classification of ocular trauma Ophthalmology. 1996; **103**: 240–3.

Woodcock MG, Scott RA, Huntbach J, Kirkby GR. Mass and shape as factors in intra-ocular foreign body injuries. *Ophthalmology* 2006s; **113**(12): 2262–9.

Maxillofacial trauma

Maxillofacial trauma

Maxillofacial trauma is a relatively common presentation to the emergency department. These injuries are important for aesthetic and for functional reasons. The facial bones and soft tissues protect the neurocranium, and severe facial trauma is an indicator of potential intracranial trauma. There is a wide range of severity depending on the mechanism of facial injury.

Mechanisms

The pattern of facial injury has steadily changed over the last 30 years. Improvements in road safety, car design, alcohol, and seatbelt legislation have all resulted in a decrease in road traffic collision injuries. However, interpersonal violence is now a factor in more than half of facial trauma cases in the United Kingdom, and alcohol consumption is a contributing factor in almost all independent studies:

- Interpersonal violence.   52%
- Road traffic collisions.   19%
- Sports injuries.   16%
- Mechanical falls/Collapse.   11%
- Industrial injuries.   2%

Initial management

Maxillofacial injuries are only addressed at the primary survey if they cause catastrophic external haemorrhage, or impact on airway, breathing, or circulation. A comprehensive assessment is undertaken as part of the secondary survey.

Airway and cervical spine control

Approximately 15% of patients with severe maxillofacial trauma will have a cervical spine injury. Care needs to be taken to prevent any further harm to the cervical spine during the management of the airway.

The major cause of death following severe maxillofacial injury is airway obstruction and it is vital to address this potential problem. A rapid assessment must be made with regard to the patient's ability to maintain and protect their own airway. The airway is at particular risk in unconscious patients with maxillofacial injuries:

- Displaced teeth, dentures, blood, and vomit may all cause airway obstruction. Debris should be cleared from the airway. Missing teeth, crowns, and dentures should be recorded and sought on a chest X-ray or CT scan to exclude aspiration.
- Uncontrolled haemorrhage represents a major hazard to the airway. Conscious patients with major facial haemorrhage may be able to maintain their airway by sitting forwards. They may lose their airway if forced to lie supine in a rigid collar.
- Major midface trauma can result in the facial skeleton shearing from the cranial base and being forced inferiorly.

This leads to airway obstruction at the level of the soft palate. The facial skeleton should be disimpacted by placing two fingers inside the mouth behind the soft palate and pulling the maxilla anteriorly.
- Bilateral mandibular fractures in elderly patients may rotate posteriorly and obstruct the airway. These 'bucket handle' fractures should be manually rotated to relieve any obstruction.
- The tongue may lose its anterior attachments in comminuted mandibular parasymphyseal fractures and fall backwards when the patient is supine. Airway adjuncts such as an oropharyngeal airway may help airway maintenance.
- Tongue swelling and loss of tone in the obtunded patient may obstruct the airway. A large silk traction suture or towel clip may help to apply traction to the tongue and open the oro-pharyngeal airway.
- Maxillofacial injuries may be associated with injuries to the larynx and trachea. Symptoms and signs are neck swelling, noisy breathing, dyspnoea, altered voice, surgical emphysema, and palpable fractures.

Circulation and haemorrhage control

The maxillofacial region is one of the most vascular areas of the body. It is supplied by branches of the carotid and vertebral artery systems, with the internal and external carotid arteries anastamosing in the orbital region. Despite this, life-threatening haemorrhage leading to hypovolaemic shock is rare in this region and the major problem posed by the bleeding is to patency of the airway:

- Bleeding from the facial soft tissues is often brisk. Blind clamping within wounds should be resisted because of the risk of damage to branches of the delicate facial nerve. Direct wound compression or regional artery pressure are safer options. The facial artery can be compressed as it crosses the lower border of the mandible just anterior to the masseter muscle. The superficial temporal artery can be compressed against the skull just anterior to the ear.
- Scalp wounds bleed profusely and vessels often remain open. The facial nerve is not at risk within the hairy scalp and it is safe to use clamps for haemostasis. A few deep sutures within the scalp can help stabilize the bleeding prior to definitive treatment.
- Tongue lacerations can be temporarily sutured with large silk sutures. Deep tissue bites are required as the tongue musculature adjacent to contused lacerations may be friable.
- Severe midface fractures can cause significant haemorrhage. The management of this is dealt with in a separate section on maxillofacial haemorrhage.

Clinical examination

Once the patient is stable and the primary survey has been completed, a thorough maxillofacial examination is carried out as part of the secondary survey. Facial injuries often have a dramatic appearance and it is important that treatment is restricted to life-threatening injuries during the primary survey.

History

A comprehensive history of the mechanism of injury is important as it alerts the clinician to the possibility of associated injuries and sequelae, which would not otherwise be apparent. If details are not available directly from the patient then it is important to ask anyone present at the incident for details such as vehicle speed, position of the patient, entrapment time, and condition of other casualties. This information helps the clinician appreciate the possibility of other associated injuries both within the maxillofacial region and systemically. As part of the general medical evaluation it is important to detail the patient's tetanus status and allergies.

Examination

The entire head and neck should be exposed and cleaned to remove dried blood and debris. Care must be taken to avoid excessive manipulation of the cervical spine where there is a possibility of instability. A systematic examination should be made from scalp to chin.

Scalp

The scalp should be examined for lacerations, bruising and haematomata. The scalp has a natural plane of cleavage between the galea aponeurotica and the periosteum of the cranial bones. Debris can be driven into this plane and may be present some distance from the wound edges. The wound edges must be elevated and irrigated copiously prior to suturing. Small children who fall over in the garden may have impacted dirt under wound edges and unless these wounds are thoroughly examined and cleaned they will later return with a wound infection.

The bony skull table should be examined through any scalp laceration and palpated. Bony depressions or steps may indicate an underlying fracture. A boggy scalp haematoma can overlie a skull vault fracture and diagnostic imaging should be considered.

Elderly patients may present with a large forehead haematoma following an unbroken fall to the ground. Tissue laxity allows this haematoma to expand and the pressure on the friable skin may cause superficial necrosis in a similar fashion to a pretibial haematoma. The possibility of an occult cervical spine fracture should be considered in this group of patients.

Eyes

The eyes should be examined early before periorbital swelling makes this difficult. Visual loss following trauma is a devastating consequence. In some cases, the original trauma leads to irredeemable visual damage; however, some pathologies such as retrobulbar haematoma are potentially salvageable. Careful clinical examination and documentation are important in order to prevent permanent visual deterioration.

The eye examination begins with a general examination of the eye and periorbita. Periorbital oedema, ecchymosis, and lacerations should be noted. Unilateral signs are seen in soft tissue injuries and orbitozygomatic fractures. Bilateral signs may indicate a middle third or anterior skull base fracture. A subconjunctival haemorrhage with no posterior border may also be noted with these fractures. Hypertelorism, an increased distance between the eyes, is seen in naso-ethmoidal fractures. An intercanthal distance >35 mm is indicative of canthal spread and >40 mm is diagnostic.

Proptosis or forward projection of the globe is an important sign, which may indicate retrobulbar haemorrhage. This is a sight threatening injury, which is potentially reversible and must not be missed. Prompt intervention is required to prevent irreversible visual loss.

Enopthalmos and ptosis are more subtle clinical signs that are difficult to see in the acute trauma case due to periorbital oedema. They are, however, important signs in the late presentation of trauma and should be noted.

A four point ophthalmic checklist is useful to prevent omission of important clinical symptoms and signs:

- *Visual acuity:* the eye must be examined and visual acuity documented. If the eye cannot be opened due to swelling then the lids should be gently opened manually. If even this is not possible, a bright light should be shone through the closed lid. Visual acuity is tested using a Snellen chart at 6 m and then at 1 m. If the patient is unable to read the chart at any distance then counting fingers, hand movement, and finally light perception are tested.
- *Pupils:* pupil size and reaction to light in both the direct and indirect reflexes are tested. Changes in pupil size may be a localizing sign in rising intracranial pressure, but mydriasis is also seen following direct trauma to the globe and in retrobulbar haemorrhage.
- *Visual fields:* ophthalmoplegia is a paralysis or weakness of one or more of the six extra-ocular muscles that control movement of the eye. The muscles are innervated by the third, fourth, and sixth cranial nerves. Nerve damage, muscle oedema, and muscle entrapment in an orbital floor or wall fracture can all cause patients to complain of diplopia. A common pattern of injury is diplopia on upward gaze with an orbital floor fracture from entrapment of the inferior rectus muscle within the fracture. Visual fields are tested by confrontation and if a problem is noted then formal testing with a Hess chart is advisable.
- *Fundoscopy:* lens dislocation and hyphaema may be seen in the anterior chamber. Retinal detachment, foreign bodies and vitreous haemorrhage may be present in the posterior chamber. Urgent ophthalmological assessment should be sought.

Retrobulbar haemorrhage

The increased pressure resulting from retrobulbar haematoma leads to occlusion of the central artery of the retina and an ischemic optic neuropathy.

There is a progressive increase in:

- Pain.
- Proptosis.
- Mydriasis.
- Ophthalmoplegia.
- Reduction in visual acuity.

Nose

Patients may complain of pain, deformity, difficulty breathing and epistaxis. The nose should be examined from the front and side for deformity. A nasal septal haematoma may cause nasal obstruction and should be specifically looked for. An untreated septal haematoma may cause necrosis of the septal cartilage and subsequent development of a saddle nose deformity. Any haematoma can be evacuated under local anaesthesia. The bridge of the nose is gently palpated between finger and thumb to detect any abnormal mobility in the nasal bones or cartilages.

Epistaxis or cerebrospinal fluid (CSF) rhinorrhoea may indicate a base of skull fracture of the cribriform plate in the anterior cranial fossa. In the supine patient lying on a trolley, the blood and CSF will pass posteriorly into the nasopharynx. Nasal intubation and the passage of nasogastric tubes should be avoided where there is an anterior skull base fracture.

Ears

Examination of the ear involves careful inspection of both the external ear and mastoid region, and otoscopy of the ear canal.

Battle's sign is bruising over the mastoid process. It is an indicator of a skull base fracture and may suggest underlying brain trauma. The pinna of the ear should be examined for a haematoma which should be aspirated under local anaesthesia. If left untreated it will lead to a 'cauliflower ear'.

CSF otorrhoea may be present with a skull base fracture and otoscopy may reveal a perforated drum or haemotympanum. Condylar fractures can lacerate the ear canal leading to bleeding from the external ear.

Facial movement and sensation

The facial nerve supplies the muscles of facial expression. The nerve exits from the skull via the stylomastoid foramen and traverses within the substance of the parotid gland within which it divides into its five terminal branches:

- *Temporal:* crosses the zygomatic arch to supply the frontalis muscle. Damage leads to forehead droop.
- *Zygomatic:* supplies the orbicularis oculi muscle, which is responsible for closing the eye sphincter. This is critical for corneal protection.
- *Buccal:* supplies the buccinator muscle and the muscles, which elevate the upper lip. Damage leads to an asymmetric smile.
- *Marginal mandibular:* emerges from the lower pole of the parotid gland and loops down into the upper neck. It supplies the lower lip depressors and damage leads to an asymmetric smile.
- *Cervical:* runs vertically downwards to supply the platysma muscle in the neck. This muscle is vestigial in humans and this nerve does not need to be repaired if damaged.

The main trunk of the facial nerve may be damaged in skull base fractures and the peripheral branches in facial lacerations and in misplaced surgical incisions. The patient should be asked to move the muscles of the upper, middle and lower thirds of the face and movements compared between sides. In order to avoid litigation, facial nerve function must be carefully documented before the administration of local anaesthetic.

The trigeminal nerve supplies sensation over the anterior face and is the motor nerve to the muscles of mastication. It has three divisions:

- *Ophthalmic:* the five terminal branches supply the skin of the upper eyelid, the forehead, and the external surface of the nose.

- *Maxillary:* the infra-orbital nerve is the continuation of the maxillary division; it emerges from the infra-orbital foramen to supply the lower eyelid cheek and upper lip.
- *Mandibular:* the three terminal branches supply the skin of the lower lip and lower cheek. It also supplies a strip of skin in front of the ear and the lower part of the temple.

Light touch sensation should be tested in the upper, middle, and lower thirds of the face and sensation compared between sides.

Lateral movements of the mandible should be tested. Fractures of the zygomatic arch may impinge on the coronoid process of the mandible leading to impaired lateral excursions. Limitation of mouth opening is seen in mandibular and midface fractures.

Mandibular fracture may cause paraesthesia or dysaesthesia of the lower lip and zygomatic fractures infra-orbital nerve paraesthesia or dysaesthesia.

Facial palpation

The orbital rims and zygomatic bones should be carefully palpated looking for surgical emphysema or bony steps. Surgical emphysema around the eyes and cheeks suggests a fracture involving the air sinuses. Bony steps at the frontozygomatic suture, infra-orbital rim, and zygomatic arch are indicative of an underlying zygomatic fracture.

The mandible should be palpated for localized tenderness, step deformities and crepitus.

Abnormal movement of the midface is a difficult clinical sign to demonstrate. The upper anterior teeth are firmly grasped between the index finger and thumb of the dominant hand, while the index finger and thumb of the non-dominant hand are used to hold the nasal bridge. Abnormal movement of the maxilla indicates a fracture at the Le Fort I, II, or III level.

Intra-oral examination

Inside the mouth, both soft and hard tissues should be inspected. Bleeding, mucosal and gingival lacerations and sublingual haematomata are soft tissue signs of possible fracture. Hard tissue signs include loose, missing, or broken teeth, abnormal jaw alignment, mobile bone segments, and displacement of the centrelines.

The occlusion or intercuspation of the teeth is an excellent indicator of fracture in the lower two-thirds of the face. The patient is asked to bite together on the back teeth and the teeth are observed as they come together. Premature contacts, steps in the occlusion and open bites are indicative of a fracture. Inability to close the anterior teeth together with premature contact of the posterior teeth is seen in bilateral condylar fractures, where there is a reduction in the posterior facial height.

The buccal mucosa should be inspected bilaterally to observe the openings of the parotid ducts, opposite the upper second molar at the level of the occlusal plane. The mucosa should be dried and the cheek firmly compressed in an anterior direction to milk saliva from the duct orifice. Clear saliva should be expressed. If there is no salivary flow or if the saliva is bloody then the duct may have been transected.

Documentation

Maxillofacial trauma often results in legal proceedings. Clear contemporaneous notes are important in the subsequent preparation of legal reports. Diagrams and clinical photographs are valuable adjuncts.

Radiographic assessment

A comprehensive clinical examination should always precede radiological evaluation of the facial skeleton. Potential airway and haemorrhagic complications must be identified and stabilized prior to transfer for diagnostic imaging. The skull has complex three-dimensional anatomy and considerable skill is required in both positioning the patient and interpreting the images in order to maximize the radiographic diagnostic yield.

Patients will present in two broad categories:
- *Unstable patients:* the minority of patients. These patients must be treated according to the principles of major trauma management. Once stable, these patients often undergo urgent CT scans of the brain and cervical spine.
- *Stable patients:* the majority of patients. Radiographic examination can be delayed until optimal conditions for imaging are achieved.

Unstable patients

If CT scans of the brain and cervical spine are requested, then consideration should be also be given to requesting fine cut CT scans of facial injuries, which can be done at the same time as they only take a few extra seconds in modern spiral CT scanners, and later return for CT scanning is often more difficult for clinical reasons. The information obtained from 2D and reconstructed 3D images is often invaluable in the management of complex facial injuries.

Stable patients

Stable patients should be imaged when they are sober and co-operative. Plain X-rays are often sufficient with CT scans normally requested following specialist review of the plain films. Suspected fractures should be imaged in two planes, preferably at right angles to one another. In pan-facial and severe facial trauma, CT scans are ordered early. For frontal sinus, orbital, and complex zygomatic trauma, CT scans are often carried out at outpatient review stage and are rarely requested acutely in the stable patient.

For descriptive purposes it is useful to divide the facial skeleton into three areas:
- *Lower third:* the mandible. These injuries require a PA mandible and an orthopantomogram. Lateral oblique views may be requested when tomography is not available.
- *Middle third:* between the occlusal plane and the superior orbital margin. This is a complex anatomical area which includes nasal, naso-ethmoid, orbitozygomatic, orbital, and maxillary fractures. Suspected fractures require occipitomental 10°, occipitomental 30°, and a lateral projection.
- *Upper third:* frontal and frontal sinus fractures. Suspected fractures require occipitofrontal and lateral projections.

The orthopantomogram (OPG) and occipitomental (OM) views are the workhorses of maxillofacial radiology and these views will be considered in greater detail.

Orthopantomogram

An OPT is a scanning dental radiograph, which includes the whole of the mandible, the maxilla, maxillary sinuses, all of the teeth and the temporomandibular joints (TMJs). Specialist equipment is required and the patient must be able to stand upright and still for 1 min, while the beam and film rotate around their head. This presents an obvious problem in the intoxicated or obtunded patient.

A common error is to regard a single OPT as an adequate film on its own to exclude a mandibular fracture. Although the beam rotates around the patient, a second view, such as a PA mandible is also required. The OPT must include both mandibular condyles.

Normal anatomical structures can sometimes be mistaken for fractures.
- Air in the oropharynx at the angle of the mandible.
- The intervertebral spaces over the mandibular symphysis, mimicking a dentoalveolar fracture.
- Calcification of the stylohyoid ligament projecting over the ascending ramus.
- The hyoid bone projecting over the posterior part of the horizontal ramus.

Occipitomental views

The OM view may be taken with standard radiographic equipment. The tube is angulated to ensure that the petrous temporal bone is not projected over the maxillary antra. Care should be taken not to rotate the head to allow for accurate comparison between the two sides. McGrigor and Campbell described four lines that allow orientation and interpretation of the OM radiograph (Fig. 18.1). A fifth line was described by Trapnell:
- *Line 1:* across the frontozygomatic suture, the superior orbital margin and the frontal sinuses.
- *Line 2:* along the zygomatic arches, zygomatic body, infra-orbital margin, and nasal bones.
- *Line 3:* across the condyles, coronoid process and the maxillary sinus.
- *Line 4:* along the mandibular ramus and the occlusal plane of the teeth.
- *Line 5:* (Trapnell's line) along the inferior border of the mandible from angle to angle.

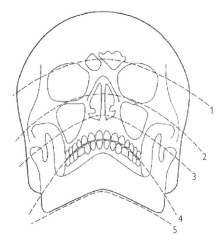

Fig. 18.1. Campbell's lines. (This image was published in Banks & Brown, *Fractures of the Facial Skeleton*, 2000, copyright Elsevier.)

Maxillofacial haemorrhage

The maxillofacial region has a rich vascular supply and even minor wounds may bleed considerably. The situation is compounded in patients taking warfarin or antiplatelet medication.

Facial lacerations

Facial aesthetics are important for the psychological well being of the patient and it is critical to achieve the optimal aesthetic result at the time of initial surgery. Brisk bleeding will often stop with local pressure, which can be applied with clean dressing gauze by the patient themselves. Lacerations around the lips may be compressed between a thumb placed in the mouth and a finger on the face. Blind application of artery forceps to lacerations should be avoided as the facial nerve or parotid duct may be damaged.

Foreign bodies, such as tooth fragments, windscreen glass and grit must be removed. If the history is suggestive of foreign body implantation, a lateral soft tissue radiograph should be taken. Minor wounds may be cleaned and sutured in the emergency department. Extensive lacerations, tissue loss, and large dirty wounds often require debridement under general anaesthetic. This is particularly important in facial abrasions where the wounds are at risk of tattooing if dirt and grit particles are not scrubbed out.

Scalp lacerations

The arteries in the scalp are surrounded by connective tissue which prevents the artery constricting if it is cut. These small arteries will continue to bleed and can lead to profuse blood loss. It is safe to use haemostatic forceps in the scalp as the facial nerve is not at risk. A tight compression bandage or large silk sutures to approximate the edges will often tamponade the bleeding. Haemostasis with bipolar diathermy is frequently necessary before wound closure. Tissue loss is unusual on the scalp. Large rotational flaps may be required to close defects because of the inelastic nature of the scalp tissues.

Nasal haemorrhage

The nose has a rich blood supply that originates from both the external and internal carotid arteries. Nasal haemorrhage following trauma is often brisk initially and it is frequently difficult to tell exactly where the bleeding is coming from. The source may range from a relatively trivial nasal fracture with minimal displacement to a pan-facial fracture with severe mid-face disruption. The haemorrhage is distressing to the conscious patient and may compromise the airway when the patient is obtunded.

Simple nasal haemorrhage may be controlled by inserting an anterior nasal pack. There are several proprietary products available, such as Merocel® nasal tampons, Rapid rhino® nasal balloons, and Epistat® nasal catheters. Ribbon gauze soaked in bismuth iodoform paraffin paste (BIPP) is a suitable alternative. Care should be taken to direct the pack along the nasal floor and caution should be exercised when packing superiorly in the nasal cavity to avoid intracranial disruption if a cribriform plate fracture is present.

Midface haemorrhage

Midface disruption often leads to significant nasal and oral haemorrhage. If the patient is intubated then the posterior pharyngeal wall and soft palate should be palpated to examine for mucosal tears and evidence of a bony fracture.

If the mid-face has been driven posteriorly then it should be disimpacted by placing two fingers inside the mouth behind the soft palate and pulling the maxilla anteriorly. This action reduces the fractures and should help stop haemorrhage. The maxilla may be unstable in this position and bilateral mouth props inserted between the upper and lower teeth will help to keep it in the correct position.

Posterior nasal haemorrhage may require the insertion of a posterior nasal pack. The Epistat® has two balloons, and is designed to provide both anterior and posterior nasal pressure. It is inserted along the nasal floor, parallel to the hard palate until the tip of the catheter is felt at the back of the soft palate. The procedure is repeated on the opposite nostril. The posterior (white) balloon is inflated with no more than 10 mL of saline. Gentle anterior traction is applied until resistance is felt and the anterior (green) balloon is filled with no more than 30 mL of saline. A 12–14G Foley catheter is an alternative method of providing posterior pressure with a BIPP pack placed anteriorly.

Occasionally haemorrhage continues despite the placement of adequate anterior and posterior nasal packs. In the intubated patient the oropharynx, nasopharynx, and mouth may be packed with ribbon gauze which applies local pressure.

Penetrating neck trauma

Diagnosis of penetrating neck trauma

Penetrating neck trauma is potentially fatal. Vascular injuries occur in 20% and aerodigestive tract injuries in 10% of cases. Initial mortality is related to exsanguinating haemorrhage, but oesophageal perforation resulting in mediastinitis can also be fatal. The phrenic nerve, brachial plexus, and cranial nerves IX–XII may all be damaged.

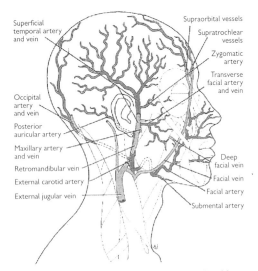

Fig. 18.2. The superficial arteries of the head. (Reproduced from Johnson & Moore *Anatomy for Dental Students*, 1997, with permission from Oxford University Press.)

External haemorrhage or expanding haematoma indicate vascular injury. Stridor, haemoptysis, hoarseness, and surgical emphysema are indicative of tracheal or laryngeal injury. Dysphagia and haematemasis indicate trauma to the digestive tract.

The sternocleidomastoid muscle divides the neck into anterior and posterior triangles. The majority of important vascular and visceral structures lie in the anterior triangle. The neck is invested in two layers of fascia, the superficial fascia, enveloping the platysma muscle, and wounds deep to this require surgical exploration in an operating theatre.

Classification of penetrating neck trauma

For descriptive purposes, the neck is divided into three zones:

- *Zone 1:* from the clavicle to the cricoid cartilage. Structures at risk are the great vessels, trachea, oesophagus, lung apices, and brachial plexus. Clinical signs may be occult. A thorough chest examination is required to exclude significant pathology, such as a pneumothorax or haemothorax.
- *Zone 2:* between the cricoid cartilage and the angle of the mandible. Injuries in this zone tend to be apparent on inspection. Important structures in this region include the carotid arteries, internal jugular vein, and laryngopharynx.
- *Zone 3:* between the angle of the mandible and the skull base. The main structures of concern in this area are the internal carotid artery, internal jugular vein, and cranial nerves. Surgical access to this zone is difficult.

Management of penetrating neck trauma

A systematic approach is required. The primary survey should identify and manage airway obstruction, breathing, and adequacy of circulation, all of which are potential problems with penetrating neck trauma. Senior surgical and anaesthetic help should be summoned immediately as loss of airway patency is a major concern and may occur suddenly. A meticulous secondary survey should identify damage to vital structures. Frequent evaluation is required because the onset of clinical signs may be delayed and their development may be progressive.

External haemorrhage should be controlled by direct pressure and blind clamping of vessels should be avoided. In the neck several cranial nerves run close to major blood vessels and these delicate structures are easily damaged. Protruding objects should not be removed and deep wounds should not be explored in the emergency department as these actions can dislodge clot or cause air embolism. Where it is difficult to control bleeding by direct pressure, a foley catheter can be inserted into the wound and inflated with saline. This manoeuvre is particularly useful in zone 1 injuries, where the catheter is inserted into the pleural cavity and can be used to compress the subclavian vessels against the first rib or clavicle.

Penetrating trauma in the oral cavity lateral to the tonsilar fossa may cause occult internal carotid artery injury. A significant bleed, which ceases spontaneously may indicate carotid injury and increased risk of subsequent carotid blow out.

Interventional radiology

Angiography is useful to evaluate stable patients with injuries, which penetrate platysma in zones 1 and 3. Four vessel angiography allows assessment of collateral circulation if carotid ligation is deemed necessary.

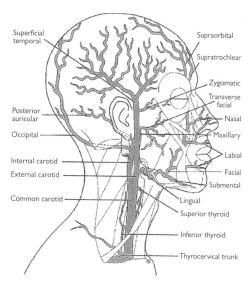

Fig. 18.3 The carotid arteries and their branches. (Reproduced from Johnson & Moore, *Anatomy for Dental Students*, 1997, with permission from Oxford University Press.)

If surgical exposure and access to bleeding vessels is difficult then selective therapeutic embolization of the damaged vessels should be considered. Care must be exercised to avoid dislodgement of clot leading to stroke or further arterial intimal damage or perforation.

Dental haemorrhage

Bleeding after dental extractions is a common emergency department presentation. In facial trauma, profuse dental haemorrhage can also occur when teeth have been loosened or avulsed. Warfarin or antiplatelet therapy may be a contributing factor. Most dental haemorrhage will stop with the application of local pressure. Congealed blood should be removed from the mouth and a thorough inspection carried out. A warm, damp saline swab should be placed in the mouth over the bleeding socket and firm pressure should be applied for 20 min, either by biting on the swab or by digital pressure. The temptation to remove the swab before this time should be resisted as this will disturb the developing clot.

If simple pressure fails to control the haemorrhage then the mucosa on either side of the socket should be infiltrated with dental local anaesthetic, which contains 1:80,000 adrenaline as a vasoconstrictor. The socket is irrigated with warm saline and packed with a resorbable haemostatic gauze, such as Surgicel®, which stabilizes the clot. The gingival margins are sutured over the socket to stabilize the haemostatic gauze and apply local pressure. Occasionally, further treatment is required, such as dental impressions to construct a thermoplastic splint, which is placed in the mouth over the teeth to apply pressure.

If bleeding is unusually brisk then a FBC, LFTs, and coagulation screen should be requested. Undiagnosed haemophiliacs and new cases of leukaemia can present with prolonged dental haemorrhage.

Tranexamic acid (an antifibrinolytic agent) mouthwash helps clot stabilization in warfarinized patients. The effects of warfarin can be reversed by giving coagulation factors or vitamin K.

Maxillofacial fractures

Skull anatomy

The skull can be divided into two main regions, the neurocranium, and the viscerocranium (Figs 18.4a,b). The neurocranium is the region of the skull that surrounds the brain and it is further subdivided into the cranial vault—the portion of the skull that overlies the brain—and the cranial base, the portion, which underlies the brain. The neurocranium consists of eight bones:

- Frontal.
- Occipital.
- Sphenoid.
- Ethmoid.
- Temporal (2).
- Parietal(2).

The viscerocranium is the region of the skull that makes up the bones of the face. The viscerocranium consists of fourteen bones:

- Maxilla (2).
- Zygoma (2).
- Nasal (2).
- Palatine (2).
- Lacrimal (2).

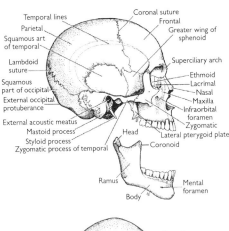

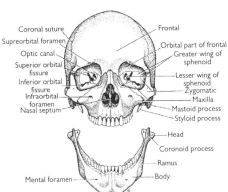

Fig. 18.4 (a,b) Bony anatomy of the skull. (Reproduced from Johnson & Moore, *Anatomy for Dental Students*, 1997, with permission from Oxford University Press.)

- Inferior nasal concha (2).
- Vomer.
- Mandible.

The clinician needs to be familiar with the normal anatomy of the facial skeleton in order to understand the types of disruption, which occur in the trauma patient.

Mandibular fractures

Diagnosis of mandibular fractures

Mandibular fractures are second only to nasal fractures in frequency of occurrence in facial trauma. The key for diagnosis and treatment is the occlusion of the teeth. Conscious patients should be asked whether or not their teeth meet in the correct position for them. A disrupted occlusion may occur with missing teeth, fractures, dislocations, and temporomandibular joint haemarthrosis. Gaps between teeth or a step in the occlusion are simple clinical signs, but more subtle signs of a fracture are a sublingual haematoma or gingival bruising or tears.

Opening of the teeth at the front of the mouth with posterior tooth contact is seen in bilateral condylar neck fractures. Bleeding from the external ear is commonly seen in condylar fractures which tear the ear canal.

A fracture involving the mandibular canal, which transmits the inferior alveolar nerve often results in paraesthesia or dysaesthesia of the ipsilateral lower lip and chin. Soft tissue ecchymosis and lacerations indicate a potential underlying bony problem. Palpation of the mandible may reveal bony steps and abnormal mobility of fracture segments.

Classification of mandibular fractures

The mandible behaves like a complete ring when it is injured. If one fracture is located then a second fracture should be sought, as one will be present in 52% of cases. An anatomical system is commonly used to describe mandibular fracture patterns:

- *Dentoalveolar 1%:* a fracture related to the tooth bearing portion of the mandible with no disruption to the remaining bone.
- *Symphysis 3%:* a vertical fracture in the incisor region between the alveolar process and the lower border.
- *Parasymphysis 17%:* a vertical fracture between the lateral incisor and the mental foramen, which extends between the alveolar process and the lower border.
- *Body 21%:* a fracture between the mental foramen and the distal aspect of the second molar, which extends between the alveolar process and the lower border.
- *Angle 36%:* a fracture between the distal aspect of the second molar and the junction of the ramus and body of the mandible, which extends between the alveolar process and the lower border.
- *Ramus 2%:* a horizontal fracture that passes between the anterior and posterior borders of the ramus or a vertical fracture from the sigmoid notch to the lower border.
- *Condylar 18%:* a fracture that runs from the sigmoid notch to the posterior border of the mandible.
- *Coronoid 2%:* a fracture that runs from the sigmoid notch to the anterior border of the mandible.

Common fracture patterns are parasymphysis and contralateral angle, parasymphysis, and contralateral condyle, and bilateral condyle and symphysis.

Radiology of mandibular fractures

The two standard views for a suspected mandibular fracture are an orthopantomogram (Fig. 18.5) and PA mandible (Fig. 18.6).

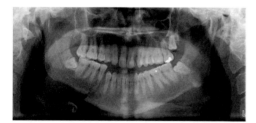

Fig. 18.5. OPG of mandibular fracture showing displacement of a right body fracture, but not showing displacement at the left angle fracture.

If patient is unable to stand for an orthopantomogram then right and left lateral oblique films give good views of the mandibular body and angle. Occasionally, a poor view of the condyle is obtained in the PA mandible film, as the mastoid process can overly the condylar neck (Fig. 18.6). A reverse Towne's projection angulates the skull to move the mastoid away from the condyle allowing better visualization. A lower occlusal projection is useful for suspected symphyseal fractures.

Zygomatic fractures

Diagnosis of zygomatic fractures

The zygoma or malar bone is commonly fractured with a lateral blow to the cheek. The zygoma articulates with the frontal, temporal, sphenoid, and maxillary bones. When it is fractured these articulations are disrupted.

The zygomatic arch may also fracture independently. Soft tissue swelling and bruising often mask the underlying bony deformity, which is much more apparent at review a few days later when the swelling has subsided. Bony tenderness at the zygomaticofrontal (ZF) suture and infra-orbital rim, and a subconjunctival haemorrhage with no posterior border are often evident. Tenderness intra-orally in the buccal sulcus in the zygomatic buttress region may be present. A step is frequently palpable on the infra-orbital margin. Infra-orbital nerve paraesthesia or dysaesthesia may be present. Markedly displaced fractures may interfere with mouth opening because the displaced zygoma impinges on the mandible. Associated mandibular coronoid process fracture may also be present. A full ophthalmic examination is essential.

Classification of zygomatic fractures

Several classifications have been proposed. The Henderson classification is clinically relevant and descriptive:

- **Type I**: undisplaced.
- **Type II**: arch fracture.
- **Type III**: tripod fracture, ZF suture undisplaced.
- **Type IV**: tripod fracture, ZF suture distracted.
- **Type V**: pure orbital blow-out facture.
- **Type VI**: isolated orbital rim fracture.
- **Type VII**: comminuted fracture.

Radiology of zygomatic fractures

- Occipitomental 10 degrees.
- Occipitomental 30 degrees (Fig. 18.7).
- Submentovertex for arch fractures.

The four key areas to be examined on the occipitomental views are the ZF suture, the infra-orbital rim, the junction of the body, and arch and the zygomatic buttress. In acute radiographs a fluid level of blood will be present in the maxillary antrum.

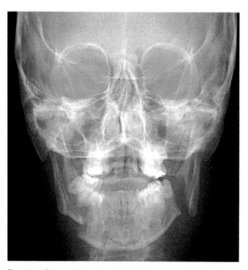

Fig. 18.6. PA mandible of mandibular fracture reveals the gross displacement of the left angle fracture

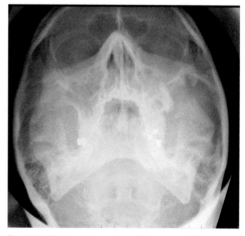

Fig. 18.7. OM view of a comminuted left zygomatic fracture.

Orbital fractures

Diagnosis of orbital fractures

The bony orbit is a four-sided pyramid composed of seven bones. The orbital floor and medial wall are the two areas where fractures commonly occur. The lateral wall and roof have thicker bony walls, and fracture of these areas requires significantly more force. The orbital floor is formed by the orbital plate of the maxilla, the orbital surface of zygoma, and the orbital process of the palatine bone at the orbital apex. The medial wall is formed by the frontal process of maxilla, the lacrimal bone, the orbital plate of the ethmoid, and the body of the sphenoid posteriorly. Orbital fat may become trapped in a fracture line leading to muscle restriction and diplopia. Injury of the infra-orbital nerve in the orbital floor leads to numbness of the cheek and side of the nose on the injured side.

A comprehensive ophthalmic examination is essential. It is vital to determine that the visual pathway is intact. The periorbital tissues are often grossly swollen and it can be difficult to open the eyelids to examine the pupil. A bright light may be shone through the lids to confirm the perception of light. Visual loss immediately following trauma has a poor prognosis for recovery, but evolving visual loss may be indicative of a retrobulbar haemorrhage and is potentially treatable.

After the acute swelling has subsided, patients may present complaining of diplopia or of a staring appearance of the eye due to enopthalmos. A Hess chart is a valuable tool in formally assessing diplopia.

Classification of orbital fractures

Pure orbital floor fractures are classified as Henderson type V zygomatic fractures. They are also seen in combination with other zygomatic and maxillary fractures.

Radiology of orbital fractures

- Occipitomental 10 degrees.
- Occipitomental 30 degrees.
- Fine cut orbital CT with coronal reformatting (Fig. 18.8).

The bony buttresses are often intact with orbital blow out fractures. A hanging teardrop of fat may be seen in some orbital floor fractures on occipitomental views. In acute radiographs a fluid level of blood will be present in the antrum.

Maxillary fractures

Diagnosis of maxillary fractures

Maxillary fractures are usually the result of high energy trauma. Patients present with typical bilateral periorbital bruising and gross facial swelling. The occlusion is disrupted and typically there is an anterior open bite with only contact of the molar teeth. A palatal mucosal tear or bruising may indicate a split palate. Assessment of the occlusion is more difficult if there is an associated mandibular fracture.

It is important to look for clinical signs of an associated skull base fracture, namely bruising over the mastoid process, CSF rhinorrhoea, and CSF otorrhoea. The maxilla may be mobile with low level fractures, but higher fractures are often impacted and immobile. Haemorrhage and airway problems are an immediate concern.

Classification of maxillary fractures

The Le Fort classification is well described. Fractures may not be symmetrical and different level Le Fort fractures may be present on each side of the face. There may also be associated zygomatic and orbital fractures.

- *Le Fort I:* horizontal fracture (Fig. 18.9a). The tooth bearing portion of the maxilla separates from the remainder of the midface. The fracture passes low in the nasal septum to the piriform aperture, crosses the lateral maxilla above the tooth apices and crosses the lower one third of the pterygoid plates.
- *Le Fort II:* pyramidal fracture (Fig. 18.9b). The fracture extends from the nasal bridge at or below the frontonasal suture and runs through the frontal process of the maxilla, lacrimal bones, and medial orbital floor. It crosses the orbital rim above the infra-orbital nerve and runs inferoposteriorly below the body of the zygoma to separate the middle third of the pterygoid plates. The fracture may involve the anterior cribriform plate and be associated with a CSF leak.
- *Le Fort III:* craniofacial separation (Fig. 18.9c). The fracture runs through the frontonasal and frontomaxillary sutures into the medial orbital wall below the optic canal. The fracture extends through the inferior orbital fissure and crosses the lateral orbital wall through the zygomaticofrontal suture and zygomatic arch. Posteriorly, the fracture separates the base of the pterygoid plates. The entire facial skeleton is therefore separated from the skull base.

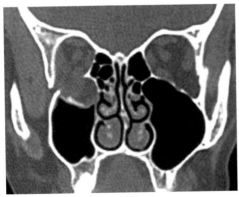

Fig. 18.8. Coronal CT scan of a right orbital floor blowout.

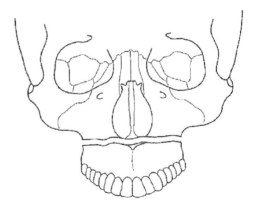

Figure 18.9(a) Le Fort I.

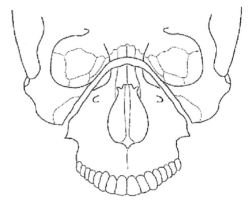

Fig. 18.9(b) Le Fort II.

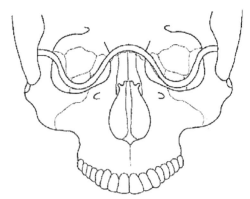

Fig. 18.9(c) Le Fort III.

Radiology of maxillary fractures
• Occipitomental 10 degrees.
• Occipitomental 30 degrees.
• Lateral projection.

The above films are useful screening tools. Fine cut CT scans of the facial bones should be obtained to allow accurate assessment of the fracture pattern to allow planning for definitive surgery.

Nasal fractures
Diagnosis of nasal fractures
The nasal bones are the most commonly fractured bones of the facial skeleton. The usual mechanism of injury is a lateral force which fractures both the nasal bones and the frontal process of the maxilla. The nasal septum is often deviated in the same direction as the bones. A frontal blow may cause telescoping of the nasal bones and septum and often results in a more complex fracture pattern. Swelling, bruising, epistaxis and nasal deviation are often present. A careful intranasal examination should be carried out to exclude the presence of a septal haematoma, which requires immediate evacuation to prevent septal necrosis and the subsequent development of a saddle deformity. In the management of midface fractures, nasal bone fractures are commonly overlooked.

Clinicians should have a high index of suspicion of nasal bone fracture in all midface injuries. Deviation of the nasal bones is best detected visually by standing behind the seated patient with their head tilted back. It is important to ascertain if the patient has a previous healed fracture of the nose. All new fractures will be tender on palpation and crepitus may be felt.

Classification of nasal fractures
• *Type I:* simple unilateral.
• *Type II:* simple bilateral.
• *Type III:* comminuted, unilateral, bilateral, or frontal.
• *Type IV:* nasal fracture and septal dislocation.

Radiology of nasal fractures
Plain radiographs such as a lateral view of the nasal bones add little to the information gleaned from a thorough clinical examination, and are not recommended.

Naso-ethmoid fractures
Diagnosis of naso-ethmoid fractures
The ethmoid bone is a single midline structure at the superior aspect of the nasal cavity. It has projections that extend into the nasal cavity, orbits, and cranium. The perpendicular plate forms part of the bony nasal septum, while the orbital plate is the major contributor to the medial orbital wall. The cribriform plate separates the anterior cranial fossa from the nasal cavity. Naso-ethmoid fractures range in severity from minimally displaced fractures where no active treatment is required to severely displaced fractures with CSF leaks and orbital sequelae.

The nasal bones telescope into the ethmoids and the bridge of the nose is impacted leading to a characteristic turning up of the nasal tip. There is a widening of the intercanthal distance and periorbital oedema and bruising are present. An intercanthal distance >35 mm is indicative of canthal spread and >40 mm is diagnostic of telecanthus. The medial canthal tendon may be avulsed from the medial wall of the orbit and diplopia may be present. Bony fragments may impinge on both the frontonasal duct which drains the frontal sinus and the lacrimal sac which drains tears. A full ophthalmic examination is essential.

Classification of naso-ethmoidal fractures
A useful clinical classification relates the size of bone fragment attached to the medial canthal tendon (MCT)
• *Type I:* MCT attached to a single large bone fragment.
• *Type II:* MCT attached to a smaller comminuted fragment of bone.
• *Type III:* MCT avulsed with gross comminution.

Radiology of naso-ethmoidal fractures
• Occipitomental 10 degrees.
• Occipitomental 30 degrees.
• Lateral projection.

The above films are useful screening tools. Fine cut CT scans of the facial bones should be obtained to allow accurate assessment of the fracture pattern to allow planning for definitive surgery.

Frontal sinus fractures
Diagnosis of frontal sinus fractures
The frontal sinuses develop throughout adolescence. The anterior table normally ranges from 4–12 mm in thickness and the posterior table 0.1–4.8 mm. Considerable force is required to fracture the frontal sinus. Patients present with

bruising, periorbital ecchymosis, subconjunctival haemor-rhage, CSF rhinorrhoea, and eye signs. A full ophthalmic examination is essential.

Classification of frontal sinus fractures

Central fractures (types I and II) involve the skull base adjacent to the paranasal sinuses, while lateral fractures involve the frontal bone and orbital roof:

- *Type I:* cribriform fracture.
- *Type II:* fronto-ethmoid fracture.
- *Type III:* lateral fracture.
- *Type IV:* complex.

Radiology of frontal sinus fractures

- Occipitofrontal.
- Lateral projection.
- Fine cut sinus CT with coronal reformatting.

Fractures of the anterior table are an aesthetic issue, but posterior table fractures may result in a dural tear. The degree of displacement of the posterior wall of the frontal sinus is a critical feature to note. Fracture displacement greater than the thickness of the bone is a strong indicator of associated dural tear and a neurosurgical opinion should be sought regarding a craniofacial repair. Damage to the frontonasal duct may lead to later problems with sinus drainage.

Displaced anterior table fractures without frontonasal duct involvement are treated with simple plating. Where the frontonasal duct is involved the sinus is treated by stripping of the lining mucosa and obliteration with bone or a bone substitute. Treatment of displaced posterior table fractures involves removal of the posterior table bone, obliteration of the frontonasal ducts, dural repair and cranialization of the frontal sinus.

Management of soft tissue injury

The rich blood supply to the head and neck results in wounds that bleed profusely. However, head and neck wounds also heal faster and tissue can survive on a very narrow pedicle which would almost certainly fail in other anatomical areas.

Type of anaesthesia

The majority of lacerations are small enough to be dealt with under local anaesthesia. This has the advantage of speed of treatment and convenience for the patient. The disadvantages of local anaesthetic are pain during the injection and distortion of the tissues making accurate alignment more difficult. Regional nerve blocks to the inferior dental and infra-orbital nerves can be helpful in preventing wound distortion.

Large lacerations require more anaesthetic and care must be taken not to exceed the maximum recommended dose. Dental local anaesthetic cartridges contain 2.2 mL of 2% lidocaine with 1/80,000 adrenaline. The maximum dosage is 7 mg/kg, which equates to 11 cartridges in a 70 kg adult. Warmed local anaesthetic should be infiltrated slowly into the tissues through the existing wound edges. Regional nerve blocks allow a large area of tissue to be anaesthetized with a small volume.

Wound cleansing

Thorough cleansing removes foreign bodies and reduces bacterial numbers. Wound cleansing should be carried out with a solution, which does not cause further tissue damage such as 5% aqueous betadine solution. A surgical scrubbing brush is ideal to remove dirt and grit. If left in a wound, dirt and grit will cause unsightly tattooing, which is difficult to treat as a secondary procedure. Outdoor injuries may have dirt and debris under the wound edges. If not removed this will lead to abscess formation and early wound breakdown. The requirement to explore and scrub a large area may necessitate the patient having a general anaesthetic.

A careful history will guide the clinician when exploring and cleansing a wound. Car crash victims may have embedded glass, which is best located by gentle probing within the wound. Chipped teeth and broken porcelain crowns can embed within the lips. A lateral soft tissue radiograph should be taken if there is a suspicion of a glass, ceramic or metallic foreign body.

Dog bites need to be cleansed along the entire length of the puncture wound. Young children are often bitten around the mouth by dogs and there may be a puncture wound, which extends all the way through the lip. The tract should be irrigated by using a blunt needle placed on a syringe prior to scrubbing the entry and exit wounds. In contrast to bites on other anatomical areas, it is acceptable and often necessary to clean and close facial bites.

Wound closure

Meticulous attention to detail is required in order to obtain the best possible results. Scar revision is always a compromise and optimal results are obtained following good primary surgery.

Tissue preservation

Tissue of dubious viability should be preserved and given the benefit of the doubt. Skin loss is uncommon and missing skin is often to be found rolled up at the edges of a wound. This skin can be unrolled over the wound and will adhere and survive much like a skin graft over the rich vascular bed.

Accurate anatomical alignment

Care must be taken to correctly align disrupted facial structures. Eyebrows, eyelids, helical rims, nostrils, and the vermillion border of the lips are critical areas where a discrepancy in tissue alignment is easily noticed.

Layered wound closure

Tension free skin closure provides optimal conditions for epithelial repair. This is achieved by approximating the deeper layers sequentially with 3-0 or 4-0 undyed vicryl sutures. Lacerations involving muscle such as full-thickness lip lacerations require the muscle layer to be repaired to restore the function of the oral sphincter.

Fine sutures and early suture removal

5-0 or 6-0 monofilament sutures should be used. Excessive tension on the final skin sutures leads to tissue necrosis and visible suture track marks. Sutures can be removed at 5–7 days and the wounds supported by tissue glue or steri-strips.

Post-operative care

The routine use of antibiotics for simple lacerations has no proven benefit. They are of use, however, in grossly contaminated wounds such as dog bites. Suture lines should be kept clean and moist with either plain petroleum jelly or antibiotic ointment, such as chloramphenicol.

After suture removal wounds should be gently massaged with moisturizing cream and protected from bright sunlight for at least 6 months. Silicon sheets and gel may be of use in the prevention of hypertrophic scar formation.

Facial nerve injuries

There is no requirement to repair injuries to the facial nerve anterior to a vertical line dropped from the lateral canthus of the eye. The facial muscles are innervated by nerve branches that enter the muscles more proximally and permanent weakness is unlikely. If the nerve is transected posteriorly to this perpendicular line then repair by a specialist using an operating microscope is indicated within the first 24 h following injury.

Parotid duct injuries

The parotid duct runs parallel to the buccal branch of the facial nerve. It is 4–5 mm in diameter and repair is possible with operating loupes. Early referral to a specialist is advised.

Retrobulbar haemorrhage

Prompt diagnosis and treatment are required to prevent visual loss. Once the diagnosis is made treatment should be instigated and time should not be wasted awaiting confirmatory tests such as a CT scan. Treatment involves both medical and surgical management to reduce intra-ocular pressure (IOP).

Medical management

- *Mannitol:* reduces elevated IOP by direct osmosis of water. Dose: 1–2 g/kg (5.0–10.0 mL/kg) of 20% solution IV over 30–60 min. The patient should be catheterized and urine output measured.

- *Acetazolamide:* inhibits enzyme carbonic anhydrase, reducing rate of aqueous humour formation, which in turn reduces IOP. Dose: 500 mg IV bolus followed by 125–250 mg IV 4–6 h.
- *Methylprednisolone:* reverses increased capillary permeability. *Dose:* 1 g/day IV as a single dose. Many other regimes have been described in the literature.
- *Timolol drops:* may reduce elevated and normal IOP by reducing the production of aqueous humour. *Dose:* 1–2 drops of 0.25–0.5% solution in affected eye bd.

Surgical management

The immediate surgical management involves a lateral canthotomy and inferior cantholysis, which can be carried out under local anaesthesia. This releases the lateral attachment of the eyelid and allows the tense globe to move anteriorly reducing retrobulbar pressure. It is a temporizing measure, which gains time prior to definitive surgical treatment.

An artery clip is inserted between the upper and lower eyelids at the lateral canthus and closed to crush the tissues. This helps with haemostasis and disperses tissue oedema, which distorts local anatomy. The canthotomy is carried out with sharp scissors and allows exposure of the Y-shaped lateral canthal tendon. The inferior cru is cut which mobilizes the lower eyelid.

Prompt surgical referral for definitive treatment of the retrobulbar haemorrhage is indicated, along with continuing medical management. There may be a window of opportunity to obtain a CT scan, while awaiting surgical review.

Dislocated mandibular condyle

The TMJ is a synovial joint with an interposing cartilaginous disc. Simple dislocation normally occurs in an anterior direction. If a condylar fracture is present, more complex dislocations may occur. Patients present with an inability to close their teeth together. Dislocation may be unilateral or bilateral.

The mandible may be reduced in the emergency department (with analgesia and sedation if necessary). Local anaesthetic can be injected around the joint capsule. Reduction of the condyle requires firm downward pressure in the molar region of the mandible, while rotating the chin region upwards. The condyle is felt to slip into place and a normal occlusion is noted. A simple bandage should be applied to prevent further dislocation until muscle tone returns.

Fracture management

Some maxillofacial fractures require immediate hospital admission and treatment, while more simple injuries can be reviewed at outpatient visit. It is important to know what the local treatment protocols are in the unit to which you are referring. Significant facial fractures require a considerable force and admission for head injury observations should always be considered.

Typical admission guidelines

- *Mandibular fractures:* fractures are painful and eating is difficult. Patients require admission for surgical management. The incidence of post-operative complications, such as infection and non-union is much less if the fracture is treated within 24 h of injury.
- *Zygomatic fractures:* a retrobulbar haemorrhage must be excluded. If there are no other injuries then the patient can be seen after 5–7 days when soft tissue swelling has subsided. Some units advocate immediate admission for treatment.
- *Nasal fractures:* a septal haematoma must be excluded. Nasal packing may be required for haemorrhage. If there are no other injuries then review after 5–7 days should be arranged.
- *Naso-ethmoidal and frontal maxillary fractures:* admission for observation and specialist review.
- *Frontal and frontal sinus fractures:* admission for observation and specialist review.
- *Pan-facial fractures:* admission for observation and specialist review.

If there is any doubt regarding the severity of the injury then caution should be exercised, hospital admission arranged, and a specialist opinion requested.

Principles of fracture management

Facial fracture management follows the same general principles of fracture management in other anatomical areas:

- Reduction.
- Fixation.
- Immobilization.
- Restoration of function.

Historically, fracture management was described as either operative or conservative. This description leads to confusion, and it is better to describe treatment as either open or closed. Undisplaced or minimally displaced fractures may not require active treatment and can be kept under close observation.

Closed reduction involved manipulation of the bones without exposure of the fracture. Open reduction involves direct visualization of the fracture. The fracture is exposed via carefully placed incisions in the mouth, skin, or a suitable skin laceration. This allows an anatomical reduction of the fracture and fixation with titanium mini-plates.

Mandibular, nasal, and zygomatic fractures are relatively common and will be discussed in detail. Complex upper and midface trauma is relatively rare, and is treated according to the same general principles.

Mandibular fractures

Treatment of mandibular fractures varies according to the severity of the fracture, the occlusion of the teeth, and the medical history of the patient.

Undisplaced fractures

Compliant patients with undisplaced fractures of a favourable pattern and no derangement of the occlusion can be managed with analgesics, soft diet, and regular clinical review. They must avoid heavy physical activity as further minor trauma may cause the fracture to displace. If there are fractures through the tooth-bearing portion of the mandible, then the fractures open into the mouth and antibiotic prophylaxis is indicated.

Displaced fractures

Displaced fractures are painful when the patient moves the mandible. Immediate pain relief can be achieved by local anaesthetic infiltration around the fracture or by an inferior dental block. A wire loop placed around the teeth adjacent to a fracture and gently tightened will reduce and immobilize the fracture temporarily and help with pain control.

Correct post-operative occlusion of the teeth is of fundamental importance in facial fractures. Several methods of holding the teeth together are available. This is termed inter-maxillary fixation (IMF). Arch-bars, wire loops, screws, circumferential wires, and brackets bonded to teeth can all be used to hold the teeth in the correct position. In patients with no teeth, their dentures can be wired or screwed to the maxilla and mandible to act as splints (Gunning splints).

Fractures immobilized in this way will usually heal in 3–6 weeks depending on the age and nutritional state of the patient. The disadvantages of this method of treatment are weight loss, poor oral hygiene, damage to the teeth and supporting structures, and poor patient tolerance. It is contraindicated in patients with airway disease, reduced mental capacity, epilepsy, and psychiatric disease.

Open reduction and internal fixation (ORIF) is much more acceptable to patients as it allows them to open their mouths and eat a normal, but soft diet. The occlusion is maintained in IMF temporarily and the fracture sites are exposed. Titanium mini-plates are used to hold the bone fragments in the correct alignment and the IMF is released. In general, the more displaced, comminuted or unfavourable the fracture, the more rigid (thicker) the titanium plate needs to be. Surgical access to condylar fractures is often difficult and there is a risk of a traction injury to the facial nerve. Bilateral condylar fractures are often treated with ORIF to the accessible fracture combined with elastic IMF to the treat the other condylar fracture.

Clear instructions regarding soft diet, jaw exercises, dental hygiene and regular clinical review are given prior to discharge. Patients should be followed up at 1–2 weekly intervals for 6–8 weeks to ensure adequate healing. Arch bars are subsequently removed. Titanium mini-plates are only removed if they become infected or cause problems.

Nasal fractures

Nasal haemorrhage and septal haematomata are dealt with acutely. Manipulation of the nasal bones can be carried out immediately under local anaesthesia, but it is more usual to review patients after 5–7 days. Any history of previous trauma must be ascertained and documented.

Simple cases can be manipulated by hand, care must be taken when instruments are used to manipulate the nasal bones and septum as it is easy to precipitate brisk nasal haemorrhage. The nose may be packed with ribbon gauze for 24–48 h, and a thermoplastic splint or plaster bolster placed over the bones for protection for 10 days.

More complex cases and cases where presentation is delayed, often require open reduction.

Zygomatic fractures

If there are no eye signs that may indicate a retrobulbar haemorrhage, patients with isolated zygomatic complex or arch fractures can be assessed after 5–7 days. They should be advised to avoid nose blowing because of the risk of periorbital surgical emphysema, which can progress to cellulitis. A previous history of trauma and deformity must be ascertained. Undisplaced or minimally displaced stable fractures do not require reduction and fixation. The indications for elevating a fractured zygoma are:
• Displaced fracture visible on radiograph.
• Facial deformity.

• Limitation of mandibular movement.
• Ophthalmic considerations.
• Infra-orbital nerve paraesthesias.

There is a small chance of unexplained visual loss after zygomatic elevation, so blindness in the contralateral eye is an absolute contraindication to treatment.

Several approaches are described for the elevation of zygomatic fractures. Gillies' temporal approach, intra-oral elevation, and percutaneous hook elevation are in common use. If the elevated zygoma is stable then no fixation is required. Unstable zygomatic complex fractures are fixed with a mini-plates placed at the zygomatic buttress, zygomaticofrontal suture or infra-orbital rim. Zygomatic arch fractures are usually unstable after simple elevation.

Elevation of a zygomatic fracture may precipitate a retrobulbar haemorrhage. Regular post-operative eye observations are mandatory.

Dentoalveolar trauma

Dentoalveolar trauma is common in childhood. The upper anterior teeth are most frequently injured. It is twice as common in boys.

Mechanisms
The majority of primary teeth injuries occur when the child is aged between 2 and 4 due to falls when co-ordination and judgment are still developing. Injuries to the permanent dentition occur most frequently at ages 7–10 due to falls, collisions, and bicycle accidents. In teenagers, dentoalveolar trauma is most commonly seen in contact sports such as rugby and soccer. Assaults and road traffic accidents, frequently associated with alcohol, are the main causes in older teenagers and young adults.

People with protruding upper incisors are more at risk of dentoalveolar trauma to these teeth.

Dental anatomy
A basic knowledge on dental anatomy is required in order to understand the management of dental trauma. A tooth is a layered structure:
- *Enamel:* hard outer layer of the crown of the tooth. It has no nerve supply.
- *Dentine:* makes up the body of the tooth. Microscopic tubules communicate with the pulp or nerve of the tooth making it sensate.
- *Cementum:* covers the root surface of the tooth. It binds the periodontal ligament to the root surface.
- *Pulp:* the nerve and blood supply of the tooth. It enters the tooth at the apex of the root.
- *Periodontal ligament:* orientated collagen fibres that attach the tooth to the alveolar bone.
- *Alveolar bone:* the bone that surrounds the roots of the teeth. When teeth are extracted this bone is slowly resorbed.

One-third of the tooth is visible in the mouth as the crown of the tooth, while two-thirds of the root anchors the tooth in the alveolar bone.

History and examination
The degree of force indicates the likelihood of damage to the teeth and underlying structure. The timescale between injury and presentation is important for deciding whether subluxed or avulsed teeth can be replanted. The patient's occlusion should be assessed and any tooth displacement, fractured crowns, or fractures of the tooth enamel recorded. All teeth and tooth fragments need to be accounted for. Inhalation of teeth and tooth fragments may occur and a chest X-ray should be considered. Lip lacerations may contain fragments of teeth, therefore, a thorough exploration should be undertaken. The mobility of the teeth should be assessed both vertically and horizontally, and the vitality of the teeth measured and recorded.

Periapical, occlusal, and panoramic radiographs can be taken to assess for root fracture, displacement, and alveolar process fracture. Photographic records are also useful.

Management of the primary dentition
There are 20 primary teeth which erupt between the ages of 6 and 24 months. The tooth germ of the permanent incisor tooth develops in the palate above the root apex of the primary tooth. Treatment of the primary dentition must not compromise the development of the permanent tooth germ. Parents should be warned to keep all traumatized teeth under close observation and to contact their dentist for regular review. All trauma to primary teeth may lead to loss of pulp vitality and an abscess may develop, which may damage the developing permanent tooth germ.
- *Enamel fracture:* the rough edges are smoothed to prevent trauma to the soft tissues.
- *Dentine fracture:* exposed dentine is sensitive; with good co-operation a protective dressing can be placed.
- *Exposed pulp:* pulpal exposure is visible by a small amount of bleeding from the tooth. Removal of the pulp and dressing is possible with good co-operation. This is seldom possible and extraction of the tooth should be considered.
- *Crown and root fracture:* fractures passing below the gingival margin will expose the pulp. Restoration is unrealistic and the tooth is best extracted.
- *Root fracture:* non-mobile teeth with undisplaced fractures can be monitored by a dentist for loss of vitality. Mobile teeth should be extracted. Any small apical fragment remaining *in situ* after removal of the tooth can be left to resorb with eruption of the permanent tooth.
- *Subluxation:* the tooth is mobile, although not displaced. Minimally mobile teeth are left in place and should be monitored by a dentist. Grossly mobile teeth may represent an airway hazard and can often be removed by finger extraction.
- *Lateral luxation:* palatal displacement of the crown often interferes with the occlusion. Labial displacement of the crown implies palatal displacement of the root and possible disruption of the permanent tooth germ. Extraction of the tooth should be considered.
- *Intrusion:* radiographs should be taken to determine the position of the root of the impacted tooth. Palatal root impaction may damage the permanent tooth and should be extracted. Labial impaction away from the developing tooth germ may be monitored and the tooth may subsequently erupt.
- *Dentoalveolar trauma:* the supporting bone in young children usually heals without the need for splinting of teeth.
- *Avulsion:* primary teeth should not be replanted due to the risk of infection and damage to the permanent tooth.

In all cases of trauma to the primary dentition parents must be warned of possible damage to the developing permanent teeth. Complications of primary tooth trauma include pulpal necrosis and pulpal obliteration. In either condition, if periapical inflammation occurs the teeth should be extracted to prevent damage to the developing permanent tooth. Trauma before 3 years of age disrupts the developing crown of the tooth, which may be hypoplastic. After this age, the developing root is disrupted and eruption may be delayed.

Management of the permanent dentition
There are 32 permanent teeth which erupt between the ages of 6 and 24 years, when the wisdom teeth erupt. The root of the central incisors takes approximately 3 years to fully form after eruption of the crown and the apex of the root remains open with a wider than normal diameter until this time.

Initial treatment of traumatized permanent teeth involves covering exposed dentine with an adhesive restoration, treating exposed pulpal tissue, maintaining tooth vitality, reduction, and immobilization of displaced teeth, and antibiotic and tetanus prophylaxis.

Definitive treatment involves stimulation of root end closure in immature teeth, root canal treatment of mature teeth, final restoration of coronal damage, and long-term monitoring.

The implications of tooth loss are a permanent gap, which will require expensive implants or crown and bridgework to correct. Many of the treatment interventions require specialist dental equipment, which is not readily available in the emergency department.

- *Enamel fracture:* the patient should consult a dentist and the tooth can be restored with a composite resin. The rough edges may be smoothed to prevent trauma to the soft tissues.

- *Dentine fracture:* exposed dentine is sensitive and should be covered with a dressing. A dentist can then place a composite resin restoration.

- *Exposed pulp:* the pulp will become necrotic if prompt treatment is not instigated. Ideally, treatment should be carried out by a dentist. Root canal treatment (RCT) is required. If the root apex is closed, the nerve is removed and a permanent RCT is placed. With an open apex either a partial pulpotomy or filling with calcium hydroxide is required in order to allow apex closure. In the emergency department, the exposed pulp should be dressed and the patient referred to a dentist immediately.

- *Crown and root fracture:* RCT is required if the pulp is involved. Restoration is difficult as the margin is below the gingival level. Orthodontic extrusion or gingival surgery is required to obtain a suitable margin.

- *Root fracture:* root fractures often occur around the middle of the root. The coronal tooth fragment should be reduced if luxated, and splinted for 2–3 weeks. Teeth with fractures in the apical third of the root are often firm and may not require splinting. The crown of the tooth should be splinted to the adjacent teeth.

- *Subluxation:* if swelling within the periodontal ligament extrudes the tooth from the socket it is the first point of occlusal contact. A minor occlusal adjustment helps with pain control and will allow periodontal swelling to subside. Splinting is required for 2–3 weeks if mobility is significant.

- *Lateral or intrusive luxation:* local anaesthetic should be infiltrated and the tooth manipulated back into the socket with firm finger pressure. Dental forceps may be required to move deeply intruded teeth. Splinting and soft diet are required for 2–3 weeks. Antibiotics and chlorhexidine mouthwash are also advisable.

- *Dentoalveolar trauma:* where alveolar fractures occur with or without tooth injury, these fractures should be reduced and rigidly splinted for 3–4 weeks if not fully stable. Splints with wire and adhesive material attached to the fracture segment teeth and adjacent stable teeth on either side may be used to stabilize the fracture. Mini-plates or IMF screws may be used to stabilize the fracture.

- *Avulsion:* avulsed teeth should be placed back in the socket as soon as possible. External resorption of the tooth may occur, but alveolar bone height and width are maintained, and this facilitates later implant placement. Viable periodontal ligament cells on the root surface are the key to success. Mature teeth with a dry storage time greater than 1 h will not have any remaining viable cells. The time beyond which success is minimal varies according to the storage medium used to transport the tooth.

Immediate first aid of the avulsed tooth

The ideal place to store a tooth is back in the socket. The tooth should be picked up by the crown, rinsed under cold water, and placed in the socket. The patient should bite on a handkerchief to keep the tooth in the socket and proceed to definitive treatment.

Milk, contact lens solution and proprietary solutions are also suitable transport media.

Tooth splinting

Avulsed permanent teeth require splintage for 7–10 days.

Methods of splinting include:

- Thermoplastic.
- Composite resin and wire.
- Orthodontic brackets and wire.
- Lead foil and cement.

Teeth with a closed apex should be root canal treated when the tooth is firm. Those with an open apex should be observed and if root apex development does not occur the root canal should be dressed with a calcium hydroxide dressing.

Splinting should allow physiological movement of the tooth within the socket. If the splint is rigid, bony ankylosis occurs. In this disorder the periodontal membrane is replaced with bone and tooth becomes fused to bone. These teeth will not erupt in the normal way in the developing dentition and are more difficult to extract at any age.

Avulsed and luxated teeth should be monitored by a dental surgeon and if any evidence of periapical inflammation, external, or internal root resorption, or tooth discolouration occurs the teeth should be root filled. Teeth in which the pulp canal becomes obliterated do not require any treatment.

Further reading

American College of Surgeons. *Advanced Trauma Life Support for Doctors: ATLS*, Faculty Course Manual. Chicago: American College of Surgeons, 2004.

Andreasen JO, Andreasen FA, Andersson L. *Textbook and Color Atlas of Traumatic Injuries to the Teeth*. London: Blackwell Munksgaard, 2007.

Banks P. (1991) *Killey's Fractures of the Mandible*. London: Butterworth-Heinemann Ltd.

Gibbons AJ. Bone screw stabilization of a dentoalveolar fracture. *J Oral Maxillofac Surg* 2007; **65**: 1439.

Greaves I, Porter K, Ryan J. *Trauma Care Manual*. Oxford: Oxford University Press, 2001.

Ward Booth P, Eppley B, Schmelzeisen R. *Maxillofacial Trauma and Esthetic Facial Reconstruction*. London: Churchill Livingstone, 2003.

Damage control

Damage control

The majority of trauma patients require standard resuscitation and clinical decision-making. Improvements in pre-hospital care and resuscitation have increased the number of severely-injured patients reaching hospital alive. There is a small group of patients with severe injuries, which are accompanied by hypovolaemic shock leading to the physiological derangement of hypothermia, acidosis, and coagulopathy. A conventional management approach is associated with high mortality in this group of patients. These patients require expedient and intensive concomitant resuscitation and surgery to reduce morbidity and mortality. This is when a damage control approach is appropriate, analogous to that described by the US navy in relation to battleships: '… the capacity of a ship to absorb damage and maintain mission integrity'.

The primary aim of damage control is to restore normal physiology before normal anatomy. Damage control surgery is defined by an abbreviated resuscitative procedure consisting of rapid control of haemorrhage and contamination, temporary closure, resuscitation to normal physiology in an intensive care unit, then return to the operating theatre for definitive repair. The initial surgery is limited to enable the patient to reach the intensive care unit alive, reduce complications, and live to fight another day.

Aggressive correction of hypothermia, coagulopathy, and acidosis are essential to reduce the morbidity and mortality associated with post-traumatic multi-organ failure.

Four stages of damage control have been described:
- *Stage 1:* recognition and resuscitation.
- *Stage 2:* initial operation.
- *Stage 3:* restoration of physiology.
- *Stage 4:* definitive surgery.

Stage 1: recognition and resuscitation

Pre-hospital management in severely-injured, bleeding patients should be prompt, and on scene times short, in an effort to reduce the time to definitive surgical haemorrhage control. Damage control is aimed at reducing the incidence of the lethal triad of acidosis, hypothermia, and coagulopathy. Once this lethal triad is established, haemorrhage control and correction of coagulopathy become more difficult.

The patient requiring damage control is identified by a combination of their mechanism of injury, and a clinical presentation of severe or progressive shock. Once the patient with severe bleeding is identified, the decision to perform damage control surgery must be made early, and must be communicated rapidly to the resuscitation and operating team. They should then move the patient to theatre immediately, expedite preparation, and facilitate abbreviated surgery with simultaneous resuscitative transfusion.

When the source of bleeding is clinically apparent then no investigations are required. When the possibility of multiple sources of bleeding are present, simple investigations to help decision-making, regarding which body cavity to enter first include chest radiograph, pelvic radiograph, FAST scanning, and insertion of intercostal drains if massive haemothorax is suspected. If a major pelvic fracture is present, then a pelvic belt or sheet should be applied to help stabilize the bones and provide a counter weight if pelvic packing is subsequently required. These manoeuvres

should be immediately available in the resuscitation room, and should be carried out as the patient is being prepared for movement to theatre. They should not delay the required surgery. To achieve this, well organized systems for trauma care are required.

Damage control resuscitation

Damage control resuscitation begins alongside initial assessment, and continues into the operating theatre and intensive care unit. Large volume fluid resuscitation following haemorrhagic trauma is associated with a transient rise in blood pressure, which may remove the clot, cause dilutional coagulopathy, dilutional anaemia, and further cooling. There is also an increased risk of pulmonary complications and multi-organ failure.

The evidence for permissive or hypotensive resuscitation in penetrating trauma, although not conclusive, is more compelling than that for blunt injury. Resuscitation targets are controversial; for penetrating injuries it is reasonable to aim at a systolic blood pressure associated with cerebration or between 70–90 mmHg, until haemostasis is achieved. It may be reasonable to aim for similar figures in blunt trauma for short periods if the patient is to be transferred to theatre or angiography and there is no associated traumatic brain injury.

The benefits of hypovolaemic resuscitation must be balanced against the risks of organ hypoperfusion and the resuscitation targets adjusted if there is no rapidly identifiable surgically correctable bleeding point. Once haemostasis has been achieved, resuscitation aims to restore tissue perfusion, of which there is currently no ideal measure.

The treatment of coagulopathy has evolved with the greater understanding of the early coagulopathy associated with trauma. For the 10% of patients who are the most severely-injured, blood and plasma have been found to be the best resuscitation fluids. By using point of care testing, warming devices, multiple blood products, and haemostatic adjuncts, all efforts are directed towards normalizing clotting, base deficit, and temperature. Clot preservation is maximized with hypotensive resuscitation, and a ratio of blood to blood products of 1:1 has been found to be associated with reduced mortality in the most severely injured. Fresh frozen plasma and packed red blood cells should be administered in approximately equal amounts during a damage control approach to resuscitation. Having a massive transfusion protocol in place ensures that blood and products are available as soon as possible.

Stage 2: initial operation

Patients with major exsanguinating injuries will not survive complex procedures since intra-operative metabolic failure, rather than failure to complete operative repair, will result in early mortality. The operating theatre can be considered to be a physiologically unfavourable environment and, therefore, treatment of abnormal physiology should be considered as more important than anatomical correction at this stage.

Communication between the surgeon and anaesthetist regarding monitoring, resuscitation, and operative findings is vital. Good vascular access should be secured, adequate suction available, and plenty of large opened abdominal packs should be to hand. The team should be aware of the clock—true damage control must not take longer than

90 min. This is not the time for complex hepatic resections or pancreatic reconstructions; simple manoeuvres are required to achieve the goals of damage control surgery:
- Haemorrhage control.
- Protection from further injury.
- Prevent contamination.

Adequate exposure is essential to ensuring damage control surgery can be performed correctly and expediently. The worst case scenario should always be prepared for, as this will save crucial time in a life-threatening situation. The patient should be positioned by the surgeon prior to scrubbing up: supine crucifix position with both upper limbs out on arm boards and the skin prepared from clavicles to knees. Patients in severe shock or with multi-system injury may require multiple vascular access and this is facilitated by having the arms in this position, still allowing full access to all body cavities and major limb vessels for proximal control. In multi-system injuries or when junctional injuries are present, the initial incision should be chosen to deal with what is considered to be the greatest threat to life first. If this decision is wrong, it may be necessary to change tack immediately.

Laparotomy

The peritoneal cavity should be entered through a long midline incision (xiphisternum to pubis) with a scalpel. Preperitoneal fat is thinnest just cranial to the umbilicus and makes an ideal place to enter the cavity and often can be breached with finger dissection alone. Using a pair of heavy scissors the peritoneum can be opened the full extent of the incision. Beware of iatrogenic injury to the left lobe of the liver, small bowel, and bladder.

The hypotensive trauma patient requires immediate control of large volume intra-abdominal haemorrhage, rather than diathermy of tiny bleeding vessels. Suction should be readily available and the first manoeuvre should be to remove all small bowel loops to allow directed abdominal packing. The easiest way to achieve this is by placing large abdominal packs in the following areas:
- *Right upper quadrant:* a hand should be placed over the right and left domes of liver. Packs should be placed over the hand above the liver. The sub-hepatic area should be packed to form a 'sandwich'.
- Right paracolic gutter.
- *Left upper quadrant:* a hand should be placed above the spleen, which should be pulled gently forward and then a pack applied over the hand and then medially.
- Left paracolic gutter.
- Pelvis.

The packs should be left in place to allow volume resuscitation to take place before removal. The temptation to 'pack and peek' (a dangerous cycle of repeated packing, bleeding and resuscitation) should be avoided. After packing, packs should be removed using a system starting in the area with the least amount of bleeding, working towards the likely site of bleeding. Empirical abdominal packing will arrest all but major arterial bleeding, and will permit a more thorough inspection of the peritoneal cavity.

Following empirical packing the priority is to identify the source of haemorrhage. If packing has failed to control major bleeding, proximal aortic control may be necessary. This is achieved by opening up the lesser omentum, followed by blunt dissection at the diaphragmatic hiatus onto the supracoeliac aorta. Digital pressure is an effective

manoeuvre and often safer than formal cross clamping when in extremis.

The aim at this stage is to formally arrest the haemorrhage. Strategy is dependent on the organ. The commonest sites of bleeding are from the liver, spleen, and mesenteric vessels.

Splenic injury

During damage control procedures, bleeding from splenic injuries should be treated by splenectomy. There is no place for splenic preservation attempts in patients at the limits of their physiological reserve. Following splenectomy the splenic bed should be packed to prevent continuous post-operative oozing of blood.

If a splenic injury is present, but not bleeding, then packing this off may be helpful to prevent re-bleeding prior to the planned re-laparotomy.

Liver injury

If the initial packing controls the liver bleeding, this should be formalized. The initial packs should be removed to identify the site of the liver injury. The assistant should then be positioned so as to compress the liver into its original anatomical shape to control bleeding. The falciform ligament and triangular ligaments should be divided to enable formal packing of the involved lobe to maintain its anatomical shape with packs placed superiorly, inferiorly, and anteriorly. In the case of the right lobe, packs may also be placed laterally.

If initial packing has not controlled the bleeding, a Pringle manoeuvre should be performed by manual compression of (or placing an arterial clamp across) the porta hepatis. If this controls the bleeding, it suggests that the hepatic artery or one of its branches has been injured. There are two approaches to this situation, and the decision taken is dependant on the resources immediately available:
- If there is early access (within 30 min) to interventional angiography either on table or in the radiology suite, the Pringle manoeuvre should be maintained and compression, mobilization of the liver and formal packing should take place as above. The patient should then have other sources of bleeding controlled before proceeding directly to interventional angiography with a view to embolization of the hepatic artery and its branches. The clamp on the porta hepatis will need to be removed as close to the time of embolization as possible.
- If immediate access to interventional radiology is not possible, the porta hepatis should remain clamped whilst the packs are removed. The liver should then be compressed and mobilized as previously. The depth of the liver injury is examined whilst the clamp is temporarily released, in an attempt to identify the arterial injury and control it by suture ligation. To minimize blood loss the number of attempts and time taken to achieve this should be limited. In between attempts, the porta hepatis should be re-clamped and the liver should be compressed manually. If successful the liver should again be compressed and packed formally. If unsuccessful in gaining rapid control of liver arterial bleeding then the liver should be compressed and packed followed by formal ligation of the hepatic artery in the porta hepatis.

If initial packing and a Pringle manoeuvre have not controlled bleeding, it is likely that an intra-hepatic caval or hepatic vein injury are the cause. Heroic surgery is usually not possible due to the rapid blood loss and high chance of exsanguination in a short space of time. The triangular ligaments should not be divided and the liver should not be mobilized, as this will open up further potential spaces and remove constraints to bleeding formed by the diaphragm and the triangular ligaments. The liver should be pushed back posteriorly to compress the inferior vena cava and the hepatic veins, which should slow the bleeding. The anaesthetist should be informed prior to carrying out this manoeuvre, so they are prepared for the decreased cardiac return and subsequent cardiac output in a patient with an already compromised circulation. Packs should now be placed anteriorly and inferiorly to maintain this position of the liver compressing the site of haemorrhage.

Bleeding from knife or bullet tracks in the liver are best managed by balloon tamponade. The easiest way to achieve this is by inserting a Sengstaken tube into the track and inflating the balloon with saline until the bleeding is arrested. This can then be left *in situ* until the subsequent laparotomy.

Mesenteric vessel injury
Injuries to these vessels are managed by clamping and ligation or direct suture ligation. If the viability of the bowel supplied by the injured vessels is doubtful, this is not the time for resection and repair. The bowel either side of the doubtful segment should be stapled off or ligated to reduce possible contamination.

Retroperitoneal bleeding
Before entering a retroperitoneal haematoma it is helpful to achieve vascular control first. For a central haematoma the aorta can be controlled at the hiatus as previously described. For lateral haematomas (likely to be due to renal bleeding), if possible control of the appropriate renal artery and vein should be obtained prior to entering the haematoma.

Central retroperitoneal haematoma
If the haematoma is central then the approach is dictated by the most likely source of the bleeding. If it is thought to be arterial, the approach should be via left medial visceral rotation, which will expose the full length of the abdominal aorta and its branches. If major venous bleeding is thought to be the most likely source then right medial visceral rotation should be performed to expose the inferior vena cava and its tributaries.

Once exposed, the source of bleeding should be identified and controlled initially digitally, and then by clamp or control with balloon catheters (Fogarty or Foley depending on vessel size) if arterial. If venous it is usually safer to compress either side of a major venous injury with a swab held in a sponge holding forceps.

A judgement then needs to be made as to the ease of formally controlling the bleeding. If the injured vessel has a simple laceration, direct suture repair is appropriate. If complicated repairs or interposition grafts are required then a choice of inserting a shunt, or ligation is most appropriate.

In general the following vessels can be ligated:
- Coeliac axis and main branches.
- Inferior mesenteric artery.
- Internal iliac arteries.
- Renal arteries.
- All major named veins.

If the superior mesenteric artery trunk is injured and a complex repair is required, flow needs to be preserved and shunting is appropriate. If one or more of the branches is injured then these can be ligated and the affected segment of bowel will need to be isolated by stapling or ligating either end of the affected segment.

The common and external iliac arterial flow should be maintained if possible by simple repair or shunting. In extremis, they can be ligated and a plan made for an early return to theatre within 6 h to complete a definitive repair to restore blood supply to the involved leg. Fasciotomies of the involved leg should be performed at the initial operation.

Lateral retroperitoneal haematoma
A lateral haematoma that is not expanding should be packed off, since entering the haematoma is likely to end in a nephrectomy. Angiography with a view to embolization is appropriate following the operation.

An expanding lateral haematoma is usually due to a renal injury. If this requires surgery for control, a nephrectomy should be expected, as there is no place for renal preservation in extremis. Before entering the haematoma, the presence of a kidney on the contra-lateral side should be confirmed. Ideally, control of the renal artery on the affected side should be gained by approaching the anterior of the aorta by mobilizing the fourth part of the duodenum to expose the aorta at the level of the renal arteries. The left renal vein traversing the aorta marks the level of the renal arteries.

If the haematoma is encroaching across the aorta an alternative approach is to use medial visceral rotation from the opposite side leaving that kidney *in situ* to access the aorta.

Once the renal artery is controlled, the colon should be mobilized from the haematoma, and the haematoma and perinephric tissues should be entered to gain access to the kidney. If control of the renal vessels is difficult then a direct approach similar to that for splenectomy is appropriate. The perinephric fascia is entered and the kidney is held in one hand to compress the bleeding and is rapidly mobilized. The renal artery and vein should be double-ligated. The ureter should be located and ligated, and the kidney removed. The renal bed should be packed to reduce continued blood loss.

On occasion a lateral retroperitoneal haematoma is due to severe soft tissue injury of the lateral and posterior abdominal wall. In this situation the affected area should be packed off and post-operative angiography, and embolization considered if packing does not give complete control.

Pelvic haematoma
Ideally a pelvic fracture will have been identified and a pelvic sling applied pre-operatively. The pelvis should be entered in the pre-peritoneal plane anterior to the lower abdominal peritoneum. This gives direct access to the true pelvis and this should be packed. Consideration should be given to proceeding to angiography and embolization if bleeding from the pelvis is not completely controlled by packing.

Subsequent abdominal exploration must be thorough, systematic, and complete to include inspection of:
- *Inframesocolic compartment*: transverse colon to rectum (careful attention should be paid to the posterior surface as injuries here are often missed).
- *Supramesocolic compartment*: liver, gallbladder, right kidney, stomach (up to oesophagogastric junction), duodenum (Kocher's manoeuvre is required to visualize fully), spleen, left kidney, both hemidiaphragms.
- *Lesser sac* (blunt dissection through greater omentum-between stomach and transverse colon): posterior wall of stomach, body and tail of pancreas.

This will ensure that all sites of bleeding, and sources of contamination are identified and controlled.

Hollow organ injuries

Simple bowel injuries can be repaired with a single layer of sutures, or skin staples with bowel mucosal inversion can be utilized to achieve this quickly. With multiple perforations, or damage to a significant length of bowel, control of contamination is best achieved through bowel interruption without resection using a linear stapler or cotton tape to ligate the bowel proximal and distal to the injury. Stomas do not need to be fashioned during the first procedure and should be avoided as the abdominal wall is likely to become oedematous placing the stoma at risk. Primary anastomosis should be avoided and reserved for a later date when bowel wall oedema has subsided and gut perfusion can be assured to reduce the risk of anastomotic failure.

Biliary contamination is reduced by drainage either by placing large drains to the area of injury, placing a t-tube in an easily accessible common bile duct injury, or placing a cholecystomy tube in a gall bladder injury. Injuries to the pancreas should be drained. Bladder injuries can be drained or primarily repaired if limited in size.

Closure

Abdominal compartment syndrome is common in these patients secondary to massive fluid shifts and bowel oedema. Most patients, especially those with packs *in situ*, will require a re-look procedure and, therefore, a form of temporary closure is the most appropriate technique. Laparostomy with saline bag cover or vacuum-pack closure devices are both effective in containing and protecting abdominal viscera. The advantage of the vacuum dressing is that it collects intra-abdominal fluid and keeps the patient dry, but unlike the saline bag does not afford visualization of the bowel to assess viability. A formal note of all packs, shunts, and instruments needs to be included on the operation note.

Vascular injuries

The main principle in patients with vascular trauma is life before limb preservation. Injuries to major vessels may be compressible or non-compressible depending on the body region injured. For compressible injuries usually involving the limbs or zone 2 of the neck, temporary proximal or direct control can be carried out by pressure or by tourniquet. Recent use of tourniquets in current conflicts in the Middle East has given favourable results in single and multiply-injured patients. Incompressible injuries need to be quickly recognized and surgical control rapidly achieved. Temporary control of incompressible bleeding at the root of the neck and in the groin may be possible with balloon tamponade by inserting a foley catheter in a wound track and inflating the balloon.

Formal control of bleeding due to vascular injuries requires proximal and distal control. Incisions should be longitudinal and extensible. A combined cavity and limb approach may be required for junctional injuries; for example, laparotomy for iliac vessel control followed by longitudinal groin and upper thigh incisions for femoral vessel control for injuries involving the groin, or median sternotomy followed by neck extension for carotid injuries in zone 1 of the neck.

The damage control procedures available to the surgeon include simple direct repair, ligation, and shunting. Direct repair should be reserved for simple lacerations that can be sutured without compromising the lumen of the vessel. The choice of shunt is dependant on availability and vessel size. If commercial shunts are not available then appropriate diameter and lengths of infusion giving sets, naso-gastric feeding tubes and thorocostomy tubes may be appropriate. Prior to insertion the shunt should be clamped in the middle. They should be inserted gently and under vision so as not to raise an intimal flap. The distal end should be inserted first as this is the most likely source of an intimal flap. Once positioned the shunt clamp should be released to ensure back flow, and then the proximal end inserted. They can be secured in position by nylon tapes before finally releasing flow.

Complicated primary repairs, such as vein patching and interposition grafts should be reserved for those with extensive vascular surgical experience and in patients with sufficient physiological reserve, and an otherwise limited injury burden. Distal fasciotomy should be carried out readily and pre-emptively to avoid limb compartment syndrome.

Thoracotomy

This may be performed as a stand-alone procedure, or combined with a laparotomy or vascular procedure. In these cases the patient is usually supine and so traditional thoracotomy approaches are limited. If it is certain that the thoracic injury is limited to the heart and proximal great vessels then a median sternotomy can be performed alone or as an extension of a laparotomy.

More usually the requirement for thoracotomy becomes apparent due to large volumes of blood in one or both pleural cavities. In this situation the simplest and most expedient approach is via an anterior-lateral approach, which can readily be extended across the sternum using a heavy pair of scissors to a clamshell incision, which has unrivalled access to thoracic structures. The pericardium should be inspected and opened to exclude tamponade. The pleural cavities should be examined to assess the source of the greatest threat to life and this should be dealt with first. Proximal vascular control of great vessel injuries can be carried out either by manual pressure or instrumentation.

Cardiac wounds

Resuscitative thoracotomy is required when the patient is peri-arrest due to cardiac tamponade. It should be considered for all penetrating wounds to the chest, epigastrium, and the root of the neck. The most straightforward approach is via a left fifth intercostal space anterior thoracotomy and then the pericardium should be opened longitudinally, avoiding the phrenic nerve, to relieve the tamponade. Depending on the position of the cardiac wound the incision may be adequate to open up the pericardium further to gain better access to the wound, or if better access is required this can be achieved by extending to a clamshell thoracotomy.

Temporary manoeuvres to control cardiac wounds include digital pressure and foley catheter insertion with gentle traction once the balloon is inflated in the cardiac chamber (remembering to occlude the lumen to prevent blood loss). Depending on the site of the wound it may be repaired by simple suturing, or if the wound is adjacent to a coronary artery then horizontal mattress sutures should be used to avoid incorporation of the coronary artery. If a coronary vessel is injured and the heart is still viable, simple ligation is the best course of action.

The posterior of the heart should be examined by gentle lifting to examine for a through and through injury. The anaesthetist needs to be forewarned when this manoeuvre is carried out.

Lung injury

In instances of massive blood loss or an air leak that precludes adequate oxygenation, damage control procedures should be carried in preference to formal repair or resection. The initial step should be to gain access to the lung hilum by dividing the inferior pulmonary ligament, taking care not to injure the inferior pulmonary vein. Hilar control can most easily be achieved by squeezing digitally. Other options for hilar control include tape ligation, lung twist, or clamping. Once hilar control is achieved, the lung can be assessed for the degree of injury and options for management decided upon.

Simple linear surface lacerations can be managed by suture ligation of obvious bleeding vessels and air leaks. Through and through injuries following penetrating trauma should be managed by tractotomy to gain access to the bleeding vessels along the course of the wound track. A linear stapler is used to open up the length of the track, followed by suture ligation of the bleeding vessels and leaking airways. If a stapler is not available the same procedure can be performed by opening up the track between two straight vascular clamps, suturing vessels in the base and under-running the lung tissue controlled with the clamps.

If sections of a lung lobe are severely injured these areas can be controlled by performing non-anatomical resections with a linear stapler or applying vascular clamps and under-running the resected margins.

The hilar control is released once the repair has been completed, and the resection margins and sutured wounds should be inspected for active bleeding or large air leak. If present, these require further simple sutures for control.

If the injury involves the majority of a lung, then control of the hilum should be maintained and a decision made as to whether to proceed to immediate pneumonectomy, or to leave this until further resuscitation has been achieved and the patient is in a better physiological condition. If there are other injuries present, delaying this is usually the best choice.

Chest wall injury

Following penetrating injuries it is easy to overlook a lacerated intercostal or internal thoracic artery injury, particularly when shock is present. A point should be made to inspect for these injuries along the course of the wound track and ligate them if an injury is identified.

Massive bleeding from a major blunt chest wall injury can be very difficult to deal with. Bleeding can be from the ribs, thoracic vertebrae, muscles, or intercostal vessels. The best approach is to pack off the injured area and apply pressure to control the bleeding, and allow resuscitation with blood and clotting factors. If bleeding is controlled then the packs should be left *in situ*.

If bleeding is not controlled, the packs should be gently removed to inspect for active arterial bleeding from muscular branches or intercostals arteries. If identified they should be ligated. Once all easily controlled arterial bleeding has been addressed the injured area should be packed again and the lung replaced in the chest to help provide further tamponade. Post-operative selective embolization (if readily accessible) is worth considering.

Tracheo-bronchial injury

Injuries involving the trachea are best dealt with by inserting a tracheal tube into the site of injury or if lower down by passing a tracheal tube across the defect. For proximal bronchial defects, one lung ventilation achieved by passing the endotracheal tube into the uninjured main bronchus can be life-saving. If difficult due to bleeding and location, this can be enabled by a joint approach by the anaesthetist and operating surgeon. Injuries of the main bronchial branches, or more distally in the lung hilum, are best dealt with by hilar clamping or non-anatomical resections when the patient is *in extremis*.

Oesophageal injury

These should be sought with penetrating injuries involving the posterior mediastinum and with severe blunt injury. Control of contamination is obtained by placement of suitable large drains and spillage can be prevented by insertion of a large bore T-tube in the oesophageal defect.

Thoracic closure

Prior to closure, chest, and pericardial drains should be placed as appropriate. Rapid closure of a thoracotomy can be achieved by interrupted sutures around adjacent ribs and mass closure of the muscles. Take care to ensure that injured or divided inter-costal and internal thoracic arteries are identified and ligated as severe bleeding can occur post-operatively if these are not ligated, once the circulation is restored.

If thoracic closure is not possible because of packing or a distended heart following repair, temporary closure can be achieved using a plastic bag technique similar to that for laparotomy.

Orthopaedics

In patients with pelvic and long bone fractures with associated other injuries (particularly head, chest, and abdominal), a damage control approach to fracture fixation leads to better outcomes. This is likely to be due to the lesser physiological insult to the patient at this critical time when they are already close to their physiological limit. Temporary fixation is obtained expeditiously by external fixation with less operating time and lower blood loss. Associated wounds are cleaned and debrided.

Initial control of bleeding from severe and mangled limb injuries can be achieved by application of a tourniquet. This can be applied pre-hospital by trained personnel, in the emergency department or in the operating theatre. The identification and ligation of major vessels can then take place. Initial soft tissue debridement should be kept to devitalized or heavily contaminated tissues, while maintaining length of skin and muscle flaps. The wounds should be left open for later review. On release of the tourniquet, it should be ensured that bleeding from larger vessels is controlled by ligation and bleeding from the soft tissues is controlled by compression bandages.

Stage 3: restoration of physiology

The patient should be moved to the intensive care unit once all life-threatening bleeding has been controlled. The circulation should be restored rapidly to normal volumes with a combination of blood, blood products (including plasma, platelets and cryoprecipitate), and crystalloid solutions. Crystalloid use should be restricted to that required to make up for using packed red blood cell transfusions and daily fluid requirements so as to minimize pulmonary complications, reduce bowel oedema, and the risk of abdominal compartment syndrome. The restoration of normal coagulation should be guided by laboratory testing and may be aided by thromboelastography. During this resuscitative process, fluids should be warmed, and warming blankets applied to restore normal temperature.

If a secondary survey has not been completed this should be performed at this stage. The timing of further imaging is dependent on the physiology of the patient and the degree of urgency required for the treatment of the suspected injury. Transfers to the radiology department should be kept to a minimum, as any transfer is a further challenge to the physiology of the patient. If all bleeding is controlled and a major head injury is suspected, this would justify an early move for CT scanning, compared with a suspected spinal injury or simple fracture, both of which can be managed with a period of immobilization without major consequences for the patient.

A tertiary survey needs to be performed in the first 48 h to identify any missed injuries. A careful plan then needs to be made for the management of all the identified injuries and for the completion of surgery.

Stage 4: return to theatre

Unplanned

An unplanned return to theatre may be required before the patient has been fully resuscitated if there is ongoing bleeding, re-bleeding, or thrombosis or dislodgement of a vascular shunt. In these circumstances, a damage control approach should again be used.

If the initial packing has failed to control bleeding, a further attempt is justified. The original packs should be removed and an assessment made as to whether they were sited appropriately, the organ involved was not compressed adequately or the bleeding was arterial in origin. In the former situations, an attempt at further packing has a good chance of success. In the case of arterial bleeding, if ligation is a straightforward option then this should be performed. If access is difficult or is likely to be prolonged, for example, with liver injuries, then packs should be replaced and the patient taken for selective embolization.

If a shunt has been dislodged this can be re-sited, or if the patient is in a good physiological condition and an appropriate surgeon is present formal repair can be considered at this time. If a shunt has thrombosed and the limb is threatened a similar approach can be taken depending on the condition of the patient and surgeon availability.

Planned

The return to theatre is ideally on a planned basis and should be carried out by the best available surgical teams. One or more procedures may be carried out during this session depending on the injury burden and the physiological reserve of the patient.

The time for this procedure varies between 6 and 72 h following the initial surgery, depending on the patient and the original injuries. For example, a shunted vascular injury, or cross-clamped or twisted lung hilum would justify an earlier return than a well controlled packed liver injury.

For an early planned return this should occur once the patient's temperature is greater than 35°C, the serum lactate is less than 2.5 mmol/L, and there is normal coagulation by laboratory testing or thromboelastography. For surgery at 24 h or later, the patient's physiology should be as close to normal as possible.

Blood, plasma, platelets, and cryoprecipitate should be available for the re-operation. The temporary closure should be removed and an assessment made as to a plan of attack. Definitive repairs that are straightforward and easily accessible should be performed prior to pack removal, as they would not get done if severe bleeding were to reoccur on pack removal. Examples include a limb vascular repair, or small bowel anastomosis prior to removal of abdominal packs. If access is difficult with packs in situ then they should be removed. Packs should be removed following soaking in saline, by gently teasing them apart and removing them. Packs should be counted against those recorded as being inserted at initial operation.

Once the packs have been removed, the packed area should be inspected for bleeding. Frequently, minor surface bleeding occurs and this may be controlled by a short period of direct pressure. If a vessel is identified as the source it can be ligated. Occasionally, massive bleeding recurs and, in this situation, the packs should be replaced and left for a further period. The development of a subsequent plan of attack may be aided by angiography and CT investigation.

Bowel continuity should be restored at the first re-operation if possible. Colostomies and ileostomies should be avoided, particularly if abdominal closure is unlikely due to bowel oedema or re-packing.

Any dead or doubtful tissue should be debrided, and abdominal or thoracic closure should be attempted. If closure of the abdomen is not possible, it may be attempted again after a further 48 h, to allow further reduction in oedema and swelling. If closure is not achieved after this, then the wound should be allowed to granulate and a split skin graft applied. If skin closure only is possible, this can be performed. In both situations a plan for formal abdominal wall reconstruction can be made for 9–12 months later.

Long bone injuries can be definitively fixed and skin cover achieved if appropriate at this stage. For severe soft tissue injuries and traumatic amputations further surgery may be required before formal wound closure is achieved.

Complications

Complications of damage control include sepsis and multiorgan failure, wound infections, intra-abdominal abscess, and enterocutaneous fistulae. Abdominal compartment syndrome may occur even when a temporary abdominal closure has been used. Complications should be managed on their merits, taking into account the patient's condition at the time they present.

Further reading

Bickell WH, Wall MJ Jr, Pepe PE, Martin RR, Ginger VF, Allen MK, et al. Immediate versus delayed fluid resuscitation for hypotensive patients with penetrating torso injuries. *N Engl J Med* 1994; **331**: 1105–9.

Borgman MA, Spinella PC, Perkins JG. The ratio of blood products transfused affects mortality in patients receiving massive transfusions at a combat support hospital. *J Trauma* 2007; **63**: 805–13.

Brohi K, Singh J, Heron M, Coats T. Acute traumatic coagulopathy. *J Trauma*. 2003; **54**: 1127–30.

Burch JM, Moore EE, Moore FA, Franciose R. The abdominal compartment syndrome. *Surg Clin North Am* 1996; **76**: 833–42.

Roberts CS, Pape H-C, Jones AL, Malkani AL, Rodriguez JL, Giannoudis PV. Damage control orthopaedics. evolving concepts in the treatment of patients who have sustained orthopaedic trauma. *J Bone Jt Surg Am* 2005; **87**: 434–49.

Dutton RP, Mackenzie CF, Scalea TM. Hypotensive resuscitation during active hemorrhage: impact on in-hospital mortality. *J Trauma* 2002; **52**(6): 1141–6.

Giannoudis PV, Pape HC. Damage control orthopaedics in unstable pelvic ring injuries. *Injury* 2004; **35**(7): 671–7.

Hirshberg A, Mattox. KL *Top Knife—the Art and Craft of Trauma Surgery*. Shrewsbury: TFM Publishing Ltd, 2005.

Hirshberg A, Mattox KL. 'Planned reoperation for severe trauma'. *Ann Surg* 1995; **222**: 3–8.

Holcomb J. Damage control resuscitation. *J Trauma* 2007; **62**: S36–7.

Johnson JW, Gracias VH, Schwab CW, Reilly PM, Kauder DR, Shapiro MB, et al. Evolution in damage control for exsanguinating penetrating abdominal injury. *J Trauma* 2001; **51**(2): 261–71.

Ketchum L, Hess JR, Hiippala S. Indications for early fresh frozen plasma, cryoprecipitate, and platelet transfusion in trauma. *J Trauma* 2006; **60**: S51–8.

Moore EE, Thomas G. Staged laparotomy for the hypothermia, acidosis and coagulopathy syndrome. *Am J Surg* 1996; **172**: 405–10.

Pape HC, Hildebrand F, Pertschy S, Zelle B, Garapati R, Grimme K, et al. Changes in the management of femoral shaft fractures in polytrauma patients: from early total care to damage control orthopedic surgery. *J Trauma* 2002; **53**(3): 452–61.

Rotondo MF, Schwab CW, McGonigal MD, Phillips GR, Fruchterman TM, Kauder DR, et al. 'Damage control—an approach for improved survival in exsanguinating penetrating abdominal injury'. *J Trauma* 1993; **35**: 375–82.

Shapiro MB, Jenkins DH, Schwab CW, Rotondo MF. Damage control: collective review. *J Trauma* 2000; **49**: 969–78.

Smith LA, Barker DE, Chase CW, Somberg LB, Brock WB, Burns RP. Vacuum pack technique of temporary abdominal closure: a four year experience. *Am Surg* 1997; **63**: 1102–7.

Paediatric trauma

Paediactric injury

Epidemiology

Injury is a major killer of children and adolescents throughout the world. Millions more children require hospital care for non-fatal injuries, many of whom are left with a permanent form of disability, often with life-long consequences.

The burden of injury is unequal, in that it falls most heavily on to the poor: the burden of trauma is greatest on children in poorer regions and countries. Overall, it is estimated that approximately 95% of all childhood injury deaths occur in low and middle income countries. Although the child injury death rate is much lower among children in high income countries, injuries are still one of the major causes of death between the age of 1 and 18 years (40% of childhood deaths).

Tragically, both the absolute numbers, and the rates of childhood injury and deaths per population, are continuing to rise in low and middle income countries, mainly as a result of urban evasion and increased motorization. It is expected that trauma will be the leading cause of childhood deaths worldwide by 2020.

Childhood injuries can be classified in a number of different ways according to whether they are deliberate or accidental. Often things are not so clear: a 3-year-old child who is run over by a car on a busy road may be classified as an accident, but if the child had been left unsupervised, the question of neglect or abuse arises. Also, in terms of intentional injury, the gradient ranges from actively intending to hurt a child on one end of the spectrum to neglect (where a child is injured through lack of reasonable supervision) on the other. Only at approximately the age of 8 years does a child become neuro-developmentally mature enough to deal with the dangers of their complex environment. Children under the age of 8, therefore, are extremely vulnerable to injuries related to traffic, drowning, and burns.

The World Health Organization (WHO) classifies injuries as shown in Box 20.1.

A recent WHO analysis indicated the injury related causes of child and death as shown in Table 20.1.

Table 20.1. Traumatic causes of childhood deaths, WHO

Road traffic collisions	26%
Drowning	20%
Burns	10%
Falls	5%
Poisons	5%
Violence	4%
Self-inflicted	2%
Others (choking, animal stings and bites, electrocution, firearm injuries and conflicts)	28%

Some key facts about childhood injury:

- Approximately 1 million children under the age of 18 years die each year from injuries.
- Injuries are a leading cause of death in children between the ages of 1 and 18 years.
- The two leading causes of childhood injury deaths are road traffic crashes and drowning.
- Intentional injuries, such as child abuse and youth violence, are also a leading cause of death, especially among older children.
- Non-fatal injuries affect the lives of between 10 and 30 million children each year.
- Children in poor families are at higher risk of injury.
- Many injuries occur in or around the home.
- The majority of injuries can be prevented.

Child injury prevention

The ecological model provides a useful framework for injury prevention efforts, as it specifies the various networks and institutions (including schools, communities, and legislative bodies) that play a role in creating a safer environment for children by the implementation of preventative strategies. The Haddon Matrix is a useful tool in this regard; it was originally developed with a focus on unintentional traffic injuries, but nowadays has been widely applied to understanding the development of the phases of any injury event Table 20.2. The matrix simultaneously identifies where best to target any interventions.

The focus of injury prevention efforts should be the environmental circumstances which lead to injury events. Environmental factors, whether from the social or physical environment, are in many cases preventable and amenable to control. For example, in many impoverished households there are no lockable cupboards to store poisonous substances (such as paraffin or cleaning agents), leaving the child at high risk of becoming poisoned.

Injury prevention advocates or representatives can play a valuable role in investigating the circumstances around, and contributors to, childhood injuries and contribute to the information available on aetiology of injuries, as well as strategies required to prevent these injuries in the future. The vast majority of childhood injuries have predictable factors and are therefore preventable.

Box 20.1. WHO classification of childhood injuries

Unintentional injuries
- Road traffic collisions.
- Falls.
- Burns.
  - Flame.
  - Scalds.
- Drowning.
- Poisoning.
- Animal bites.

Intentional injuries
- Interpersonal violence.
- Homicide.
- Sexual violence.
- Self-harm (attempted suicide).
- Self-mutilation.
- Legal interventions.
- War.

Table 20.2. The use of the Haddon matrix in a 3-year-old child who was involved as a pedestrian in a motor vehicle crash, in a developing world setting.

Injury phases	Aetiological dimensions			
	Child and parental factors	Agent (vehicle, toy, etc.)	Physical environment	Sociocultural environment
Pre-event	Lack of supervision	Ineffective brakes	Dawn, poor street lighting	Informal township, no pavements (street is playground)
Event	Child distracted by stray dog	Speeding, intoxicated minibus driver	Busy township traffic, Thursday afternoon rush	Party mood among all people; long weekend coming up
Post-event	Parents unknown and uncontactable	Minibus not really damaged, driver left to continue work	No nearby clinic available	Parents poor and live far from hospital, no transport money available to visit the child

Psychological trauma

Trauma is an event that causes an influx of sensations that overwhelm the coping capacity of the ego or conscious mind. All childhood injuries constitute traumatic events, and the intensity and meaning of the sensations that have to be endured can be overpowering. It should be recognized that the younger a child is, the lesser the distinction between body and mind, and therefore, relative minor physical injuries or surgical procedures can lead to post-traumatic stress disorder. The younger the child involved in trauma the more serious the potential consequences can be.

Short cuts in paediatric trauma

Dealing with injured children is difficult for emergency personnel; the stresses of emergency interventions are amplified by the need to individualize every step. Not only does one have to consider the anatomical, and physiological differences between adults and children, but also the variation in size from infants to preteens. The range of interventions required can be daunting. Children need different drug dosages to be administered and different sizes of equipment. This is in addition to the emotional stress that dealing with an injured small child brings for staff.

A number of tools are available to assist with the management of injured children, all of which can help to reduce the stress of the situation. The most reliable of these are height- or weight-based. Accurate weight assessment is important, as medications are calculated by a formula per kg of body weight; equipment size is determined by patient size (and, therefore, weight) and resuscitative interventions, such as defibrillation energy or blood transfusion volumes are also calculated by weight in kg. Inaccurate weight estimation leads to inaccurate drug and fluid dosages, and incorrect equipment sizing.

Length-based formulae require measurements that may take up valuable time before resuscitation, and consume precious human resources. However, these formulae are believed to be more accurate than those based on age or weight.

The ideal formula for estimating weight should be one that is:

- Easy to remember.
- Easy to calculate (particularly in stressful situations).
- Able to provide a reasonable weight estimate to deliver clinically appropriate effects—so as not to under-or over-resuscitate.

- Accurate for both sexes.
- Accurate across different age-groups.
- Accurate across different ethnic groups.
- Validated for the local population.

Age-to-weight formulae

Age-to-weight formulae are most commonly used, and include Advanced Paediatric Life Support (APLS), Best Guess, and Luscombe and Owens formulae. They are based on the relationship between age (in completed years) and weight. Age-based formulae do not require any resources such as measuring tools or tables, and can be used in all environments. They require easily obtainable information and minimal training. Their use allows for pre-planning before a critically-injured child's imminent arrival, including preparation of essential equipment and drugs.

One of the main problems with age-based formulae is the variation in size of different sexes at different ages, related to the timing of the onset of the growth spurt. The effect of this is that in older children there is a wider spread of weights. Earlier pubertal onset in modern populations (predominantly in girls) may also emphasize the variability between the sexes. In the older age group of children, females tend to be heavier than males. Ethnicity may also impact on age-based formulae in certain populations.

The rising obesity epidemic with increasing weight-for-age in children, mostly in developed countries, has also had an impact on the usefulness of age-to-weight formulae.

The three formulae in most common use are:

APLS formula

This is taught on APLS courses across the world, and is used from age 1–10 years:

$$Wt \ (kg) = 2 \ (Age + 4)$$

It has been found to underestimate weight in UK samples over recent years, but has also been shown to be a reasonable estimate in other countries.

Best Guess

The Best Guess formula was derived and validated in Australia, and has not been tested outside of that country:

$$<12 \ months: Wt \ (kg) = (Age \ in \ months + 9)/2$$
$$1–4 \ years: Wt \ (kg) = 2 \times (Age) + 5$$
$$5–14 \ years: Wt \ (kg) = 4 \times (Age)$$

Luscombe and Owens

Again, this formula is for 1–10 years of age, but was developed on the premise that the APLS formula underestimates weight.

$$Wt\ (kg) = (3 \times Age) + 7$$

Length-based formulae

Much of the research has moved to length-to-weight formulae. The advantage of such formulae is that there is less variation with body habitus; they are thought to be more accurate and may show less variability with age. However, they do rely on physical measurement, which needs to be accurate, often involving training and needing accurate measuring tools. Measurement can also be time-consuming in emergency situations.

Broselow Tape

The Broselow–Luten® tape was developed in the early 1980s by Dr Jim Broselow, an Emergency Physician, as a resuscitation aid. It is a colour-coded tape, which is placed next to the patient. The child is measured from head to toe, and by length is assigned to a specific weight class.

The usefulness of the tape extends beyond weight estimation, as the colour-coded weight classes also list dosages of commonly used resuscitation drugs and the sizes of resuscitation equipment, such as endotracheal tubes and suction catheters.

The tape is supported by the Broselow system, which consists of pre-packaged colour-coded drugs and equipment for simplified resuscitation.

Its use is limited to children under 145 cm (35 kg). Children taller than this are treated as adults with the appropriate drugs and equipment. It has previously been shown to be accurate at estimating drug dosages, but it was derived from the 1977 NCHS data, meaning that it may not be as accurate in 2008.

Technical problems exist with the tape: training is required to use it correctly; accurate positioning of the tape is required in relation to the child (with the red end at the head); accurate measurement of length and accurate interpretation of results in terms of correct colour-coded block are required for effectiveness.

Management of the injured child

The successful management of the injured child requires an organized team approach, with a designated team leader, frequent review of the response to the treatment, and adherence to a structured initial approach and decision making.

Differences from adult trauma

The injured child differs from an adult in three main respects.

Type and pattern of injuries

Childhood injuries differ from those in adults in four main ways:
- Blunt trauma predominates.
- Multiple system injuries are common.
- Severe injuries are more often concealed than revealed.
- Non-accidental injuries are common.

Paediatric physiology

Children are not little adults. They have different physiological normal ranges and different physiological responses to injury.

Normal physiological ranges for blood pressure, heart and respiratory rate are provided by a variety of texts—most are at odds with other sources and none have a convincing evidence base. However, the ranges quoted by APLS are easy to learn, are widely used, and provide a useful guide for identification of abnormal values. These are shown in Table 20.3.

Table 20.3. Physiological normal ranges (APLS, ALSG, Manchester)

Age	Heart rate	Respiratory rate
<1	110–160	30–40
1–2	100–150	25–35
2–5	95–140	25–30
5–12	80–120	20–25
>12	60–100	15–20

Ventilation: high oxygen consumption, low functional residual capacity, therefore increased right to left shunting.

Circulation: increased physiological reserves, so vital signs are often normal despite significant fluid loss.

Shock with a low blood pressure is a pre-terminal event in children. Adequate perfusion is maintained for a long period, but if the underlying pathology goes unchecked, circulatory collapse occurs and resuscitation is often futile.

Anatomical features

Important anatomical differences include
- *Small size:* requires appropriate resuscitation equipment and techniques (e.g. venous access).
- Fluid volumes and drug dosages should be calculated according to weight.
- Relatively large head, which is frequently injured.
- *Thin integument plus high surface weight ratio:* risk of rapid temperature loss, and increased oxygen demand.

- *Immature upper respiratory tract:* obligate nose breathing under 6 months of age.
- Soft bones with poor protection of the viscera.
- Open epiphysis with a high incidence of growth plate injuries until adolescence.

Primary survey and resuscitation

This follows the <C>ABCDE approach. Resuscitation is concurrent with the primary survey. Problems are treated as they are found.

<C> Control of catastrophic external haemorrhage

Although rare, where present, life-threatening external haemorrhage must be controlled as the first stage of resuscitation.

A Airway with cervical spine control

- Supplemental oxygen should be administered early using a well fitted face mask with reservoir bag.
- In case of stridor or central cyanosis, a check must be made for inhaled foreign body, and appropriate manoeuvres performed to eject the object.
- It is essential to avoid over extension of the neck, particularly in infants (kinking of the trachea, possible cervical spine injury) and pressure on floor of mouth (tongue falls back easily).
- A properly-sized oropharyngeal airway should be inserted only if the gag reflex is absent.
- For endotracheal intubation, a straight laryngoscope blade is appropriate for children aged under one year; an uncuffed endotracheal tube (ETT) of an appropriate size to allow a small air leak should be chosen.
- Needle cricothyroidotomy may be chosen if the upper airway is compromised.
- Manual in-line cervical immobilization must be maintained, until the cervical spine can be cleared or triple immobilization (hard collar, blocks, and tape) is in place.

B breathing with oxygen

- Breathing should be assessed clinically using the parameters of respiratory rate, colour, auscultation, and pulse oximetry (oxygen saturation should be over 95%).
- When ventilation is inadequate, aspiration of vomit or foreign body must be excluded, an ET tube in the oesophagus, tension pneumothorax (clinical diagnosis), flail segment, rupture of the diaphragm, or splinting of diaphragm from acute gastric dilatation must also be considered and excluded.
- The most common cause of respiratory failure is a depressed level of consciousness from a head injury.
- A prophylactic intercostal chest drain should be considered on the side of injury if the patient requires mechanical ventilation.

C circulation with haemorrhage control

- Haemorrhage should be controlled by splinting fractures and direct pressure over external bleeding:
  - the normal systolic blood pressure in a child is 80 plus (2 × age) mmHg;
  - the pulse is often a better indicator than blood pressure, which is well maintained until the child suddenly decompensates;

- trends in pulse rate and blood pressure are more useful than single values;
- emergency department thoracotomy is not indicated in blunt trauma;
- fluid loss is assessed using peripheral colour, temperature, and capillary refill time;
- blood pressure and haemoglobin levels are poor guides for degree of blood loss;
- IV fluid replacement must not be delayed until vital signs deteriorate. Intravenous access can be through peripheral cannulae, femoral vein, saphenous vein cut down (ankle), or intra-osseous (tibial) infusion. Central venous catheterization is best avoided due to the high morbidity (unless CVP measurements required);
- blood must be taken for cross-match, FBC, blood gas;
- IV fluid replacement should commence with 10 mL/kg balanced salt solution (lactated Ringers or normal saline); this should be repeated as needed up to 40 mL/kg and followed as soon as possible with packed red blood cells; immediate O negative blood is seldom necessary.

Failure to respond to fluid resuscitation may be due to:
- Pneumothorax.
- Cardiac tamponade.
- Myocardial contusion.
- Exsanguinating intra-abdominal bleeding.

Response to resuscitation is monitored using the parameters of heart rate, respiratory rate, blood pressure (BP), urine output, and Hb.

D disability
Closed head injury is common in children. There are, however, many causes of a reduced level of consciousness (always remember to check the blood glucose level).

An early baseline assessment of neurological status is essential. The AVPU scale is appropriate initially (is the patient alert, responding to vocal stimuli, early painful stimuli, or unresponsive?). The Children's coma score is an alternative; pupils should be assessed for size, equality, and response to light; the patient's posture should be noted.

E exposure
The patient should be fully exposed. It should be remembered that the patient has a front and back, and two sides. If it has not been done already, a log roll should be performed at this stage.

Further tests
A chest X-ray and pelvic X-ray are adjuncts to the primary survey, when clinically indicated. A lateral cervical spine X-ray gives further information, but should be delayed until time-critical interventions have been performed. A naso- or orogastric tube, and urinary catheter may be necessary at this stage. If not considered already, analgesia should be given according to requirement, e.g. morphine 0.1–0.2 mg/kg titrated by slow iv infusion.

Secondary survey
This is a top to toe, back and front detailed examination for evidence of injury:
- All clothing should be removed to avoid missing injuries, but excessive heat loss must be avoided by the use of warming blankets, overhead heaters, and an appropriate ambient temperature.
- Monitoring of vital signs must continue while examining for injuries.

Head and neck
- Primary injury is irreversible. Secondary injury is common and can be prevented by adequate resuscitation, oxygenation, and controlled ventilation.
- *Raised intracranial pressure:* it is necessary to watch for SIADH (low plasma sodium, high urinary specific gravity).
- *Intra-cranial haematoma:* clinical signs are subtle compared with adults. A careful watch is necessary for changes in level of consciousness and abnormal behaviour.
- *Basilar skull fractures involving anterior cranial fossa:* there is a small, but clinically significant risk of bacterial meningitis. The use of prophylactic antibiotics is still controversial. CSF culture should be performed early if signs of meningeal irritation develop.
- Indications for CT scan are similar to adults.
- Non-penetrating cervical spine injuries are uncommon. If C-spine X-rays are normal, but there is suspicion of injury, a CT of the upper C-spine should be considered. Significant cord injury can occur without fractures (SCIWORA; see Chapter 11). It is essential to be familiar with anatomic variants in children if unnecessary errors are to be avoided.

Chest
- The majority of injuries are minor, with rib fractures and small pulmonary contusions.
- Most pleural collections are small effusions and should be drained only if clinically indicated (splinting, dyspnoea, underlying atelectasis).
- Ruptured diaphragm and cardiac contusion are less common than in adults, but life-threatening. Diagnosis is clinical, and radiographical. A high index of suspicion is important.
- Supplemental oxygen is mandatory whether the patient is symptomatic or not.
- IV morphine (see above) should be considered for rib fractures.

Abdomen
- The stomach should be deflated before physical examination using a gastric tube.
- Intra-peritoneal haemorrhage from solid organ injury is often self-limiting. Vital signs should be regularly monitored—circulatory shock will precede abdominal distension. Surgery is indicated for massive or ongoing haemorrhage heralded by haemodynamic instability.
- Ultrasound and CT are used to further define intra-abdominal injuries, depending on the resources available.
- Increasingly angio-embolization is being used instead of surgery for definitive haemorrhage control.
- *Ruptured viscus and peritonitis:* surgery is based primarily on clinical impression with deterioration in signs (free air is seen on the initial radiograph in less than 10%).
- IVP is necessary for all children with macroscopic haematuria or loin mass/tenderness suggesting significant renal injury.
- Diagnostic peritoneal lavage is not indicated in the vast majority and compromises subsequent clinical examination.

Musculoskeletal

- The epiphysis (cartilaginous growth plate) is the weakest part of the musculoskeletal system—growth plate fractures are common; sprains and ligament injuries are rare before adolescence.
- It is essential to beware of compartment syndrome following the reduction of supracondylar fractures of the humerus or fractures around the knee joint (pain on extension of the wrist, or dorsiflexion of the foot). Early fasciotomy of all compartments should be performed if suspected.
- *Open fractures:* early debridement and systemic antibiotics are the cornerstones of preventing bone and soft tissue sepsis.
- *Possible vascular injury:* on-table angiography followed by exploration and repair if indicated.

Burns

Children are more likely to be burnt in conditions of social disruption, poor socio-economic infrastructure, poor adult supervision, or latent child abuse. Children are inquisitive by nature and their environmental exploration places them at higher risk for all types of burn injury.

The three major categories of burns are:

- Thermal.
- Chemical.
- Electrical.

The most frequent causes of burn injuries in children are scalding (being burnt by boiling water, cooking oil, hot bath water, hot beverages, and foods); flame (house fire, open fire, experimentation with fire); contact (cooking appliances, heaters); electrical (low voltage with open wires, high voltage overhead wires and substations); chemical (unsafe storage practice for household acids and alkali, oven cleaner, drain cleaner, detergents), and sun exposure (without appropriate sunscreen protection).

Systemic effects of burns include

- Increased capillary permeability with subsequent fluid loss leading to hypovolaemia and shock.
- Cardiac suppression.
- Hypothermia.
- Anaemia.
- Susceptibility to infection.
- Renal failure due to hypoperfusion and myoglobinuria.
- Catabolic metabolism with increased energy expenditure.
- Respiratory distress due to carbon monoxide or cyanide poisoning, sepsis, or multi-organ failure.

The assessment of the burn wound is critical to the management of the burnt child, and after the primary survey needs to be accurately determined. This is key to successful fluid resuscitation. The proportional body surface area of children differs significantly from adults, and appropriate children's burn charts should be utilized.

A modified Parkland's formula is recommended for burn resuscitation:

3.5 mL/kg/% body surface area

Half should be given within the first 8 h from the time of the burn; the other half in the subsequent 16 h. In addition, maintenance fluids are required:

- *First 10 kg:* 100 mL/kg/day.
- *11–20 kg:* 50 mL/kg/day.
- 21 kg +: 20 mL/kg/day.

For practical purposes there are only two types of burns—those that heal spontaneously and those that don't.

Burns healing spontaneously:

- Epidermal burns (first degree burns) are pink, painful and swollen, and heal within 2–3 weeks. They are analogous to severe sun burn.
- Superficial partial thickness burns are pink to red, painful, swollen, with a blistered, loose epidermis; they are weeping wounds and will heal within 1–2 weeks.

Burns which do not heal spontaneously:

- Deep partial thickness burns are painful with a thin layer of parchment (dead tissue on the surface, blotchy red in colour, with blisters and weeping wounds).
- Full thickness burns are less painful; they have a dry surface, which appears parched, brown, or charred depending on the agent that caused the burn wound.

Escharotomies may be required for circumferential burns.

Transfer to a specialized burns unit is indicated in:

- Patients with deep burns greater than 5% of total body surface area.
- Burns of special areas: face, hands, feet, genitalia, perineum, and major joints.
- Electrical burns.
- Chemical burns.
- Inhalational injury.
- Circumferential burns.
- Burns with associated trauma.
- Suspected child abuse.
- Any patient that cannot be managed at the referring facilities.

Non-accidental injury

Child abuse and neglect can be broadly defined as being maltreatment of children by parents, guardians, or other caregivers. It occurs amongst all income, cultural, and language groups. The smaller the child, the higher the risk of fatality or serious injury. Health care workers and other professionals who work with children should make the detection, treatment, and reporting of child abuse a priority in the list of responsibilities. It is vital for the medical treatment to take a holistic approach to the ongoing needs and safety of the child.

Suspicion for non-accidental injury should exist where:
- There is a delay in seeking medical care.
- The history is unforthcoming, vague, or inconsistent with type or degree of injury.
- There are multiple hospital attendances for minor complaints.
- There are obvious suspicious injuries—cigarette burns, bruising away from bony prominences, perianal, dorsal or genital injuries.
- Multiple injuries are found at various stages of healing or incidentally diagnosed (by skeletal survey for instance).
- There are diagnostic features such as bucket-handle fractures.

Types of child abuse

Physical abuse or non-accidental injury can be defined as injuries inflicted by the care-giver.

Sexual abuse is the use of a child for sexual gratification. It should be noted that the differentiation is much broader than child rape. Besides sexual intercourse, it also includes:
- Touching, fondling, or licking of genitals or breasts.
- Masturbation of a child by an adult or vice versa, and masturbation of an adult in the presence of a child.
- Body contact with adult genitals.
- Exhibitionism.
- Pornography including photography and erotic talk.

Nutritional neglect leading to failure to thrive or severe malnutrition is most commonly seen within the first 2 years of life. It is estimated that approximately 50% of all failure to thrive in this age category is due to maternal neglect.

Intentional drugging or poisoning takes place when parents give a prescribed drug or alcohol, which is harmful to the child.

Medical care neglect occurs when the child suffers from disease or injury, and the condition worsens without the parents seeking medical attention. Safety neglect is present when there is a gross lack of supervision especially in the younger age categories.

Emotional abuse can be defined as repeatedly blaming the child for incidents. or continuous belittling or rejection of the child by his or her caregivers. Severe verbal abuse and berating are common. This is a difficult condition to prove.

Organized abuse is a form of organized crime and often involves multiple victims and perpetrators.

It is generally thought that socio-cultural income group plays an important role in the incidence of child abuse. However, many studies indicate that abuse occurs amongst all income categories, and all cultures. Younger children are at greatest risk since they are more demanding, completely defenceless, and non-verbal. A third of physical abuse takes place under the age of 6 months, another third under the age of 3, and a third above the age of 3.

Non-accidental injuries are events resulting from deliberate actions by a person against a child, which intentionally threatens and actually inflicts physical harm. Accidental injuries result from events that are usually unforeseen and that cause external trauma to the body. The events are usually not of such a nature that they are intended to harm anyone.

Causes of child abuse and predisposing factors
- Parents or caregivers who were abused themselves as children.
- Alcoholism and drug abuse.
- Up to 10% of abusers have severe psychiatric problems.
- Breakdown of family structure.
- Socialization.
- Poverty.
- Unemployment.

Typical characteristics of abusers include being the primary caregiver, being financially or otherwise stressed, or being an under-achiever with low self-esteem. During the history-taking and examination they are often jealous, manipulative, and intervening.

Child abuse should be suspected when there is evidence of
- Unexplained injuries.
- Discrepant histories.
- Alleged self-inflicted injuries.
- Alleged third party inflicted injury.
- Repeated injuries.
- Sexualized behaviour.
- Sexually transmitted diseases.

The role of the healthcare worker
The healthcare worker must ensure that they:
- Recognize child abuse.
- Complete accurate documentation of the extent of the clinical findings, physical, and psychological.
- Institute the appropriate treatment for injuries sustained.
- Report the case to the appropriate authorities. Good communication is vital.

Typical clinical findings
- Typical physical findings in child abuse are shown at Box 20.2.

Box 20.2. Typical findings in child abuse

Skin

- Skin lesions can occur everywhere.
- Bruises on the buttocks and lower back are often related to punishment.
- Bruises on the cheek may be due to being slapped.
- Other typical findings in child abuse are slap marks, pinch marks, and circumferential bruises.
- Defining the age of injuries is difficult. Most skin lesions have an initial red collar followed by a reddish purple period within 24 h, which then gradually progresses to a predominantly purplish colour over the next week. Discolouration to yellow green brown is due to degradation of Hb and occurs over 1–3 weeks, depending on the depth of the bruise.

Burns

Approximately 10% of physical abuse involves burns. Typical lesions found in child abuse are cigarette burns and stocking–glove injuries in toddlers as a result of hot water immersion (especially in the absence of splash injuries).

Head injuries

- The spectrum of head injury can range from mild trauma to lethal extradural and subdural haematoma.
- Skull fractures are commonly seen in children due to child abuse.
- Although often associated with skull fractures, inflicted subdural haematomas may also be a result of shaking. The rapid acceleration and deceleration of the head appears to tear bridging veins with a result in bleeding and subdural haematomas, often bilaterally. Retinal haemorrhages are nearly always present in these cases. Fundoscopy is to be done in any child with unexplained loss of consciousness in order to look for retinal bleeds.

Skeletal injuries

- Fractures in small children are rare. In all patients under the age of 3 years presenting with a fracture without adequate history, child abuse should be considered.
- Approximately ¼ of physical abuse cases have skeletal lesions. Two-thirds are fractures involving the long bones, and the fractures can be spiral or transverse.
- Certain fractures are almost pathognomonic for child abuse, such as a chip fracture (corner fracture of the long bones). The corner of the metaphyses is usually torn off the periosteum during wrenching injuries to the long bones. Approximately 10 days after an injury, calcification of the sub-periostal bleeding will give rise to the classical double cortex line.
- In all children with suspected child abuse, a skeletal survey is strongly advocated. A skeletal survey compromises a combination of radiographs of the chest, skull and extremities (A–P views). A radionuclear bone scan is a more sensitive method to pick up old injuries, but is unreliable under the age of 1 year.

Differential diagnosis

The most important differential diagnoses are:

- *Birth trauma:* this should be evident from the birth history.
- *Congenital syphilis:* chronic periosteal reaction combined with metaphyseal widening and positive blood tests.
- *Osteogenesis imperfecta:* multiple fractures, blue sclera, osteopaenia.
- *Ricketts:* renal disease, bowed long bones, blood abnormalities.
- *Scurvy:* poor wound healing, bleeding gums, petechiae.
- *Bleeding disorders:* haemophilia, meningococcaemia, idiopathic thrombocytopaenic purpura.
- *Skin diseases:* impetigo, chicken pox, scalded skin syndrome.

Management

Child abuse is a family problem and effective treatment should involve the co-operation of a multidisciplinary child abuse management team with the representatives from the Child Protection Services, the courts, the Police Departments, Rape Crisis Centres, Hospitals, and the Mental Health Services.

Health-care workers should be aware that their input should be limited to their profession and expertise. Careful management should be followed in order to spare the child having to repeat statements to different agencies. The management of the child via social worker and a child psychologist is highly recommended. The important task of the social worker is not only interviewing, but also reuniting the child with his or her family when appropriate.

It is important during the treatment of the child to stress that he or she is not to blame for the abuse. Specific reactions, such as guilt, anxiety, phobia, anger, and depression should be appropriately addressed.

Child abuse cases represent a big responsibility for a managing physician. However, compassionate medical treatment with proper and legally acceptable documentation will go a long way in dealing with such cases.

Epiphyseal injuries

Children's bones have a very active periosteum, which tends to tear on the convex side of a fracture, but remains intact on the concave side and assists with fracture reduction. The periosteum contributes to vigorous callus formation and active bony healing, meaning that non-union of fractures is rare in children.

Typically, ligaments are stronger than the epiphyseal plates and, therefore, fractures tend to be commoner than sprains and strains. In addition, a reasonable degree of remodelling occurs with young children's bones and, therefore, larger degrees of deformity are often accepted, especially with metaphyseal fractures.

Unlike adults, children have active growth in the epiphyses and these are the areas prone to fractures. There are two types of epiphysis—traction epiphyses (base of fifth metatarsal, tibial tuberosity, anterior iliac spine) tend to be affected by avulsion injuries; pressure epiphyses occur at the end of long bones and are responsible for longitudinal growth.

Fractures of the pressure epiphysis are classified by the Salter Harris system (Fig. 20.1):

- *Type I:* separation of the epiphysis from the shaft.
- *Type II:* displacement of the epiphysis with a small triangular segment of metaphysis (Thurston Holland sign).
- *Type III:* separation of part of the epiphysis.
- *Type IV:* separation of part of the epiphysis with a segment of metaphysis.
- *Type V:* crush injury of the epiphyseal plate.

Type II injuries are the commonest, accounting for up to 75% of all epiphyseal fractures; severity increases from 1 to 5.

Type I injuries are uncommon, and diagnosis can be very difficult as the degree of displacement may be minimal. Comparative X-rays of the unaffected side may be helpful. Cases where a fracture is clinically suspected, but X-rays appear normal should be treated as a fracture. Disturbance to growth is uncommon with type 1 injuries.

Type II injuries also have a good prognosis, as long as good alignment of the fracture segments is achieved.

Type III injuries are intra-articular. Failure to achieve good alignment will result in problems with bony growth and potential articulation issues. Specialist referral is recommended, although adequate reduction does not always prevent growth disturbance.

Type IV injuries are dealt with like type III: they are associated with growth disturbance and articulation problems, and need specialist referral—surgical fixation may be necessary.

Type V injuries are the rarest but the most serious. They typically occur at the knee or ankle. Like type I, they are difficult to diagnose on X-ray (as there is often no displacement), although the child will usually present with obvious signs and symptoms of a fracture. MRI may confirm the diagnosis. Even with appropriate initial treatment, growth failure usually occurs—specialist consultation is essential.

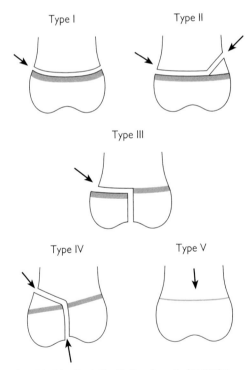

Fig. 20.1. Salter Harris Classification of growth plate injuries.

Pitfalls in the management of paediatric trauma

The main pitfalls in the management of the paediatric trauma patient are:
- Not following basic principles.
- Not totally undressing and examining the patient.
- Under-estimating shock due to compensatory mechanisms.
- Missing concurrent multiple injuries.
- Attributing circulatory shock to head injury. Although this is a possibility in a very small child with a relatively large head, it is unusual and a cause for shock always has to be searched for.
- Not communicating adequately with the parents or carers.

Further reading

Advanced Paediatric Life Support. *Advanced Paediatric Life Support.* Manchester: BMJ Publishing, 2005.

Hall DMB, Elliman D (eds). *Health for All Children,* 4th edn. Oxford: Oxford University Press, 2003.

Harrison VC. (ed.) *Handbook of Paediatrics for Developing Countries,* 6th edn.Oxford: Oxford University Press, 2004.

Nicol A, Steyn E (eds). *Handbook of Trauma for Southern Africa.* Oxford: Oxford University Press, 2004.

McRae R. *Practical Fracture Treatment.* London: Longman, 1994.

van As S, Naidoo S (eds). *Paediatric Trauma and Child Abuse.* Cape Town: Oxford University Press Southern Africa (Pty) Ltd, 2006.

World Health Organization. *Child and Adolescent Injury Prevention. A WHO Plan of Action.* Geneva: World Health Organization, 2006.

Trauma in pregnancy

Trauma in pregnancy

Emergency care of a pregnant woman with physical trauma poses several unique challenges. Indeed, any female patient of reproductive age should have a pregnancy test performed early during trauma evaluation in the Emergency Department. Physical trauma during pregnancy is a relatively common event. It occurs in up to 7% of pregnancies and the frequency increases with advancing gestational age. More than half of these incidents occur during the third trimester.

Mechanisms of injury vary according to the environment. In western countries, motor vehicle collisions account for up to 60% of all trauma, falls approximately 20%, domestic violence and sexual assaults for around 10%. Pregnant patients involved in motor vehicle collisions who do not use seatbelts are at increased risk of maternal and foetal fatality. Among pregnant women, restraint use averages 24–46%. Many pregnant women still believe that the belt may cause foetal injuries. Public information programmes are vital in the dissemination of information regarding injury prevention. Even minor trauma is associated with adverse pregnancy outcomes, with preterm labour occurring in 8% of cases, placental abruption in 1–5%, and foetal death in 1%.

Life-threatening (major) trauma occurs in less than 0.1% of pregnancies and causes maternal death in approximately 9% of cases. Foetal injuries occur in isolation in 5% of cases. The foetal death rate ranges from 20% to 61%, and reaches 80% when there is evidence of maternal shock. Placental abruption occurs in up to 66% of cases. Major trauma with head injury or haemorrhage remains the main cause of maternal death during pregnancy.

In the USA, over-exertion (particularly in the last trimester) is one of the mechanisms of injury that may result in early delivery and adverse maternal outcomes.

Blunt trauma

Blunt trauma may cause multiple life-threatening injuries to the mother. Intra-abdominal haemorrhage, pelvic fracture, and uteroplacental vascular injuries are the most common major injuries. Pelvic fractures add a significant risk of substantial hidden blood loss. The gastrointestinal tract appears to be protected by the gravid uterus and is rarely injured. The maternal abdominal and uterine walls protect the foetus, but blunt trauma may still result in foetal skull fractures and intracranial haemorrhage. Once other life-threatening injuries have been defined, placental abruption remains by far the greatest concern.

Penetrating trauma

In penetrating abdominal trauma, foetal mortality ranges from 40% to 70%, whereas maternal mortality ranges from 5% to 10%. It is often quoted that the foetus protects the mother. As a matter of fact, mortality is lower for pregnant women with penetrating injuries than for non-pregnant women with similar penetrating injuries. Cases of direct penetrating foetal trauma following the intra-vaginal route with no maternal organ disruption have also been reported.

Domestic violence and sexual assault

Domestic violence frequently goes unreported. It may afflict up to 30% of pregnant women and may be associated with an astonishing 5% foetal death rate. Prevalence of sexual assault varies enormously according to setting, from 3% in industrialized countries, such as the USA, to as much as 13% in developing countries. In some African countries up to 70% of pregnant women are physically abused, and of these 80% present with physical injuries.

Independent predictors of foetal mortality and morbidity

Following trauma, foetal-neonatal death does not necessarily correlate with severity of maternal injury. In a large prospective study conducted in a heterogeneous group of pregnant women evaluated for minor trauma, none of the most commonly used objective measures evaluated for minor trauma, including a positive Kleihauer-Betke (KB) test (which is indicative of the presence of foetal-to-maternal haemorrhage), fibrinogen less than 200 mg/dL, more than 5 contractions per h, abdominal pain, anterior placenta, or direct abdominal trauma were predictive of adverse outcomes.

Retrospective cohort studies have shown that increasing ISS (as well as trauma during the early phase of gestation) predicts a poor long-term foetal outcome, with an increased risk of both preterm delivery and low birth weight. Data from the American College of Surgeons National Trauma Data Bank were examined by multivariate logistic regression analysis to identify independent risk factors in pregnant trauma patients. Injury Severity Score (ISS) higher than 15, Abbreviated Injury Score higher than 3 of either head, abdomen, thorax, or lower extremities, and Glasgow Coma Score lower than 8 were all independent risk factors for foetal loss. Reportedly, maternal serum lactate and increasing base deficit also may predict poor foetal outcome.

Pathophysiological considerations

Foetus

The changes occurring both in the foetus and in the mother need to be considered. The foetus is especially susceptible to the teratogenic consequences of radiation and drugs during the early phases of embryogenesis and is considered to become independently viable only after the 24–26th week. Relevant anatomical and physiological changes that occur in pregnancy are listed in Table 21.1.

Uterus

The uterus becomes an intra-abdominal organ at 12 weeks, and, as it enlarges, displaces abdominal contents upwards, reaching the costal margin at between 34 and 38 weeks. The diaphragm may be elevated as much as 4 cm, with accompanying displacement of associated thoraco-abdominal organs, altering interpretation of physical examination and radiographic findings. When patients are supine, the enlarged uterus may compress the inferior vena cava and decrease venous return, and the supine hypotension syndrome may develop. Positional changes in blood pressure are also well documented.

Maternal foetal unity

The maternal cardiopulmonary system also adapts to pregnancy. By the second trimester, a mild increase in resting heart rate and decreased systolic blood pressure are accompanied by moderate hypocapnia caused by increased minute ventilation. Foetal haemoglobin has a higher oxygen affinity than maternal haemoglobin. Progesterone and increased carbon dioxide (CO_2) production are main forces behind the condition known as hyperpnoea of pregnancy. This condition results in a reduction in arterial CO_2 tension ($PaCO_2$) from 40 mmHg to 34 mmHg and an increase in arterial oxygen tension (PaO_2) from 60 mmHg to 100 mmHg. This exaggerated gradient between the mother and the foetus facilitates efficient gas exchange. With the decreased $PaCO_2$, the expecting mother also experiences respiratory alkalosis and the oxyhaemoglobin dissociation curve is thus shifted to the right, again facilitating delivery of oxygen to the foetus. Maintenance of adequate oxygen levels in the mother is therefore essential, and all pregnant trauma patients should have supplemental oxygen.

Increases in maternal blood volume (by 50%) and relatively smaller increases in red blood cell volume (by 30%) create the relative physiological anaemia of pregnancy with expected haematocrit values between 30 and 35% in the third trimester. Cardiac output increases during the second trimester, an increasing portion of which is shunted to the developing foetus and uterus. Mild increases in heart rate and mild decreases in blood pressure may be noted, but should never be attributed to pregnancy alone without first excluding all other potential sources of shock such as bleeding.

Other physiological changes include delayed gastric emptying, and increased gastro-oesophageal reflux due to decreased gastrointestinal motility and laxity of the lower oesophageal sphincter. Following trauma, aspiration is therefore more common and early gastric decompression is warranted. Diaphragmatic elevation must be considered when insertion of an intercostal drain is necessary, and it is safer to place the tube one or two interspaces higher than usual.

Table 21.1. Relevant physiological changes associated with pregnancy

Parameter	Non-pregnant	Pregnant
Cardiovascular		
Heart rate	70–80 bpm	↑ 10–15 bpm
Cardiac output	4.5 L/min	↑ to 6 L/min (↑ 30%)
Systolic blood pressure	110 mmHg	↓ by 5–15 mmHg
Haematology		
Blood volume	4000 mL	↑ by 30–50%
Plasma	2400 mL	↑ to 3700 mL
Red blood cells	1600 10^{12}/L	↑ to 1900 10^{12}/L
Haemoglobin	12–16 g/dL	↓ to 10–14 g/dL
Haematocrit	37	↓ to 32–34%
White blood cells	4.5–10 10^9/L	↑ to 5.0–14 10^9/L
Respiratory		
Oxygen demand		↑ by 20%
Tidal volume	500 mL	↑ by 40% (700 mL)
Residual volume	1200 mL	↓ by 40% (720 mL)
Respiratory rate	12–20 breaths/min	↑ to 25 breaths/min
pH	7.38–7.44	↑ 7.41–7.46
$PaCO_2$	40 mmHg	↓ to 30 mmHg
PaO_2	60 mmHg	↑ to 100 mmHg

bpm = beats per minute.

$PaCO_2$ arterial carbon dioxide tension.

PaO_2 arterial oxygen tension.

Diagnostic imaging

Especially during the later stages of pregnancy, clinical examination of the abdomen is unreliable at detecting significant intra-abdominal injuries. This is due to progressive stretching of the parietal peritoneum and consequent dilution of afferent neural input. Interposition of omentum and small intestines between the parietal peritoneum, and any intra-abdominal process may also contribute. Diagnostic imaging is, therefore, a critical tool in the assessment of traumatic injury occurring during pregnancy, since it offers the opportunity to obtain key diagnostic elements about both the mother and the foetus. Non-ionizing radiation imaging and especially ultrasonography (US) are most valuable in this context since they are free from the risks inherent with ionizing radiation. However, on occasion X-rays will be necessary to exclude major injury. When they are performed, it is important to shield the pregnant uterus as extensively as possible, keeping it in mind that the cumulative radiation dose adsorbed by the foetus should be as low as possible. However, in the trauma setting, concern about ionizing radiation exposure should not prevent medically indicated maternal diagnostic or therapeutic radiological procedures from being performed. Whenever feasible, the pregnant patient needs to be informed and consented regarding the diagnostic and treatment options. Importantly, radiation-induced foetal risks are highest very early in gestation, when the patient herself may well be unaware of the pregnancy.

Ionising radiation imaging

Although cumulative exposure to fewer than 5 rad (50 mGy) has not been associated with any increased risk of foetal loss or birth defects, even a 1–2 rad exposure is known to increase the chance of developing leukaemia during childhood. A chest radiograph will cause minimal foetal exposure (0.00007 rad); an abdominal CT will expose the foetus to 2–5 rad. Both chest and head CT are much safer with exposure of 0.1 rad and 0.05 rad when shielding of the foetus is performed.

Trauma series

As mentioned, plain films cause minimal foetal exposure. Trauma series should be performed as clinically indicated to exclude life-threatening maternal injury. Shielding of the foetus and a judicious request for further plain films should be considered.

CT

In head trauma CT should be performed as clinically indicated. CT also represents the gold standard in assessing blunt abdominal trauma, but ultrasound (and in particular FAST) may avoid the need to go on to CT. CT of the abdomen should be reserved for patients with suspicion of pelvic, retroperitoneal or lumbar spine injury.

Angiography

Angiography and interventional radiology play an important role in assessing and controlling haemorrhage from solid organ and pelvic trauma. It should be performed as clinically indicated in the pregnant trauma patient.

Non-ionizing radiation imaging

Ultrasound and magnetic resonance imaging (MRI) are safe to use in the pregnant patient as they do not expose the foetus to ionising radiation.

Focused assessment with sonography for trauma (FAST)

FAST is the first-line diagnostic examination in torso trauma. It is widely used as a quick and reliable tool for the bedside assessment of trauma patients with suspicion of intra-peritoneal bleeding or cardiac tamponade. In pregnant trauma victims, FAST has shown 83% sensitivity for free intra-peritoneal fluid. Moreover, both the presence and rate of the foetal heart can be identified. Documented foetal heart beat in a peri-mortem trauma patient is an indication for a peri-mortem caesarean section, when the gestation is 24 weeks or more.

Some authorities have recommended that all female trauma patients of reproductive age should undergo FAST initially, with the secondary intent to screen for pregnancy. The technique should include normal assessment of the four areas (cross-reference radiology chapter), followed by identification of the foetal heart, and estimation of the foetal age and gestation.

Formal ultrasound

Formal US is a very useful tool in the evaluation of foetal gestational age, foetal heart rate, and foetal activity. However, even in expert hands ultrasound may miss up to 50% of subchorionic haemorrhage or a retroplacental clot typical of placental abruption. The difficulty in picking up placental abruption with US represents one of the greatest challenges in imaging trauma in pregnancy as the attending team may receive false reassurance from a normal US study.

MRI

Although logistically demanding, improvements in MRI techniques have widened the indications for the assessment of foetal brain malformations and maternal injuries. The placenta, as the organ that mediates oxygen delivery from the maternal circulation to the foetus, can also be assessed by MRI. However, there is little evidence supporting the use of MRI for trauma in pregnancy. The Eastern Association for the Surgery of Trauma (EAST) does not recommend MRI use during the first trimester.

Other diagnostic tools

Diagnostic peritoneal aspiration and lavage (DPA and DPL)

Despite the decline in this investigation, in the haemodynamically unstable patient, when FAST examination is equivocal or not possible, DPA can be used to diagnose intraperitoneal haemorrhage.

When the patient is haemodynamically normal, but bowel injury is suspected, DPL may be considered. This method has an accuracy of 92% in detecting bowel injuries, but is rarely used today.

After the first trimester, if DPL is to be performed, an open, supra-umbilical technique must be used in order to avoid injury to the gravid uterus.

Cardiotocography (CTG)

The role of early foetal heart monitoring cannot be overemphasized. Maternal perfusion is preserved at the expense of uterine perfusion and, in fact, foetal hypoxia with subsequent foetal bradycardia (the 'mammalian diving reflex') may well be the first indicator of maternal haemorrhage.

Once maternal life-threatening injuries have been defined and managed, the presence of foetal distress (decelerations and bradycardia on CTG) and uterine contractions may indicate placental abruption. CTG should be started as soon as possible, and most authors agree on a 24-h period of monitoring. Indications of placental abruption (which can occur up to 72 h post-injury) are more than one uterine contraction every 15 min, an abnormal foetal monitor strip, uterine tenderness, vaginal bleeding, rupture of the membranes, or any serious maternal injury.

Patients presenting after worrying mechanisms of injury (motorcycle collisions, pedestrian, or those ejected from motor vehicles), or those with minor trauma should also be monitored for at least 24 h (with at least 4 h of CTG monitoring).

Kleihauer–Betke testing

The KB test is able to detect foetal-to-maternal haemorrhage. It uses differences in the colorimetric properties of foetal and maternal erythrocytes to measure presence and proportion of foetal red blood cells in the maternal blood. After abdominal trauma a degree of foeto-maternal haemorrhage is detected in about 50% of patients, especially in the presence of an anterior placenta.

To prevent maternal sensitisation with Rh antigen (present in the foetus since the 6th week of gestation) administration of a standard dose of anti-Rh immunoglobulin within 72 h is standard of care in all unsensitised Rh-negative pregnant women who have undergone even minor abdominal trauma. The role of KB (if repeated in the days following trauma) is to diagnose large foeto-maternal haemorrhages that may require additional doses with anti-Rh immunoglobulin.

According to recent studies, a positive KB test (with concomitant foetal distress) may also be indicative of a life-threatening haemorrhage in the foetal circulation, as well as accurately predicting preterm labour and placental abruption. For this reason, the EAST group recommends that KB analysis is performed in all pregnant patients who are of more than 12 weeks gestation.

Management of trauma in pregnancy

The greatest challenge in managing trauma in pregnancy is early and accurate diagnosis and treatment. Obstetricians are skilled in dealing with the pregnant patient, but uncomfortable with trauma, and traumatologists are used to dealing with trauma, but are uncomfortable with pregnancy. There is, therefore, a requirement for a truly multi-disciplinary team. Facilities for rapid caesarean section should be readily available.

Before measures can be taken to appropriately manage the pregnant trauma patient, the diagnosis of pregnancy needs to be made. An appropriate physical examination, and serum or urine pregnancy testing should be undertaken in all female trauma patients of reproductive age. FAST may also play a role as screening tool.

Trauma team

Recently, it has been suggested that pregnant patients with no physiological, mechanistic, or anatomical criteria for trauma team activation would be best managed by expeditious evaluation by an emergency physician, and a rapid referral to the obstetric service for foetal heart monitoring and ultrasound. However, pregnant patients need a lower threshold for activation of a multi-disciplinary trauma team, as adverse outcomes may complicate any kind of trauma, and these can not always be reliably predicted.

The haemodynamically unstable patient

When faced with an injured pregnant patient, all efforts should focus on the mother, rather than the foetus, as rapid resuscitation of the mother will optimize foetal haemodynamics and final outcome.

Maternal assessment should follow standard trauma protocols, with a few extra elements that need consideration. In relation to primary assessment, expansion of the gravid uterus after the 20th week requires left lateral displacement of the uterus (which compresses the inferior vena cava in the supine position—the supine hypotension syndrome) to improve blood flow to both the mother and the foetus. This can also be achieved by tilting the patient to the left by approximately 35 degrees using a wedge, or if still on a long spine board tilting the whole board. The patient should be tilted as an entire unit maintaining spinal immobilization. Alternatively, in pregnant trauma patients with potential spinal injury it can be beneficial to maintain the patients supine, but manually displace the uterus to the left until spinal injury has been ruled out.

With this in place, control of the airway, optimization of ventilation and perfusion, and early haemorrhage control should be the priorities. Fluid resuscitation must be tailored to the modified haemodynamic state in pregnancy, and vital signs interpreted with this in mind.

The following points should be considered:

- Administration of high flow O_2.
- Resuscitation of the mother first.
- If the gestation is >24 weeks, tilting into the left lateral position or manual displacement of the uterus to left will be required.
- Early intubation should be considered due to the risk of aspiration.
- Chest tubes should be placed higher than in the non-pregnant patient due to the elevated diaphragm.
- Rh-negative blood should be used.

Trauma laparotomy

The haemodynamically unstable mother with free abdominal fluid demonstrated by FAST (or DPA) requires a trauma laparotomy. The usual principles apply, namely a warm environment and active re-warming devices, appropriate assistance, several laparotomy sponges (packs) to assess and stop bleeding, early contamination control, and an early shift to damage control surgery when necessary. However, aortic clamping should be avoided in order to maintain placental circulation.

Uterine rupture is a rare condition that should be dealt with by primary repair with absorbable simple or running sutures. Packing may be required in case of uncontrolled haemorrhage from the uterus, and in the case of total destruction of the uterus, hysterectomy may be required. Injury to the ovaries may require oophorectomy. The successful use of a temporary abdominal closure with the vacuum pack technique has also been reported.

Pelvic trauma

Foetal mortality associated with maternal pelvic trauma varies between 9% and 35%. In the haemodynamically unstable, non-pregnant patient with severe pelvic trauma and a negative FAST scan, pelvic stabilization with a pelvic binder or external fixation, and haemorrhage control with angio-embolization is the current standard. There are limited reports on safety and efficacy of angio-embolization for acute pelvic haemorrhage in pregnant patients. Direct injuries to the foetus (most often fractures of the skull) and placental abruption are other feared complications following pelvic fractures. Fixation of unstable fractures of the pelvic ring with percutaneous osteosynthetic techniques has been reported to result in favourable pregnancy outcome and successful vaginal deliveries in up to 75% of injured mothers.

Emergency Caesarean section

In haemodynamically unstable patients, the presence of foetal distress (decelerations and bradycardia at CTG or US) will further dictate decision making. Caesarean section in haemodynamically unstable mothers is indicated either to control haemorrhage (in placental abruption or uterine rupture) or, sporadically, to enable the exposure and control of non-obstetric intra-abdominal bleeding. Overall reported survival rates are around 45% for the infants and 72% for the mothers.

Once the haemodynamic status of the mother has improved, foetal distress may be the initial presenting symptom of placental abruption or uterine rupture. These two conditions, plus a gestation age of 24 weeks or more, are indications for emergency caesarean section.

Peri-mortem Caesarean section

When faced with a severely injured mother who is not responding to resuscitation attempts, a peri-mortem caesarean section may save the life of the foetus. The decision to carry out a peri-mortem caesarean section and the procedure itself must be performed without delay. From the onset of an unresponsive maternal cardiac arrest the foetus must be delivered within 10 min. Foetal heart beat must be documented on Doppler, FAST, or CTG and the foetus must be older then 24 weeks (therefore viable). The procedure should be performed in the ED, while maternal cardio-pulmonary resuscitation (CPR) is continued. Effective CPR can be achieved with bimanual cardiac compressions through a thoracotomy without cross-clamping the aorta. No preparation or draping is necessary.

A generous midline incision is performed through all layers of the abdominal wall. For hysterotomy, a midline longitudinal incision is performed with a scalpel and extended caudally with scissors while the non-dominant hand protects the foetus. Placenta, bladder, and other structures can be incised as all collateral damage will be repaired later should the mother survive. Once delivered, the mouth and nose of the newborn are suctioned holding the head down, the cord is clamped and cut, and the infant is resuscitated as necessary. A foetal survival rate greater than 60% with favourable neurological outcome has been reported. Maternal revival after peri-mortem caesarean section has also been reported in a few instances, presumably due to relief of vena cava compression.

The criteria for ED caesarean section (all must apply):
- Uterine size above umbilicus.
- Foetal heart beat documented (Doppler, FAST).
- Maternal CPR not longer than 10 min.

Keys to efficient foetal delivery are:
- Continued CPR of the mother.
- Not clamping the aorta.
- Large midline vertical incision through all layers (xipho-pubic).
- Large midline vertical incision through upper uterine segment.
- Suctioning, cord clamping, and early transfer of the infant to neonatal intensive care.

The haemodynamically normal patient

For the haemodynamically normal pregnant patient, the following should be ascertained:
- Length of gestation.
- Any complications during gestation.
- Previous pregnancies, deliveries, miscarriages.
- Whether the foetus moved following the injury?

It is important that there is no delay in the correct diagnosis and initiation of treatment is prompt. There are several anatomical and physiological modifications that occur in pregnancy, and it is important to be aware of these changes to avoid errors in assessment and management. Increased blood volume and enhanced cardiac output of the pregnant patient can easily mask hypovolaemia. As much as 30% (2 L) of maternal blood volume can be lost before haemodynamic instability is suggested by tachycardia and hypotension.

Secondary survey

The secondary survey is carried out as normal. With regard to vaginal examination, this is usually performed by an obstetrician or gynaecologist. Blood in the vagina may suggest placental abruption or physical violence. Any fluid other than blood needs to be tested for pH (pH around 7 may indicate amniotic fluid (from traumatic rupture of membranes), whereas a pH around 5 is indicative of normal vaginal secretion). The fornix requires thorough speculum examination (possibly under general anaesthesia) to exclude perforations that would mandate a laparotomy to identify possible bowel injuries.

When sexual assault is reported or suspected, forensic medicine procedures should also be followed.

Specific conditions

Penetrating abdominal trauma

Most authors advocate exploratory laparotomy whenever the peritoneum is penetrated, although some have suggested conservative management for low-velocity penetrating injuries, proposing laparotomy for worsening maternal symptoms. Laparotomy is relatively well tolerated and is preferable to the sequels of a delayed diagnosis. In the haemodynamically normal patient with an anterior abdominal stab wound, peritoneal bridging can be diagnosed either by local wound exploration under local anaesthesia, or by diagnostic laparoscopy. Local wound exploration is particularly effective in the thin and co-operative patient.

Placental abruption

Placental abruption is the second most common cause of foetal mortality in trauma. The incidence varies between 20 and 50%, and can be even higher in those who survive major trauma, while it is in the order of 1–5% in minor trauma.

Even minor abdominal trauma may compress and deform the elastic myometrium. This may exert a shearing force on the fibrous and rigid placental villi, which can rupture small placental sinuses, causing small retroplacental clots. The high local concentration of thromboplastin in trophoblastic tissue may lead to the expansion of the clot. If this process continues, eventually a complete placental separation can occur.

The early stages may be totally asymptomatic. Clinical findings may include abdominal cramps, uterine tenderness, amniotic fluid leakage, and maternal hypovolaemia out of proportion to visible bleeding. Up to 2 L of maternal blood can accumulate in the uterus and cause maternal shock (uterus will be larger than expected based on gestational age). Only 35% of clinically significant placental abruptions manifest with vaginal bleeding.

Placental abruption involving more than 50% of the placenta is frequently associated with foetal death. It is also noteworthy that placental abruption can lead to a consumptive coagulopathy.

Both screening and diagnosis of placental abruption can be achieved by long term (4–24 h) CTG monitoring revealing uterine activity or abnormal foetal heart rate. Ultrasound and the KB test are poor predictors of placental abruption.

Uterine rupture

Uterine rupture is rare, but carries a grave outcome for the foetus. It occurs in less than 1% of blunt abdominal trauma in pregnancy, but is associated with almost 100% foetal mortality and 10% maternal mortality (in most cases due to concomitant maternal injury). It is most frequent and usually anterior in patients with a previous uterine scar.

Asymptomatic myometrial defects may lead to rupture later in pregnancy, particularly during labour.

Clinical findings of uterine rupture include:

- Subtle or marked uterine tenderness.
- Bladder injury.
- Maternal hypotension.
- Palpation of foetal parts.
- Amniotic fluid embolism.

Traumatic rupture of membranes

Rupture of membranes secondary to trauma requires a careful search for concomitant injuries, with prolonged foetal monitoring strongly advocated, since the incidence of concomitant placental abruption is high. In the absence of maternal or foetal compromise, it is usually managed in the same way as spontaneous rupture of membranes.

Foetal maternal haemorrhage

Foetal maternal haemorrhage (FMH) occurs with the passage of foetal blood into the maternal circulation. It frequently occurs in pregnant women who have suffered injury, but it may also occur in other non-traumatic circumstances. The reported incidence of FMH in trauma patients is 8–30%, and for pregnancies not complicated by trauma it is 2–8%. Anterior placental location and uterine tenderness are associated with an increased risk.

FMH occurs more commonly after 12 weeks of gestation when the uterus rises out of the pelvis and becomes susceptible to direct trauma. FMH can lead to foetal anaemia, foetal paroxysmal tachycardia, foetal exsanguination, pre-term labour and foetal death. Maternal Rhesus sensitization occurs in 70% of Rh-negative women following the transplacental passage of as little as 1 mL of Rh-positive blood.

All unsensitized Rh-negative pregnant patients who present with a history of abdominal trauma should receive a prophylactic dose of Rhesus immunoglobulin regardless of KB testing results. A 300 µg dose will be protective against exposure to as much as 15 mL of foetal red cells. The KB test is then repeated at 24–48 h to investigate for continuing FMH.

The first immunoglobulin dose must be administered within 72 h to prevent erythrocyte alloimmunization and the development of *erythroblastosis foetalis* during subsequent pregnancies.

Amniotic fluid embolus

This is a rare cause of disseminated intravascular coagulopathy (DIC). More commonly, DIC is seen in conjunction with placental abruption and a retained dead foetus.

Post-exposure prophylaxis (PEP) following sexual assault

When a pregnant woman, as any other individual, is victim of a sexual assault, an additional element of concern is that she may have been exposed to one or more infectious pathogens as a consequence of the crime. The infectious agents that should be considered are described in Table 21.2. The patient ideally needs to be assessed and treated by a specialized team who are trained to provide psychological support, to counsel about emergency contraception if appropriate, and also to offer anti-infective prophylaxis.

Current guidelines, particularly those issued by the Centres for Disease Control and Prevention in the USA suggest that appropriate broad-range PEP should be offered to all the victims of sexual assaults.

Deep vein thrombosis prophylaxis

Pregnancy is a characterized by a state of hypercoagulability. This, combined with the insult of trauma, predisposes the pregnant trauma patient to venous thrombo-embolic disease. Prophylactic low molecular weight heparin,

Table 21.2. Some infections that may be acquired as a result of sexual assault and prophylaxis options

Infection	Level of risk	Options for prophylaxis
Bacterial vaginosis	High	Antibacterial drugs[1]
Neisseria gonorrhoeae	Intermediate	
Chlamidia trachomatis	Intermediate	
Trichomonas vaginalis	Intermediate	
Treponema pallidum	Low	
Human immunodeficiency virus	Low	Antiretrovirals[2]
Hepatitis B virus	Low	HBV immune globulin Vaccination (3 doses) Antiviral drugs[3]
Hepatitis C virus	Very low	None currently available
Herpes simplex virus type 2	?	None currently available
Human papillomaviruses	?	Vaccination?[4]
Haemophilus ducreyi (chancroid)[5]	Generally low	Antibacterial drugs
Calymmatobacterium granulomatis (granuloma inguinale)[5]	Generally low	
Chlamidia trachomatis serovars L1, L2, L3 (lymphogranuloma venereum)[5]	Generally low	

[1] Certain antibacterial regimens are effective against multiple infections. The regimen recommended by CDC includes ceftriazone 125 mg im, metronidazole 2 g per os, and azithromycin 1 g per os in single doses. In pregnant women, avoid doxycycline and use metranidazole only after the first trimester.

[2] In pregnant women, efavirenz, as well as other drugs that may unfavourably impact on the baby, should be avoided.

[3] HBV prophylaxis should be given only to persons who have no documented previous immunity. Vaccine alone is believed to protect adequately and should be administered within 24 h from assault.

[4] Vaccination against selected human papillomaviruses has been introduced only in recent years and is currently administered to preadolescent girls only. Given its success in this population, it should also be evaluated as a potential PEP tool.

[5] Extremely rare in industrialized countries.

pneumatic compression devices, and early ambulation are of paramount importance to avoid the complication of deep vein thrombosis.

Conclusion

After injury during pregnancy, the key to a successful outcome for both the mother and the child is prompt, and adequate initial assessment and resuscitation of the mother. All patients with minor trauma should be admitted to hospital for at least 24 h and receive 4 h CTG monitoring. Those with major trauma always require careful foetal monitoring. If maternal resuscitation fails, an urgent perimortem caesarean section may save the life of the foetus.

Frequently asked questions

Will the seat belt hurt my baby?
Correct placement of the lap belt is under the pregnant abdomen over the bony prominences of the pelvis with the shoulder harness placed between the breasts. An incorrectly placed lap belt over the dome of the uterus increases the risk of uterine and foetal injury. If driving, the woman should sit at least 10 inches from the steering wheel. The wheel should be tilted towards the chest and away from abdomen. Airbags should not be disabled.

Can I exercise?
Physical activity during pregnancy is beneficial within sensible limits. However, in the last trimester, increased body weight in conjunction with hormonal changes lead to increased joint laxity and hypermobility, placing the pregnant woman at increased risk of injury.

Further reading

Aboutanos SZ, Aboutanos MB, Malhotra AK, Duane TM, Ivatury RR (2005). Management of a Pregnant Patient with an Open Abdomen. *J Trauma* 2005; **59**: 1052–6.

American College of Obstetricians-Gynecologists. Practice Bulletin. Clinical Management Guidelines for Obstetrician-Gynecologists. *Obstet Gynecol* 2006; **107**: 957–62.

Bochicchio GV, Haan J, Scalea TM. Surgeon-performed focused assessment with sonography for trauma as an early screening tool for pregnancy after trauma. *J Trauma* 2002; **52**: 1125–8.

Cahill AG, Bastek JA, Stamilio DM, Odibo AO, Stevens E, Macones GA. Minor trauma in pregnancy—is the evaluation unwarranted? *Am J Obstet Gynecol* 2008; **198**: 208–15.

Centers for Disease Control and Prevention. Sexual assault—Sexually transmitted diseases treatment guidelines *2006*. Available at: www.cdc.gov/std/treatment/2006/sexual-assault.htm

Dhanraj D, Lambers D. The incidences of positive Kleinhauer-Betke test in low-risk pregnancies and maternal trauma patients. *Am J Obstet Gynecol* 2004; **190**: 1461–3.

Eastern Association for the Surgery of Trauma. EAST Practice Management Guidelines Work Group. Diagnosis and Management of Injury in the Pregnant Patient. Available at: http://www.east.org/tpg/pregnancy.pdf.

Greene W, Robinson L, Rizzo AG, Sakran J, Hendershot K, Moore A, et al. Pregnancy is not a sufficient indicator for trauma team activation. *J Trauma* 2007; **63**: 550–5.

Ikossi DG, Lazar AA, Morabito D, Fildes J, Knudson MM. Profile of mothers at risk: an analysis of injury and pregnancy loss in 1,195 trauma patients. *J Am Coll Surg* 2005; **200**: 49–56.

Mattox KL, Goetzl L. Trauma in pregnancy. *Crit Care Med* 2005; **33**: 385–9.

McCollough CH, Schueler BA, Atwell TD, Braun NN, Regner DM, Brown DL, et al. Radiation exposure and pregnancy: when should we be concerned? *Radiographics* 2007; **27**: 909–18.

Muench MV, Baschat AA, Reddy UM, Mighty HE, Weiner CP, Scalea TM, et al. Kleihauer-Betke. Testing is important in all cases of maternal trauma. *J Trauma* 2004; **57**: 1094–8.

Pearlman MD, Tintinalli JE, Lorenz RP. A prospective controlled study of outcome after trauma during pregnancy. *Am J Obstet Gynecol* 1990; **62**: 1502–10.

Schiff MA, Holt VL. The injury severity score in pregnant trauma patients: predicting placental abruption and fetal death. *J Trauma* 2002; **53**: 946–9.

Sperry JL, Casey BM, McIntire DD, Minei JP, Gentilello LM, Shafi S. Long-term fetal outcomes in pregnant trauma patients. *Am J Surg* 2006; **192**: 715–21.

Burn injuries

Burn injuries

Definition

A burn is an injury from thermal, electrical, chemical or radiation energy resulting in the loss of some or all of the layers of the skin.

Burn injury is common, but fortunately most burns are minor and cause only inconvenience. Every year, however, a significant number of patients suffer burns that will have a dramatic effect on the rest of their lives. In the United Kingdom, around 300 people die of burns every year. In less developed countries, death or severe injury from burns is much more common.

Functions of the skin

The skin is the largest organ of the body. In order to appreciate the problems associated with damage to this organ, one must be aware of the key functions which have the potential to be disrupted:

- *Thermoregulation.* vasodilatation or constriction, under neural and paracrine control, allow dissipation, or conservation of body heat. Loss of this function, and destruction of sweat glands, contribute to the impaired thermoregulation seen in burns.
- *Barrier to water loss.* the tightly packed cells of the stratum corneum of the epidermis act as an efficient barrier to water loss. If this barrier is lost, interstitial fluid can escape as exudate. This protein-rich exudate is an ideal culture medium for micro-organisms.
- *Barrier to infection.*
  - *physical*—intact skin is a mechanical barrier to bacterial invasion;
  - *immunological*—as well as white cells from its blood supply, Langerhans cells are present in-between the keratinocytes. These capture and process microbial antigens, and present them to T-cells.
- A physical barrier from trauma.
- *Psychological:* the appearance of the skin, particularly of the face and hands, is very important in social interaction and psychological well-being.
- *Sensation:* touch, pain and temperature sensation allow the patient to experience the outside world.
- *Protection from radiation:* loss of melanocyte-derived pigmentation will prevent radiation induced injury. Sun protection is therefore vital until normal pigmentation returns.

Management priorities

Stop the burning

If the patient is still on fire, needless to say the fire needs to be extinguished. Burning clothes must be extinguished or removed. For chemical burns, stopping the burning can only be achieved by removing the chemical.

Cool the wound

It has been well demonstrated in animal studies that cooling the burn wound can lessen the degree of damage (Fig. 22.1). Applying cold tap water for 10 min will reduce the temperature of the injured tissue back to within physiological limits. Of course, the temperature of water from the cold tap varies from country to country, and from season to season. Cooling for more than 10 min is not necessary. Clean water is preferable to dirty water, but dirty

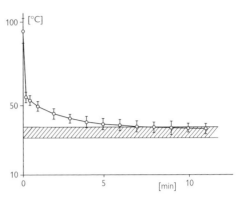

Fig. 22.1. Effect of cold water on burn wound temperature (Moserova 1973).

water is preferable to no water. If more than 30 min has passed since the time of the burn, cooling is not likely to have any effect on the degree of injury as the damage will already be done, but cooling will still be soothing for the patient. Care must be taken to ensure that the patient does not become hypothermic. Children are at particular risk of hypothermia. Sheets and blankets may be used to protect the patient against hypothermia. Once the burn is cooled, protection with cling film should be applied.

There is no place for the use of the various gel dressings in the cooling of burns. These dressings, much loved by the people that sell them, are much less effective than cold water at cooling, and can act as a heat sink, prolonging the thermal injury.

Determine the mechanism of injury

If the patient is conscious, a full history of the mechanism of the injury must be obtained. An experienced burn surgeon will often make the treatment plan based on the history, with examination of the patient merely adding confirmation.

At temperatures as low as 45°C, denaturation of proteins and other vital cellular molecules causes first cellular dysfunction, then cellular death. As the insult continues, the depth of the damage increases.

Young children are more susceptible to the effects of burn injury. They have thinner skin and are less aware of the dangers around them. Sadly, they are also may be subject to deliberate harm.

Scalds

Scalds are caused by contact with hot liquid or steam. They are more common in children. Typically, an inquisitive toddler sees something interesting above it, just within reach. They grab the kettle or pan, and suffer a cascade burn to the face, neck, shoulder, and chest (Fig. 22.2). It is very worthwhile eliciting an exact history. The depth of the burn will depend on how hot the liquid was, how thick or sticky, and how good the first aid was. Tea with milk added seldom produces a deep burn.

Flame burns

These are more common in adults and are nearly always deep dermal or full thickness.

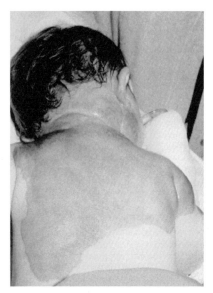

Fig. 22.2. A typical scald in a toddler.

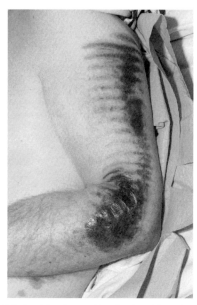

Fig. 22.4. Burn injury from prolonged contact with a radiator.

Flash burns

These are caused by brief exposure to intense thermal radiation. They are limited to exposed skin.

Contact burns

These result from brief contact with a very hot surface (e.g. an iron; Fig. 22.3), or prolonged contact with a less hot surface (e.g. a patient who collapses against a radiator; Fig. 22.4). Prolonged contact can cause very deep burns.

Chemical burns

These burns occur when the skin is exposed to a reactive chemical substance. The degree of damage depends on the type, quantity, and the concentration of the agent, and the timing and effectiveness of the first aid. Chemical injury to the eye is particularly serious and needs urgent wash-out and ophthalmological referral.

Strong acids tend to cause 'coagulative necrosis', as denatured protein forms a hard eschar, limiting further penetration of the acid.

Hydrofluoric acid (HFl) produces burns that are very painful. This acid is commonly used by industry as a cleaning and etching agent. As this acid is poorly dissociated, the hydrogen ion often only produces a superficial burn, but with stronger concentrations full thickness burns can occur. The fluoride ion penetrates the skin, binding with calcium. This causes pain, and can cause significant hypocalcaemia. Penetration of the skin is easier at certain sites (e.g. subungual), and in areas previously affected by minor abrasion, as the incomplete keratinization offers less protection. Death has occurred after a HFl burn of just 2% total body surface area (TBSA). In cases of burn from HFl over 50% in strength, or burn of over 5%TBSA from HFl of any strength, it is recommended that the patient undergo ECG monitoring, and serum calcium levels should be measured.

Strong alkalis cause 'colliquative necrosis'. The slough formed is softer, and allows deeper penetration of the tissues. The burn has a 'soapy' appearance, due to the saponification of the triglyceride fats.

Management The simplest and most widely available form of treatment is dilution with water. The speed of such dilution is important, as once the chemical is bound to the tissues water will be ineffective.

A few chemicals have specific antidotes which are recommended for use. One example of an antidote is calcium gluconate gel, which is used in the treatment of hydrofluoric acid burns, and which should be available at the workplace where this acid is used. Recently, universal antidotes, such as diphoterine have been recognized as effective treatment for a variety of chemical burns. Such amphoteric compounds are able to bind to the chemical agent so strongly that even when the chemical is bound to the tissues it can still be removed.

Electrical burns

Kouwenhoven described the six factors that determine the extent of an electrical injury:
• The type of current (AC or DC).
• The voltage.

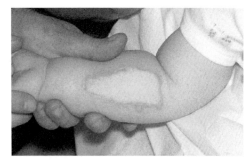

Fig. 22.3. A contact burn from an iron.

- The current.
- The duration of exposure.
- The resistance.
- The pathway of the current.

The heat produced (and, therefore, the damage) is more dependant on the current than the resistance. Therefore, tissues with a lower resistance (such as blood vessels and nerves) will heat up more than tissues with a high resistance (such as bone), and will sustain more damage.

Low voltage injuries occur from sources less than 1000 V, and are commonly sustained in the home. The burns are usually small, but can penetrate to deep structures. A 12-lead ECG should be performed, as dysrhythmias can occur. If the ECG is normal and if there has been no loss of consciousness, further dysrhythmias are unlikely to develop.

High voltage injuries are more commonly obtained in the work place and can produce devastating injuries. In between the entry and exit wounds, serious muscle and nerve damage can occur. This terminology is not particularly accurate in the face of alternating current, and it is more accurate to describe a 'contact point with electrical source' and a 'contact point with the grounding site'. Fasciotomies may be necessary, and renal impairment from rhabdomyolysis must be sought and treated. These injuries are often associated with flash or flame burns. Fractures and dislocations may also be present, caused either by tetanic muscle contractions or by falling or being thrown. Demyelination of the spinal cord, cataracts, and seizures are all possible sequelae from these injuries.

Lightning may cause burns from the direct passage of current (over 10 million V) through the body, from the vaporization of water in the (often) wet clothing, or from the ignition of clothing. The current may come directly from above, or via a side strike from a nearby object, such as a tree. A direct strike has a mortality rate of about 30%. Lichtenberg figures are fern-like patterns of erythema, which usually resolve within 24 h of injury, but if present are pathognomonic of lightning injury.

Frostbite
Although not technically a burn, the mechanism of injury in frostbite is similar—molecular and cellular damage leading to tissue disruption. Hypothermia should be treated with rapid, active rewarming. Anti-inflammatory and analgesic medication should be given. Care of the affected part is usually conservative, with a priority to prevent infection until demarcation takes place.

Inhalational injury
The presence of an inhalational injury will worsen the chances of survival following burn injury. Fibre optic bronchoscopy is more accurate than clinical examination alone in diagnosing the extent of any inhalational injury, and can help remove debris.

The airway can be affected by burn injury in the following ways:

Thermal injury to the upper airways
This is caused by the heat of the air that the patient was exposed to. The lips, tongue, oral, and pharyngeal mucosa swell and the patency of the airway can be threatened. This swelling can occur rapidly. High flow oxygen should be administered. If upper airway swelling is suspected, the most senior airway physician available should assess the patient immediately, as intubation becomes increasingly difficult as the swelling increases. The need to transfer

the patient to a distant unit will lower the threshold for intubation.

The endotracheal tube should not be cut short due to the propensity for tissues to swell. Once in place, the tube must be secured, as loss of the tube once the swelling has fully developed would be potentially disastrous, particularly if it occurred in the back of an ambulance. The tube may be secured by using ribbon tape or ideally by wiring the tube to a tooth.

Chemical injury to the lower airways
Smoke from fires, particularly where man-made substances are burned (carpets, curtains, furniture), contains many chemicals, which will dissolve in the fluid of the mucous membranes lining the lower airways to form acids and alkalis. These will produce a chemical burn, and along with the inhaled soot, will cause irritation, and inflammation.

Systemic intoxication
The two main culprits are:
- *Carbon monoxide (CO)*: this colourless, odourless gas results from the incomplete oxidation of carbonaceous material. The affinity of haemoglobin for CO is 240 times that for oxygen. The presence of carboxyhaemoglobin (HbCO) will reduce the oxygen carrying capacity of the blood, and even small amounts of carbon monoxide can result in a significant reduction in the oxygen carrying capacity. For example, if the carbon monoxide concentration in the air is just 0.1%, the blood would contain equal amounts of oxyhaemoglobin and HbCO. The affinity of cardiac myoglobin for CO is even higher, exacerbating the situation. Symptoms will increase as the HbCO levels (expressed as a percentage of the total haemoglobin available) increase (Fig. 22.5).

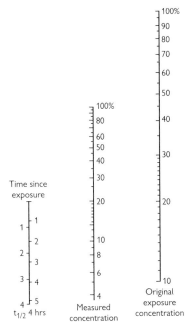

Fig. 22.5. Carboxyhaemoglobin extrapolation nomogram.

Blood should be taken for HbCO levels as soon as possible, and extrapolation backwards will allow an estimation of the HbCO levels at the time of the injury (see Table 22.1). The half-life of HbCO is 4 h. This is reduced to 45 min if 100% oxygen is given, and this is the recommended treatment. The role of hyperbaric oxygen therapy is controversial.

• *Hydrogen cyanide (HCN):* combustion of nitrogen containing polymers, often found in man-made fibres, will produce HCN. HCN inhibits cytochrome oxidase, preventing cellular utilization of oxygen. Symptoms include headache, nausea, loss of consciousness, convulsions, and ultimately death. HCN is metabolized by the liver. Although specific antidotes are available, they are themselves toxic and, hence, they are not commonly used.

Do not forget to examine for other injuries

Large burns can appear dramatic, but attention must be given to excluding other life-threatening injuries. People suffering from burn injuries may have sustained other injuries from extrication (e.g. jumping from a window), direct injury (e.g. from falling masonry) or blast injury. A full secondary survey, including trauma series X-rays, should be undertaken if appropriate.

Table 22.1. Symptoms of HbCO exposure

HbCO levels	Symptoms
0–10%	No symptoms
10–20%	Headache, confusion
20–40%	Nausea, fatigue, disorientation
40–60%	Hallucination, convulsion, coma
>60%	Death

Assessment of the extent of burn

Assessment of the area of cutaneous burn is expressed as a percentage of the Total Body Surface Area (%TBSA). The four most common ways of estimating this value are:

Palm of the hand = 1%TBSA

It is the hand of the patient including the thumb, not the examiner, that must be used. Oriental patients have proportionally smaller hands, representing approximately 0.75%TBSA.

Wallace's rule of nines

Although simple to remember, the inaccuracy of this assessment is amplified in children, who have proportionally bigger heads and smaller legs than adults. This method can be used in conjunction with the 'palm = 1%' rule, e.g. if all of one upper limb apart from one palm's worth is burned, then the burn is 8% TBSA (Fig. 22.6).

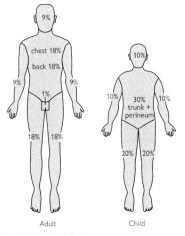

Fig. 22.6. Wallace's rule of nines.

Lund and Browder charts

These offer a more accurate breakdown of the various body parts. Charts reflecting different ages are available (Fig. 22.7).

Serial halving

This is a useful tool in the pre-hospital assessment of burns, as it allows staff to quickly determine the severity of the burn, and to take decisions about which hospital the patient should be taken to.

Assessment of the depth of burn

It is unusual to find that a burn that is uniform in depth. More commonly, some areas (those closest to the source of injury) are deeper, surrounded by more superficial burns. Assessment of burn wound depth is important as it dictates the best treatment, as well as predicting the ultimate outcome.

In 1953 Douglas Jackson (from the Birmingham Accident Hospital) described a classification system for burn injury,

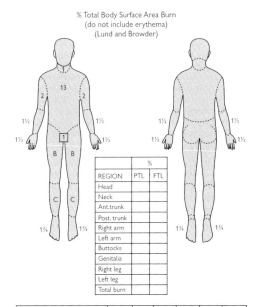

% Total Body Surface Area Burn
(do not include erythema)
(Lund and Browder)

REGION	% PTL	% FTL
Head		
Neck		
Ant.trunk		
Post. trunk		
Right arm		
Left arm		
Buttocks		
Genitalia		
Right leg		
Left leg		
Total burn		

AREA	Age 0	1	5	10	15	Adult
A-1½ OF HEAD	9½	8½	6½	5½	4½	3½
B-1½ OF ONE HEAD	2¾	3¼	4	4½	4½	4¾
C-½ OF ONE LOWER LEG	2½	2½	2¾	3	3¼	3½

Fig. 22.7. Lund and Browder Chart.

which is still in use today. He described three zones: the central area of the burn consists of coagulated tissue, and is clearly dead and unsalvageable. Surrounding this is an area he called the 'zone of stasis', where cells have been injured to a certain extent but may survive if conditions are optimal (Fig. 22.8). Suboptimal conditions, such as infection, reduced nutrition (e.g. in hypoperfusion states or oedema), desiccation, or other co-morbid factors may tip the balance in favour of necrosis or apoptosis for the cells in this layer. Outside this is the 'zone of hyperaemia', which is affected by the release of numerous inflammatory mediators by the dead and dying cells.

- *Epidermal burns:* in these burns, only the epidermis is injured, with no dermal loss. Erythema is evident, but no blistering. This erythema should not be included in the estimation of the %TBSA involved.
- *Superficial dermal burns:* these blister, but the blistering may not develop immediately. The roof of the blister consists of dead epidermis and dermis. When the

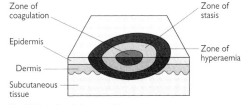

Fig. 22.8. Jackson's burn model.

blister roof is missing, the burn appears red, is tender, and blanches when touched (use a sterile wound swab) (Fig. 22.9).

- *Mid-dermal burns:* the deeper adnexal structures, such as hair follicles and sweat glands (which are lined with epidermal cells), are preserved, so healing can still take place without scarring (Fig. 22.10).
- *Deep dermal burns:* these burns appear white, as dead dermal collagen is visible (Fig. 22.11). Red patches of fixed staining may be present, representing haemoglobin trapped in thrombosed capillaries. There is no blanching and these burns are insensate.
- *Full thickness burns:* all of the dermis is burned (Fig. 22.12). The skin has a leathery appearance, and is insensate. The skin feels firm or hard to the touch.

Laser Doppler Imaging (LDI) currently offers the gold standard in determining the depth of a burn. It uses Doppler to detect and measure the movement of haemoglobin (and, therefore, the circulation of blood) within the upper layers of the skin and allows accurate prediction of healing times. These machines are currently very expensive and, hence, tend to be located in bigger, well-funded burn centres.

Fluid resuscitation

Capillary leak occurs after burn injury, due to a local and systemic inflammatory response. Mediators including histamine are responsible for the disruption of the normal capillary barrier separating the intravascular and the interstitial compartments. In small burns, this capillary leakage is confined to the burned areas. In burns of over about 25% TBSA, the systemic spread of inflammatory mediators means that this leakage also occurs throughout the body, in unburned sites. To prevent hypovolaemic shock following burn injury, it is recommended that intravenous fluid resuscitation be commenced in burns of 10% or over in children, and in burns of over 15% in adults. Two large bore cannulae should be inserted, ideally through unburned tissue in the upper limbs. Fluid balance should be monitored and catheterization may be necessary to measure urine output.

Because the fluid lost following burn injury is to some extent predictable, various formulae have been developed to guide fluid replacement. In the UK, the formula in most common use is the Parkland formula, which recommends administration of Hartmann's solution at 4 mL/kg/%TBSA over 24 h. Half of this volume should be given over the first 8 h and the second half over the next 16 h. It must be remembered that this is a guide only, and should be tailored to the clinical state of the patient. The urine output

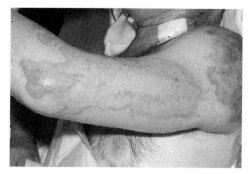

Fig. 22.10. Mid-dermal burn.

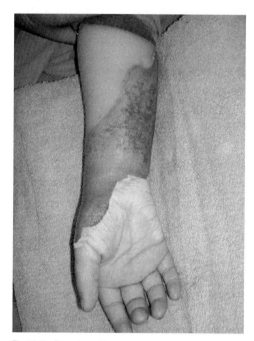

Fig. 22.11. Deep dermal burn.

is a simple representation of tissue perfusion, and should be maintained at between 0.5 and 1.0 mL/kg/h in adults, and between 1.0 and 1.5 mL/kg/h in children. Persistent metabolic acidosis may also indicate inadequate resuscitation.

Circumferential burns

As deep dermal or full thickness burns dry out, the burned skin shrinks and becomes rigid. If the burn is circumferential around a limb, this results in a tight leathery band around the limb. At the same time, oedema as described above will make the soft tissues swell. These two factors add up to reduce tissue perfusion in the limb. As capillary pressure (16–32 mmHg) is much lower than arterial blood pressure, significant reduction in tissue perfusion can occur despite a palpable (or audible on Doppler) pulse. It is sometimes difficult to assess the limb distally for the

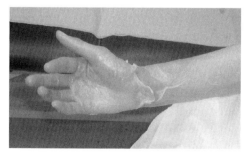

Fig. 22.9. Superficial dermal burn.

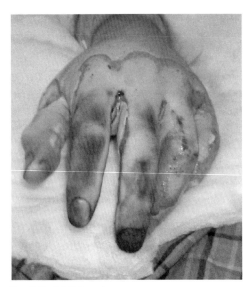

Fig. 22.12. Full thickness burn.

adequacy of the circulation, as the limb is burned, and soot and blister debris may obscure the examination. It is important to spend time cleaning off the debris, get good light, and examine the limb in detail. Capillary refill time should be sought in unburned (or superficially burned) areas. Unburned areas may sometimes be found between fingers and toes. Elevation of the limbs may reduce the swelling sufficiently in cases where the constriction is not fully circumferential, or the burns are not full thickness. Otherwise incision through the constricting eschar (escharotomy) will be required. If the patient is being transferred to a distant burn centre, escharotomy should be performed prior to transfer.

Circumferential full thickness burn around the chest may inhibit chest wall movement, and hence reduce respiration. If the patient is being ventilated, the pressures required to maintain ventilation will be seen to increase. This situation also requires escharotomy. Young children, who rely on diaphragmatic movements for ventilation, may require escharotomy of the abdomen to allow this.

Escharotomy

Like all operations, the best location in which to perform these is in an operating theatre, where there is adequate space, lighting, and assistance, as well as access to diathermy and dressings. The site should be prepared aseptically. The surgeon should be experienced in performing escharotomies and, hence, in the majority of the developed world these will be performed by burn surgeons in burn centres. If there are difficulties with transporting the patient (such as is the case in rural Australia or in many third world countries), then escharotomy may need to be performed as a limb saving emergency.

Limbs

It is recommended that the eschar is released using medial and lateral incisions, with the limb placed in the anatomical position.

Chest

If facilities (theatre, staff, experience, time) allow, these constrictions may be treated more efficiently by performing an escharectomy (removal of the eschar), rather than simply releasing it. Full thickness burns require excision, and this technique is practised in some of the larger burn centres (Fig. 22.13).

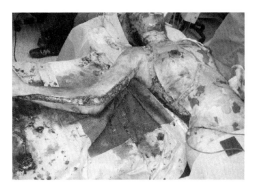

Fig. 22.13. Limb and torso escharotomies.

Mortality data

Mortality and morbidity from major burns has improved over the past 30 years, primarily as a result of better resuscitation, earlier wound closure, better control of infection, and dedicated intensive care support. A large study from the USA showed that the three most important risk factors for death following burn injury were age over 60 years, burns over 40% TBSA, and the presence of inhalational injury. The mortality rate was dependent on the number of these risk factors pre-sent, as shown in Table 22.2.

Table 22.2. Risk factors for death following burn injury

No. of risk factors present	Mortality rate (%)
0	0.3
1	3
2	33
3	90

Non-accidental injury

It is unfortunate that vulnerable patients of all ages are subject to deliberate injury from those who are closest to them. Typically, young children are the commonest group affected, but all age groups of vulnerable patients can suffer in this way. Clinicians should always be suspicious of burns in these groups, particularly if there is:
- Delay in presentation.
- Inconsistency in histories given to different health workers.
- Discrepancy between the pattern of injury and the history as described.
- Circumferential distal limb injuries with no splash marks.

A detailed history should be obtained and recorded, good quality photographs taken, and the patient should be referred to a specialist centre that has the facilities, time and expertise to investigate further.

Analgesia

Burns can be very painful, and this pain will increase the hypermetabolic response to the burn injury. Initially, the pain from a burn can be treated by cooling the burn with cold tap water. After this, covering the burn with cling film will help to reduce pain. However, administration of analgesia should not be delayed and many patients will require intravenous opiate analgesia to control their initial symptoms.

Application of dressings

Before any dressings are applied, the wound must be cleaned with soap and water. Clingfilm will protect the wound from further contamination, as well as helping prevent further evaporative and heat loss. It must be applied in sheets and not wrapped around a limb or torso. It is also easy to remove by the burn centre staff. Antimicrobial dressings are prone to stain the burn wound, particularly creams such as flamazine and flammacerium, and as such may make assessment of the depth of the injury difficult. These should, therefore, not be applied until the wound has been assessed by the burn surgeon. Rarely (in the developed world), it may be impossible to get the burn wound seen at a burn unit within 24 h. In these circumstances, preferably after consultation with the burn unit, dressings with antimicrobial activity may need to be applied.

The use of prophylactic antibiotics is not recommended.

Feeding

In major burns patients a nasogastric tube should be inserted to decompress the stomach. Burn injury results in a hypermetabolic state, more so than any other trauma. Enteral feeding has been shown to be protective to the gut mucosa, preventing bacterial and endotoxin translocation, and should be started as soon as possible. It is also the best prophylaxis against stress ulcers. Parenteral nutrition should be avoided in burns if at all possible as the complication rate is very high.

Tetanus

Like any wound with tissue damage, burns are prone to tetanus and suitable prophylaxis needs to be sought, after the wound has been cleaned.

Toxic shock syndrome

This is a rare life-threatening condition. It is occasionally seen after a burn of any size, after infection with microorganisms which produce 'super antigens', which can activate T-cells directly, without the need for antigen presenting cells. The clinical features are high fever, shock, vomiting, diarrhoea, rash, disseminated intravasclar coagulation, and ultimately multi-organ failure. Patients should be resuscitated and transferred to a specialist burn centre.

Transfer principles

In the UK, there has been rationalization and centralisation of burn services in order to concentrate and develop expertise. The National Burn Care Review has produced guidelines for which burns need to be referred for specialist assessment and management. These are summarised in Fig. 22.14.

If the patient has other injuries, ideally the patient should be transferred to a hospital that has all the relevant specialties on site. This may not be feasible, and discussion with the relevant clinicians will be needed in order to prioritize the injuries. For example, a small burn with a serious head injury will be best served by transportation to a neurosurgical unit, whereas a big burn with a broken ankle should go to the burn centre.

Transportation

After consulting the burn centre, the most appropriate mode of transport for the patient should be selected. Air transport should be considered for a long distance transfer. Unless a retrieval team is being sent by the receiving unit, the well-being of the patient is the responsibility of the referring unit until they are delivered to the burn centre. The patient should be kept warm during the transfer. All documentation, including details of any treatment (including fluid) given, should be sent with the patient. If there is any concern about the airway, or the burn is major, the patient should be accompanied by a doctor who has the appropriate skills. Helicopter transfers, although quicker, are not without problems. Noise, limited space, and the inability to heat the cabin are all disadvantages.

Referring the Acutely Burned Patient to a Burn Unit or Centre

Key Question: Is the injury large and/or complex (including patient factors)?

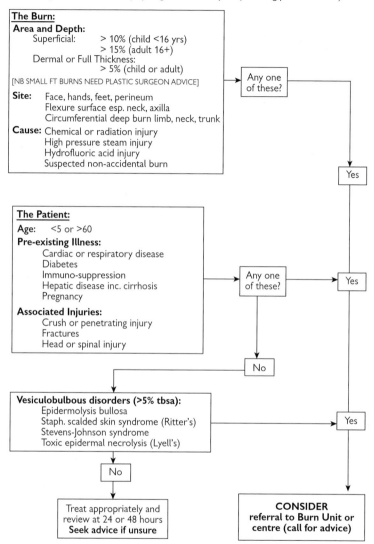

Fig. 22.14. Burn referral guidelines.

Further reading

Clark CJ, Campbell D, Reid WH. Blood carboxyhaemoglobin and cyanide levels in fire survivors. *Lancet* 1981; **1**: 1332.

Emergency management of severe burns (EMSB) course. Details can be found at www.britishburnassociation.co.uk.

Jackson DM. The diagnosis of the depth of burning. *Br J Surg* 1953; **40**: 588–96.

Kouwenhoven WB. Effects of electricity on the human body. *Ind Med Surg* 1949; **18**: 269.

La Hei ER, Holland AJ, Martin HC. Laser Doppler imaging of paediatric burns: burn wound outcome can be predicted inde-pendent of clinical examination. *Burns* 2006; **32**: 550–3.

Moritz A, Henriquez FC. Studies of thermal injury II. *Am J Pathol* 1947; **23**: 695–720.

Moserova J, Prouza Z. Standard non-contact burn. Subcutaneous temperature dynamics during a thermal injury. *Acta Chir Plast* 1973; **15**: 247–57.

Ryan CM, Schoenfeld DA, Thorpe WP, Sheridan RL, Cassem EH, Tompkins RG. Objective estimates of the probability of death from burn injuries. *N Engl J Med* 1998; **338**: 362–6.

Smith JJ, Malyon AD, Scerri GV, Burge TS. A comparison of serial halving and the rule of nines as a pre-hospital assessment tool in burns. *Br J Plast Surg* 2005; **58**: 957–67.

Penetrating torso injury

Penetrating injuries

Penetrating injuries are infrequent in the UK, although there has been a significant recent increase in major urban areas. As they are uncommon, there is a lack of experience among clinicians in the UK in dealing with these injuries, which mandates that a cautious standardised approach is taken with all patients sustaining such injuries.

The common forms of penetrating injuries involve stabbing with knives and other sharp implements (such as screwdrivers and bicycle spokes), impalement following falls or road traffic incidents, and gunshot wounds. Patients with penetrating injuries may present with normal vital signs and little clinical abnormality, but may harbour significant and life-threatening injuries. Each patient should therefore be assumed to have the worst possible injury; a comprehensive assessment and management plan that actively identifies or rules out the presence of serious injury is necessary, before a plan for the treatment of identified injuries is implemented.

Pre-hospital management

Penetrating injuries require surgical input more frequently than those following blunt trauma and transport to a centre where definitive, sometimes life-saving management is available is imperative. However, multi-system injury requiring a balanced approach to maintaining airway, cerebral perfusion, and other organ systems is not usually present in penetrating injuries. More often the situation is of bleeding from one or more sites which requires rapid control of haemorrhage to save life. For this reason the pre-hospital approach for penetrating injuries should be to spend as short a time on scene as possible and carry out only immediately life-preserving interventions (scoop and run). Minimal or no intravenous fluids are required, particularly with short transport times in urban areas. If the implement causing the injury remains *in situ* (or impalement has occurred), this should not be removed at the scene. If impalement has occurred to a fixed object, such as a railing or street furniture, this should be divided outside the body and the portion causing penetration be left *in situ*.

It is helpful to know something about the aetiology of the injury in order to anticipate likely injury patterns. Knowledge of the type and length of the blade used can help, but often the force used and depth of insertion is not evident. The injuries sustained following shootings are influenced by the degree of energy transfer, velocity of weapon, distance from the victim, and the type of bullet (round), but frequently this information is not available. More importantly, the injuries identified should be treated on their merits, as they are identified.

It is important to note that when gunshot wounds are present, and there are two wounds, it should never be assumed that a bullet has entered and exited the body, no matter how obvious this would seem.

In-hospital treatment

Given the invidious nature of many penetrating injuries the approach should be based on the assumption that all patients with a penetrating injury will require advanced intervention until proven otherwise. This may include endotracheal intubation, tube thoracostomy, interventional radiology, or surgery.

The clinical findings on initial assessment, the early physiological measurements, and the response to resuscitation are important indicators to the appropriate course of management.

Patients usually fit into three main categories:

- Initial physiological derangement that is not improved, or improves only temporarily, with resuscitation; or gross physical signs of injury. The majority of these patients will require early intervention, depending on the site of the wound and the results of rapidly performed basic investigations.

- Initial physiological derangement that improves, or remains stable, with basic resuscitation, or equivocal clinical signs. A significant proportion of these patients will require a procedure following focused investigation and active observation.

- Minimal physiological derangement or physical signs suggestive of minor or no significant injury. Large numbers of these patients will require simple wound care and suturing, but only after careful clinical evaluation, appropriate investigation and a period of observation has ruled out the need for intervention. This will prevent avoidable morbidity and mortality with missed injuries.

Resuscitation room decision-making requires careful initial assessment, allied to good judgement, and experience. Early senior surgical input is vital to assist with this, forming the main link with the patient as they progress through further assessment, investigation if required, surgery, critical care, and ward care. At all stages the surgeon needs to keep answering the question 'does the patient need an operation?'

In general, penetrating wounds should not be probed either digitally or with instruments, as this is unlikely to give useful information, will be painful for the conscious patient and, most importantly, may dislodge blood clot precipitating further bleeding.

For some victims of penetrating injury the primary pathology is blood loss due to external haemorrhage. The quickest and simplest way to deal with this is to identify the site, and apply direct manual compression (or a tourniquet for some limb injuries). The focus in management should be to identify the cause of the problem and put in place a plan to deal with it. For example, in the management of shock, the approach should be to identify the cause, treat the cause (while using a hypotensive resuscitation policy until the haemorrhage has been controlled), and then to rapidly restore the circulation and blood components if necessary.

Patients presenting in refractory shock, partial responders or gross physical signs

Catastrophic external bleeding

Patients with significant external haemorrhage usually present with evidence of shock. Sites of external haemorrhage should be identified and direct pressure should be applied to control this. For sites of penetrating injury causing incompressible bleeding, for example, the supraclavicular fossa, a Foley catheter may be inserted into the wound, and the balloon inflated to provide compression (see Chapter 19). Following completion of the initial assessment, limb wounds that require compression, or a tourniquet should be taken to the operating theatre for surgical exploration, but surgical control of non-compressible haemorrhage in the torso should usually take precedence over limb injuries.

Neck injuries

20% of knife wounds and 35% of gunshot wounds to the neck require surgery. Penetrating wounds of the neck presenting with stridor, a change in voice, or a wound that is bubbling indicate airway involvement. This can be due to a direct injury to the airway, a nerve injury, the effects of a haematoma, or oedema. If airway signs are present, early intubation by an experienced clinician is required with a surgeon on standby to perform a surgical airway if intubation fails. Occasionally, a direct wound to the airway is apparent, and in this situation a suitable tracheal tube can be directly inserted into the airway via the wound.

Patients who are shocked from injuries elsewhere that require immediate surgery, should undergo early intubation to facilitate safe transfer to the operating theatre or, in the case of acute deterioration, attention can be focused on dealing with the cause.

Once the airway is secured and initial assessment is complete, the patient should be managed depending on their clinical state and the site of the wound.

Patients with zone 1 and 2 injuries (see Chapter 16) who are haemodynamically unstable should be taken to theatre for surgical exploration. Shocked patients with zone 3 injuries (due to difficult and limited surgical access) are best served by rapid transfer to the interventional radiology suite for angiography followed by embolization, balloon tamponade or stenting of the injured vessel depending on site and access. Surgery is necessary if these are not available. Hard signs of major vessel injury include pulsatile bleeding, ongoing bleeding, and expanding haematoma.

Resuscitative thoracotomy

Patients in extremis or who lose cardiac output within 10 minutes of medical support, and who have wounds to the chest, require immediate resuscitative thoracotomy. Tension pneumothorax is ruled out by performing initial open thoracostomies in the fifth intercostal spaces in the anterior axillary line bilaterally and ensuring any air is released by inserting a finger into the wound. If air escapes under pressure and the patient improves, intercostal tubes should be inserted and the initial assessment continued. If no air escapes or no improvement occurs, massive blood loss or cardiac tamponade is likely to be the cause. Cardiac tamponade should be suspected in the case of penetrating chest trauma and thoracotomy in the resuscitation room should be performed. The surgeon opening the chest should be able to perform damage control on lung and great vessel injuries. There is no role for needle pericardiocentesis, except in a smaller institution where no surgical capability exists. Survival following resuscitative thoracotomy for penetrating injury is in the region of 10–20%.

When resuscitative surgery is required for combined thoracic and abdominal injury then resuscitative thoracotomy should be carried out as above. If the chest problem has been addressed and cardiac output has returned, the descending thoracic aorta should be identified and simply compressed by digital pressure. If appropriately skilled personnel are present, a clamp can be applied. This will facilitate vital organ perfusion whilst reducing blood loss in the abdomen. The patient should then be transferred to the operating theatre for immediate laparotomy and haemorrhage control, following which the thoracic aorta can be released.

If the loss of cardiac output is due to isolated abdominal injury there are two approaches, both have which have led to reports of successful outcomes. The first is to do an immediate left thoracotomy and control the descending aorta prior to laparotomy. This allows access to the heart to enable direct massage, and reduces abdominal blood loss. The other option is to proceed immediately to laparotomy and to compress the supracoeliac aorta (which can be done digitally), to obtain haemorrhage control. The benefit of this approach is quicker direct access to the site of bleeding.

Thoracic injuries

Separating out breathing and circulation problems in the chest following penetrating injury is not particularly helpful, as problems with either may manifest with similar clinical findings. Examples include shock caused by tension pneumothorax or cardiac tamponade, and co-existing conditions such as haemothorax and pneumothorax. Most penetrating injuries of the chest (about 75%) can be managed with careful assessment and tube thoracostomy. The torso should be inspected carefully front and back (and in the axillae) for evidence of wounds. Wounds involving the costal margins and the upper abdomen often involve both the chest and abdominal cavities. Cardiac injury should be suspected with any penetrating injury occurring from the clavicles to the costal margin between the nipples anteriorly and between the medial borders of the scapulae posteriorly. They should also be suspected with the majority of gunshot injuries to the chest. Bullet entry points in one-half of the chest can result in the projectile fragments embedding almost anywhere including the other side of the chest and the abdomen, with a trail of disruption along their trajectory.

Clinical examination of the chest should be performed, but classic signs of pneumothorax, haemothorax, and cardiac tamponade may not be present or detectable in a busy resuscitation room, particularly when shock is present. For this reason, a high index of suspicion and a rational approach are needed with rapid access to initial investigations, such as chest radiography, ultrasound, and computed tomography, with management options including tube thoracostomy, interventional radiology, and thoracotomy.

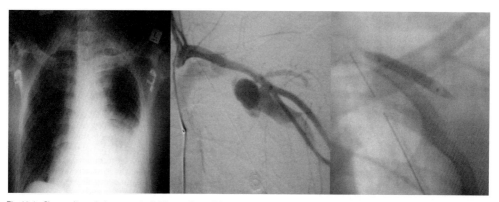

Fig. 23.1. Chest radiograph demonstrating left haemothorax following stabbing to left supraclavicular fossa. The middle picture demonstrates a subclavian arteriovenous fistula with contrast extravasation and the picture on the right demonstrates an angioplasty balloon inflated at the site of the injury to control bleeding. Surgical exploration then followed.

For patients presenting with difficulties in breathing, tachypnoea, or shock, the likely causes are tension pneumothorax, bleeding in the chest (or abdomen), and cardiac injury. These patients may require early surgery and the clinical findings and initial investigations are used to determine which cavity should be opened first.

A tension pneumothorax should be treated with immediate tube thoracostomy. If there is little or no improvement following this, a check should be made to ensure the tension has been relieved. If this is confirmed, the most frequent cause of persistent shock is bleeding (either in the same side of the chest or involving a different site) or cardiac tamponade. If this is the case, a rapid re-evaluation to find the cause is required. If the tension is not relieved, a further drain should be inserted. If there is still difficulty with ventilation, then the possibility of an injury to the tracheo-bronchial tree should be considered, requiring intervention such as selective intubation of the unaffected bronchus, and surgery.

An early chest radiograph (preferably erect) is a useful adjunct to diagnosis, and this can be obtained as the assessment of the patient continues. A supine chest radiograph may not clearly demonstrate a pneumothorax or haemothorax, and in the presence of haemothorax will demonstrate a generalized increase in opacification on the affected side as the blood in the pleural space spreads evenly across the posterior of the chest.

Ultrasound can be useful in the identification of significant haemothoraces, pneumothoraces, haemopericardium, and bleeding in the abdomen in appropriate hands.

If there is any doubt as to the exact diagnosis, and if physiological compromise does not improve, an intercostal tube thorocostomy should be performed on the suspected side(s) of injury. The contents of the drain (air or blood), and the patients physiological response will guide further management. If air is released and the patient improves, then initial assessment may continue. With tracheobronchial injuries the pneumothorax is likely to re-accumulate and a further drain should be inserted. Mediastinal air on the chest radiograph is a helpful sign in this regard. If there is continuing respiratory compromise or tension pneumothorax does not resolve, then immediate surgical intervention is required to control the injury.

If blood is released and the patient's condition improves, then the initial assessment should continue, with close monitoring of vital signs and output from the drain. Resolution of a haemothorax can be assessed with further chest radiographs. If the patient does not improve then a rapid re-assessment should search for other causes of shock, such as cardiac tamponade or bleeding in the abdomen. The volume of blood collected in the drain and the ongoing blood loss should be used as a guide to the indication for thoracotomy. This decision should also take into account the physiological state and response of the patient. It is possible for a large volume of blood to be retained in the chest and only a small volume to be apparent in the drain, misleading the clinician as to the cause of the shock. A repeat chest radiograph can help with decision-making in this situation.

Definitive management can either take place in the operating theatre or the interventional radiology suite, depending on resources available and the nature of the injury. If the injury involves the clavicular, supraclavicular and axillary regions, and there are hard signs of vascular injury or evidence of brachial plexus injury, with no cardiac tamponade, then it is likely that the shock is caused by bleeding from the subclavian or axillary vessels. If an interventional suite and appropriate personnel are immediately available, rapid and relatively straightforward haemorrhage control can be achieved by radiological insertion of a balloon across the site of the injury. Surgery can then proceed in a more controlled way with the balloon being used as a guide in what is often a difficult area due to the anatomy and possible distortion by a haematoma (see Fig. 23.1). A further option is that an endovascular stent may be placed across the injury, but in this situation there is a high chance of subsequent stent failure and thrombosis due to kinking, bony impingement and stent breakage.

If cardiac tamponade is identified clinically or on ultrasound, and the patient is not in extremis, they should be moved to the operating theatre for thoracotomy and repair of the cardiac injury via a median sternotomy or left thoracotomy, depending on the presence of other injuries to the chest and the surgical expertise available.

Evidence suggests that the outcome for operating theatre thoracotomy is much better than for emergency room thoracotomy. This may be partly due to bias, as a patient who survives to theatre may be in a better clinical condition, but without doubt the more controlled environment of theatre, and the availability of familiar equipment and operating staff will make a difficult and harrowing situation easier for the surgeon.

Thoraco-abdominal junctional injuries

The most difficult group of patients presenting with severe shock and penetrating injuries are those with injuries around the costal margin. These may involve either the thoracic or abdominal cavities, or sometimes both, and choosing the appropriate cavity for initial exploration may be vital if a good outcome is to be achieved. The choice should be made on the basis of information from initial clinical evaluation and investigations.

If cardiac tamponade and a large haemothorax are excluded by a combination of examination, chest radiograph, insertion of tube thoracostomy on the side of injury, and ultrasound, then a laparotomy should be performed.

If cardiac tamponade is present with suspected bleeding in the abdomen, the cardiac tamponade should be addressed first via whichever approach the surgeon is comfortable with and then a laparotomy should be performed.

If there is evidence that there is bleeding in the chest and abdomen, then a 'best guess' as to which cavity contains the most serious injury should result in that cavity being entered first. The sources of bleeding identified should be treated by damage control, before proceeding to open the other cavity, again using damage control principles. In the event that the wrong cavity is opened first, the surgeon should proceed immediately to the unopened cavity.

For example, a patient may present with a gunshot wound to the right costal margin, and blood in the right side of the chest and in the abdomen on initial assessment and investigation. If on opening the chest, it is found that the blood is welling up through a diaphragmatic laceration then the surgeon should rapidly open the abdomen prior to closing the chest to deal with the likely liver injury. In this situation it is likely that the liver will be the most life-threatening source of bleeding. The surgeon should aim to deal with all sites of bleeding at the first operation.

Abdominal injuries

Patients presenting in shock with a penetrating injury involving the abdomen should have an initial assessment of the neck, chest, and limbs, as well as the abdomen. It should be emphasized that the back, flanks, groins, perineum, and buttocks should all be inspected for wounds. Wounds of the upper thigh may involve the abdomen. If there are combined injuries, the priorities for treatment should be decided by what is likely to be the most life threatening injury. Direct pressure may be applied to limb, groin, and neck injuries. Haemothoraces can usually be managed initially with a chest drain and close monitoring of the drain output, while the patient undergoes damage control laparotomy. Patients with isolated abdominal injuries still require assessment and management of the airway and chest prior to the laparotomy.

Patients presenting with peritonitis should undergo early laparotomy. Abdominal rigidity may, however, be related to the wound or muscle haematoma. In appropriate patients who are physiologically suitable, and where there is doubt about the exact nature of the injury, a CT scan may be helpful. Laparotomy is indicated in the presence of shock, peritonitis, evisceration, and in most gunshot wounds.

Patients presenting in shock that improves following resuscitation

Neck injuries

Patients with penetrating injuries to the neck who fall into the second and third categories (who improve after initial resuscitation, have stable signs, or have little or no signs) should go on to have a CT scan of the neck and upper thorax with contrast. This will define any significant injuries and surgery can be planned to follow if necessary. For example, a carotid artery injury with an intimal flap can either be stented or surgically repaired. Injuries to the airway and oropharynx, with minimal swelling, disruption of tissue plains or surgical emphysema, can be managed with an active conservative approach. This involves 12–24 h of close observation and re-examination, with repeated assessment confirming that the patient does not require urgent surgery. Patients with oesophageal injuries require surgical exploration and repair. Patients who are found to have a nerve injury may initially be treated expectantly, with formal exploration and repair if required at a later date once the haematoma and swelling have resolved.

Thoracic injuries

Patients with chest injuries that present with shock and adverse physical signs, that improve with a period of resuscitation and chest drainage, can be managed with a more considered approach. A large number of these patients will eventually settle with conservative management. However, that fact that the patient was displaying signs of shock should alert the clinician to the possibility that surgery may be required. The clinical assessment and initial investigations should be carried out as previously described. Patients with pneumothoraces and haemothoraces should be managed with tube thoracostomy, and their progress subsequently monitored using clinical parameters, physiological observations, output into the drains, and repeated radiographs. Patients with simple pneumothorax require a period of observation as an in-patient until air leakage stops and the lung is fully re-expanded (assessed by repeat chest X-ray), at which point the drain may be removed. Repeat chest radiographs that show no resolution to the pneumothorax should prompt reassessment. Those drains that continue to bubble and do not achieve lung re-expansion may be a sign of bronchial disruption causing a persistent air leak.

Patients with haemothoraces should undergo further evaluation with contrast-enhanced CT of the thorax. This will give information about the track of the wound, the injured structures and the ultimate requirement for surgery. Evidence of ongoing bleeding from major vessels should lead to early interventional radiology or vascular surgery depending on the site and available expertise. Daily review of the drain output and chest radiograph should be undertaken to ensure resolution of the haemothorax. If a single drain does not sufficiently remove the haemothorax or there is radiological evidence of persisting haemothorax, a second drain should be placed in an appropriate position clinically or with radiological guidance. If the haemothorax has not resolved after 5–7 days, consideration should be given to using thoracoscopic washout (or mini-thoracotomy) to fully evacuate the blood, due to the risk of subsequent empyema.

Other injuries requiring further evaluation by CT and possible surgical intervention include the presence of mediastinal air (indicating oesophageal or airway injury), and impalement injuries, so that appropriate preparation can be put in place prior to surgical removal. The injured structures can frequently be defined based on the identified track of the wound.

Thoraco-abdominal junctional injuries

Patients with injuries at the costal margin should undergo thoraco-abdominal CT scan to look for evidence of intra-abdominal injuries, including injuries to the solid organs, gastro-intestinal tract, and major blood vessels. The presence of a laceration to the diaphragm needs to be considered in injuries around the left costal margin. If a left diaphragmatic laceration is overlooked, it may lead to late presentation of strangulation of prolapsed abdominal organs. On the right side, the diaphragm is protected by the liver, and prolapse of intra-abdominal contents is much less likely. Frequently, the chest radiograph and CT scan show no evidence of apparent diaphragmatic injury, but it should be suspected in the presence of a pneumothorax or haemothorax with co-existing evidence of sub-diaphragmatic injury.

A useful approach is to admit the patient and inspect the diaphragm at laparoscopy the following day. If present, the diaphragmatic laceration can be sutured and the abdominal cavity inspected for the presence of bile or faeces, indicating a bowel injury requiring repair. This is often preferable to doing an immediate laparoscopy, when finding a small laceration to the bowel can be technically very difficult.

Abdominal injuries

Patients with abdominal injuries who initially present with shock and who improve following resuscitation, or those with equivocal signs, should be managed with an active conservative approach (investigation and careful repeated evaluation of the patient by a senior member of the surgical team). It should be emphasized that patients who improve with resuscitation, but continue to bleed, are liable to sudden decompensation.

As well as palpation, inspection of all wounds is crucial, including inspection of the axillae and perineum for evidence of entry and exit wounds in both stab and gunshot injuries. All patients should have a rectal examination, and urinalysis to check for haematuria. When pelvic injury is suspected, for example, in the presence of buttock and perineal lacerations, sigmoidoscopy should be performed to rule out a rectal injury.

Blood in the rectum is an indication that the bowel has been breached and is an indication for laparotomy. Haematuria on urinalysis is an indication that there is renal tract injury, and this warrants further investigation in the form of CT. Ultrasound may indentify free fluid in the abdomen, but does not differentiate between blood and other fluids, such as bowel content, so does not necessarily indicate the need for emergency laparotomy (for example, in isolated liver injury with controlled haemorrhage).

The trajectories of ballistic fragments within body cavities are highly unpredictable. Bullets entering the abdominal cavity may easily enter the chest. A plain abdominal radiograph might help to identify the trajectory and residual fragments (one of the few indications for plain abdominal X-ray in the emergency department). The history from the patient is often unreliable, as they may say they heard only one gunshot, but have clinical evidence of more.

Most gunshot injuries involving the abdomen require laparotomy. Exceptions to this are when the bullet wound tracks can be demonstrated to be tangential to the abdominal wall, and in injuries involving the right upper quadrant. In both cases, the patient should be stable enough following initial resuscitation to undergo further assessment with CT. In those with tangential wounds the ballistic track will be confirmed on CT.

In the case of right upper quadrant gunshot wounds, if the CT shows a clear wound track involving the liver, that is no longer bleeding, or if there is contrast extravasation which can be treated by angio-embolization, then laparotomy can potentially be avoided. However, if the CT demonstrates that there are associated gastro-intestinal or vascular injuries, or if the patient deteriorates clinically, then laparotomy should be undertaken.

The initial presence of shock, equivocal abdominal signs, haematuria, or intra-abdominal free fluid is an indication for further investigation. The best investigation is contrast-enhanced CT, which identifies the majority of patients in this group who require surgery. However, the patient needs to be in a reasonably stable condition to tolerate the transfer to, and time taken for CT, and in cases of doubt the patient should undergo exploratory laparotomy.

Experienced radiologists using modern multi-slice CT achieve very high diagnostic accuracy. Wound tracks, peritoneal penetration, solid organ injuries, bowel injuries, and vascular injuries can all be defined (see Fig. 23.2). Contrast extravasation (contrast 'blush') on CT indicates ongoing bleeding. Small volumes of free intra-peritoneal air are sometimes indicative of bowel injury, but air may have entered via the external wound so it is not absolutely diagnostic. If the CT shows either gastro-intestinal tract injuries or active contrast extravasation, intervention is necessary in the form of laparotomy or interventional radiology (in the case of isolated solid organ injury and some vascular injuries).

However, CT is not 100% sensitive at detecting injury, and, in particular, injuries to the gastro-intestinal tract, ureter and bladder may not be identified. Patients with non-bleeding solid organ injuries may re-bleed following investigation. All patients with equivocal signs, or whose vital signs improve after resuscitation, should therefore be admitted for active conservative management after their CT scan. The development of further shock or peritonitis during this period indicates the need for laparotomy.

To ensure that active conservative management is safe, with reduced working hours for doctors and more frequent handovers, it is prudent for both the doctor leaving and the one taking over to examine the patient together, so that changes in the patient's condition can be appreciated and that the management plan and indications for intervention are fully understood.

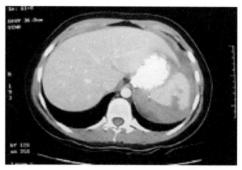

Fig. 23.2. CT scan of splenic injury and surrounding haematoma from stab.

Patients who are physiologically normal

Thoracic injuries

The vast majority of these patients have no major structures injured. However, careful evaluation taking into account clinical findings and chest radiography should be performed. If the injury could involve the heart then ultrasound is a useful addition to the investigations. If no abnormalities are identified from this evaluation then the patient should be observed for a period of 6 h. A small number of these patients may develop a pneumothorax or haemothorax during this time, and if present this should be treated by tube thoracostomy. If there is no deterioration during this time, they can be safely discharged.

Abdominal injuries

Patients with abdominal injuries who appear well, with no immediate indication for surgical intervention, can usually best be managed with an active conservative approach. Abdominal stab wounds may seem innocuous but can cause significant occult injury (Fig. 23.3).

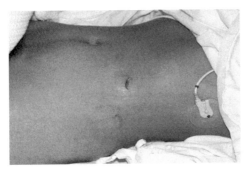

Fig. 23.3. Abdominal stab wound.

The key question is whether or not there has been intra-abdominal injury requiring surgery. For example, of patients with peritoneal penetration following stabbing, only 40% have an injury requiring laparotomy.

The most straightforward approach to patients with anterior abdominal stab wounds, demonstrated to be safe and practical, is to carefully assess and examine the patients, and admit them for close observation and repeated examination. They should be kept nil-by-mouth for the first 12 h. At 12 h the vast majority of patients with gastrointestinal injuries will have declared themselves with clinical features of peritonitis; they can then proceed to laparotomy. If at 12 h they remain well, they should be fed and continue under observation for a further 6–12 h. At the end of this period if they still have no signs they can be safely discharged. If there is any doubt at this stage, or if signs are equivocal, CT can be performed.

Some surgeons advocate wound exploration to triage anterior abdominal stab injuries. However, this can be a difficult procedure under local anaesthetic, particularly in obese or muscular patients. Even if the wound track is successfully followed and peritoneal penetration is demonstrated, only 40% require surgery, so patients still need to be admitted for observation to avoid significant numbers of unnecessary laparotomies.

CT is not an ideal investigation for these patients for reasons already discussed. There is a low diagnostic yield in patients with abdominal stab injuries with no clinical signs, and early sensitivity for detecting bowel injury is poor. Patients therefore still need to be admitted for active observation as above. The longer the period between injury and CT scan, the more sensitive it is in detecting significant injury.

Laparoscopy has been advocated, but the best time to perform this procedure is after a period of several hours, by which time bile or faeces will be evident if a bowel injury is present. If performed early, laparoscopy may be falsely negative, as it is technically difficult to accurately visualize the whole bowel, and with small lacerations bowel content may not initially leak out.

Stab wounds involving the flanks, back, and buttocks represent a different challenge as the thick muscles make clinical assessment unreliable. The significant injuries sustained from stabbings to these areas frequently involve retroperitoneal structures or pelvic structures, and physical signs from these injuries manifest late, with bleeding or sepsis leading to morbidity and mortality. For these reasons, after careful initial assessment patients with flank, back, and buttock stab injuries should undergo CT. In addition, patients with buttock wounds should undergo sigmoidoscopy to rule out rectal injury.

The injuries identified following these investigations should be treated on their merits, with different surgical emphasis. For example, a renal laceration that is not actively bleeding may be managed conservatively; an inferior vena cava injury should be surgically repaired; a low rectal laceration following a buttock stab injury should undergo a rectal washout and defunctioning colostomy. Patients with a wound track clearly limited to the back or flank muscles, and are not actively bleeding, can undergo local wound care and be safely discharged. For all others, and where there is any doubt about the extent of the wound, they should be admitted for a period of active observation.

Summary

All patient with penetrating torso injuries should be suspected of harbouring life-threatening injuries until their clinical state, targeted investigations, and appropriate observation have proven otherwise.

Patients in refractory or transiently responding shock, or those with gross physical signs, need rapid identification of the cause by clinical assessment and simple well-directed investigations before undergoing rapid surgery. For those patients who initially respond to resuscitation, a more considered approach is possible with active conservative management. The clinical team responsible for the patient needs to be vigilant, looking for injuries identified by investigation, physiological change, or development of clinical signs indicating the need for surgical intervention. Patients presenting without evidence of shock or physical signs also require careful assessment and observation, to ensure that significant injuries are not missed.

Further reading

Biffl WL, Kaups KL, Cothren CC, Brasel KJJ, Dicker RA, Bullard MK, et al. Management of patients with anterior abdominal stab wounds: a Western Trauma Association multicenter trial. J Trauma 2009; **66**(5): 1294–301.

Demetriades D, Rabinowitz B. Selective conservative management of penetrating abdominal wounds: a prospective study. Br J Surg. 1984; **71**: 92–4.

Friese RS, Coln CE, Gentilello LM. Laparoscopy is sufficient to exclude occult diaphragm injury after penetrating abdominal trauma. J Trauma 2005; **58**(4): 789–92.

Garner J. The early hospital management of gunshot wounds. Part 1: head, neck and thorax. Trauma 2005; **7**: 143–154.

Leppaniemi A, Haapiainen R. Occult diaphragmatic injuries caused by stab wounds. J Trauma 2003; **55**(4): 646–50.

Pham TN, Heinberg E, Cuschieri J, Bulger EM, O'Keefe GE. Gross JA, et al. The evolution of the diagnostic work-up for stab wounds to the back and flank. Injury 2009; **40**(1): 48–53.

Pryor JP, Reilly PM, Dabrowski GP, Grossman MD, Schwab CW. Nonoperative management of abdominal gunshot wounds. Annl Emerg Med 2004 Mar; **43**(3): 344–53.

Shanmuganathan K, Mirvis SE, Chiu WC, Killeen KL, Scalea TM. Triple-contrast helical CT in penetrating torso trauma: a prospective study to determine peritoneal violation and the need for laparotomy. Am J Res. American Am Journal of Roentgenology Roentgenol 2001; **177**(6): 1247–56.

Sugrue M, Balogh Z, Lynch J, Bardsley J, Sisson G, Weigelt J. Guidelines for the management of haemodynamically stable patients with stab wounds to the anterior abdomen. Aust NZ Journal of Surgery Surg 2007; **77**(8): 614–20.

Tsikitis V, Biffl WL, Majercik S, Harrington DT, Cioffi WG. Selective clinical management of anterior abdominal stab wounds. Am J Surg 2004; **188**(6): 807–12.

Whitfield C, Garner JP. The early management of gunshot wounds Part II: the abdomen, extremities and special situations. Trauma 2007; **9**(1): 47–71.

Ballistic and blast injuries

Pathophysiology of ballistic wounding

Physics of projectile motion

Ballistics is the study of the motion of projectiles. Bullets fired from a gun have three phases of ballistic motion beginning with events within the barrel through to the interaction with the target, or terminal ballistics. If the target is living tissue then the subject is known as wound ballistics. All forms of injury occur because of transfer of energy to the victim and ballistic wounding is no exception. It is, perhaps, the archetypal example of energy transfer causing injury. The energy of a moving missile—its kinetic energy (KE)—is given by the equation:

$$KE = \tfrac{1}{2}MV^2$$

where M = the mass of the missile and V = its velocity.

Some of the available energy is transferred to the target when the missile interacts with it and this transferred energy performs work on the tissues. Assuming there is no loss of mass, the amount of energy transferred to a target is dependent on the change in velocity between the incident missile (V_i) and that on exiting the target (V_e), thus the energy transferred to the target is:

$$KE = \tfrac{1}{2}M(V_i^2 - V_e^2)$$

and it also follows that if the missile does not exit the target then $V_e = 0$ and the missile's total incident energy has been transferred to the target. This concept of energy transfer is crucial and has replaced the old nomenclature based solely on velocity—the terms high and low velocity injury are now obsolete, although the only easily available method of comparing the wounding potential of different sorts of weapons remains the available energy—and, therefore, velocity—at the muzzle. Table 24.1 compares the available energies of a selection of well known weapons and ammunition.

Table 24.1. Available energies of commonly known ammunition types

Ammunition type	Mass (g)	Velocity at muzzle (m/s)	Kinetic energy (J)
0.22 short pistol	1.8	280	71
0.38 Smith & Wesson	9.4	220	227
0.44 Remington Magnum	15.6	440	1510
AK-74	3.45	900	1397
M-16	3.56	965	1658
AK-47	8.0	700	1960

Differences between weapon types

Handguns

These are generally regarded as low available energy weapons that can produce only low energy transfer wounds. The obvious exception to this is Magnum ammunition, which is lengthened handgun ammunition to accommodate an additional charge of gunpowder in the base, increasing muzzle velocity and available energy substantially; in this instance, the magnum round is 3 mm longer than the standard, but has nearly four times the available energy and leaves the muzzle with more available energy than a Russian military assault rifle (AK-74).

Rifles

Rifles generally have a longer barrel than handguns and a greater available energy at the muzzle. The grooves on the inside of the long barrel—the rifling—serve to spin the bullet as it leaves the muzzle, an effect that tends to stabilize the bullet in flight. This stabilization takes up to 50 m of flight to become maximal and, thus, close-range rifle wounds represent the interaction of an unstable bullet with the tissue and produce a different wound, typified by earlier energy deposition and significant superficial tissue damage. High available energy rifles may produce either high or low energy transfer wounds.

Shotguns

These fire a cartridge packed with small lead pellets varying from 1 mm diameter (birdshot) to 10 mm buckshot loads. After leaving the muzzle the individual spherical pellets spread out in a conical fashion and rapidly loose velocity and, therefore, available energy. At close range, however, the pellets act as a single large mass and retain most of their velocity, producing high energy transfer wounds which typically demonstrate significant tissue disruption and shredding. Beyond 50–70 m most shotgun pellets will not penetrate skin. Shot dispersal is inversely related to barrel length and is further limited by a constriction of the barrel diameter near the muzzle called the 'choke'–sawing off the barrel shortens it and removes the choke allowing greater spread at close range of pellets with greater velocity. Possession of a shotgun with a barrel less than 24 inches in length is prohibited in UK.

Despite the lack of precise definition, the categorization into low and high energy wounds is probably still valid and is based on the wound morphology and mechanism of production. Low energy transfer wounds limit tissue damage to the path of the missile, whereas high energy-transfer wounds generate tissue damage distant from the path of the missile.

Mechanism of wound production

Energy is transferred to the medium through which the missile is travelling as it is retarded by the drag imparted to it. The drag is dependent on the square of the velocity, the presented area of the missile and the density of the medium, thus a missile with a high velocity loses velocity—and, therefore, transfers energy—faster in a given medium than one with a low velocity. Wounds are generated in tissue by three principle mechanisms:

Cutting or laceration
A region of extremely high pressure develops at the front edge of the projectile as it travels through tissue, which disrupts the tissues ahead of the projectile. This is a direct and permanent effect.

Stress wave
A stress wave will be generated by the contact of the projectile on the body wall. It is a very short duration, high-pressure compression wave that travels at about the speed of sound in the medium. As the projectile continues on its path through tissues, it pushes tissue at each instant and generates a stress wave. It is possible that this intense pressure wave may cause tissue damage, such as long bone fracture after close passage of a high energy projectile.

Radial energy dissipation
Radial dissipation of energy from the projectile causes a short duration, low-pressure shear wave that pushes away the surrounding tissues to form a temporary cavity. It is an indirect effect of the projectile transit and is discussed in detail below. It accounts for most indirect trauma observed in high energy wounds from projectiles that remain intact. Heating of the tissues adjacent to the track of the projectile track also occurs. This is only of the order of 1 or 2°C and is of no clinical consequence.

The temporary cavity
The formation of a temporary cavity is a dynamic event that occurs because of the radial dissipation of energy, by a low frequency, relatively low-pressure wave. The forces cause radial displacement of material that reaches maximum extent after the passage of the projectile. The formation of the cavity begins in earnest about 1 ms after the passage of the projectile. It has been estimated that over 80% of the total energy transfer that occurs after a projectile strikes tissue is utilized in temporary cavitation. The cavity expands to reach its maximum volume about 4 ms after passage of the projectile; this may be after the missile has exited the target (Fig. 24.1A,B).

The temporary cavity then collapses in an asymmetrical fashion because of the elastic energy in the displaced tissues. This triggers a rebound phenomenon and one or more subsequent cavities may form and collapse—the temporary cavity pulsates. The *size* of the temporary cavity is largely dependent on the magnitude of energy transfer and may be up to 30 times the diameter of the projectile responsible. The *shape* of the cavity is rarely uniform throughout its length for bullets and the changing shape is a reflection of non-uniform transfer of energy as the projectile passes through the target. During growth and pulsation of the temporary cavity, the internal pressure is sub-atmospheric, and contamination is introduced into the medium, principally through the bullet's exit wound. This contamination becomes distributed throughout the

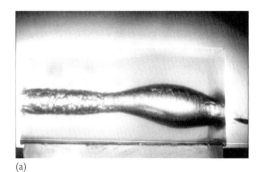

(a)

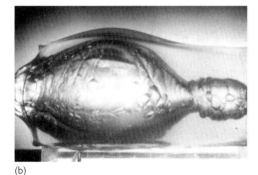

(b)

Fig. 24.1. Temporary cavitation in a 30-cm long gelatine block used as a tissue simulant, in a still from a high-speed film. In (a) a 7.62 mm NATO rifle bullet has traversed the gelatine from left to right and can be seen exiting the right edge of the block with high yaw (base first). The temporary cavity expands and in (b) has reached its maximum dimensions well after passage of the missile. © Copyright, Dstl 2009.

greatest volume of the cavity and will remain at some distance from the permanent wound track that is evident after final cessation of temporary cavitation. This has implications for the debridement of high energy transfer missile wounds.

Wound morphology
A skeletal muscle wound has three components: the permanent cavity, surrounded successively by zones of extravasation and then a rim of 'concussion'. The high pressures in front of the projectile form the permanent cavity. It contains pieces of detached tissue, blood clots and any foreign material that has ingressed. The zone of extravasation extends for a centimetre or so beyond the permanent cavity and contains shredded muscle, ruptured small blood vessels and a resultant haemorrhagic slough. Microscopically, it is characterized by necrotic myocytes, extravasated erythrocytes and the beginnings of an inflammatory infiltrate of neutrophils that increases over the first 72 h or so from wounding. This zone of extravasation is thought to be the result of the strain imparted by temporary cavitation, but the tissues involved are not *de facto* necrotic. The band of frankly dead tissue is generally less than 5 mm in diameter around the permanent cavity and this has important implications for wound debridement.

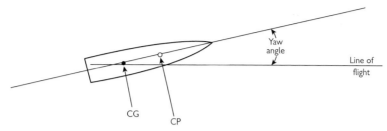

Fig. 24.2. A diagram to illustrate the concept of yaw. CG = centre of gravity CP = centre of pressure, an idealized point about which the whole of the retarding force of drag can be said to act.

Outside the extravasated muscle lies the zone of concussion, which may extend radially for a further 3 cm or so, and represents macroscopically normal muscle with microscopic evidence of injury, such as small interstitial haemorrhages, atypical myocyte morphology, and some degree of vascular congestion. An initial severe vasoconstriction in this zone is quickly replaced by a marked dilatation in keeping with a marked inflammatory reaction in the tissues nearby.

Factors that modify energy transfer

Energy transfer is dependent on the drag inflicted on the missile as it traverses the tissue and drag is proportional to the square of the velocity and presented area, as well as tissue density. When a missile leaves the muzzle of a gun it is unstable as a result of the asymmetric flow of exhaust gases around the missile, and oscillates about its long axis in a process known as yaw (Fig. 24.2).

This oscillation is damped as the projectile flight progresses and is minimal after approximately 25–50 m, so a missile hitting a target beyond this distance will be relatively stable and enter point first. The increased density and drag of the target tissue destabilizes the missile again and the projectile begins to yaw. As it oscillates it presents a larger surface area and deposits energy at a greater rate. This produces a wound track that is initially no more than the diameter of the missile with the region of greatest energy deposition and cavitation deeper within the tissue at the point where the presented area is greatest that equates to where the angle of yaw has reached 90 degrees (Fig. 24.3).

Instability remains and the bullet now flips to travel base first. Yaw is not solely associated with bullets, as fragments in flight or tissue will also yaw, but modern weapons systems are designed to ensure anti-personnel fragments are generally uniform in shape and mass; as a consequence, yaw changes the fragment's presented area little, with minimal consequences on the rate of energy transfer. If presented area was the sole determinant of energy transfer, the wound track produced could be expected to be a tunnel of fairly uniform dimensions throughout its length, but as retardation is also proportional to the square of the velocity, drag and thus energy transfer are highest when

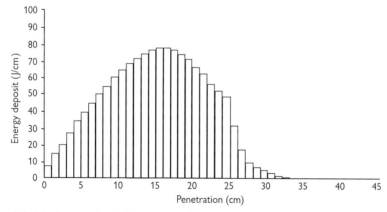

Fig. 24.3. A graph depicting the energy deposited per centimetre of wound track (J/cm) at various stages of penetration for a standard NATO 5.56 mm military rifle bullets. The location of the peak energy deposit is where the bullet has achieved 90-degree yaw. At 30 cm the bullet has deposited virtually all its energy; in comparison a 7.62 mm rifle bullet has greater available energy and is more stable in both air and tissue and deposits energy more gradually throughout the wound track. © Copyright, Dstl 2009.

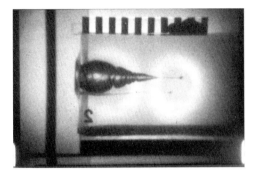

Fig. 24.4. An image from a high-speed film of the track produced in gelatine by a high available energy ball bearing. Maximum energy transfer occurs early in the track. A sphere will have no change in presented area during the penetration process and so this factor does not contribute to the distribution of energy, unlike the situation with bullets. Drag is proportional to V^2 and so the forces are highest immediately upon impact. © Copyright, Dstl 2009.

the fragment's velocity is greatest, early in the track. Fragments tend to dissipate most energy just after impact in the proximal track, followed by a fairly steady decline in energy transfer along the length of track as the projectile reduces speed (Fig. 24.4).

Factors that modify wound production

Interaction with intermediate targets

Any intermediate interaction with things such as vegetation or vehicles, renders a previously dynamically stable projectile unstable, with a concomitant increase in the angle of yaw. The jacket of the bullet may also be damaged or distorted. If the projectile then strikes tissue before stability is re-established the presented area at impact will be increased (Fig. 24.5).

This will result in early, more proximal, energy transfer along the track. A large superficial wound will be produced and, dependent on the amount of residual energy, penetration is likely to result in a large channel of laceration because of the larger surface area. Temporary cavitation may occur close to the surface, further exacerbating the degree of superficial mechanical damage.

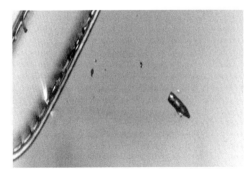

Fig. 24.5. The interaction of bullets with materials may induce yaw and damage to the bullet. This bullet has struck wire mesh and has emerged with high yaw (about 40 degrees when the image was taken), and evidence of damage to the jacket. Subsequent impact upon tissue will lead to enhanced energy transfer, and possibly disruption of the bullet, weakened by the defect in the jacket. © Copyright, Dstl 2009.

Projectile design

The presented area of a projectile, which influences the drag forces upon it, is increased by yaw, but may also increase by either deformation or fragmentation. Military bullets are specifically designed to remain intact without fragmentation or deformation throughout the course of the tissue track to comply with the Hague Convention of 1899. This is achieved by enclosing the soft lead or lead/steel core in an outer casing of copper or copper alloy, known as a metal jacket. Several circumstances are recognized in which the bullet may extrude the core from the base or disrupt—impacts against a dense bone such as the femur or pelvic ring are one such example. The effect of fragmentation is to increase energy transfer and consequently the formation of both a larger permanent wound track and temporary cavity. The generation of secondary projectiles produces sidetracks to the additional cavities; the result is a much greater degree of tissue destruction. Deformation without fragmentation tends to increase surface area and result in a permanent cavity greater than the calibre of the bullet with an associated increase in temporary cavitation.

No prohibition on the use of projectiles *specifically designed* to fragment or deform is in force in civilian life and bullets that increase presented area in this way are actually deemed desirable in many situations. By mushrooming the soft core on impact and increasing presented area, energy transfer is dramatically increased in the proximal wound track. The benefits are two-fold; high energy transfer is achieved early in the wound track, avoiding the potential for a fully jacketed bullet to traverse the target without entering its yaw cycle and, secondly, the bullet is more likely to have limited penetration, reducing the chance of it exiting the target and injuring others.

Properties of the target tissue

The properties of the target tissue, such as density, elasticity, and the presence of a restraining capsule, influence the type and severity of mechanical damage inflicted by a projectile. Lung parenchyma has a density approximately one-tenth that of bone and a high elasticity. As energy transfer is a function of the retardation applied to a projectile, and drag is proportional to tissue density, a high energy bullet traversing lung parenchyma may transfer little energy. Coupled with its ability to withstand the stretch imparted by temporary cavitation by virtue of its elasticity, lung tissue damage after a gunshot wound to the chest may be surprisingly limited.

Conversely, the liver is a highly vascular, relatively inelastic organ encased within a connective tissue capsule. A projectile penetrating hepatic tissue will be significantly retarded by the dense tissue and the proportion of energy transferred high. This results in the formation of a large temporary cavity, but the inelastic nature of the liver parenchyma determines that the liver is torn by the cavitation, rather than stretched; the confining capsule serves only to restrict the temporarily displaced tissue and exacerbate the degree of tissue disruption (Fig. 24.6). Even relatively low energy transfer wounds to the liver may have serious clinical consequences due to the enormous vascularity of the organ and its propensity for significant haemorrhage after minor trauma.

The densest tissue in the body is compact bone and it provides a high degree of retardation to a projectile. Unsurprisingly, the consequences of a projectile hitting bone in terms of energy transfer are notable. Low energy projectiles may produce a simple fracture on impact and

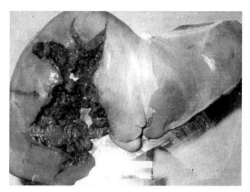

Fig. 24.6. A high energy transfer wound to liver with gross hepatic parenchymal disruption.

dissipate all their energy in doing so, whereas high energy transfer leads to severe comminution of bone, a large temporary cavity, and the potential for serious damage to the relatively fixed soft tissues. The bullet itself may fragment after impact and the energy transfer may accelerate the comminuted bone fragments, forming secondary projectiles. The metallic and bone fragments contribute to the extensive tissue disruption often seen in these wounds (Fig. 24.7). Long bone fractures may also occur without direct impact of the projectile on bone principally due to the temporary cavity, and the high pressure stress waves generated by close passage of a high speed projectile, but the morphology of these fractures is markedly different with little in the way of comminution.

The projectile-target interaction is often not as idealized as portrayed in experiments with gelatine blocks, simply because living targets present a heterogeneous target morphologically, and in terms of density and tissue strength. A projectile encounters tissues of different densities and elasticity along its path, and these characteristics affect energy transfer and mechanical damage inflicted.

Wound track length
Indirect tissue damage is dependent primarily on energy transfer, and the length of projectile track in tissue has an important influence on wound formation. If a stable, high energy projectile hits with low yaw and describes only a short track within tissue, such as traversing the forearm, it is unlikely that the projectile will have had sufficient track

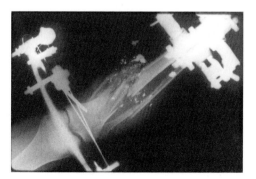

Fig. 24.7. A fracture from a high energy transfer bullet. Gross comminution has occurred and the resultant bone fragments may be accelerated as secondary missiles. This fracture has been stabilized by external fixation.

to enter its yaw cycle. The projectile will exit the tissue with low yaw and, as a consequence, energy transfer is also likely to be low. This would be different if the bullet had struck hard, compact bone, but the bones of the hands and feet, which are relatively soft and mobile, may not exert a notable effect on energy transfer. If the wound track length is sufficiently long to allow the projectile to enter its yaw cycle, and this distance will vary between projectiles of differing mass, size, shape, or construction, then high energy transfer and significant tissue damage may occur. In cases with a long wound track, such as projectile traversing the abdomen, the bullet may complete its entire yaw cycle and exit, if at all, through a small wound. In this instance, the projectile will have dissipated all or virtually all of its energy within the abdominal cavity and the degree of tissue damage may be considerable.

Entry and exit wounds
Penetrating wounds plainly have an entry site, but not necessarily an exit wound. Additionally, the unwary may make unwise assumptions regarding the degree of internal injury, based on the small size of the entry and exit sites. The size of the entry wound is dependent upon the angle of incidence of the projectile and its presented area, and in the case of bullets with minimal yaw, a small hole of diameter just less than the bullet will be present. The degree of incident stability will determine how early the projectile enters its yaw cycle within the tissue and if this is soon after impact, the temporary cavity may encompass the entry site, leading to gross superficial tissue injury.

If a projectile expends all its energy within the body, there will be no exit wound. The converse is that the absence of an exit wound implies transfer of all available energy and for a high energy projectile strike, considerable tissue injury within the body can be expected under these circumstances. The size of the exit wound is determined in part by the degree of residual energy possessed by the projectile and the proximity of the exit wound to the point of maximum cavitation; thus, the length of wound track is one determinant of exit wound size. In general terms, few assumptions about the degree of internal injury, and the appropriate medical management should be made solely on the appearance of the entry and exit wounds, and little time should be wasted in trying to identify which is the entry and which is the exit wounds. Small entry and exit wounds may occur with high energy transfer internally.

Mechanical damage and clinical consequence
Transfer of energy to the tissues performs work and causes mechanical damage, and the chapter so far has discussed those factors that will affect the degree of damage caused. In the clinical context, it is important to recognize that significant clinical consequences may ensue from minimal energy transfer and limited tissue damage. A high available energy missile wound tangentially through the buttocks may cause massive muscle damage and present with large ragged wounds overlying significant muscle necrosis. The degree of energy transfer has been high, and the mechanical damage marked, but after debridement the clinical consequences are likely to be minimal. Conversely, a low energy transfer fragment that enters an intercostal space before penetrating the left ventricle of the heart will transfer little energy and cause insignificant tissue damage, but the clinical consequence of the penetrating cardiac injury and cardiac tamponade may be fatal. The degree of injury that a tissue can withstand before serious clinical consequences ensue is dependent on the tissue type and function, and is largely independent of the wounding process.

Presentation and initial management of ballistic wounds

Unsurprisingly, as the level of energy transfer and wound production is dependent on so many variables, the clinical presentation of gunshot wounds can be extremely varied. The initial management, however, should follow a standard systematic approach, such as that described by the <C>ABCDE method. The application of this approach to ballistic wounding is no different to any other trauma situation with one or two caveats. In gunshot wounding there is a much greater likelihood of catastrophic haemorrhage, especially from major vessel injury in junctional areas and this must be controlled as the priority. In addition, the potential need for resuscitative laparotomy or thoracotomy as part of the primary survey to control life-threatening torso haemorrhage must also be recognized.

Head wounds

High energy transfer wounds to the head and brain are poorly tolerated as temporary cavitation within the brain is restrained by the bony calvarium; the cerebral tissue is disrupted, rather than stretched and substantial loads are transferred to the bones of the skull. This initially tries to stretch under the pressure loading, but the capacity for the skull to strain is limited. Continued pressure loading leads to fractures of the skull vault, often along the osseous suture lines which are points of weakness. Very high energy transfer magnifies this effect and effectively totally disrupts the skull (Fig. 24.8). These are clearly unsurvivable injuries.

Low energy transfer wounds to the head, however, can be eminently survivable; the low energy missile may dissipate all its energy in fracturing the bone to enter the skull and thus not actually penetrate brain tissue at all. In potentially survivable ballistic head wounds the priority is the prevention of secondary brain injury by optimization of oxygenation, ventilation, and perfusion. In isolated gunshot wounds to the head there is no indication for immobilizing the cervical spine. Hypovolaemic hypotension is rare in isolated head injury and, if present, profound hypotension usually indicates significant and probably fatal brain disruption. The exception to this is in paediatric ballistic head injury, where significant haemorrhage may ensue from scalp wounds, although this is usually clinically obvious. A full neurological examination should identify lateralizing signs and systemic antibiotic treatment is indicated. The imaging of choice is a CT scan to delineate bony injury, the degree of cerebral contusion or disruption, and the accumulation of intracranial haematoma. In the presence of a deteriorating patient, CT scanning should be deferred in favour of exploratory craniotomy by a neurosurgeon.

The neck

Gunshot wounds to the neck are uncommon, mainly due to its relatively protected position, but may present with injuries impacting on any part of the <C>ABCDE algorithm. Catastrophic external haemorrhage can usually be controlled by digital pressure; if this fails then gentle insertion of a Foley urinary catheter, inflation of the balloon and traction should suffice. The security of the airway may be compromised by direct injury or compression from haematoma or bleeding. Airway injury is suggested by air bubbling into the wound, hoarseness, respiratory distress, haemoptysis or subcutaneous emphysema, and if there is an obvious airway injury an endotracheal tube may be inserted directly as a temporizing measure. Patients with a high suspicion of laryngotracheal injury should undergo fibre optic bronchoscopy and intubation over the bronchoscope. Surgical airways should be avoided if possible unless the site of injury is known and the airway can be confidently sited below.

The lung apices are at risk of penetration and pneumothoraces should be decompressed; persisting large air leaks after tube thoracostomy suggest major airway injury. Haemorrhage may be controlled as described above. All penetrating neck wounds should undergo chest radiography looking for subcutaneous emphysema indicative of an airway injury or pneumothorax. Disruption of the column of air may indicate the site of laryngotracheal penetration. Unstable patients after resuscitation should undergo operative exploration of the neck. Stable patients should have the airway, great vessels, and aerodigestive tract assessed for integrity using a combination of endoscopy and angiography or colour flow Doppler. Conservative management of suitably investigated stable patients with ballistic wounds to the neck is safe.

Thoracic injury

The thorax presents a large surface area for penetrating missile injury in civilian life, but such injury is now uncommon in a military context because of the advent of personal protective equipment (body armour). The thoracic contents may also be injured without a thoracic entry wound as the missile may enter from the root of the neck above or through the diaphragms below. An anterior wound between the nipples laterally, and between costal margin and clavicles with systemic hypotension should prompt thoughts of penetrating cardiac injury (PCI). The signs of pericardial tamponade (Kussmaul's sign, Beck's triad) may be absent or difficult to elicit, but where the suspicion of penetrating cardiac injury persists the extent and urgency of investigation is directed by the degree of haemodynamic stability.

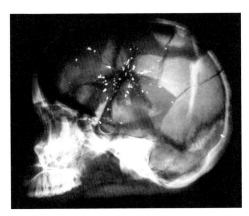

Fig. 24.8. The consequences of the interaction of a high energy 5.56-mm bullet with a skull model. The model comprised a dried human skull filled with gelatine, covered with chamois leather. The bullet had also penetrated a helmet. The bullet has disintegrated—undoubtedly a consequence of the helmet penetration. The formation of the large temporary cavity resulting from the high energy transfer has led to disruption of the cranium. © Copyright, Dstl 2009.

Patients suffering PCI with vital signs at scene or in the Emergency Department who suffer cardiac arrest or become agonal despite maximal resuscitation should undergo emergency thoracotomy and cardiac repair. Shotgun injuries, which have a tendency to shred tissues, or multi-chamber penetration, may not be amenable to repair. Unstable patients despite resuscitation, but who are not agonal with PCI should be transferred immediately to the operating theatre for emergency thoracotomy, with a six-fold improvement in survival over ED thoracotomy.

Stable patients with suspected PCI should be investigated with echocardiography, FAST scanning, or a subxiphoid pericardial window all acceptable alternatives, depending on local availability and expertise. A sub-xiphoid window should be performed in the operating theatre with the staff and patient prepared to convert to thoracotomy or median sternotomy if the window is positive. Pericardiocentesis is imprecise and potentially dangerous. A clotted haemopericardium will not be aspirated, giving a false negative result, whereas decompressing a cardiac tamponade without control of the bleeding point may precipitate catastrophic decompensation.

Non-cardiac penetrating thoracic injury has a much lower morbidity and mortality than injury to the heart, and most can be treated simply. The airways may be injured below the neck, with intrapleural injury causing pneumothoraces, whereas extrapleural airway injury will cause subcutaneous emphysema or pneumomediastinum. Tracheal disruption may present as airway obstruction. Pneumothoraces should be treated by tube thoracostomy with failure of re-expansion, excessive bubbling or increasing dyspnoea suggesting a major bronchial injury. Penetrating injury of the chest not involving the airways will still produce pneumothoraces (tension or simple), which should be treated appropriately. Similarly haemorrhage from either lung parenchyma or intercostal vessels should be treated by chest tube drainage after establishment of wide bore venous access and assessment by chest radiography. Prolonged or excessive drainage of blood should prompt consideration of thoracotomy although the outcomes after emergency lung resection for trauma are poor.

Abdomen

The abdominal viscera may be injured by a ballistic wound anywhere between the level of the 4th intercostal space down to the inguinal ligaments both front and back, and may also be injured by missiles breaching the peritoneum via the back and buttocks, the perineum and external genitalia, or trans-diaphragmatically from the thorax, thus, all these areas must be examined for wounds. Presentation may be anywhere along the spectrum of haemodynamic stability, from normality to catastrophic cardiovascular collapse; similarly abdominal signs may range from being absent to frank peritonism. Haemodynamic collapse unresponsive to resuscitation coupled with either abdominal signs or an obvious abdominal gunshot wound is an indication for resuscitative laparotomy without delay. In less extreme circumstances, the abdominal examination should be supplemented with adjunctive investigations to try and answer the questions:

- Has the abdomen been breached?
- Have the abdominal viscera been injured?
- Does the patient require laparotomy?
- If so, how quickly?

The relative merits of the potential adjunctive investigations (DPL, FAST, CT, laparoscopy) are discussed in Chapter 12.

Experienced trauma centres are now moving away from a policy of mandatory laparotomy for ballistic injury of the abdomen and have reported successful selective non-operative management (SNOM) in up to 30% of penetrating abdominal gunshot wounds. This approach relies upon a haemodynamically stable patient with low suspicion of bowel injury that is readily available for repeated clinical assessment. The SNOM approach may be augmented by angiography and angio-embolization. In centres that deal with low volumes of penetrating abdominal trauma or gunshot wounds, a policy of mandatory laparotomy for intraperitoneal ballistic injury remains the safe option.

Extremity injury

Extremity injury presents the possibility of four types of injury; vascular, neurological, bony and soft tissue—all of which may contribute to the pattern of morbidity. Mortality from extremity gunshot wounds is uncommon unless there is a major vascular injury in the incompressible junctional areas, such as the groins, axillae, or root of neck. With this in mind, vascular assessment of the limb takes priority, remembering that significant proximal vascular injury may be present even in the presence of a distal pulse, and seeks to identify hard signs of vascular injury (Table 24.2).

Table 24.2. The hard and soft signs of major vascular injury

Hard signs	Soft signs
Pulseless cold pale limb	History of active bleeding
Expanding haematoma	Penetrating injury close to major vessel
Palpable thrill or audible bruit	Non-expanding haematoma
Active bleeding	Neurological deficit

The detection of pulses may be enhanced by the use of a hand-held Doppler machine. The presence of hard signs of vascular injury suggests a threat to limb viability and an ischaemic time beyond 6 h results in permanent tissue necrosis. Limbs with hard signs should be explored surgically unless swift access to angiography (either percutaneous, CT, or magnetic resonance) is available. Surgical exploration may be augmented by on-table angiography, or the success of intervention recorded by a post-surgery angiogram. In those with soft signs of vascular injury, non-invasive assessment with either colour flow Doppler or CT angiography allows an accurate delineation of potential vascular injury and allows conservative non-operative management of these cases.

Damage to the peripheral nerves is often hard to identify in the early post-injury period in a patient who may have multiple injuries, such as limb fractures or ischaemic limbs that preclude accurate delineation of the neurological status. Injured nerves found at surgical exploration should be repaired if the surgical expertise is available or, if not, both ends of the nerve should be marked with a non-absorbable suture for later delayed repair or nerve grafting.

Nowhere is the need to differentiate low energy transfer wounds from high energy ones more important than when considering ballistic fractures. As civilian surgeons have been confronted with an ever increasing number of gunshot wounds, the dogma of mandatory surgical debridement of ballistic fractures has been replaced by an evidence-based shift towards conservative management of low energy transfer fractures. Local wound care and oral antibiosis are sufficient coupled with appropriate stabilization for the bony injury.

High energy transfer fractures are notable for the high degree of bony comminution and associated soft tissue injury; these are usually heavily contaminated wounds and debridement is essential coupled with bony stabilization and assurance of vascular integrity. Such wounds should receive penicillin as clostridial prophylaxis, as well as ongoing coverage with a cephalosporin (and gentamicin if severe anaerobic contamination is expected). Tetanus prophylaxis should be ensured.

The need for soft tissue exploration and debridement again relates to the degree of energy transfer with low energy transfer wounds being suitable for local wound care without formal debridement. High energy transfer typically generates a large temporary cavity that sucks in debris and contamination, which becomes lodged in the tissues distant from the resulting permanent wound track and will necessitate debridement. These wounds should be left open and a second look operation planned; if all is well then delayed primary closure may be possible. Alternatively, plastic surgical skills for tissue transfer to obtain soft tissue coverage may be needed.

Blast injury

The physics of explosions

An explosion is a physical, chemical, or nuclear process that rapidly liberates large amounts of energy in the form of high pressure shock waves. Explosives release their energy in a very short space of time, so the energy per unit time (i.e. the *power*) is huge, although the overall energy released may be significantly lower than slower chemical releases of energy such as combustion of carbon fuels.

The energy is released by the process of detonation, which breaks down the chemical bonds within the explosive in an exothermic reaction. As the temperature increases and exceeds conductive losses, heat production increases exponentially. At this stage the process is contained, increasing the pressure within the explosive. This pressure, in the form of a wave, propagates through the explosive until the induced shock wave is travelling faster than the speed of sound and traverses the remaining explosive almost instantaneously, rapidly liberating energy in the form of a shock wave, gaseous products, and thermal energy. Detonation waves typically act over only a few microseconds and travel at speeds of up to 8 km/s for high explosives, such as trinitrotoluene (TNT). Low explosives are compounds such as gunpowder, which don't actually detonate, but deflagrate, i.e. the decomposition is propagated by a flame front, rather than a pressure wave at a much slower rate (up to approximately 400 m/s). The blast effects of such explosives are therefore reduced.

When the detonation wave reaches the explosive-air interface it generates a shock (blast) wave, compressing a rim of the surrounding air around the ball of explosive products. The cloud of very hot, highly energized gaseous products of explosion expands rapidly and the rim of compressed air remains attached to the gaseous products. As the gases expand, they quickly cool and slow down and when subsonic, the rim of compressed air containing the pressure pulse detaches through the atmosphere. The blast wave therefore consists of the high pressure shock wave closely followed by the passage of energized heated gas products when close to the explosion, but further out it is the pulse pressure alone.

The pressure changes induced by the blast wave are usually described as those at a single point over time, where there is a virtually instantaneous sharp rise in pressure within the air surrounding the blast rapidly attaining its *peak (static) over-pressure*. As the blast wave propagates through the surrounding atmosphere the magnitude of the pressure wave decreases in proportion to the cube of the radius of its sphere of expansion. Over-expansion, because of an inertial effect in air is followed by rarefaction and pressures below ambient pressure *(the under-pressure)*, which then returns to ambient atmospheric pressure. This waveform is known as a Friedlander wave and represents the pressure changes of a simple blast wave, or one that does not interact with obstacles or constraints, such as walls or buildings, which complicate the wave pattern produced as well as the effects (Fig 24.9).

Passage of the blast wave also accelerates the air it traverses and this mass movement of air is known as the blast wind or *dynamic over pressure* and is different from the hot gaseous products that form part of the initial blast wave.

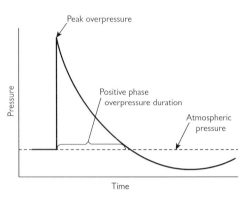

Fig. 24.9. Diagrammatic representation of the pressure changes over time at a single fixed point during passage of the blast wave.

Mechanisms of blast injury

Since 1940 the effects of blast injury have traditionally been divided into four categories (Table 24.3). A fifth, quinary, mechanism has been recently described as a hyperinflammatory response to a specific constituent (penta-erythritol-tetra-nitrate) of a suicide bomb in Tel Aviv. This mechanism is not yet universally accepted and has not been reported elsewhere.

Primary blast injury

Primary blast injury (PBI) is the effect of the blast wave on the body tissues and is the effect least well recognized by clinicians. In general terms, the incidence and degree of primary blast injury depends on both the level of peak over-pressure endured and the duration of exposure to it. The body can withstand moderate blast over-pressures for longer before injury occurs compared with higher levels of blast over-pressure, which can be tolerated for much shorter durations. Table 24.4 gives examples of the likely effects of a 4-ms exposure to various levels of blast over-pressure, bearing in mind that detonation of 1 Kg of TNT

Table 24.3. The four mechanisms of injury from explosions

Type of blast injury	Mechanism of injury
Primary	Interaction of the blast wave with the body
Secondary	Energized fragments from the bomb itself or environmental debris accelerated by the blast wind
Tertiary	Physical displacement of the body by the blast wind including tumbling and impact with stationary objects; crush from building collapse caused by the blast wind
Quaternary	All other miscellaneous effects that may include the psychological effects of the explosions, burns and inhalational injury

Table 24.4. Likely effects of 4 ms exposure to various blast over-pressures

Over-pressure (kPa)	Probable effect
7	Damage to standard buildings and windows break
14	Slight risk of perforation of tympanic membrane
100	50% chance of tympanic membrane rupture
275	Reinforced structures suffer significant damage
480	50% chance of marked pulmonary damage
900	50% mortality risk

generates a peak over-pressure of about 1300 kPa at a distance of 1m which falls away to 280 kPa at 2 m.

Transfer of energy to the body in PBI

A shock wave is coupled into the target when it strikes, and primary blast injury is the effect of the blast wave at the air–body interface. The effects are greatest where the differential in tissue density is greatest, such as the tissue–air junctions in the ear, lung, and intestines. Solid organs including the skin are relatively resistant to energy transfer from blast and a seriously blast-injured casualty may have no outwardly visible stigmata of injury.

When a blast wave strikes a human body two different types of energy wave are generated:

- Stress waves of high amplitude and velocity, which propagate through the body at speeds greater than the speed of sound in that medium.
- Shear waves of low-velocity and long-duration.

The stress waves couple across the density interface causing intense local forces over a short time duration resulting in microscopic damage, rather than macroscopic lacerations. Three mechanisms are thought to be responsible for the tissue damage:

- A proportion of the incident compressive wave is reflected as a tension wave across the reflecting boundary, such as the wall of a hollow viscus, and as tissues are weaker in tension than compression, the surface of the tissue breaks up, a phenomenon known as *spalling*.
- The compressive wave may cause the hollow structure to implode—the passage of the over-pressure contracts contained air bubbles and when the overpressure then falls, the bubbles rapidly expand again, causing a series of 'mini-explosions'.
- The difference in pressure across the wall of a hollow organ may be sufficient to rupture a delicate membranous tissue, such as the tympanic membrane.

Tissues of different densities will move differentially under the influence of the transverse shear waves, which results in tearing of organs at points of attachments, such as the small bowel mesentery and retroperitoneal colon, and shearing of solid organs, such as liver and spleen, typically at points of their capsular attachments.

Reflex physiological responses to blast waves

Thoracic, but not abdominal, blast exposure results in a reflex triad of hypotension, bradycardia, and apnoea, which are mediated, at least in part, by a vagally conducted pathway. The hypotension begins within 2 s and blood pressure takes between 1½ and 3 h to return to normal; the bradycardia has a latent period of approximately 4 s, returning to normal within 15 min. The apnoea is often difficult to assess experimentally, but seems to last for less than 30 s, although it is possible that some of the immediate deaths that occur after blast exposure without external signs of injury are, in fact, due to a prolonged apnoea. Also apparent is the lack of response to hypotension by increased systemic vascular resistance despite a diminished systolic pressure and cardiac index. The fall in cardiac index occurs in the presence of a normal heart rate and stroke volume suggesting myocardial impairment that can last many hours after blast exposure; the vasodilator response may be due to a rapid, massive, release of nitric oxide from the pulmonary circulation with the potential to cause a widespread maldistribution of microcirculatory blood flow.

The incidence of primary blast injury

This is difficult to determine exactly as the diagnosis is usually not considered by the unsuspecting physician unfamiliar with its protean manifestations and accurate data collection in the aftermath of a large explosion may be difficult. Militarily, anecdotal reports of men dying after shell bursts without any external injuries date back to the First World War, but the documented incidence is surprisingly varied. The Americans report only two cases of PBI during the whole of the Vietnam War, but there was a reported incidence of 51% in 1300 survivors of explosive munitions in the Balkans conflict between 1991 and 1994. Three-quarters of these were auditory blast injury, 28% had pulmonary PBI, and there was a 16% incidence of abdominal blast injury.

In the civilian environment there have been several large scale terrorist explosions in the last 10 years; the Oklahoma City bomb in April 1995 killed 168 people with three deaths attributed to 'traumatic shock', whilst 13 fatalities had internal thoracic injury with no external signs of injury. Of the 701 injured survivors, 13 were admitted to hospital with pulmonary contusions, Pneumothorax, or ARDS, compatible with primary blast injury of the lungs, in addition to a group of survivors who were noted to be hypotensive after the blast without external injury. The Madrid train bombs killed 177 instantly and injured more than 2000, with an incidence of primary blast lung injury of 63% amongst the critically-ill immediate survivors; the British Army's experience in Northern Ireland reported a very low incidence of pulmonary PBI amongst survivors and an incidence of 16% in those fatally injured.

Not all explosions or bombings are from international terrorism. In the 10 years to 1997 the Federal Bureau of Investigation investigated 17,579 bombings, 427 related deaths, and 4063 injuries in the United States. Similarly, industrial accidents may also generate the full range of blast injuries.

Secondary blast injury

Acceleration of bomb casing, contents, or environmental debris by the explosion and subsequent blast wind produces a barrage of highly energized projectiles, which produce penetrating ballistic wounds as described earlier in this chapter. The injury produced is a function of the energy transferred to the target, and its clinical consequences dependent on the type and location of the tissue involved. Military ordnance contains preformed fragments of uniform mass and dimension, usually steel spheres or ball bearings, and so their pattern of energy deposition within tissues occurs earlier on in the wound track (when their velocity is greatest) with limited cavitation followed by a fairly steady decline in energy transfer along the length of track as the projectile reduces speed. Terrorist devices, with a much greater variation in fragment size, or energized environmental debris, present a different wound pattern. The large presented area of these fragments at impact ensures a large initial energy transfer, which frequently results in a gaping superficial wound; if it retains sufficient energy the fragment can continue to penetrate tissue, yaw, and produce a pattern of deep injury similar to that from high energy bullets.

The energy of the blast wave falls off in proportion to the third power of the distance from the explosion whereas energized fragments lose energy, by drag, in a linear fashion, thus they retain more energy for longer than the blast wave and thus the lethal radius for secondary effects is always greater than that for primary blast injury in air. In practice, this means that anyone close enough to the centre of an explosion to incur significant primary blast loading is likely to be killed outright from massive secondary (and tertiary—see below) blast injury.

A new secondary blast threat is now represented by the potential for disease transmission. At least three survivors of suicide bombings in the Middle East have been penetrated by bone fragments of the bomber, one of whom was Hepatitis B positive. There have been no reports to date of actual disease transmission, but the Israeli Medical services currently recommend Hepatitis B vaccination for all close range survivors of suicide bombings.

Tertiary blast injury

This is an effect produced by the blast wind. Unsheltered individuals are physically accelerated by the dynamic overpressure, which may throw them into solid objects creating mainly blunt injuries. Blast winds may achieve speeds of up to 160 km/h and human fatalities from tumbling induced by the blast wind start at wind speeds of 80 km/h; ground impact speeds of 35 km/h are sufficient to kill half of those so affected. It is estimated that 70% of survivors of the atomic detonations at Hiroshima and Nagasaki suffered injury from either flying debris or being bodily displaced.

Traumatic amputation has traditionally been described as a tertiary effect, but this is not entirely accurate. Limbs are not ripped off through a joint by the passage of the blast wind; the coupling of the primary blast wave into the bone causes intense local force generation and fracture, typically through the upper or lower third of an extremity long bone. Subsequent passage of the blast wind then serves to disconnect the soft tissues and disconnects the limb at the fracture site. Irrespective of whether it is considered a primary or tertiary effect, traumatic amputation remains uncommon in survivors, and is a marker of severe blast exposure. In an analysis of over 3000 survivors of explosions the incidence of traumatic amputation in survivors was only 1.2% as those sufficiently close to the detonation to suffer such an injury usually succumb to overwhelming primary and secondary effects.

Quaternary blast injury

This catch-all category encompasses all effects of the blast not considered in the first three classes. Probably the commonest of the quaternary effect are psychological trauma, burns, and crush. The burns suffered in blast injury are usually superficial flash burns to the exposed skin, so hands and faces are particularly affected. Victims sufficiently close to the centre of the explosion to suffer significant thermal injury are usually killed by a combination of primary, secondary, and tertiary injuries. Certain explosive devices are augmented with inflammable material such as napalm or petrol, which are specifically designed to increase the thermal injury component of the blast effect.

Psychological injury after bomb explosions is commonplace amongst survivors, bystanders, and witnesses, and the population in general who become scared to continue their normal daily activities for fear of becoming victim to the next explosion. Rescuers and emergency service personnel are not immune to this aspect of blast injury.

Crush injury, may also contribute significantly to the death and injury toll from bomb explosions as the dynamic over-pressure causes building collapse—most of the injuries in the Old Bailey Bombing in London in 1973 were by this mechanism.

The literature also contains reports of other less common quaternary injuries, including inhalation of infected dust.

Clinical and pathological effects of explosions

Blast injuries affect most body systems with many similar pathological changes throughout; this widespread effect means that blast injury can present to clinicians of a wide range of specialities.

Lung injury

Upper respiratory tract damage, such as bruising of the mucosa lining the airways with the marks corresponding to the cartilaginous rings of the trachea, may serve as an indicator of primary blast injury elsewhere. In the lungs proper, the deposition of energy by the stress wave traversing the thorax tears the delicate interalveolar septa causing haemorrhage into the alveoli and bronchioles. At post-mortem a spectrum of severity is noted from scattered small petechial haemorrhages to large areas of confluent haemorrhage. If the blast load has been particularly severe then tears of the parenchyma are apparent. Damage is greatest in areas of concentration of the stress wave such as the costophrenic angles, adjacent to the mediastinum and in the intercostal spaces that produces a striped appearance, which is often erroneously referred to as rib markings. Tearing of superficial alveoli and pleura give rise to pneumothoraces, and if there is underlying parenchymal damage, haemothoraces as well.

Microscopically, there is a widespread capillary dilatation, as well as tearing of the fragile capillaries resulting in haemorrhagic congestion of the lung spaces. There is separation of the capillaries from their supporting connective tissue structures creating perivascular spaces, which fill with blood appearing as 'ring haemorrhages' on light microscopy. The formation of traumatic alveolar-venous fistulae is common and results in air emboli, which contribute to the extra-pulmonary pathology of PBI. There is also ultrastructural evidence that the changes of pulmonary blast injury, such as blebbing of the epithelial cell membrane and increased pinocytosis, evolve and increase over the 24 h following blast exposure.

These pathological features present clinically with well-recognized, but disparate signs, symptoms and radiographic features (Table 24.5).

Cardiac effects

Cardiac blast injury appears to cause limited macroscopic damage in the form of petechiae, or direct valvular or myocardial rupture, but the majority of cardiac pathology arises from the effects of coronary artery emboli and the effect on cardiac function. Coronary emboli may provoke arrhythmias, ischaemia, or frank myocardial infarction and is a likely cause of many of the immediate deaths that are attributed to primary blast injury. In addition, there is experimental evidence to suggest that thoracic blast exposure can adversely affect the innate contractility of the heart, with a decrease in cardiac index and poorer response to fluid resuscitation.

The ear

The ear is specifically designed to transmit acoustic waves, and thus blast waves affect the ear because of the pressure differential across the delicate membrane. The tympanic membrane will rupture at overpressures as low as 35 kPa and half will have ruptured by the time the overpressure reaches 104 kPa, although the orientation of the ear to the blast wave is important. The majority of people exposed to blast suffer some degree of hearing loss, with the incidence of permanent sensorineural hearing loss ranging between 30–50%. Tympanic membrane rupture, typically of the pars tensa, is a common accompaniment to blast exposure, but correlates poorly with the presence of blast injury elsewhere and is of no use as a predictive marker. A study of nearly 650 survivors of explosion exposure, reported 193 with evidence of blast injury. Three-quarters had isolated eardrum rupture, none subsequently developed other blast injuries, whilst nearly 10% of cases with pulmonary blast injury had intact tympanic membranes. Higher blast over-pressures will disrupt the middle ear ossicular chain as well. The inward positive pressure of the blast wave implants keratinized squamous epithelium through the tympanic membrane perforation into the middle ear and generates cholesteatoma later on. The incidence is up to 20% with subtotal perforations and increases according to size of perforations. Otological assessment

Table 24.5. The signs, symptoms and radiographic features of pulmonary primary blast injury (blast lung).

Symptoms	Signs	Radiographic features
Dyspnoea	Tachyopnoea	Bilateral butterfly infiltrates
Cough—initially dry progressing to frothy	Cyanosis	Interstitial infiltrates (linear peribronchial lucencies)
Haemoptysis	Dullness to percussion	Pneumothorax Pneumomedisatinum Haemothorax Subcutaneous emphysema
Retrosternal chest pain	Decreased breath sounds Widespread coarse rhonchi Haemo/pneumothorax Retrosternal emphysema (in pneumomedisatinum) Retinal vessel emboli Hypoxia	

should note hearing loss, otalgia, vertigo (which is uncommon after blast injury), ear canal bleeding suggestive of TM perforation, and perforation itself which is slit like or punched out and may have tiny clots attached to the edge; purulent mucorrhoea indicates secondary infection of the middle ear.

The abdomen

The different effects of long and short duration blast waves can be more easily discerned in the abdomen than elsewhere. Short duration stress waves deposit energy by spalling at the mucosal surface (air-tissue interface) of the intestines in a similar manner to alveolar wall disruption. If the blast over-pressure is sufficiently large then direct perforation of the bowel occurs. At lesser over-pressures mural contusions of varying degrees occur, their extent spreading from mucosa to serosa. These lesions are histologically similar to the damage caused by blunt abdominal trauma and are at risk of delayed perforation up to 2 weeks after injury. The solid abdominal organs, retroperitoneal colon, small bowel mesentery, and testicles are injured by the long duration shear waves generated by the gross displacement of the abdominal wall. The injuries are typically tearing of the capsules at points of fixation and attachment, generating subcapsular haematoma or with higher over-pressures, parenchymal laceration. Abdominal blast injury is regarded as rare after air-blast, but its incidence increases in explosions in enclosed spaces and in underwater detonations (see below). The presentation is varied and the patient may initially complain of little or no abdominal symptoms; others may present with abdominal pain, nausea and vomiting, gastrointestinal bleeding, haematemesis, rectal pain, and tenesmus, and testicular pain. Examination may reveal frank peritonism if perforation has already occurred, but more usually abdominal pain and vague tenderness. Bowel sounds may be absent and signs of hypovolaemia may represent concealed gastrointestinal haemorrhage.

Limbs

Extremity orthopaedic injury in survivors is generally due to secondary effects, with traumatic amputation rare, except after landmine injury (see below). Fragment injury depends on the type of munitions used as the degree of penetration will be related to the fragment size and mass.

Central nervous system

Head injury is a leading cause of blast related mortality, usually from secondary or tertiary mechanisms. Neurological effects in survivors are less common and have been less easy to discern, although historical descriptions of paralysis or neuraesthesia of the lower limbs date back to the First World War. Minor histological changes have been described in blasted brains, but correlation with neurological symptoms is vague; some of these symptoms may be related to cerebral emboli. Recent evidence from the American military suggests that many primary blast survivors are likely to exhibit the effects of mild traumatic brain injury, with a wide range of symptoms including sleep disturbance, attention deficits and behavioural changes, such as anxiety, emotional outbursts, and depression. Experimental evidence confirms neuronal degeneration and associated decrement of performance of both motor activity and higher cognitive function after whole body primary blast exposure.

The eye

Given its small presented area, the eye is particularly vulnerable to blast injury, especially penetrating fragment injury. Very occasional reports of presumed primary ocular blast injury occur with vitreous haemorrhage and commotio retinae producing reduced visual acuity.

Principles of management

Management of blast injury can usefully be separated into that for the individual and the management of the mass blast casualty situation that focuses on triage. In an individual likely to have been exposed to a significant blast, assessment begins with a full history and examination, bearing in mind that they may well have some degree of hearing loss. Examination should specifically assess the tympanic membranes and look for fragment wounds over the whole body; pulse oximetry gives a rapid indication of hypoxia, which may be augmented by arterial blood gas assessment if there is any suspicion of primary blast lung injury. This should be coupled with a plain chest radiograph, which is likely to show the typical features of pulmonary infiltrates on presentation if blast lung is present. Thoracic CT, if available, is more sensitive for the early detection of pulmonary contusion. Haemopneumothoraces are treated by tube thoracostomy, and there should be a low threshold for intubation and ventilation for those with evidence of significant blast lung injury. Avoidance of further lung injury uses a low peak inspiratory pressure ventilation regime, with permissive hypercapnia; high frequency ventilation is preferred. Fluid resuscitation of hypotensive blast victims is problematic. Thoracic blast may have triggered the reflex hypotension described earlier or it may be due to undiscovered haemorrhage. Aggressive fluid resuscitation may overload a blast damaged heart. If there is any suspicion of air embolism, high flow oxygen therapy should be instituted immediately—the definitive treatment is hyperbaric oxygen therapy.

Tympanic membrane injury rarely requires urgent treatment. The patients should be told to avoid immersing the head in water or probing the ear canal. Grossly contaminated ear canals should be gently cleaned and topical antibiosis commenced; specialist follow-up is indicated because of the longer-term risks of non-healing of TM perforations and implantation cholesteatoma.

The decision for laparotomy is based on standard clinical grounds, such as peritonism, pneumoperitoneum on imaging with abdominal signs, diaphragmatic rupture, or persistent gastrointestinal bleeding. Aside from surgical management of frank gastro-intestinal perforations there is considerable evidence for the prophylactic excision of mural haematomas greater than 2 cm in diameter in the colon and 1.5 cm in the small bowel as these are highly likely to perforate subsequently, sometimes up to 14 days after initial injury.

Penetrating fragment wounds are managed along conventional lines, with local cleaning and antibiotics if superficial, or formal debridement if there is suspicion of high energy transfer injury. Crush injury may require high fluid loading to prevent the nephrotoxic effects of rhabdomyolysis and invasive monitoring may be required if there are concerns about overloading a failing heart or waterlogging already-injured lungs.

Special situations

The discussion so far has centred on the effects of unrestrained simple blast waves, which is clearly not always going to be the case. Certain special situations will alter the wave pattern, and thus the injuries produced. The management remains largely unchanged once the specific injuries have been recognized.

Enclosed spaces

Explosions in enclosed spaces reflect the energy at junctions of walls and solid objects in an additive manner meaning that the power of the blast wave may be many times more in some areas of the room than others. There is a significantly increased chance of dying, suffering primary blast injury and receiving more severe injuries in an enclosed space explosion. Conversely, the reflection of the blast wave may also create protected areas where the over-pressure is reduced and injuries minimal.

Enhanced blast weapons

These use the blast wave itself, rather than secondary and tertiary blast effects to engage the enemy. They produce a blast wave of lower peak pressure, but longer duration over a wider area than conventional explosives and markedly increases the potential for primary blast injury. There are virtually no secondary or tertiary effects. Primarily military ordnance, they have been widely used by the former USSR in Chechnya and Afghanistan and are available in portable shoulder launched versions.

Underwater blast

Water transmits the pressure wave of an explosion much better than air and so the primary blast effects are greater than an air detonation; conversely, the water acts as a significant drag on the fragments propelled as a secondary effect and so they have a much shorter lethal radius. The injury distribution is therefore skewed towards primary blast injury in underwater blast. As the abdomen is in the water and the thorax often above it, there is a relative preponderance of abdominal primary blast injury. In addition, the incident wave is mainly reflected at the air-water boundary (the surface) in an additive manner, meaning that below the surface the power of the blast wave is greater still. The mass movement of water, representing the analogous process to the blast wind in air detonations, is translated into a water ram effect and the abdomen again suffers blunt trauma resulting in an increase of solid organ injury, such as ruptured spleen and liver.

Landmines

Despite the worldwide ban on their usage, landmine injuries remain common because of the enormous number of residual mines. A landmine is a small explosive device containing 20–200 mg of high explosive designed to be buried just below the ground or if mechanically distributed to lie on the surface, and is triggered by either trip wire or direct contact. Detonation releases the shock wave, hot gaseous products of explosion, the blast wind, and fragments of a standard explosion. The shock wave is coupled into the limb and leads to microvascular injury, stripping of soft tissue and stress fractures of the long bones. Shock wave effects may be discernible as proximal as the upper thigh and demyelination of peripheral nerves may occur for up to 30 cm above the level of gross tissue injury. Over the short distances involved the flow of energized gaseous products strips, and erodes soft tissues and induces substantial torsion and bending stresses on the limb, which may already have been fractured by the shock wave. The dynamic over-pressure may detach the limb at the site of fracture. Whilst not designed to be a fragmentation weapon, both the flow of gaseous products and the blast wind serve to implant environmental debris, small fragments of mine case, soil and destroyed footwear for a significant distance up the injured limb, infiltrating along the tissue planes separated by the shock wave and gaseous products and contaminating the limb beyond the level of visible destruction. The upward flow of fragments also constitutes a threat to ocular integrity and is a common cause of penetrating eye injury. The overall effect of a combination of these mechanisms is gross destruction of the lower limb, which may require amputation at a high level to gain soft tissue coverage free from contamination. The contralateral limb is usually less severely affected, although soft tissue damage and contamination from penetrating debris are common.

Summary

Blast and ballistic injuries are still uncommon occurrences for most UK clinicians, but the changing social and international political climate now means that they are increasing in incidence and an understanding of the underlying pathophysiological mechanisms allows a rational management strategy to be implemented. Penetrating ballistic injury is a function of the amount of energy transferred to the tissues, and can be broadly divided into high and low energy transfer wounds. Tissue damage in low energy transfer wounds is usually confined to the track itself, whereas distant tissue damage from temporary cavitation is the hallmark of high energy transfer. This distant tissue injury must be remembered when surgical debridement is undertaken. The level of mechanical damage imparted by a ballistic wound is not necessarily synonymous with its clinical importance and even relatively minor wounds of vital structures, such as the heart, eye, or brain can have serious if not fatal consequences.

Blast injuries are subdivided into four classes of mechanism, of which secondary, tertiary, and quaternary are easily understood with management strategies little different from the analogous wounds from non-blast causes. Primary blast injury is often unsuspected, but has manifestations across most body systems. Rupture of the tympanic membranes is the commonest primary blast injury, but is usually of little clinical consequence; pulmonary blast injury generates lung lesions akin to blunt traumatic pulmonary contusions, and the clinical course and management is largely the same.

Further reading

Special issue. Wounds of conflicts. *J R Army Med Corps* 2001; **147**(1).

Bellamy RF, Zajtchuk R (eds). Conventional Warfare: Ballistic, Blast and Burn Injuries. In: Zajtchuk R (ed.) *Textbook of Military Medicine*. Washington DC: Department of the Army, Office of the Surgeon General, and Borden Institute, 1991.

Bellamy RF. The causes of death in conventional land warfare: implications for combat casualty care research. *Mil Med* 1984; **149**: 55–62.

Benzinger T. Physiological effects of blast in air and water. In: *German Aviation Medicine, World War II, Vol 2*. Washington DC: US Dept Air Force; pp. 1225–59.

Cernak I, Savic J, Malicevic Z, Zunic G, Radosevic P, Ivanovic I, et al. Involvement of the central nervous system in the general response to pulmonary blast injury. *J Trauma* 1996; **40**(3 Suppl): S100–4.

Clemedson CJ, Hultman HI. Air embolism and the cause of death in blast injury. *Mil Surg* 1954; 114(6): 424–37.

Cooper GJ, Dudley HAF, Gann DS, Little RA, Maynard RL (eds). *Scientific Foundations of Trauma*. Oxford: Butterworth Heineman, 1997.

Cullis IG. Blast waves and how they interact with structures. *J Roy Army Corps* 2001; **147**: 16–26.

de Ceballos JP, Turegano-Fuentes F, Perez Diaz D, Sanz Sanchez M, Martin-Llorente C, Guerrero-Sanz JE. The terrorist bomb explosions in Madrid, Spain—an analysis of the logistics, injuries sustained and clinical management of casualties treated at the closest hospital. *Crit Care* 2005; **9**: 104–11.

Greaves I, Porter K, Garner JP (eds). *Trauma Care Manual*, 2nd edn. London: Hodder Arnold, 2009.

Guy RJ, Kirkman E, Watkins PE, Cooper GJ. Physiologic responses to primary blast. *J Trauma* 1998; **45**(6): 983–7.

Horrocks CL. Blast injury Biophysicis, pathophysiology, and management principles. *J Roy Army Corps* 2001; **147**: 28–40.

Leibovici D, Gofrit ON, Stein M, Shapira SC, Noga Y, Heruti RJ, et al. Blast injuries: bus versus open-air bombings- a comparative study of injuries in survivors of open-air versus confined-space explosions. *J Trauma* 1996; **41**(6): 1030–5.

Mellor SG. The relationship of blast loading to death and injury from explosion. *World J Surg* 1992; **16**: 893–8.

Scott JB (ed.) Hague Convention. *Declaration III. Laws of War: Declaration on the Use of Bullets Which Expand or Flatten Easily in the Human Body*. Hague Conferences of 1899 and 1907. A series of lectures delivered at the John Hopkins University 1908. Vol II—Documents Baltimore: John Hopkins Press, 1909.

Sellier KG, Kneubuehl. *Wound Ballistics and the Scientific Background*. Amsterdam: Elsevier Science BV, 1994: 109.

Simpson BM, Grant RE. A synopsis of urban firearm ballistics: Washington DC model. *Clin Orthop* 2003; **408**: 12–1.

Trimble K, Clasper J. Anti-personnel mine injury: mechanism and medical management. *J Roy Army Corps* 2001; **147**: 73–79.

Zuckerman S. Experimental study of blast injuries to the lungs. *Lancet* 1940; **2**: 219–24.

Chemical, biological, and radiation injuries

Introduction

Hazardous materials (HazMat), including toxic industrial chemicals, present a significant risk and challenge to emergency services and medical staff. HazMat incidents may involve casualties that are contaminated and require special plans to be in place. Chemical, biological, and radiological agents also are cause for concern because of their potential use by terrorists against both military and civilian targets.

Where there has been an accidental release, this is referred to as a HazMat incident, while a deliberate release of hazardous materials is referred to as a CBRN (chemical, biological, radiological, and nuclear) incident, the difference being the intent to cause harm. For medical staff, the differentiation is often academic as the agent used (e.g. chlorine) causes the same clinical effects.

Historical context

The use of CBRN agents dates back to antiquity and indeed legend—Hercules dipping his arrows into the toxic blood of the Hydra. In the middle ages, the bodies of plague victims were catapulted into the siege city of Kaffa. An unintentional consequence of this may have been the spread of the Black Death across Western Europe resulting in millions of deaths.

An early example of the investigation into the causation of a biological incident or outbreak was demonstrated by Dr John Snow. He identified the pattern of disease (epidemiology) during a cholera outbreak in London and its association with a local water pump. He then went on to remove the pump handle to prove his theory and limit the outbreak (hazard management).

The use of chemical warfare agents during World War I demonstrated not only the clinical impact of their use, with high morbidity and mortality, but also the psychological impact. The first agents used, chlorine, phosgene, and cyanide, highlighted the overlap between chemical weapons and industrial hazards. Mustard, also used in WWI, and the later organophosphate derived nerve agents, were developed solely for military use.

The end of WWII saw the first deployment of a nuclear weapon over Hiroshima, a true weapon of mass destruction (WMD). Casualties not only died from the effects of blast and thermal burns but also high levels of radiation. This cohort of casualties led to the baseline data for the effects of high levels of radiation (acute radiation syndrome) and has since been used as a reference for other ionizing radiation incidents. In 1986, the world saw the consequences of unsafe working practices at Chernobyl with the acute and long-term effects of a nuclear reactor accident. Bad working practices were also a contributing factor to the Bhopal incident, leading to the release of methyl isocyanate over the local residential area leading to significant loss of life and continuing morbidity.

The current requirements for the preparedness for an incident involving HazMat/CBRN come from a number of scenarios—the management of an individual casualty, an industrial accident, a transportation accident, a terrorist event involving a CBRN agent or causing the secondary release of hazardous materials.

Concepts of CBRN exposures

Contamination/contagious (2C's)
- External contamination, including clothing, skin, and hair.
- Internal contamination. Routes for internal contamination include inhalation, ingestion, inoculation (through penetrated skin), transcutaneous (through intact skin), eyes, and mucosa.
- Wound contamination.
- Contagiousness is an infectious state where a patient may present a continuing hazard to responders leading to person-to-person spread.

Persistency
- Non-persistent agents are generally light gases and vapours (carbon monoxide, cyanide gas).
- Persistent agents are generally liquids and solids, including airborne particles (sulphur mustard, VX nerve agent, anthrax spores, radioisotopes, such as caesium, uranium, plutonium).

Effects of exposure to CBRN agents and trauma (4I's)
- Intoxication (chemical and biological toxins); this may be a recognized pattern of symptoms due to a toxic substance (toxidrome).
- Infection (live biological agents); this may be a fever with a recognized pattern of infection (syndromic approach).
- Irradiation (radiation/nuclear); this may be the presentation of either cutaneous radiation injuries (radiation burn) or early effects of high dose radiation (prodromal syndrome including nausea, vomiting diarrhoea, and erythema).
- Injuries (trauma); these are conventional injuries and the pattern recognition would be consistent with the <C>ABC approach to the management of trauma.

Recognition of a CBRN/HazMat event

Safety triggers for emergency personnel (STEP) 1-2-3
- *One casualty:* proceed as usual.
- *Two casualties:* use caution and report.
- *Three or more casualties:* do not approach.

Pre-warning/health surveillance/intelligence
- Hazard identification/labelling (See Table 25.1).
- Threat briefs (pre-planning).
- Community risk registers (pre-planning).
- Missing hazard reports (hazard management).
- Unusual cases reported (case reporting).
- Illness pattern surveillance (epidemiology).

Detection, identification and monitoring (DIM) equipment
- Chemical detectors.
- Chemical mass spectrometry.
- Radiation contamination monitors (Geiger counters).
- Radiation dosimeters.
- Radioisotope identification (gamma spectroscopy).
- Biological sampling (culturing and polymerase chain reaction (PCR) detection).

Chemical syndrome (toxidrome) recognition
- Multiple casualties—see STEP 1-2-3.
- Sudden onset—cyanide
- *Cholinergic (nerve agents):* miosis, excessive secretions, convulsions, respiratory distress.
- *Opiate:* miosis, respiratory depression, reduced level of consciousness.
- Non-thermal burns.

Unusual illnesses
- Single case of an eradicated or extremely rare illness (smallpox).
- Single or multiple cases of a non-endemic illnesses or inconsistent travel histories (viral haemorrhagic fevers, plague, any anthrax presentation).
- Case presentation suggesting deliberate poisoning/release or weaponization (thallium, polonium-210, inhalational anthrax, ricin).
- Multiple cases of common illness with no obvious common pathway/epidemiology (malicious release of salmonella).

Laboratory confirmation
Laboratory confirmation may be by direct visualization of the causative biological agent, or by one of a number of techniques including PCR identification, antigen specific identification, toxicological screening, and assay or biological markers for CBRN exposure, examples include red blood cell acetylcholinesterase levels for nerve agents, cytogenetics for radiation and antibody levels for biological agent exposure.

Table 25.1. Hazard identification

CLASS	SYMBOL	DEFINITION
1		**EXPLOSIVE** Subgroups 1.1 – 1.6 1.1 – Mass explosion hazard 1.4 – No significant hazard
2		**GASES** Subgroup 2.1 – 2.3 2.1 – Flammable 2.2 – Non-flammable 2.3 – Toxic
3		**FLAMMABLE LIQUIDS**
4		**FLAMMABLE SOLIDS** Subgroups 4.1 – 4.3 4.1 – Flammable solid 4.2 – Spontaneous combustion risk 4.3 – Release of flammable gas on contact with water
5		**OXIDISERS (5.1) ORGANIC PEROXIDES (5.2)**
6		**TOXIC (6.1) INFECTIOUS SUBSTANCES (6.2)**
7		**RADIOACTIVE SUBSTANCES**
8		**CORROSIVE SUBSTANCES** (includes chlorine, sodium hydroxide, sulphuric acid)
9		**MISCELLANEOUS** Includes asbestos, CS spray

Incident management

Types of emergency situations

Classification by causation
- Natural causes, including earthquake, tsunami, flooding, natural fires, heat waves, epidemic, and volcanoes.
- Man-made including transportation accidents, war, terrorism, industrial accidents, and mass gatherings.

Classification by time scale/onset
- *Big bang:* these incidents usually result from an overt event, such as an explosion, but include non-explosive causes, such as a gas leak or obvious chemical release. The response is usually concentric around a single or multiple discrete incident scene(s).
- *Rising tide/slowly emerging threat:* this is often due to a covert release or event with a latent period or, in the case of a biological incident (epidemic), an incubation period. There will be no specific incident scene, but an affected area or region subject to potential controls such as quarantine (restriction of movement).
- *Over the horizon:* this is an event that has an indirect effect on services or response. This may be due to an indirect increase in demand for services (population movement due to war/famine in another region) or a restriction on resources due similar reasons (effect of fuel strike on emergency service provision).

Types of incident (size)
- *Major incident:* an incident where contingencies plans are required to compensate for the extra demand on finite resources (compensated response).
- *Mass casualties/fatalities:* an incident resulting in a large number of casualties/fatalities. This may require the rationing of resources for casualties unlikely to survive (expectant).
- *Catastrophy:* an incident that often leads to mass fatalities and compounded by a failure of the responding infrastructure and agencies (uncompensated response). Examples include the 2004 tsunami and Hurricane Katrina.

Concepts of major incident management

METHANE report
- *Major incident:* STAND BY/DECLARED.
- *Exact location:* this may be a grid reference or road junction.
- *Type of incident:* including MVC, explosive incident, rail crash, riot.
- *Hazards:* this part of the report has a direct effect on the safety component of the Major incident response. Some hazards are implied by the type of the incident (MVC, and risk of glass, fire, and sharp objects), while other hazards will need to be specifically identified and reported (hazardous transport). This is a key factor in defining a CBRN/hazardous materials incident, while using a conventional major incident response template.
- *Access:* this maybe a rendezvous or access point usually leading into an established or improvised one-way system (circuit).
- *Number of casualties:* this may include a provision breakdown of triage types and possible fatalities. This allows for the early notification of hospitals. The report of no casualties is also important so that hospitals are stood down.
- Emergency services on scene or required.

See Fig. 25.2.

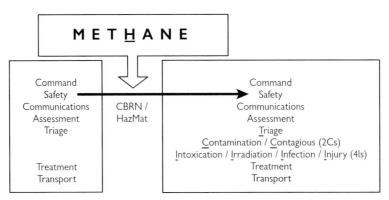

Fig. 25.2. METHANE flow chart.

Areas of an incident scene
- *Inner cordon:* an inner boundary usually controlled by Fire Service around a potentially hazardous area.
- *Outer cordon:* an outer boundary surrounding the incident response infrastructure, usually controlled by the Police.
- *Hot zone:* a non-permissive area where a significant hazard exists (contamination, fire arms).
- *Warm zone:* a semi-permissive area allowing limited treatment and decontamination, but preventing definitive care.
- *Cold (clean) zone:* an area outside the inner cordon allowing full access to casualties usually at casualty clearing stations (CCS).

Triage

Concepts of CBRN triage

For any major incident, including CBRN, with casualties, there is a requirement to allocate resources on a priority basis. This ensures that the casualties with the greatest need are treated first with the finite resources available.

The allocation of resources is based on the sorting or triage of casualties. In addition, casualties exposed to a toxic insult can be labelled as mild, moderate, and severe, based on the known effects of specific agents. There are a number of triage methods both for conventional and CBRN triage.

Triage/severity categories

- *T1—immediate/severe (RED):* these are casualties with respiratory or cardiovascular compromise, or other need for immediate life-saving treatment or intervention.
- *T2—urgent/moderate (YELLOW):* These patients may have a neurological deficit or other reason to be non-ambulatory.
- *T3—delayed/minor (GREEN):* these patients are generally walking, but not asymptomatic.
- *T4—expectant (palliative—BLUE):* this is a category only used in a mass casualty or catastrophic incident and limits intervention to palliative treatment in order to conserve resources to patients that have a significant chance of survival.
- *Dead (BLACK/WHITE):* in a CBRN incident the definition may vary from a trauma only incident due the differing aetiology of respiratory arrest usually used to declare a casualty dead.

Triage methods

- Algorithm/flowchart.
- Scoring systems.
- Injury severity.
- Clinical assessment.
- Signs of specific toxicity.

Zonal triage (see Fig. 25.3)

- *Signs of life:* no respiratory ± cardiac (ECG) activity.
- CBRN triage sieve (before decontamination) using an algorithmic system.
- CBRN triage sieve (after decontamination—see below).
- CBRN triage sort using a physiological scoring system.
- Triage for surgery based on best prognosis and injury severity.
- Triage for ICU, the use of the expectant (T4) may be a factor for ICU admission.

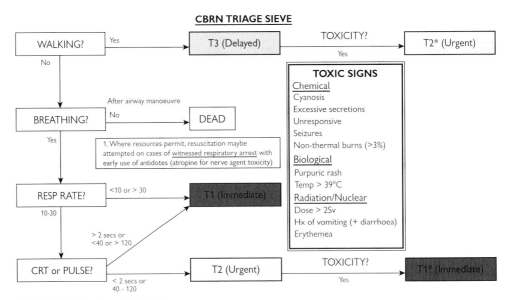

Fig. 25.3. CBRN triage sieve. © S. A. Bland.

Principles of CBRN casualty management

Hot/warm zone casualty management

Safety
A hazard assessment must be performed so that selection of correct personal protective equipment can be made (see Table 25.2). Time in the hot zone should be minimized for both casualties, who should be evacuated to the warm zone, and rescuers.

Injury pattern or syndrome recognition
Potential problems include blast injury, penetrating and blunt injuries, environmental illness (heat/cold/altitude/diving-related), and psychological problems (acute stress reactions and the worried well).

A CBRN Quick Look should take place (see next section—'Chemical agents').

Life-saving interventions (LSIs)
These will follow the generic <C>ABCD management paradigm. Tourniquets should be applied for catastrophic haemorrhage and the airway managed using basic techniques.

Antidotes, including nerve agent auto-injectors, should be administered using self or buddy aid.

Decontamination
Casualties should be exposed sufficiently to treat them (face, iv, or io access points); this means undressing them to the skin followed by full decontamination, wet/dry (military option).

Evacuation to a more permissive environment
Evacuation should take place in the sequence:

> Hot zone → Warm zone → Cold or Clean zone

Cold/clean zone casualty management

Diagnosis
A history should be taken and a clinical examination and appropriate investigations performed.

Supporting scientific (DIM) information should be sought.

Supportive management as required
This is likely to include:
- Oxygen.
- Establish definitive airway.
- Fluids.
- Analgesia.
- Broad spectrum antibiotics (benzylpenicillin, cefuroxime).

Definitive management as indicated
Definitive management includes:
- Agent specific antidotes.
- Disease specific antibiotics, such as ciprofloxacin and doxycycline for anthrax and rickettsia, respectively.
- Surgery.

Table 25.2. Personal protective equipment

Class	Description
A	Self-contained breathing apparatus in a gas-tight suit
B	Self-contained breathing apparatus in a splash-resistant suit
C	Splash-resistant suit with self- or power-ventilated respiratory protection
D	Standard precautions (includes airborne protection with high protection particulate filtered face mask (FFP3/N95)

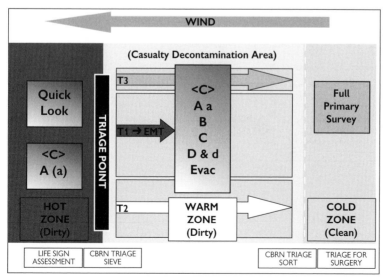

Fig. 25.4. Casualty management zones.

Chemical agents (including industrial and military threats)

Classification

There are a number of classification systems for chemical agents, both of industrial and military origin.

Chemical asphyxiants
- Cyanides.
- Carbon monoxide.
- Methaemoglobin formers.

Nerve agents
- Organophosphate nerve agents.
- Other neurotoxic chemicals of note.

Lung damaging (pulmonary) agents
- Chlorine.
- Phosgene.
- Other lung damaging chemicals of note.

Vesicants (blistering) agent/chemical burns
- Sulphur mustard.
- Lewisite.
- Acid burns (including hydrofluoric acid).
- Phosphorous burns.

Incapacitants
- CS and other riot-control agents.
- LSD/anticholinergics (atropine/BZ).
- Opiates including fentanyl analogues.

Diagnosis of chemical agents

CBRN 'Quick Look'
This can be applied to casualties within the contaminated area (hot/warm zone) as a rapid assessment. The examples given are not exhaustive (see Table 25.3).

Respiration
- Normal.
- Fast/distressed (nerve agents, pulmonary agents).
- Shallow/reduced respiratory drive (opiate).
- Apnoea (opiate, severe cyanide).
- Kussmaul type (lactic acidosis, cyanide).

Eyes
- Normal.
- Pinpoint (opiate, nerve agents).
- Dilated (anticholinergics).

Skin
- Normal.
- Pink/flushed (CO, early cyanide).
- Cyanosed (late cyanide, methaemoglobin).
- Pallor (shock).
- Erythema/blistered (early/late onset vesicants).

Secretions (and other bodily fluids)
- Normal.
- Dry (anticholinergics).
- Excessive (nerve agents, pulmonary agents).

Chemical Primary Survey

The Chemical Primary Survey can be applied to casualties following decontamination and uses the ABCD approach (see Fig. 25.6).

Table 25.3. CBRN quick look

	CBRN QUICK LOOK								
	Nerve Agent	Cyanide	MetHb	Pulm Agents	Vesicant/acid	Botulinum	Atropine/BZ	Opiate
Respiration	↑↑	↑↑/↓	↑	↑↑	↑	↓	N/↑	↓
Pupils	Pinpoint	N/dilated	N	N	N/red	Dilated	Dilated	Pinpoint
Skin	Sweaty	Pink or cyanosed	Cyanosed	Normal or Cyanosed	Erythema	Dry	Dry	N
Secretions	↑↑	N	N	↑	N/↑	↓	↓	N
Other	Fasiculation Fitting	Sudden onset	Chocolate blood		Mustard (delayed)	↓ Paralysis, no CNS effects	CNS effects	CNS effects

Chemical asphyxiants

Cyanides

Mechanism of action (chemical asphyxiant)
Interaction of the cyanide (CN^-) molecule with intracellular enzymes such as cytochrome-A_3 leading to the inhibition of intracellular respiration. This causes a profound lactic acidosis and dysfunction of organs that are particularly dependent upon aerobic respiration.

Principle routes of exposure
- Inhalation (hydrogen cyanide).
- Ingestion (cyanide salts).

Incident management
Hospital Personal Protective Equipment
Chemical PPE (Level C or above) should be considered if there is an off gas hazard from ingested salts.

Decontamination
- Non-persistent in gaseous form.
- May be persistent as ingested cyanide salt.

Clinical approach
History: key points
- Sudden onset (seconds) (key feature).
- May be identifiable source or release device.
- Plastics fire.
- Occupational access to cyanide (jeweller, chemical industry).

CBRN Quick Look
- *Resp:* rapid, Kussmaul, apnoea.
- *Eyes:* normal, dilated.
- *Skin:* normal, pink, cyanosed.
- *Secretions:* normal.

Examination: key points
- Initially pink then cyanosed.
- Rapid breathing followed by respiratory arrest.
- Arrhythmias.
- Fitting.
- Coma.
- Death.

Supportive management
- Airway support.
- High flow oxygen.
- Ventilatory support.

Antidotes
- Oxygen.
- Sodium (amyl) nitrite followed by sodium thiosulphate.
- Dicobalt edentate—cobalt donor.
- Hydroxycobalamin (vitamin $B_{12}a$)—cobalt donor.

Carbon monoxide (CO)

Mechanism of action (chemical asphyxiant)
High affinity for haemoglobin compared with oxygen. Reduction in oxygen binding capacity and oxygen delivery causing tissue hypoxia. Possible interaction with intracellular enzymes.

Principle routes of exposure
Inhalation.

Incident management
Hospital personal protective equipment
No specific PPE required.

Decontamination
Non-persistent, therefore no decontamination requirement once removed from hazardous area.

Clinical approach
History: key points
- May be identifiable source (boiler/heater) (key feature).
- May be sudden or insidious onset.
- Recent cold weather spell.
- Mild symptoms include nausea, vomiting, headaches, vertigo, poor concentration, depression.

CBRN Quick Look
- *Resp:* normal, apnoea.
- *Eyes:* normal, dilated.
- *Skin:* normal, pink (cherry-red—usually terminal).
- *Secretions:* normal.

Examination: key points
- Patent airway, no secretions.
- Reduced conscious level.
- Cerebellar signs.
- Altered gait.
- Coma.
- Cherry pink skin colour.
- Death.

Supportive management
- Airway support.
- High flow oxygen.
- CPAP/IPPV.

Antidotes & definitive management
- Oxygen.
- Consider referral to Hyperbaric Units. Referral criteria include: loss of consciousness, pregnancy, neurological signs. Hyperbaric treatment remains controversial.

Methaemoglobin formers

Mechanism of action (chemical asphyxiant)

Methaemoglobin formers, such as nitrites (poppers), nitrates, and other industrial chemical, oxidize the ferrous (Fe^{2+}) iron in haemoglobin to ferric (Fe^{3+}), thus forming methaemoglobin. This results in a reduction in the oxygen binding capacity of red blood cells and oxygen delivery causing tissue hypoxia (Fig. 25.5).

Principle routes of exposure

• Inhalation (amyl nitrite/poppers).
• Ingestion.
• Intravenous (prilocaine).

Incident management

Hospital personal protective equipment
Depends on causative agent/chemical.

Decontamination
Depends on causative agent/chemical.

Clinical approach

History: key points
• Exposure to causative agent.
• Recreational drug use.
• Cyanosis resistant to oxygen therapy (key feature).

CBRN Quick Look
• *Resp:* normal, rapid.
• *Eyes:* normal.
• *Skin:* cyanosis (key feature).
• *Secretions:* normal.

Examination: key points
• Cyanosis ('Smurf syndrome').
• Agitation.
• Tachypnoea (30% MetHb).
• Possible hypotension.
• Reduced conscious level.
• Coma.
• Death (associated with 60%+ MetHb).

Supportive management
• Airway support.
• High flow oxygen.

Antidotes and definitive management
Methylene blue ('Smurf juice') IV.

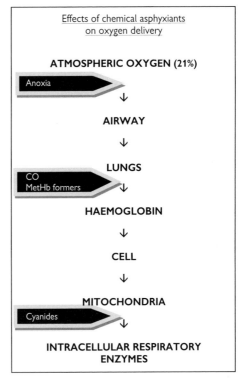

Fig. 25.5. Effects of chemical asphyxiants on oxygen delivery.

Nerve agents

Organophosphate nerve agents

Mechanism of action

Inhibition of the enzyme acetylcholinesterase leading to a cholinergic crisis. This causes:

- Increased acetylcholine at the neuromuscular junction leading to a depolarizing paralysis.
- Increased acetylcholine across CNS synapses leading to seizures and CNS dysfunction.
- Increased acetylcholine across autonomic synapses and end organs leading to autonomic overstimulation, predominantly parasympathetic.

Military nerve agents (G and V agents) are far more toxic than the organophosphate pesticides (OPPs).

Principle routes of exposure

- Inhalation (most G agents, such as sarin).
- Ingestion (OP pesticides).
- Percutaneous (VX).
- Eyes [G-agents (local effect), VX/OPPs (systemic)].

Incident management

Hospital personal protective equipment
Chemical personal protective equipment.

Decontamination
Depends on the agent and its persistency, but includes the removal of any obvious liquid contaminant and clothing, rinse-wipe-rinse, and monitoring for any continuing absorption especially if ingested. Consider gut decontamination for ingested OPPs.

Clinical approach

History: key points
- Exposure to causative agent.
- Mass casualties/STEP 1-2-3.
- Occupational history if OPPs (farmer).
- Dimmed vision, eye pain.

CBRN Quick Look
- *Resp:* rapid, distressed, wheezing, apnoea.
- *Eyes:* pinpoint (key feature).
- *Skin:* sweating, possible fasciculations.
- *Secretions:* excessive with vomiting and incontinence (key feature).

Examination: key points
- Quick Look features are diagnostic.
- Bradycardia.
- Bronchoconstriction, high airway pressures.
- Seizures.
- Reduced conscious level, coma.
- Peripheral neuropathy (delayed)—OPPs.

Supportive management
Airway support including suction

Antidotes and definitive management
- Oximes (pralidoxime, obidoxime, HI-6).
- Atropine.
- Benzodiazepines.

Other neurotoxic CBRN type agents

Acute

Spasm forming
- Strychnine.
- Tetanus toxin (biological).

Non-depolarizing paralysis
- Botulinum toxin (biological).
- Tetrodotoxin (biological).
- Neurotoxic snake venoms(biological).

Chronic

Peripheral neuropathies
- Lead.
- Thallium.
- Organophosphate intermediate syndrome (OPPs).

Lung damaging (pulmonary) agents

Chlorine

Mechanism of action (lung damaging)
Chlorine reacts with water to form hydrochloric acid. Effects are relatively rapid with immediate discomfort to airway and eyes. Local effects in the lung may be due to direct effect on cell membrane integrity and increasing alveolar permeability. This leads to a non-cardiogenic pulmonary oedema.

Principle routes of exposure
Inhalation.

Incident management
Hospital personal protective equipment
No specific PPE is required once casualty removed from hazard. Beware basements and other low areas as heavier than air.

Decontamination
Non-persistent, therefore, no decontamination requirement once removed from hazardous area.

Clinical approach
History: key points
- History of exposure to chlorine (swimming pool, mixing cleaning products).
- Painful eyes and airway, usually rapid onset.
- Cough.
- Onset usually within 6 h.

CBRN Quick Look
- *Resp:* cough, normal, rapid, distressed.
- *Eyes:* normal.
- *Skin:* normal, cyanosed (pre-terminal).
- *Secretions:* frothy sputum (key feature).

Examination: key points
- As above.
- Oxygen desaturation, responds to oxygen.
- Type 1 respiratory failure.

Supportive management
- Airway support.
- High flow oxygen.
- CPAP/IPPV (with PEEP).
- Fluid resuscitation especially if using high PEEP.

Antidotes and definitive management
None.

Phosgene

Mechanism of action (lung damaging)
Phosgene affects the lung indirectly by causing free radical formation and an inflammatory response. There may be a mixed clinical picture of non-cardiogenic pulmonary and acute acquired respiratory distress syndrome (ARDS). A worse outcome has been associated with physical exertion after exposure. Phosgene accounted for the majority of chemical deaths in WW1. Phosgene is more toxic than chlorine by an order of magnitude.

Principle routes of exposure
Inhalation.

Incident management
Hospital personal protective equipment
No specific PPE required once casualty removed from hazard. Beware basements and other low areas as heavier than air.

Decontamination
Non-persistent, therefore, no decontamination requirement once removed from hazardous area.

Clinical approach
History: key points
- History of exposure to phosgene.
- Smell of 'freshly mown hay'.
- Exposure may be asymptomatic.
- Delayed onset of up to 24 h (dependant on concentration and duration of exposure).

CBRN Quick Look
- *Resp:* cough, normal, rapid, distressed.
- *Eyes:* normal.
- *Skin:* normal, cyanosed (pre-terminal).
- *Secretions:* frothy sputum (key feature).

Examination: key points
- As above.
- Oxygen desaturation, responds to oxygen.
- Type 1 respiratory failure, maybe Type 2 component.
- Greater lung involvement/shadowing than chlorine radiographs.

Supportive management
- Airway support.
- High flow oxygen.
- CPAP/IPPV (possible protective ventilation strategy).
- Fluid resuscitation especially if using high PEEP.

Antidotes and definitive management
- Consider post-exposure steroids (inhaled/systemic).
- Animal model suggests N-acetylcystine may have a protective effect.

Vesicants (blistering) agents

Sulphur mustard

Mechanism of action
The mechanism of mustard is not clearly understood, but is thought to be due to a number of reactions. Mustard is an alkylating agent, and is thought to damage DNA and the cell membrane causing cell death as well potential carcinogenesis. Sulphur mustard is also a weak cholinergic and may cause glutathione depletion.

Principle routes of exposure
- Percutaneous.
- Inhalation.
- Eyes.

Incident management
Hospital personal protective equipment
Chemical PPE.

Decontamination
- Persistent hazard, rapid decontamination (within minutes). Removal of obvious liquid contamination and clothes, then rinse-wipe-rinse. Consider hypochlorite (0.5% bleach) solution. Blister fluid is not a significant chemical hazard—treat as biological hazard.
- Consider cooling skin, may reduce damage.

Clinical approach
History: key points
- Smell of garlic.
- Exposure to a brown-coloured liquid, similar to diesel.
- *Delayed onset of effects (hours)*, dependent on concentration and duration of exposure (key feature).
- Effects warm and moist areas (eyes, armpit, groins).

CBRN Quick Look
- *Resp:* normal.
- *Eyes:* slow onset inflammation.
- *Skin:* slow onset erythema.
- *Secretions:* normal.

Examination: key points
- Slowly developing blisters (over 24 h).
- Vesicles that develop into bullae.
- 4% mortality during WW1.
- Potential airway compromise.
- Potential ARDS.
- Monitor for leucopenia.

Supportive management
- Treat as thermal burns initially.
- Mydriatic eye drops/vaseline to eye lids.
- Potential laser ablation treatments.
- Overall good skin and ophthalmic healing with conservative management.

Antidotes and definitive management
- None except rapid decontamination.
- Skin laser ablation therapy demonstrated in animal models (improved healing rate).

Lewisite (arsenicals)

Mechanism of action
The toxicity of lewisite is due to arsenic. Unlike mustard, symptom are rapid and there is a greater associated mortality. Toxicity is local (rapid onset) and systemic due to absorption of arsenic. Arsenic has multiple sites of action including the cardiovascular and renal (nephropathies) system, peripheral nervous system (neuropathies), and haemolysis.

Principle routes of exposure
- Percutaneous.
- Inhalation.
- Eyes.

Incident management
Hospital personal protective equipment
Chemical PPE.

Decontamination
Persistent hazard, rapid decontamination (within minutes). Removal of obvious liquid contamination and clothes, then rinse-wipe-rinse. *Blister fluid is a significant chemical hazard.*

Clinical approach
History: key points
- Rapid onset of symptoms (key feature).
- Respiratory feature if inhaled.
- Associated systemic features.

CBRN Quick Look
- *Resp:* normal, possible pulmonary oedema.
- *Eyes:* rapid onset eye pain.
- *Skin:* rapid onset of painful chemical burns.
- *Secretions:* normal.

Examination: key points
- Rapid onset of symptoms.
- Silvery-grey lesions.
- Multi organ failure.
- *High mortality* (key feature).

Supportive management
- Apply antidote ointments (see below).
- Supportive eye care/antidote ointment.
- Potential long-term ophthalmic complications/scarring.

Antidotes and definitive management
Heavy metal chelating agents including dimercaprol [British Anti-Lewisite (BAL)/dimercaptosuccinic acid (DMSA)].

Acids (including hydrofluoric)

Mechanism of action

The toxic effect of most acids is due to the local effect of high hydrogen ion (H^+) concentration. However, hydrofluoric acid has systemic toxicity due to the effect of fluoride ions (F^-) on circulating calcium levels. The resulting hypocalcaemia will lead to hypotension, cardiac dysrhythmias, and cardiac arrest. HF burns of less than 5% may be lethal.

Principle routes of exposure

Percutaneous.

Incident management

Hospital personal protective equipment
Chemical PPE.

Decontamination
Immediate on scene decontamination with water on scene and application of HF antidote (calcium gluconate gel).

Clinical approach

History: key points
- Rapid onset of symptoms (key feature).
- Usually occupational history of HF use.

CBRN Quick Look
- *Resp:* normal.
- *Eyes:* normal.
- *Skin:* rapid onset of painful chemical burns.
- *Secretions:* normal.

Examination: key points
- Rapid onset of symptoms.
- ECG changes and hypotension.
- High mortality if significant area of HF burn.

Supportive management
- Apply antidote gel (calcium gluconate).
- Supportive care, fluids.

Antidotes and definitive management
- Calcium chloride iv.
- Calcium gluconate local infiltration.

Phosphorous burns

Mechanism of action

White phosphorous (WP) is used widely in flares and some munitions. It burns spontaneously in air, and causes both thermal and chemical burns. The latter is due to the formation of phosphoric acid.

Principle routes of exposure

- Percutaneous.
- Inhalation.

Incident management

Hospital personal protective equipment
- Burns kit.
- Chemical PPE.
- Fire protection equipment for residual WP.

Decontamination
- Persistent hazard, continuous water irrigation.
- Prevention of WP reigniting.

Clinical approach

History: key points
- Rapid onset of symptoms (key feature).
- Handling munitions or flares.
- Thermal burns.

CBRN Quick Look
- *Resp:* normal, possible thermal burns.
- *Eyes:* possible smoke, thermal injuries.
- *Skin:* thermal, chemical burns.
- *Secretions:* normal.

Examination: key points
Burns associated with exposure to WP.

Supportive management
- Copious fluids.
- Management of burns, using Parklands burns formula.

Antidotes and definitive management
- Irrigation with isotonic sodium bicarbonate solution.
- CAUTION: Copper sulphate is NOT recommended due to the potential for absorption and copper toxicity.

Incapacitants

Mechanism of action

There are a number of incapacitating agents. However, they all share the same ability to cross the blood–brain barrier to exert their effect, compromising the central nervous system (CNS). Some agents such as the opiates, including the fentanyl analogous, depress the CNS. Others including LSD and the centrally acting anticholinergics (atropine, BZ) tend to cause stimulation and CNS dysfunction.

Principle routes of exposure
Inhalation.

Incident management
Hospital personal protective equipment
Chemical PPE as required, agent specific.

Decontamination
Removal from environment, if gas/vapour.

Clinical approach
History: key points
- Altered conscious level (depressed/elevated) (key feature).
- Anticholinergic features with central effects.

CBRN Quick Look
- *Resp:* depressed (opiates).
- *Eyes:* pinpoint (opiates), dilated (anti-cholinergics).
- *Skin:* red, flushed (anticholinergics), cyanosed (severe opiate).
- *Secretions:* dry (anticholinergics).

Examination: key points
- Pupils.
- Secretions.

Supportive management (opiates)
Ventilatory support (opiates).

Supportive management (stimulants/anticholinergics)
- Observation and reassurance.
- Sedation (anticholinergics).
- Avoid physical restraint.

Antidotes and definitive management
- Naloxone (opiates).
- Physostigmine (anticholinergics).

CS & other riot-control agents

Mechanism of action
Under international conventions, riot-control agents (RCA) are not considered chemical weapons and are used widely in law-enforcement. Their mechanism of action is a mild to severe local irritation of the mucosa (mainly eyes and airway).

Principle routes of exposure
- Eyes.
- Inhalation.

Incident management
Hospital personal protective equipment
- Stand upwind from casualties (mild cases, low numbers).
- Chemical PPE (severe cases, large numbers).

Decontamination
- Aeration in fresh air.
- Removal of clothes in severe cases.
- Caution: avoid warm/hot water decontamination (reactivation).

Clinical approach
History: key points
- Rapid onset of symptoms (key feature).
- Civil disturbance.
- Police arrest.

CBRN Quick Look
- *Resp:* mild irritation, potential exacerbation of asthma.
- *Eyes:* mild-severe irritation (reversible).
- *Skin:* mild irritation.
- *Secretions:* normal, tears.

Examination: key points
- Improvement in fresh air.
- Absence of chemical burns/erythema.

Supportive management
Nebulizers, as required.

Antidotes and definitive management
Supportive management only.

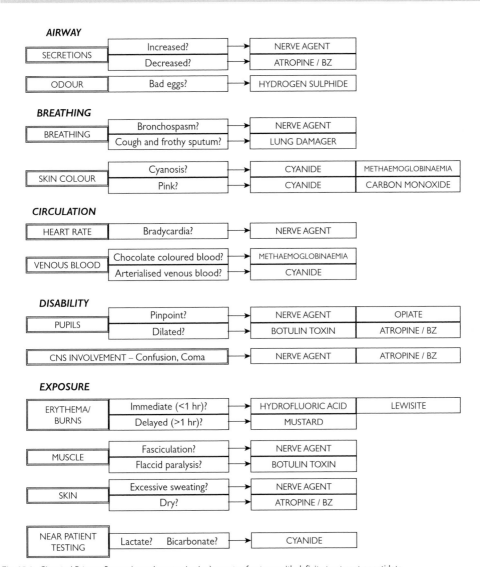

Fig. 25.6. Chemical Primary Survey (post-decontamination): agents of note or with definite treatment or antidote.

Note: the list is not exclusive, but highlights signs and symptoms more specific to CW & toxic industrial chemicals with specific and antidotal treatment.

Biological agents

Introduction
Biological agents can be classified into two groups, namely live agents and toxins.

Live agents
Live agents have the ability to self-replicate in the right environment and may also have the ability to produce disease causing toxins. Following an exposure to a live agent there will be an asymptomatic (latency) period, the incubation period. As the infection becomes established there may be a prodromal phase with flu-like symptoms including fever, myalgia, and fatigue. Live agents may be susceptible to antimicrobials, such as antibiotics. Examples of live biological agents with examples of the disease caused are:
- Bacteria (anthrax, plague, salmonella).
- Viruses (smallpox, viral haemorrhagic fevers, influenza).
- Rickettsias (typhus, Rocky Mountain spotted fever).
- Protozoa (amoebic dysentery, malaria).
- Chlamydia (psittacosis).

Toxins
A toxin can be considered to be a chemically active agent of biological origin. Therefore, it does not self-replicate and is non-transmissible; however, decontamination may be required. Biological toxins may be derived from microbes, or be of animal or plant origin. Examples include botulinum, snake/scorpion venom, or digitalis from foxglove. Toxins will generally have a shorter *latency* period (hours to days) compared with the longer *incubation period* of a live agent, which may be weeks and, in some cases, months (viral hepatitis, HIV). Some live agents will also produce toxins as part of the infection (tetanus, anthrax, botulinum). However, some toxins can be used and spread without needing a live agent (botulinum, ricin, staphylococcal toxin). Antimicrobials will not provide protection from a specific toxin, although they may combat the causative live agent if present. Treatment of toxin-related illnesses is generally based on supportive management and, in some causes, anti-toxins using immunoglobulin against specific toxin antigens, examples include botulinum and tetanus immunoglobulin.

Properties of biological agents
Pathogenicity is used to describe live agents that have the ability to cause disease (pathogens). Biological agents can be categorized broadly into *lethal* or *non-lethal, transmissible* or *non-transmissible. Transmissibility* reflects the ability of a live agent to spread from person to person. *Infectivity* differs from transmissibility as it reflects the ease an agent can establish an infection either from another person, animal, or environment. This is quantified as the infective dose to infect 50% of the exposed population (ID_{50}). For example, tularemia is extremely infectious requiring only 10–50 organisms, while anthrax spores require 10^4–10^5 spores to establish an infection. However, both are virtually non-transmissible directly from an infected patient to another human. Some patients may therefore be infected, but not infectious/contagious. Malaria is another important disease that is not transmissible from human to human, and requires an animal *vector,* in this case the mosquito.

Epidemiology
Biological incidents can occur for a number of reasons— natural outbreaks (pandemic flu, measles, plague), sudden population migration or failure of infrastructure (cholera), natural disasters (dysentery, cholera), and deliberate disease (plague, anthrax, salmonella). Unlike explosive incidents or most chemical releases, biological incidents are usually covert or slowly evolving due to the longer latency (incubation) period. The predicted casualty pattern and magnitude depends on a number of parameters including the type of agent release, infectivity, virulence, and transmissibility. In some cases, outbreaks are self-limiting because of the severity, rapid onset, and transmissibility. These outbreaks are said to *burn themselves out.* However, with modern transportation, there remains a high risk of outbreaks becoming multi-focal and even pandemic [Influenza, 1918–1919 and Severe Acute Respiratory Syndrome (SARS), 2003].

Examples of casualty patterns include:
- *Point release with no person-to-person transmission*: this pattern appears as a normal distribution peak around an average incubation period. A food poisoning outbreak or release of a toxin would be a good example. Intermittent cases following the main peak may be seen for more persistent organisms that may be re-aerosolized, such as anthrax spores.
- *Continuing release* leading to intermittent cases over a longer period of time. This would be suggestive of a compromised food chain such as a ruptured or tainted water supply (cholera) or a person-to person spread via an asymptomatic carrier (typhoid, sexually transmitted diseases).
- *Person-to-person spread*: this shape of the epidemic curve depends on the infectivity of the agent and incubation period. In general, the curve will increase exponentially. However, a peak may be seen in the curve that equates to the incubation period of each wave of the outbreak. Examples include smallpox, pneumonic plague, and influenza.

Biological agents and trauma
Following any traumatic event, but especially after a blast injury, there is potential for the transmission of blood-borne viruses. While there is limited evidence, studies have suggested that some viruses such as hepatitis B may be present in biological shrapnel. This has implications for any survivors that are injured by bone fragments from a suicide bomber or co-victim. Prophylactic treatment for hepatitis B (accelerated course) should be considered for casualties at risk. The HIV virus is much less likely to be viable and post-exposure prophylaxis (PEP) may be contraindicated in a traumatized patient. Toxins may also be implicated in the potential deterioration of trauma patients. Specific agents of concern include botulinum and ricin. Specific guidance depends on the incident and risk, but follow-up of casualties is suggested during rehabilitation and this should include counselling and further clinical risk stratification. Advice was provided by the Health Protection Agency for victims of the 7/7 London Bombings in 2005.

Syndromic approach to biological casualties

Syndromic presentations

Many of the biological agents can be grouped into specific syndromes. The syndromes they present with often reflect the route of exposure and some agents, such as anthrax, may present with more than one syndrome (inhalational, intestinal, and cutaneous).

Live agents, irrespective of their manifest syndrome generally have a flu-like prodromal phase with a characteristic fever and myalgia. Some illnesses may be limited to just this phase before resolution. The six main syndromes are shown in Fig. 25.7 with examples of causative agents. Some toxins will also present with recognizable syndromes, although they may not necessarily have a prodromal phase.

There are a few agents, both live and toxins, which have no single system presentation and may present with multiple organ involvement. These agents usually act at the intracellular level. For example, ricin acts as a protein synthesis inhibitor and presents with systemic inflammatory response syndrome (SIRS) and multi-organ failure (MOF).

Typical symptoms and signs associated with each syndrome include:

- *Respiratory*: cough, chest pain, haemoptysis, shortness of breath, cyanosis.
- *Cutaneous*: rash including erythematous, maculopapular, vesicular, pustules, and purpura (non-blanching).
- *Gastrointestinal*: nausea, vomiting, diarrhoea, dysentery, abdominal pain.
- *Haemorrhagic*: purpura, bruising, bleeding.
- *Neurological (peripheral)*: paraesthesia, hyperaesthesia, pain, flaccid paralysis, tetany, signs of respiratory failure.
- *Neurological (central) due to meningitis, encephalitis or space occupying lesion (abscess)*: neck pain, photophobia, altered consciousness, hallucinations (visual), convulsions, hyperreflexia, paralysis.

Sepsis

Following an exposure to a biological agent, a patient may become infected, and exhibit the signs and symptoms of a specific syndrome. As the infection elicits an immune response, there will an inflammatory reaction. In severe cases this will meet the criteria for Severe Inflammatory Response Syndrome (SIRS); in the presence of infection this is termed sepsis.

Management of septic patients, irrespective of a natural or malicious intent follows the guidance set by the Surviving Sepsis campaign. Priorities include:

- Early goal driven therapy.

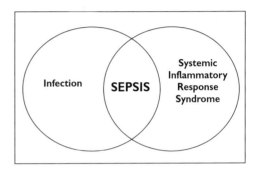

- Source identification (septic screening).
- Early empirical antibiotic therapy (<1 h).
- Refine antibiotic therapy according to microbiological results.
- Intensive care treatment bundle including, low tidal volume ventilation and euglycaemic control.

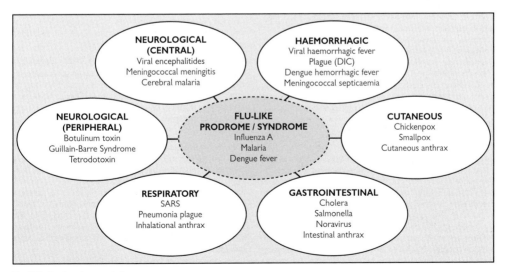

Fig. 25.7. Syndromic presentations.

Biological agents of concern

Centre for Disease Control and Prevention (CDC) Threat Classification

The Centre for Disease Control and Prevention (CDC) provides a useful classification for biological agents that may cause concern based upon likelihood and consequence. Some are naturally a threat, while others have the potential to be released deliberately or weaponized.

Class A biological agents

These agents are classed as high priority due to:
- Being easily disseminated or transmitted from person-to-person.
- Having a high mortality rates and have the potential for major public health impact.
- Having the potential to cause public panic and social disruption.
- Requiring special action for public health preparedness.

Anthrax

This is an infection with three forms, inhalational (mediastinitis), intestinal, and cutaneous, due to the spore forming *Bacillus anthracis*. Inhalational and intestinal anthrax are associated with a high lethality. There is no significant risk of person-to-person spread. Treatment is typically with ciprofloxacin. A vaccine is available.

Botulism

This is a peripheral neurological syndrome with flaccid descending paralysis, anticholinergic features and CNS sparing. The syndrome is due to a toxin, which has seven forms and is derived from *Clostridium botulinum*. There are three types of botulism due to aetiology; wound, food-borne, and infantile. Botulinum toxin may also be weaponized. The management is early treatment with polyvalent antitoxin and supportive management, including ventilatory support. Differential diagnosis includes the Miller-Fisher variant of Guillain–Barrè syndrome.

Plague

This disease, which is still endemic in some areas of the world, is caused by the bacteria *Yersinia pestis*. It has two forms, bubonic and pneumonic. The former is a vector-borne disease passed by flea bite, while the latter is passed from person-to-person. Symptoms include painful swollen, haemorrhagic lymph nodes (buboids) in the bubonic form. The pneumonic form includes a productive blood-stained cough. Death is frequent and due to sepsis and disseminated intravascular coagulopathy (DIC). Treatment includes antibiotics and supportive management.

Smallpox

This disease has now been eradicated through a WHO global immunization programme, but remains on the CDC threat list. The disease, due to a variola virus, had a major and minor form with famous victims including Elizabeth I. The more severe major strains had a high mortality rate with little definitive treatment. The rash associated with the disease is vesicular and may become haemorrhagic or pustular. The lesions tend to be more peripheral than the lesions of chicken pox, which tend to be on the trunk. Patients are infectious prior to the rash and the infection is highly contagious with an air-borne hazard. Management of an epidemic would involve a rapid mass immunization programme as the current global immunity is likely to be very low.

Tularaemia

This illness caused by the highly infectious *Francisella tularensis* has a very low ID_{50} of only a few organisms, making it ideal for weaponization, although it is naturally occurring in many regions of the world. There is no person-to-person spread. The onset of symptoms may be slow with mild non-specific symptoms and fever. If untreated, the disease may be fatal with progression to DIC and acute respiratory failure. Treatment includes doxycycline.

Viral haemorrhagic fevers (VrHF)

There is a range of VHFs, many from the *filoviridae* and arena virus (Lassa, Machupo) family. Many of the VHFs are vector-borne and are not transmissible. Ebola and Marburg are notable as they may be passed on by exposure to body fluids and potential air-borne spread. Death is due to haemorrhage, sepsis, and multi-organ failure. Treatment is supportive but there are vaccines to some VHFs (yellow fever).

Class B biological agents

These agents:
- Are moderately easy to disseminate.
- Result in moderate morbidity rates and low mortality rates.
- Require specific enhancements of CDC's diagnostics capacity and enhanced disease surveillance.

Brucellosis

This is a zoonotic bacteria infection with domestic animals such as sheep and goats as the natural reservoir. Transmission to humans is by inhalation of aerosolized or ingested infected meat. It has a relatively long latency period, 1–4 weeks, and is only moderately lethal (<6%). Treatment is with doxycycline and rifampicin.

Epsilon toxin of Cl. perfringens

This is a neurotoxin derived from *Cl. perfringens*, the causative agent of gas gangrene. The alpha-toxin has also been suggested as a possible pulmonary toxin.

Food safety threats (Salmonella, E. coli O157, Shigella)

There are a number of microbes that cause gastroenteritis that are acquired from food. In severe cases, they may be fatal, but are generally incapacitating. Person-to-person spread may occur, but limited by simple hand hygiene and standard precautions.

Glanders

This is a severe localized infection at the sites of exposure, skin, mucosa, and pulmonary lesions. The bacillus, *Burkholderia mallei*, is predominately found in horses, donkeys, and mules. In severe cases, the human version may also cause an overwhelming sepsis leading to death, if untreated. Treatment includes long-term antibiotic therapy with amoxicillin/clavulanate or doxycycline. The skin lesions (pustules) may be mistaken initially as smallpox, while the microscopic appearance is similar to *Y. pestis* (plague).

Melioidosis

Burkholderia pseudomallei, causes a disease in animals and humans with a wide range of symptoms and findings. Infection is generally from exposure to an aerosol and may lead to a significant pneumonia with cavitations. Treatment is difficult and requires long-term therapy.

Psittacosis

An atypical pneumonia caused by *Chlamydia psittaci* from infected birds. It has a varied clinical course including fever, headache and lower/upper respiratory tract infection. Treatment is with the macrolides and person-to-person spread is unlikely.

Q fever

This is a self-limiting incapacitating disease with pulmonary features due to the zoonotic rickettsia *Coxiella burnetii*. The organism is relatively persistent in the environment and can be aerosolized. The main reservoirs are sheep, cattle, and goats. Treatment is with doxycycline. Differential diagnosis includes the atypical pneumonias. There is no person-to-person transmission.

Ricin toxin

This toxin is derived from the castor oil plant. It prevents protein synthesis by inhibiting messenger RNA transcription. A SIRS response may be noted, but casualties will present with multi-organ failure and local inflammation at the route of exposure (pulmonary, percutaneous). There is no specific antidote, although research continues into an effective antitoxin. This was the toxin used to assassinate the Bulgarian dissident Georgi Markov. There is no person-to-person transmission of the toxin.

Staphylococcal enterotoxin B (SEB)

This is an exotoxin from the bacteria *Staphylococcus aureus*. The toxin is a common cause of sudden onset self-limiting food poisoning. It has the potential to be weaponized and as an aerosol may cause pulmonary complications and death. There is no person-to-person transmission of the toxin.

Typhus fever

There are a number of rickettsial species that cause a range of similar diseases with varying mortality from <1% to 40%. The vector is either a flea tick or louse, and associate with poor living conditions. This disease was a common cause of death during military campaigns during the Napoleonic era. There is no person-to-person spread.

Viral encephalitis

There are a number of zoonotic viruses from the alphavirus family (Venezuelan equine encephalitis, eastern equine encephalitis and western equine encephalitis) that have the potential to be aerosolized. Usually found in equine animals (horse, mule, and donkey) and passed on to humans by an act as simple as a bite. This disease has a low fatality rate (<1%), although this maybe higher in the paediatric population. Symptoms include flu-like symptoms and a central neurological syndrome with photophobia, headache, and neck stiffness. It is an incapacitating agent as there is usually a significant period (months) of recovery.

Category C biological agents

Emerging pathogens that could be engineered for mass dissemination in the future because of:
• Availability.
• Ease of production and dissemination.
• Potential for high morbidity and mortality rates, and major health impact.

This group of emerging infectious diseases, includes the Nipah virus and Hantavirus.

Radiological and nuclear hazards

Introduction

There are a number of potential scenarios that may lead to exposure to ionizing radiation. Most countries in the world use radiological sources within the fields of science, industry, and medicine. Accidental exposures do occur due to a failure, lack of control, and safety measures, or failure of local infrastructure. The latter includes abandoned radiotherapy clinics or collateral damage to a science lab during times of conflict. Radiological sources of varying strength are moved through a number of transportation systems and subject to the same hazards as other traffic. Radiological sources may also be used deliberately, either overtly or covertly. The most likely overt release would be a radiological dispersal device (RDD) or *dirty bomb*. A recent example of an exposure to a covert radiological source was the use of polonium-210 to kill Alexander Litvinenko, London 2006. Radiological incidents may also involve trauma.

Definitions

It is important to understand the difference between the term *radiological* (CB**R**N) and *nuclear* (CBR**N**). A *radiological incident* in the most general terms refers to any incident where a hazard from ionizing radiation exists. A *nuclear incident* refers to an incident that involves the nuclear fission process or materials. A non-nuclear radiological incident is likely to involve only a single radioisotope, an element with radioactivity. Nuclear incidents will produce over 300 fission products—a mixture of intermediate weight radioisotopes including strontium, caesium, and iodine. The term *nuclear material* may be used to refer to fissile material (uranium and plutonium), fission products, or spent reactor fuel rods.

Properties of ionizing radiation

There are four main types of ionizing radiation, although neutrons are usually only associated with the nuclear process:

- *Alpha particles* are charged helium nuclei. They only travel short distances (3 cm in air) and cannot penetrate further than the outer layers of skin. Damage is only caused if internalization occurs (by ingestion or inhalation). They are, however, the most damaging due to their weight and double positive charge.
- *Beta particles* are essentially electrons and, therefore, carry a single negative charge. They can penetrate skin and will cause damage if taken internally. They will travel about 3 m in air or about 5 mm in tissue.
- *Neutrons* are non-charged particles and usually only occur during the fission (nuclear) process. They are highly penetrating and, when they interact with biological tissue, are very damaging.
- *Gamma/X-ray radiation* has no mass or charge, but is at the high energy end of the electromagnetic spectrum. With no mass, it has a very long range and is difficult to shield against requiring thick layers of lead or concrete. X-rays may be generated using high voltage electricity and do not always require a radioactive source.

Measurements of radiation

Radiation may be measured in a number of ways. Using SI Units, absorbed radiation can be measured as joules of energy absorbed per kilogram mass; this unit is the Gray (Gy). The equivalent dose or Sievert (Sv) reflects the more damaging effects of some forms of radiation, alpha, and neutrons. A Sievert is a relatively large amount of radiation and it is usual to use microsieverts (μSv) and millisieverts (mSv). To put these units into a perspective, illustrative radiation doses are given in the Table 25.4.

Table 25.4. Illustrative radiation doses

Illustrative radiation doses	
Chest radiograph	< 20 μSv
Polar flight – UK to Japan	50–70 μSv
Annual UK background dose	1–2 mSv
Annual UK occupational dose limit	20 mSv
Threshold for Acute Radiation Syndrome	0.5–2 Sv
LD50/60* without treatment	3.5 Sv
LD50/60* with treatment	5–6 Sv

*LD50/60 is lethal dose for 50% population at 60 days.

Health effects of ionizing radiation

Ionizing radiation causes its health effects by its interaction with DNA and other intracellular components. At low levels, there is damage to the DNA increasing the chance of mutation and cancer, if DNA self-repair fails. The greater the dose of radiation, the greater the chance of cancer and this is termed a *stochastic* or probability effect.

At very high levels (>2 Sv or 1000 times annual background radiation), radiation causes cell death. This is called a *deterministic* effect as there is a threshold level and the effects are very predictable beyond this level. The most sensitive tissues are those that have the highest cell turnover (bone marrow and gastrointestinal mucosa). Death is generally due to infection or coagulopathy, both due to bone marrow suppression. The failure of different systems (haematological, gastrointestinal, and cerebrovascular) due to due to increasing radiation levels is called *Acute Radiation Syndrome* (ARS). This occurs after an initial prodromal stage (nausea, vomiting ± diarrhoea) lasting a few hours and then a latency period of a few days.

Local gamma irradiation to tissue may cause a cutaneous syndrome with erythema, loss of hair, and deeper necrosis. Whole body irradiation may not occur and bone marrow function is likely to be preserved.

Radiation protection

The principles of radiation protection are:

- *Time*: reducing the time a person is near a radioactive source reduces the dose proportionally.
- *Distance*: dose rate and distance are related by the *inverse square rule*; doubling the distance reduces the rate to a quarter.
- *Shielding*: by increasing the shielding this proportionally increases the protection.

Radiological and nuclear incidents

Types of casualties
Following a radiological or nuclear incident there may be a number of casualty sub-groups.

Contaminated casualties
These casualties will present a contact hazard to emergency responders. Internal contamination may also have occurred. Standard precautions with high specification particulate face mask filters will provide significant protection without the reduction in manual dexterity that occurs with chemical PPE. Lead aprons as used in radiology will provide additional protection if there is a significant radiation source or *shine*.

Irradiated casualties
Irradiated casualties are not a hazard to emergency responders unless they are also contaminated. There may be no presenting symptoms and exposures range from negligible through to beyond the threshold for ARS (>2 Sv).

Conventional casualties (injuries)
Conventional casualties may occur due to initial activation of the delivery device or may be incidental. The management of conventional injuries including life-saving interventions (LSIs) should take priority over decontamination, although they are likely to be in parallel.

Contaminated wounds
Conventional casualties may have localized contamination of the wounds. Simple wound irrigation should be provided as soon as possible, but full wound decontamination may require surgical debridement.

Combined injuries (conventional and irradiation)
Casualties with combined injuries following a significant dose of radiation (>2 Sv) are likely to do worse. This is due to the increase probability of infection and coagulopathy following the onset of ARS. For this reason, these patients may need to be prioritized for surgery.

Psychological casualties
There may be a significant number of psychological casualties and they need to be factored into any contingency plan. The severity ranged from minor (and often appropriate) anxiety through to acute stress reactions. At very high levels of irradiation (>8 Sv), neurovascular complications may also be seen.

Casualties following a nuclear detonation
The energy released following a nuclear detonation results in a predictable pattern of injury and irradiation. The release of energy includes ionizing radiation, blast, and thermal energy. The proportion of the effect of each type of energy depends on the yield and effectiveness of the weapon. Conventional injuries are due to the following features of the detonation:
- Flash leading to retinal damage due to the intense light.
- Thermal burns due to the intense thermal radiation.
- Blast injuries.
- Irradiation due to the ionizing radiation either during the initial release or as fallout.

Casualty management
Management of radiological casualties including nuclear can be broken into the various stages of the incident management.

Pre-hospital management
Radiological incident management should follow similar procedure as other HazMat and conventional incidents using the CSCATTT paradigm. Priorities for casualty management as this stage will be:
- Life-saving interventions (LSIs).
- Remove from any continuing radiation exposure.
- External decontamination (removal of clothing and rinse-wipe-rinse).
- Documentation of any radiation dose estimation or prodromal symptoms (nausea, vomiting, erythema, diarrhoea) (see Table 25.5).

Emergency Department management
- As above.
- Management of any traumatic injuries.
- Assess risk of internal contamination.
- Serial full blood counts, monitoring lymphocytes for any early fall suggesting ARS with HLA sampling, if at risk.
- Anti-emetics such as ondansetron, as required.
- Triage for early surgery.

In-patient hospital management
- 24-h cytogenetics for accurate biodosimetry.
- *Removal of internal contamination*: decorporation using antidote (chelating agents), physical methods, and blocking agents (stable iodine).
- Supportive management of severe ARS cases with antibiotic therapy and nutrition.
- Substitution therapy to replace blood products.
- Stimulation therapy using cytokines such as colony-stimulating factors.
- Stem cell/bone marrow transplantation.

Table 25.5. Prodromal symptoms

Dose	Expected effects	Prodromal	Probability
<1 Gy	Below threshold	−/±	Unlikely
1–2 Gy	Mild	+	Probably
2–4 Gy	Moderate	++	Severe
4–6 Gy	Severe (LD$_{50}$)*	++	Severe
6–8 Gy	Very severe	++	Severe
>8 Gy	Lethal	+++	Severe
>20 GY		+++	Severe

*In absence of medical treatment.

Further reading

CDC website. Available at: http://www.cdc.gov.

Defence CBRN Centre Winterbourne Gunner course materials.

Department of Health Emergency Planning website. Available at: http://www.dh.gov.uk/emergency_planning.

HPA (Radiological Protection Division) website. Available at: http://www.hpa.org.uk.

HPA CBRN Handbook. Available at: http://www.hpa.org.uk.

International Atomic Energy Agency. *Diagnosis and treatment of radiation injuries*, Safety Reports Series, No.2. Vienna: IAEA, 1998.

Major Incident Medical Management and Support course. Available at: http://www.alsg.org.

Surviving Sepsis campaign and guidelines. Available at: http://www.survivingsepsis.org.

Critical care issues in trauma

Some would say as long as the air is going in and out, and blood going round and round, all is well in the world. We therefore start this chapter with sections on ventilation and perfusion, with further sections covering acidosis, hypothermia, and the systemic inflammatory response to trauma.

Ventilation

Maintenance of adequate oxygenation is essential in both the initial and subsequent management of the critically ill trauma patient. Patients with severe life-threatening, or multiple injuries will often require a period of assisted or artificial ventilatory support to ensure adequate delivery of oxygen to tissues.

Pathophysiology of lung injury caused by trauma

Direct injury to the lungs can be caused by penetrating or blunt trauma to the thorax, both of which are often treated conservatively. Immediate injury and subsequent organ failure is often accompanied by a systemic inflammatory response (SIRS) which can worsen the already compromised lung function. Acute lung injury (ALI) and the acute respiratory distress syndrome (ARDS) can ensue.

Serious extra-thoracic injuries can also precipitate ALI and ARDS, prevent mobilization and increase the risk of a pneumonic process. The mainstay of non-operative treatment in major trauma is supportive, with the aim of minimizing the pulmonary and systemic consequences of the original injury.

Indications for ventilatory support

Ventilation, although used primarily to treat acute respiratory failure, can also be indicated in the facilitation of patient extraction and transfer, the maintenance of an appropriate arterial CO_2 partial pressure in the setting of traumatic brain injury, and as a consequence of a need for an artificial airway or emergency surgery.

The initiation of ventilatory support is a clinical decision supported by the use of bedside adjuncts and point of care testing, such as pulse oximetry and arterial blood gas analysis. Often it arises as a consequence of a decision to intubate for airway protection.

Mechanical ventilation allows:
- *Manipulation of alveolar ventilation (Va):*
  - V_a is the volume of gas entering the alveolus per minute: V_a = tidal ventilation (V_t) – dead space ventilation $(V_t–V_a)$ × respiratory rate (RR);
  - for the same minute volume $(V_t × RR$ per min) rapid shallow breathing will result in a reduced alveolar ventilation compared with slow deep breathing as the proportion of dead space ventilation per breath is greatly increased;
  - all carbon dioxide comes from the alveoli, thus arterial CO_2 concentration is inversely proportional to alveolar ventilation at a fixed rate of CO_2 production.
- *Increased oxygenation:*
  - by increasing maximum inspired oxygen concentration delivered to the alveoli (FiO_2);
  - improved ventilation/perfusion (V/Q) matching in the lungs, by recruitment of collapsed or damaged lung (increased functional residual capacity) and increased lung compliance.

Box 26.1. Indications for ventilation in trauma patients

Acute respiratory failure
- Thoracic trauma:
  - Contusion;
  - Flail chest.
- Ineffective ventilation as consequence of other severe injuries.
- Coma.
- Neuromuscular paralysis.

Traumatic brain injury
Transfer of potentially unstable patients
- Imaging.
- Theatre.
- Pre-hospital.

Need for artificial airway protection
- Severe maxillofacial injuries.
- High risk of aspiration.
- Neck haematoma.
- Laryngeal or tracheal injury.
- Acute stridor.
- Burns.

Increased metabolic demands
- Burns.
- Multiple trauma.

- *Reduced work of breathing:* by mechanical expansion against the natural elastic recoil of the lung and chest wall, and overcoming the resistance to the flow of gases throughout the respiratory tree.
- *Stabilization of the chest wall and improved respiratory mechanics:* in the situation of multiple rib fractures or flail chest

The decision to use non-invasive ventilation or invasive ventilation depends upon patient factors, clinical expertise and available equipment.

Non-invasive ventilation (NIV)

Non-invasive ventilation has become a standard therapy for an increasing variety of pathologies and is now in common use in most critical care environments. NIV provides ventilatory support to a patient without the need for an artificial airway. It can provide improved pulmonary mechanics, augment alveolar ventilation, and allow partial unloading of respiratory musculature.

The term non-invasive ventilation describes several different techniques. The most commonly used in the UK are continuous positive airways pressure (CPAP) and non-invasive positive pressure ventilation (NIPPV, also known as BIPAP). Both methods are usually administered by a mask, although CPAP can also be successfully delivered by a nasopharyngeal airway or helmet, which may improve patient compliance and comfort.
- CPAP provides a constant pressure through the respiratory cycle, but does not provide direct volume change except via an indirect improvement in lung compliance.
- NIPPV (BIPAP) provides a step pressure change during the respiratory cycle, between IPAP (inspiratory

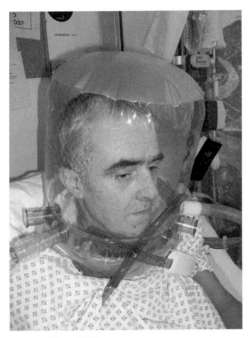

Fig. 26.1. Helmet CPAP.

positive airways pressure) and EPAP (expiratory positive airways pressure). The pressure differential between IPAP and EPAP will augment alveolar ventilation, if synchronized with the patient's respiratory effort. The EPAP is equivalent to CPAP in this mode.

NIV has a number of potential advantages over invasive ventilation, (see Table 26.1), but its usefulness may be limited in the situation of acute trauma, as it is frequently contraindicated and requires a number of patient prerequisites before it can be safely applied and used (Box 26.2).

CPAP has been used successfully in patients with isolated thoracic trauma causing hypoxemia and respiratory distress, and NIPPV in the management of ongoing hypoxaemia after major trauma after an initial period of mechanical ventilation and subsequent extubation. All the techniques described to date provided adequate analgesia via either a thoracic epidural or intravenous opiate via a

> **Box 26.2.** Contraindications to the use of NIV
> - Craniofacial trauma or facial burns.
> - Upper airway obstruction.
> - Inability to protect airway/high risk of pulmonary aspiration.
> - Haemodynamic instability.
> - Life-threatening hypoxaemia.
> - Lack of patient co-operation/agitation.
> - Reduced level of consciousness.

patient-controlled analgesia (PCA) system. This would seem essential for effective and optimal use of NIV in thoracic trauma.

In its guidelines regarding the use of NIV in acute respiratory failure the British Thoracic Society (BTS) makes the following recommendations for the use of CPAP in chest wall trauma, although the level of available evidence is weak:

- CPAP should be used in patients with chest wall trauma who remain hypoxic despite adequate regional anaesthesia and high flow oxygen (level C evidence).
- NIPPV should not be used routinely (Level D evidence).
- In view of the risk of pneumothorax, patients with chest wall trauma who are treated with CPAP or NIPPV should be monitored on the ICU (Level C evidence).
- Apnoea or severe respiratory insufficiency.
- Untreated pneumothorax.

Despite the increasing use of NIV in the acute trauma situation the main role for NIV will remain in the subsequent critical care, after stabilization and resuscitation has been achieved.

Invasive ventilation

The aims of mechanical ventilation are to provide maximal effective gas exchange with the minimum amount of iatrogenic complication. Ventilation can be either volume controlled or pressure controlled, both having specific advantages and disadvantages (see Table 26.2 and Fig. 26.2).

In volume controlled ventilation (intermittent positive pressure ventilation [IPPV], synchronous intermittent mandatory ventilation [SIMV]):
- Minute ventilation is a product of a set tidal volume and respiratory rate.

Table 26.1. Advantages and disadvantages of non-invasive ventilation

Advantages	Disadvantages
Avoids intubation and invasive ventilation	Airway is unprotected
Reduced incidence of trauma to airway	Mask can be uncomfortable and claustrophobic
Reduced incidence of ventilator associated pneumonia	No direct access to bronchial tree for suctioning/toilet
Reduced sedation requirements	
Reduced incidence of ventilator induced lung injury	
Allows intermittent ventilation	
Ease of application and removal	
Patient can eat, drink and communicate	
Patient co-operation with nursing and physiotherapy care	

Table 26.2. Advantages and disadvantages of volume and pressure controlled ventilation

Pressure-controlled ventilation	Volume controlled ventilation
Reduction of peak airway pressures	Potential for high airway pressures and barotrauma
More homogenous ventilation due to decelerating flow characteristics between over and under distended alveoli	Less homogenous distribution of gas. Flow characteristics allow preferential flow into over-distended alveoli, with reduced ventilation of collapsed compartments, causing volutrauma
Better compensation for air leaks	Cannot compensate for air leaks
Potential for hypo and hyper ventilation due to acute changes in lung compliance	Guarantees a precise minute ventilation and therefore an arterial partial pressure of carbon dioxide
Used in standard management of trauma requiring invasive ventilation	Used in management of traumatic brain injuries, and often the default mode for ventilators in the emergency department and transport ventilators

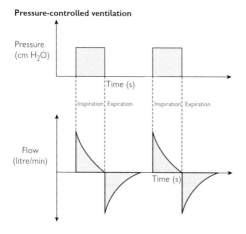

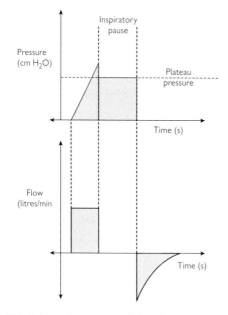

Fig. 26.2. Volume and pressure controlled ventilation.

- Peak airway pressures are dependent upon the compliance of the lung. The lower the compliance the higher the pressure achieved for the same tidal volume delivered.
- Maintains constant alveolar ventilation and, therefore, a constant arterial carbon dioxide concentration.
- Flow of gas into lungs remains constant throughout respiratory cycle.
- Most ventilators in the emergency department will provide volume controlled ventilation.
- In the SIMV mode the ventilator will attempt to match any inspiratory effort with the ventilatory effort to the patient.

In pressure controlled ventilation (biphasic positive airway pressure [BIPAP]):
- Tidal volume is determined by the set pressure differential (ΔP) between positive end expiratory pressure (PEEP), peak airway pressure (PAW), and compliance of the lung. A compliant lung will receive a greater tidal volume than a non compliant lung for the same ΔP.
- Peak airway pressures are therefore determined by the user.
- Alveolar ventilation can change with changing compliance of the lung, thus arterial carbon dioxide concentrations can also change.
- The flow of gas into the lungs is highest at the beginning of the breath and decelerates as the pressure differential decreases (decelerating flow).
- Patients can breathe spontaneously throughout the respiratory cycle at either of the set pressures. Often this spontaneous ventilation is augmented with assisted spontaneous breathing (ASB).

Complications of invasive ventilation
Although mechanical ventilation is undoubtedly life-saving, it exposes the patient to numerous potential risks and complications, which usually increase with the duration of ventilation. Safe mechanical ventilation requires monitoring of the equipment and also monitoring of the patient to a minimum level as determined by the patient's current physiological stability. A summary of the complications of mechanical ventilation can be seen in Box 26.3.

Ventilator-induced lung injury
Ventilator-induced lung injury (VILI) occurs when the act of mechanical ventilation causes direct damage to the lung and is caused by the transmission of high transpulmonary pressures and volumes (barotrauma and volutrauma) to the alveoli causing increased vascular permeability,

Box 26.3. Complications of mechanical ventilation

Damage to airway
Damage to teeth and vocal cords, pressure necrosis, tracheal stenosis.

Damage to lungs
- Ventilator-induced lung injury.
- Ventilator-associated pneumonia.
- Barotrauma.
- Oxygen toxicity.

Cardiovascular compromise
- Increased intra-thoracic pressure:
  - Reduction in preload and reduced cardiac output;
  - Increase in afterload and reduced cardiac output;
  - Reduction in renal blood flow;
  - Reduction in splanchnic blood flow;
  - Increase in intracranial pressure.

Equipment
- Failure.
- Disconnection.
- Cross contamination.

Other
- Critical illness myoneuropathy causing diaphragmatic and peripheral muscle weakness.
- Drug side effects e.g. sedatives and analgesics.
- Iatrogenic – incorrect use of ventilator.

Table 26.3. Strategies used to prevent VAP

Non-pharmacological	Pharmacological
Hand-washing and infection control	Prophylactic administration of oral and intravenous antibiotics (selective decontamination of the digestive tract)
Semi-recumbent positioning of patients	Oral antisepsis
Subglottic suctioning	Enteral feeding
Oral hygiene	Prophylactic treatment of neutropenia
Humidification of airway gases	
Postural changes	
Cuffed endotracheal tubes	
Avoidance of high gastric volumes	

alveolar fluid accumulation, and atelectasis. The shearing forces applied during repeated opening and closing of collapsed alveoli can amplify this injury and the subsequent inflammatory response (atelectrauma). Gas exchange is impaired and functional recovery limited, prolonging the period and degree of ventilation necessary. High oxygen concentrations also cause direct damage to the lungs via free radical production and absorption atelectasis.

The term protective lung ventilation is used to describe a series of techniques designed to limit the incidence of barotrauma, volutrauma (pressure limited/volume limited ventilation) and atelectrauma (open lung ventilation) and thus VILI.

Restricted tidal volumes (6 mL/kg) have been shown to reduce mortality in ARDS when compared with higher tidal volumes and pressures (12 mL/kg), and the use of high levels of PEEP and recruitment manoeuvres (actively inflating collapsed alveoli with high pressures), although not associated with a mortality benefit have been shown in a porcine ARDS model to stabilize alveoli and reduce VILI. The use of a similar protective ventilation strategy in major trauma patients may reduce the risk of subsequent multi-organ failure.

Ventilator-associated pneumonia
Ventilator-associated pneumonia (VAP) is a nosocomial pneumonia developing in a patient who has received mechanical ventilatory support for over 48 h. Trauma is an independent risk factor for the development of VAP and is associated with increased mortality, length of ICU stay, and cost. Diagnosis of a VAP is commonly made by new pulmonary infiltrates on CXR and one of neutrophilia, pyrexia, positive microbiology, or worsening oxygenation.

Various strategies have been used to prevent VAP (Table 26.3) and, if necessary, treatment should be directed against the more virulent Gram-negative organisms (and MRSA) with broad spectrum antibiotics, rapidly de-escalated to targeted monotherapy, for a limited administration period of 8 days.

Cardiovascular instability
A high intrathoracic pressure transmitted from the lungs to the thoracic cavity can impede both filling of the right heart (preload) and emptying of the left (afterload). This is more pronounced in the shocked patient and with the induction of anaesthesia.

Acute lung injury and acute respiratory distress syndrome
Acute lung injury (ALI) and acute respiratory distress syndrome (ARDS; Fig. 26.3) form a spectrum of lung diseases caused by a variety of direct and indirect pathologies. They are characterized by inflammation of lung parenchyma, non-cardiogenic pulmonary oedema and reduced lung compliance, causing both increased dead space and shunting.

The following features define ALI and ARDS:
- *ALI:*
  - acute onset;
  - PaO_2/FiO_2 ratio < 300 mmHg (40 kPa);
  - no evidence of LVF;
  - bilateral infiltrates on CXR.
- *ARDS:* PaO_2/FiO_2 ratio < 200 mmHg (26.7 kPa).

ARDS develops in approximately 10% of all trauma ICU admissions, and is more common in patients with pulmonary contusions, traumatic brain injury, ISS > 25, and in patients who have received a massive transfusion or have multiple orthopaedic injuries. The presence of ARDS is associated with an increase in morbidity, length of ICU stay, and hospital costs. Any increased mortality in this group is now thought to be a reflection of severity of injury, rather than the presence of ARDS itself.

Management of ARDS includes treatment of the precipitating causes, protective, and open lung ventilation strategies, and systemic support including enteral nutrition.

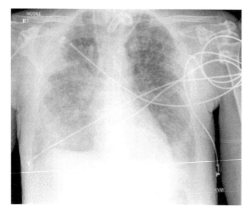

Fig. 26.3. CXR showing features of ARDS.

Independent lung ventilation (ILV)

Independent lung ventilation (ILV) is a technique in which both the right and left lungs are managed independently. An anatomical and physiological separation is achieved by the use of a double-lumen endobronchial tube (see Fig. 26.4). ILV is achieved by one lung independent ventilation (OLIV) or two lung independent ventilation (TLIV).

OLIV ventilation is used to isolate a healthy lung from an injured one, allowing surgical access, and to prevent cross contamination of blood, or infection between the two. The healthy lung only is ventilated, whilst the other will collapse, resulting in significant shunting and hypoxia. OLIV is usually used as a short-term damage control measure in severe pulmonary haemorrhage.

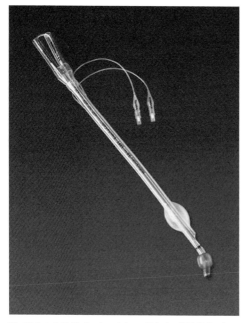

Fig. 26.4. Left Mallinckrodt endobronchial tube. © Mallinkrodt Broncho-Cath™.

TLIV allows independent ventilation of both lungs by separate ventilators, which work either synchronously or asynchronously, and allow differing modes of ventilation to be used for each lung. TLIV has a role in the management of complex pulmonary contusion, bronchopleural fistula, and bronchial injury.

Pulmonary contusion

A unilateral contusion will cause a reduction in lung compliance on the side affected, thus normal ventilation will preferentially ventilate the uninjured lung. This can lead to over-distention of alveoli, causing VILI and worsening shunt via capillary compression diverting blood back through the damaged and less ventilated lung. TLIV allows optimal recruitment and restrictive ventilatory strategies to be achieved in both lungs.

Bronchopleural fistula (BPF)

TLIV can be used to reduce the gas flow to and, therefore, the subsequent air leak from the fistulous lung. This is achieved by minimizing the volume and pressure delivered to the damaged lung, which when used with other management techniques, such as low pressure pleural suction can accelerate the rate of closure. The use of high frequency oscillatory ventilation (HFOV) has also been described in the management of BPF.

Tracheobronchial injury

TLIV has been used in the immediate post-operative period to protect the bronchial anastomosis.

Novel techniques for the management of ALI and ARDS

Various strategies have been described as adjuncts or alternatives to mechanical ventilation in the event of therapy failure or to reduce the side effects of conventional ventilation. Unfortunately, clinical trials are yet to show a mortality benefit for any of the techniques described below.

Prone ventilation

Prone ventilation is thought to work by improve lung volumes, optimizing V/Q matching and diaphragmatic function. Oxygenation has shown to be improved in 60–70% of patients.

Inhaled nitric oxide

By selectively vasodilating ventilated alveoli, V/Q matching is improved resulting in an increase in arterial oxygenation of up to 25%, which can persist for 4 days.

Partial liquid ventilation

Perflurocarbons can recruit collapsed alveoli and may have anti-inflammatory properties. Recent trials have shown both an increase in ventilator days and complications with their use compared with conventional therapies.

Extracorporeal membrane oxygenation (ECMO)

Oxygenation and carbon dioxide clearance are achieved by an extracorporeal system, allowing minimal conventional ventilation and lung recovery. Case reports have described the use of extracorporeal membrane oxygenation (ECMO) in trauma, and a large single-centre UK trial has just finished recruiting and is due to report (CESAR).

Novalung

The novalung is an extracorporeal device that allows almost complete removal of CO_2, thus allowing the prioritization of protective ventilation. Its successful use has been described in major trauma; however, no randomized clinical trials as yet support its use on a more routine basis.

Surfactant
Installation of exogenous surfactant into the lungs of patients with severe ARDS has been shown to improve oxygenation in animal trials and certain patient groups.

Steroids
As the lung undergoes repair from ARDS, collagen and fibrin may be deposited, causing permanent damage. Steroids may help to modulate this process if used at the correct time in the course of the illness, although this is only supported by small trials and concerns over harm have been recently been raised.

High frequency oscillatory ventilation
HFOV is characterized by the rapid delivery of small tidal ventilations and the use of high airway pressures, preventing over-distension and cyclical derecruitment of the alveoli, which may have theoretical advantages over mechanical ventilation in ARDS.

Perfusion

Introduction

The human body has a unique ability to maintain a constant blood flow to a specific organ over a wide range of perfusion pressures, without the central control of the autonomic nervous system. Termed autoregulation, this homeostatic phenomenon is thought to occur by both metabolic and myogenic mechanisms. During a period of decreased perfusion, vasodilator metabolites accumulate (H^+, CO_2, lactate) resulting in local vasodilatation and an increased blood flow. Increasing blood flow washes out the vasodilator metabolites and vasoconstriction occurs. The myogenic mechanism involves changes in the basal tone of blood vessels, and the effect of stretch and relaxation by increased or decreased blood flow, and thus subsequent vasodilation or vasoconstriction.

In health, flow can be maintained over a range of mean arterial perfusion pressures (60–160 mmHg). Autoregulatory processes are reset in persistently hypertensive patients, thus the ability to maintain flow occurs across a higher perfusion pressure range (e.g. 80–180 mmHg). In these patients a 'normal' mean arterial pressure of 60 mmHg may result in reduced flow to compromised organs (Fig. 26.5).

Whist most organs in the body show some degree of autoregulation, it is most clearly observed in the heart, kidney, and the brain.

Permissive hypotension

In the vast majority of critical care trauma patients the therapeutic goals are to maintain and optimize organ perfusion, minimize further insult, and prevent organ failure. This process often involves aggressive fluid resuscitation and the use of vasoactive drugs. In a situation of uncontrolled haemorrhage it may be appropriate in selected patients to allow a period of controlled hypotension until surgical intervention and haemostasis can be achieved.

Cerebral perfusion

Regulation of cerebral blood flow

Normal cerebral blood flow CBF is 750 mL/min, and is maintained over a wide range of MAP (50–150 mmHg) (Fig. 26.6) and variable partial pressures of O_2 (PaO_2) and CO_2 ($PaCO_2$).

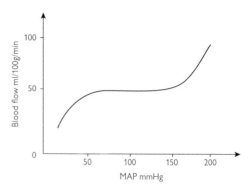

Fig. 26.6. Autoregulation of cerebral blood flow.

CBF is markedly increased when the PaO_2 falls below 6.7 kPa. Hypercapnia causes an increase in CBF via cerebral vasodilatation and hypocapnia causes a decrease in CBF via vasoconstriction. A reduction of $PaCO_2$ from 5.3 to 4 kPa reduces CBF by 30% with no further reduction of CBF when the $PaCO_2$ falls below 3.3 kPa. Flow changes induced by changes in $PaCO_2$ occur within 2 min, with chronic adaptation occurring within 36 h (Fig. 26.7).

Primary and secondary brain injury

At the point of primary brain injury, damage to tissues and blood vessels occurs triggering the initiation of complex metabolic cascades in the minutes to days following injury. Increases in intracellular calcium and sodium, increased release of the excitatory neurotransmitter glutamate, disruption of the blood–brain barrier, and reduced protein synthesis can eventually cause neuronal cell death. Whilst contributing to worsening of the primary injury, these processes may cause cerebral oedema and raised intracranial pressure (ICP), further damaging salvageable areas of the brain, which surround the primary injury.

Periods of hypoxia, hypotension, hypo- or hyperglycaemia, and hyperpyrexia cause secondary insults to damaged areas of brain, and have been independently shown to lead to increased morbidity and mortality after traumatic brain injury (TBI).

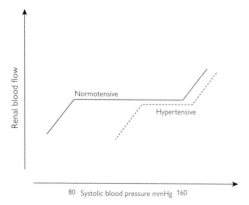

Fig. 26.5. Autoregulation in normotensive and hypertensive patients.

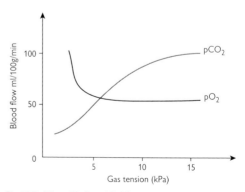

Fig. 26.7. Effect of PaO_2 and $PaCO_2$ on cerebral blood flow.

Cerebral perfusion pressure (CPP)

Autoregulation of cerebral blood flow becomes disrupted after TBI, thus flow becomes directly dependent upon pressure. Drugs such as opiates and anaesthetic agents also contribute to impaired autoregulation. Cerebral perfusion pressure can be defined as:

$$CPP = MAP - ICP - central\ venous\ pressure\ (CVP)$$

Maintenance of an adequate cerebral perfusion pressure is fundamental in the management of TBI and prevention of secondary brain injury. The Brain Trauma Foundation recommends a CPP between 50 and 70 mmHg in TBI.

Intracranial pressure monitoring is indicated in all salvageable patients with a severe TBI (GCS 3–8) and an abnormal CT scan. An adequate CPP can be achieved by manipulating MAP, ICP, or CVP.

Manipulation of ICP

The Monro–Kellie Doctrine

The skull is a rigid box with incompressible structures, therefore ICP depends upon the volume of the contents within-brain (80–85%), blood (5–7%), and CSF (5–12%). An increase in any of the three constituents causes an increase in intracranial volume. As intracranial volume increases, CSF is absorbed into the spinal canal and venous circulation, and the venous sinus becomes compressed to compensate. As compensatory mechanisms are overwhelmed small changes in intracranial volume cause large increases in ICP (Fig 26.8).

As ICP rises, CPP, and CBF fall contributing to ischaemia, and causing structural distortion, which can eventually lead to brain stem herniation.

Clinical signs of raised ICP

Raised ICP can present as headache, nausea and vomiting, confusion and coma. Papilloedema may be present, and as ICP continues to rise, hypertension, and bradycardia (Cushing's reflex) may occur. Fixed pupillary dilation due to third nerve compression is a late sign implying impending brain stem coning and is a medical emergency.

Treatment of raised ICP

Treatment and investigation of raised ICP should be initiated at a pressure of 20 mmHg. Both clinical and brain CT findings may guide subsequent treatment. Treatment strategies involve removal of one of the three intra-cerebral components, which may or may not be the pathological cause, thus reducing pressure within the cranial vault.

Removal of blood

- Surgery: acute subdural, extradural, and intracerebral haematomas may be removed via a burr hole, or formal craniotomy.

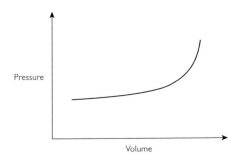

Fig. 26.8. Relationship between intracranial volume and intracranial pressure.

- PaO$_2$: hypoxaemia after TBI is associated with an increase in secondary brain injury, and a marked increase in mortality and decrease in favourable neurological outcome. Furthermore, CBF increases markedly below a PaO$_2$ of 8 kPa, which can contribute to a raised ICP. SpO$_2$ should be kept above 92% and PaO$_2$ above 8kPa.

- PaCO$_2$: CBF is related in a liner fashion to PaCO$_2$. A high PaCO$_2$ will cause an increase in CBF and a rise in ICP. A low PaCO$_2$ will cause a reduction in CBF and a reduction in ICP. Thus hyperventilation can be used as an interim measure to treat impending brain stem herniation. The reduction in CBF may conversely contribute to secondary brain injury, thus PaCO$_2$ should be maintained between 4 and 4.5 kPa.

- MAP: both pre- and in-hospital hypotension have been shown to have a deleterious influence on outcome after TBI. CPP should be maintained at 50–70 mmHg and a systolic blood pressure of <90 mmHg avoided.

- Hypothermia: reduction in core temperature from 35 to 33°C reduces both the cerebral metabolic requirement for oxygen (CMRO$_2$) and the ICP markedly. Although used routinely in many neurosurgical centres as a secondary therapy, current evidence does not conclusively support a positive influence on morbidity and mortality.

- Sedation: short-acting sedatives and opiates such as propofol and alfentanyl reduce CMRO$_2$, CBF, and ICP. A high ICP, refractory to treatment, may respond to administration of benzodiazepines (midazolam) or barbiturates (thiopentone). The pharmacokinetics of these drugs, particularly thiopentone, mean that the effects are prolonged and thus compromise clinical examination and brain stem death testing. Despite widespread use, there is no evidence to support the prophylactic use of barbiturates or convincing evidence that they improve outcomes.

Removal of CSF

External ventricular drains (EVD): an EVD may be sited to remove CSF if hydrocephalus is present or likely to develop.

Removal of cerebral oedema or cell water

Hyperosmolar therapy: mannitol given to a haemodynamically stable, euvolemic patient in doses of 0.25–1 g/kg, is effective in reducing ICP. Mannitol works by initially improving blood flow characteristics and thus oxygen delivery to the brain. Subsequently, an osmotic effect reduces intracellular water. Hypertonic saline (5%, 2 mL/kg) is another effective therapy, which may preserve MAP better than mannitol; however, there is less evidence to support its use as a first line agent. Plasma osmolalities should be measured when using hyperosmolar therapy – a plasma osmolality of 320 msom/L, suggests further administration will be ineffective and may cause harm.

Removal of brain

Contusionectomy or lobectomy may be appropriate in selected patients.

Removal of bone

Decompressive craniectomy: removal of a cranial bone flap allows reduction in ICP. Ongoing concerns over poor neurological recovery in survivors have prevented this from becoming routine practice. A large RCT, the DECTRA (Early Decompressive Craniectomy in Patients with Severe Traumatic Brain Injury) study is currently recruiting patients to address this issue. There is also the potential to intro-duce infection, worsening brain injury and outcome.

Manipulation of MAP

- *Fluid resuscitation:* hypotensive patients should be resus-citated to specific targets, using sodium-containing flu-ids. Hypo-osmolar fluids containing dextrose should not be used as they expand the intracellular compartment and can worsen cerebral oedema.
- *Vasopressors and inotropes:* if an adequate CPP is not achieved with fluid resuscitation, a vasopressor (e.g. noradrenaline) should be commenced. Dobutamine may be an appropriate choice of drug in cases of neurogenic left ventricular failure, or with signs of worsening or inadequate oxygen delivery.

Manipulation of CVP

- *Head up tilt:* patients should be sat up at 30–45 degrees to encourage venous drainage from the brain. Patients with associated spinal injuries should have the bed tilted appropriate to their injury.
- *Avoidance of venous congestion:* pressure from endotra-cheal tube ties, cervical collars, or sand bags should be avoided where possible (or released in the sedated patient), improving jugular venous drainage.

Other treatment

- *Seizures:* clinically-observed seizure activity should be treated. The use of prophylactic anticonvulsants may also be appropriate in patients with a raised ICP and a high risk of seizures (Box 26.4). Sub-clinical seizure activ-ity may manifest as a surge in ICP, and EEG is invaluable in assisting the formulation of a diagnosis and response to treatment. Anticonvulsant doses should be titrated to therapeutic plasma levels and their clinical effects.
- *Steroids:* the use of steroids is not associated with a reduction in ICP and high dose methylprednisolone causes increased mortality in patients with a TBI. Use is not recommended.

Outcome after TBI

Box 26.4. Risk factors for developing post-traumatic seizures (PTS) after traumatic brain injury (TBI)

- Glasgow Coma Score <10.
- Cortical contusion.
- Depressed skull fracture.
- Subdural haematoma.
- Epidural haematoma.
- Intracerebral haematoma.
- Penetrating head injury.
- Seizure within 24 h of injury.

The overall mortality after severe brain injury (presenta-tion Glasgow Coma Score 3–8) is 30–50%. Most recovery occurs within the first 6 months, although further recovery can continue for up to 24 months after injury. Prognosis after TBI can now be accurately predicted by validated sta-tistical models which also helps allocate health care resources more effectively.

Intra-abdominal pressure

Intra-abdominal hypertension (IAH) and abdominal com-partment syndrome (ACS) have recently been recognized as independent risk factors for the development of organ failure and carry an increased mortality in a critically ill trauma population (see Chapter 12).

Aetiology and clinical consequences

Excess fluid accumulation may be *primary* due to increased free fluid (e.g. blood or ascites) or *secondary* due to devel-opment of oedematous tissues (e.g. after massive crystal-loid fluid resuscitation).

There are a variety of consequences of IAH including decreased venous return and cardiac output, increased systemic vascular resistance, and diaphragmatic splinting which can cause difficulty in mechanical ventilation and alveolar atelectasis. IAH is also known to reduce renal and mesenteric perfusion, especially when intra-abdominal pressures are greater than 20 mmHg.

Penetrating and blunt abdominal trauma have been shown to carry a risk of developing IAH in up to 50% of patients and ACS in up to 36%. Burns, emergency surgery, massive fluid resuscitation, and hypothermia are risk fac-tors commonly seen in the critically injured trauma patient.

Effective measurement and treatment of IAH is associ-ated with improvements in patient survival. As in other systems the concept of perfusion pressure (MAP – IAP), may be more useful clinically than single values. Intra-abdominal pressure (IAP) is commonly measured via transmission through a partially full bladder, which is then read by direct pressure transduction or a modified uri-nary catheter. If a patient is identified at being at risk of developing IAH then serial measurements should be performed.

Management of raised IAP

The appropriate management of IAH and ACS is patient-specific but can be based around the following techniques, and useful treatment algorithms were published in 2007 by the World Society of the Abdominal Compartment Syndrome (WSACS):

- *Maintenance of abdominal perfusion pressure:* main-tenance of an APP at 50–60 mmHg has been shown to improve survival and discriminate between survi-vors and non-survivors in trauma, medical, and surgical populations.
- *Adequate sedation and analgesia:* may reduce the risk of ventilator asynchrony and abdominal muscle tone, thus reduce IAP.
- *Neuromuscular blockade:* can reduce IAP in mild to mod-erate IAH, but maybe less effective in ACS. The benefi-cial effects of reduced IAP must be balanced against the risk of prolonged use of neuromuscular blockers, and thus can be used as a short-term measure only, pending definitive treatment.
- *Decompression and prokinetics:* ileus is common in criti-cally ill trauma patients. Evacuation of gastric and colonic contents by improving normal peristalsis or by manual decompression may reduce size of viscera and reduce IAP.
- *Fluid resuscitation:* excessive fluid administration is asso-ciated with the development of secondary ACS and a worse survival. The maintenance of an adequate intra-vascular volume and, thus, organ perfusion is crucially important in the treatment of IAH. Over-resuscitation

should be avoided by careful monitoring of the patient at high risk of developing ACS, and consideration should be given to the use of a colloid or hypertonic crystalloid-based resuscitation strategy.

- *Percutaneous catheter decompression:* percutaneous catheter insertion into fluid collections performed under radiological guidance has been successfully described in the management of ACS in burns patients.
- *Abdominal decompression:* a laparotomy can be life-saving when the IAH is refractory to medical treatment and organ failure is present or developing. Often surgeons will leave the abdomen open if the patient is at high risk of developing ACS. This technique has been shown to improve survival.

Renal perfusion

Both renal blood flow (1200 mL/min) and glomerular filtration rate (120 mL/min) are autoregulated over a wide range of mean arterial pressures (Fig. 26.9). As perfusion pressure increases the resistance to flow also increases. With both the afferent and efferent arterioles capable of vasoconstriction and vasodilatation, blood flow and filtration pressures in the glomerulus can be manipulated independently.

Although autoregulation is effective in controlling local renal blood flow, the kidney remains highly vulnerable to external influences such as hypovolaemia or sympathetic induced renal artery vasoconstriction. Acute kidney injury (AKI) can occur despite intact autoregulatory mechanics and an adequate perfusion pressure in the face of reduced renal blood flow from another cause. AKI occurs in 18% of all trauma patients, and is associated with a doubling of risk of death. AKI after trauma is more common in the elderly and those with greater co-morbidity and injury severity.

Treatment of AKI and acute renal failure (ARF)

The mainstays of treatment of a trauma patient with ARF are to ensure adequate renal blood flow and perfusion whilst minimizing other contributory insults. The most common cause of ARF after major trauma is acute tubular necrosis (ATN). The tubular cells are highly metabolically active and, therefore, very vulnerable to even brief periods of hypoperfusion and hypoxia. As the tubular cells are continually replacing themselves, if the initial insult is removed and delivery of oxygen is restored, eventual recovery is likely.

Resuscitation with fluids and vasopressors should be goal-directed with a target of normal to high mean arterial

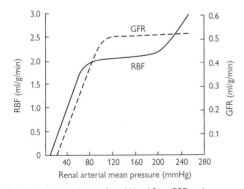

Fig. 26.9. Autoregulation of renal blood flow (RBF) and glomerular filtration rate (GFR).

pressure. Removal of nephrotoxic drugs should be attempted where possible, and consideration should be given to addressing post-renal causes of ARF such as a hydronephrosis or raised IAP. An ultrasound scan should be requested where necessary. On occasion, renal replacement therapy, such as continuous veno-venous haemofiltration (CVVH), or haemodialysis (HD), will be necessary to support the patient through a period of inadequate renal function. There is no evidence to support the use of 'renal dose' dopamine or loop diuretics in the management of ARF.

Renal prostaglandins attenuate the effects of sympathetic vasoconstriction to a degree by causing afferent arteriole vasodilation. Non-steroidal anti-inflammatory drugs (NSAIDs) block the cyclo-oxygenase enzyme involved in prostaglandin production thus can contribute to the development of ARF in a kidney at risk. NSAIDs should therefore generally be avoided in most critically ill trauma patients, although their potent analgesic and anti-inflammatory properties are a very useful adjunct to other therapies in the right patient, for example, in patients with isolated chest injuries.

Coronary perfusion

Coronary blood flow is determined by a number of factors, both physiological and pathological. Normal coronary blood flow at rest is 250 mL/min, with a 70% extraction of the delivered oxygen; therefore, oxygen debt can only be met by increased coronary perfusion. The main determinant of coronary perfusion is mean aortic root pressure, as the coronary arteries arise near the cusps of the aortic value. Coronary perfusion pressure (CoPP) can be determined by:

$$CoPP = MAP - LVEDP$$

The left ventricular end diastolic pressure (LVEDP) is determined by systemic vascular resistance (SVR), ventricular wall stress, and the efficiency of left ventricular function to eject blood. A patient who has attempted to compensate for shock by intense peripheral vasoconstriction and tachycardia will have greater left ventricular oxygen demands in generating the work required for adequate flow against a high SVR. Tachycardia will compromise coronary perfusion by reducing time for diastole and therefore time for coronary blood flow to occur (Fig. 26.10). As LVEDP is elevated and MAP reduced, myocardial perfusion may be inadequate.

If myocardial oxygen demand exceeds myocardial oxygen delivery then ischaemia will occur, causing myocardial pump dysfunction, a reduced cardiac output and ultimately myocardial cell death. Myocardial infarction or cardiac failure will eventually result.

The heart maintains an adequate blood flow over a range of pressures by local autoregulation and the subsequent alterations in coronary vessel calibre. External factors such as the sympathetic nervous system will maintain coronary perfusion pressure during periods of stress at the expense of increased myocardial work, with the net effect usually being increases in coronary blood flow. The ability to adapt to changes in myocardial perfusion pressure is severely compromised by coronary stenosis. A patient with severe myocardial disease will not be able to maintain adequate coronary perfusion in the face of a major insult such as trauma. A vicious cycle of hypoperfusion, increasing tachycardia and increasing oxygen demand ensues.

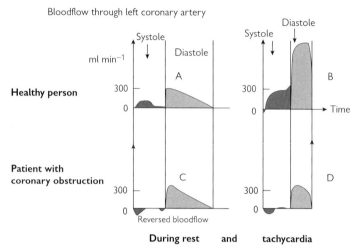

Coronary Bloodflow in Health & Disease

Bloodflow through left coronary artery

Fig. 26.10. Coronary perfusion throughout the cardiac cycle.

Management of patients with an acute coronary syndrome after trauma is profoundly difficult and involves careful manipulation of perfusion pressures, oxygen delivery and the reduction of myocardial oxygen demand by optimizing MAP, heart rate, and cardiac rhythm. Combinations of coronary and systemic vasodilators, inotropes, antiplatelet agents, and occasionally percutaneous coronary intervention (PCI) may be appropriate in selected patient groups. The advice of a cardiologist may often prove invaluable.

Hypothermia

Definition

Hypothermia is defined as a core temperature below 36°C. Core temperature is generally taken to be the temperature of blood perfusing major organs, such as the brain, liver, and heart. The traditional classification of hypothermia was originally developed to describe hypothermia relating from environmental exposure. A new classification has been suggested for the trauma victim as the prognosis in this group is now known to be markedly worse (see Table 26.4).

Table 26.4. Traditional and revised trauma classification of hypothermia

Degree of hypothermia	Traditional classification (°C)	Trauma classification (°C)
Mild	32–35	34–36
Moderate	29–32	32–34
Severe	20–28	<32

Accidental and therapeutic hypothermia

Most trauma patients have secondary accidental hypothermia or an unintentional decrease in body temperature due to an impaired thermoregulatory response. On occasion, overwhelming environmental factors can lead to hypothermia in an otherwise normal patient. This is termed primary accidental hypothermia.

Therapeutic hypothermia is the active and deliberate cooling of a patient for a potential clinical benefit.

Incidence and prognosis of hypothermia in trauma patients

Hypothermia after trauma can occur in patients of any age, in any climate and in any season. The incidence of hypothermia in patients presenting to the emergency department following trauma has been reported to be between 10 and nearly 50%, increasing with duration of entrapment and severity of injury. In patients who are matched for severity of injury and other confounding variables, hypothermia has been shown to be an independent predictor of mortality. Failure to re-warm to normothermia during resuscitation is also associated with a worse outcome.

Causes of hypothermia in trauma patients

To maintain a normal core temperature in an ambient environment the human body must generate heat by consuming oxygen. In patients in whom oxygen delivery and consumption is limited by shock, insufficient heat production occurs and hypothermia ensues. The trauma patient also has an impaired hypothalamic thermoregulatory response. The normal homeostatic mechanisms such as shivering occur at lower core body temperatures than normal and may even be abolished completely. Environmental, individual and medical factors can also contribute to the development of hypothermia (Box 26.6).

Decreases in temperature during the course of initial assessment and resuscitation are common and can contribute to increased patient morbidity and mortality. Hypothermia during resuscitation can occur in up to 92% of patients, and is often due to radiant heat loss between body and room air.

Box 26.6. Contributing factors to the development of hypothermia in trauma patients

Reduced ability to conserve or produce heat
- Extremes of age
- *Drugs:*
  - tricyclic antidepressants;
  - alcohol;
  - benzodiazepines.
- *Central nervous system disorders:*
  - head injury;
  - spinal cord injuries;
  - mental illness.
- *Co-morbidity:*
  - diabetes mellitus—hypo or hyperglycaemia;
  - severe cardiac, respiratory, renal, or hepatic impairment;
  - malnutrition.
- Anaesthesia (regional and general).

Increased heat loss
- Environmental conditions
  - immersion;
  - exposure.
- Major burns
- Administration of cold fluids and blood products
- Anaesthesia (regional and general).

Pathophysiology of hypothermia

Hypothermia has numerous adverse effects upon all organ systems, summarized in Table 26.5. Hypothermia, together with acidosis and coagulopathy, make up the *lethal triad* in trauma patients. One of the most deleterious effects of hypothermia in the trauma victim with potential clotting factor depletion is a functional coagulopathy. Platelet function is directly depressed and both the prothrombin and activated partial thromboplastin times are prolonged in proportion to the severity of hypothermia, due to reduced enzymatic reaction rates and function. All these effects are directly reversible with the correction of core body temperature to normal. It is important to note that the coagulation profile may be reported as normal if corrected to 37°C for laboratory testing and, therefore, the patient's core temperature must be stated on the laboratory request form.

Mild hypothermia causes an increase in cardiac output to meet increased oxygen demands of shivering. In the patient with intact thermoregulatory responses shivering can increase oxygen consumption by up to 400%.

As moderate or severe hypothermia develops, cardiovascular depression occurs, causing reduced oxygen delivery, a blunted response to endogenous and exogenous catecholamines, and hypotension. Arrhythmias are common with atrial fibrillation, ventricular fibrillation, and asystole occurring spontaneously with falling body temperature. The oxyhaemoglobin dissociation curve is displaced to the left resulting in further impairment of oxygen delivery to hypoxic tissues.

Cerebral function becomes depressed with increasing hypothermia. Clinically, this may present as confusion,

Table 26.5. The major physiological effects of hypothermia

Temperature °C	Cardiovascular	Respiratory	Coagulation	Neurological	Metabolic	Haematological	Endocrine
Mild (35–32°C)	Increased cardiac output, vasoconstriction	Tachyponea, bronchorrhoea	Impaired platelet function, reduced enzymatic rate and function in clotting cascade, DIC	Confusion, ataxia, inappropriate behaviour, reduction in cerebral blood flow and cerebral oxygen demand	Shivering, increase in oxygen consumption, gluconeogenesis	Increased haematocrit, immunosupression	Reduced insulin secretion and increased resistance causing hyperglycaemia
Moderate (32–28°C)	Atrial fibrillation, reduced cardiac output, bradycardia	respiratory depression, leftward shift of oxygen dissociation curve		Coma, pupillary dilatation	Shivering abolished, decrease in oxygen consumption, reduction in hepatic metabolism of drugs		
Severe (<28°C)	Ventricular arrhythmias, increased blood viscosity	Apnoea (24°C)		Hyporeflexia	Metabolic acidosis		

ataxia, inappropriate behaviour, or slowed speech. Coma, pupillary dilatation, and loss of deep tendon reflexes are common below 30°C with electrical activity ceasing around 20°C. Other effects of hypothermia include hyperglycaemia, reduced hepatic metabolism of drugs, and impairment of the immune response to injury, predisposing patients to the risks of secondary infection and impaired healing of wounds.

Prevention and treatment of hypothermia

Treatment of hypothermia should begin with the prevention of further heat loss. Most trauma patients are incapable of spontaneously rewarming to normothermia, and will require active and continued warming. Hypothermia should be corrected as quickly as possible in conjunction with any ongoing resuscitation.

Rewarming should be undertaken by the use of both passive and active methods, of which the active rewarming can be both external or internal (see Box 26.7).

External warming can help prevent ongoing heat losses, but transfers little energy to the patient. If the patient is vasoconstricted, a core to peripheral thermal gradient will exist and heat will not be transferred until the peripheral temperature is raised to at least that of the core. External warming techniques are inefficient because there is limited body surface area contact with the warming device and in the case of conductive air warmers the low density of air does not transmit a great deal of heat. The administration of warm fluid is crucial in the treatment and prevention of hypothermia. Blood products and crystalloids should always be warmed before they are administered, and modern counter current warming systems can infuse 5–8 kcal heat/L/min. Body cavity lavage is a highly effective method of transferring heat to the patient, but is invasive and often contraindicated in the trauma patient.

Extracorporeal circulatory rewarming is the most effective method of restoring a patient to a normal core temperature. Cardiopulmonary bypass and CAVR have been used successfully in severely hypothermic trauma patients. CAVR does not require a pump or systemic heparinization, and is driven by the patient's own blood pressure. Venovenous techniques may be also be used in stable patients on the intensive care unit. During rewarming there may be a period of 'reperfusion shock' as various metabolites, such as potassium and lactic acid return to the systemic circulation from poorly perfused vascular beds, causing vasodilatation, hypotension, and myocardial depression. This can be precipitated by movement of the patient's limbs during re-warming.

Box 26.7. Passive and active re-warming techniques

Passive re-warming techniques
- Providing removal from cold environments.
- Adequate patient coverage with blankets and recovering after examination.
- Increasing ambient room temperature.

External active warming techniques
- Heated blankets.
- Convective air blankets.
- Reflective blankets.
- Radiant heat sources.
- Airway gas warming.

Internal active warming techniques
- Administration of warmed intravenous fluids
- Peritoneal lavage
- Pleural lavage
- Extracorporeal circulatory warming
  - cardiopulmonary bypass;
  - continuous arteriovenous rewarming (CAVR);
  - venovenous techniques.

Therapeutic hypothermia

Cerebral blood flow reduces by 7% per degree decrease in core body temperature (°C) with an associated reduction in both the cerebral metabolic rate ($CMRO_2$), and often a dramatic reduction in intracranial pressure, which can improve oxygen delivery and reduced oxygen consumption in the injured brain. Recent studies have shown survival and outcome benefits after the use of moderate (32–34°C) induced hypothermia in patients who have suffered an out of hospital VF arrest, and many hospitals now also actively cool other types of cardiac arrest survivor. This neurological protection may have a role in certain groups of trauma victim.

Recent evidence suggests that in patients who have suffered a traumatic brain injury, hypothermia may improve neurological outcome and improve mortality, at the risk of an increased incidence of pneumonia. Other studies have looked at the role of therapeutic hypothermia in the treatment of acute spinal cord injury and haemorrhagic shock, and although there maybe some potential benefits, specific patient groups have yet to be identified.

In summary, the overall role of therapeutic hypothermia in the trauma victim remains unclear and thus aggressive rewarming continues to be considered best practice.

Acidosis

Introduction
Acidosis describes a state of increased hydrogen ion concentration in blood plasma. A patient is usually said to be acidotic when the pH of arterial blood is less than 7.35. Acidosis in the trauma patient is used clinically as a marker of shock, severity of injury, and as a guide to the response to resuscitation.

Components of acid-base balance
The acid-base balance of blood depends upon three independent factors:
- *Respiratory component:* where the arterial blood partial pressure of carbon dioxide ($PaCO_2$) is directly proportional to alveolar ventilation (Va).
- *Metabolic component:* as a result of metabolic activity producing hydrogen ions (H^+) and renal retention and excretion of H^+ and bicarbonate ions (HCO_3^-).
- *Buffering capacity of blood:* the ability of plasma to maintain a neutral pH despite the addition or removal of hydrogen ions. Body buffer systems include:
  - carbonic acid/bicarbonate;
  - haemoglobin;
  - plasma proteins;
  - phosphate.

Models of acid-base balance
The Henderson–Hasselbach model
Classically acid-base disorders have been described by the Henderson–Hasselbach model, which describes the derivation of pH by the relationship between the concentrations of dissociated and undissociated acid or base.

In the bicarbonate buffer system, carbon dioxide and water forms carbonic acid, which dissociates to form bicarbonate and hydrogen ions:

$$CO_2 + H_2O \lessgtr H_2CO_3 \lessgtr H^+ + HCO_3^-$$

The hydrogen ion concentration (and pH) is related to the balance between respiratory and metabolic systems:

$$pH \sim [HCO_3^-]/PaCO_2$$

Table 26.6. Causes of elevated and normal anion gap metabolic acidosis

Elevated anion gap metabolic acidosis	Normal anion gap metabolic acidosis
Lactic acidosis	Loss of bicarbonate • Small bowel fistula • Renal tubular acidosis
Ketoacidosis • Diabetes • Alcohol abuse • Starvation	Excess chloride administration eg NaCl 0.9%
Poisoning • Methanol • Ethylene glycol • Propylene glycol • Aspirin • Iron • Paraldehyde	Drugs • Carbonic anhydrase inhibitors • Spironolactone • Total Parenteral Nutrition
Uraemia	Hyperparathyroidism

Anion gap
The anion gap (AG) is a concept based upon the law of electrochemical neutrality of total cations (positive ions) and anions (negative ions) in plasma:

$$[AG] = ([Na^+] + [K^+] - [Cl^-] + [HCO_3^-]$$

Potassium is usually ignored as the actual changes in clinical practice compatible with life are usually small. In health there are more unmeasured anions (albumin, PO_4^{2-}, SO_4^{2-}) compared with unmeasured cations in the plasma and, therefore, the AG is usually positive, a normal range being 8–12 mEq/L.

The calculation of the AG is useful clinically in determining the differential diagnosis of metabolic acidosis.

The Stewart model
The Stewart model of acid-base balance emphasizes the importance of dependent versus independent variables in determining pH (Table 26.7).

Stewart showed that the concentration of the dependent variables was directly determined by the three independent variables:
- *Strong ion difference (SID):* The SID is the difference between the sums of strong cations and strong anions in plasma:

  $$[SID] = [Na^+] + [K^+] + [Ca^{2+}] + [MG^{2+}] - [CL^-] - [other\ strong\ anions]$$

- *$[A_{TOT}]$:* $[A_{TOT}]$ is the total plasma concentration of weak non-volatile acids; inorganic phosphate (Pi), serum proteins, and albumin:
  $$[A_{TOT}] = [Pi_{TOT}] + [Pr_{TOT}] + albumin.$$
- $PaCO_2$.

This means metabolic disturbances can no longer be viewed as a consequence of changes in bicarbonate concentration as bicarbonate is a dependent variable. Metabolic changes occur through alterations in SID and changes in $[A_{TOT}]$.

SID changes as the plasma concentration alters or there are changes in the concentration of strong ions, such as chloride or inorganic acids, such as lactate. A_{TOT} is mainly determined by the concentration of albumin which acts as a weak acid, and phosphate, which if very high can contribute to the acidaemia of renal failure.

In a similar way to the clinical application of AG, the calculation of SID and the strong ion gap (SIG) allows metabolic acidosis to be classified and causes determined:

Table 26.7. Dependent and independent variables in the Stewart Model of acid-base balance

Dependent variables	Independent variables
$[H^+]$	Strong ion difference (SID)
$[OH^-]$	$[A_{TOT}]$
$[HCO_3^-]$	$PaCO_2$
$[CO_3^{2-}]$	
$[HA]$	
$[A]$	

$$[SIG] = [SID] - [A_{TOT}] \text{ and } [HCO_3^-]$$

The SIG is less than 4 mEq/L in health. It can be calculated from plasma blood biochemistry and an arterial blood gas, usually in a critical care environment. The calculation of SID and SIG is not used routinely in clinical practice in the UK, but there has been recent resurgence of interest, which may lead to its greater use.

Base excess and deficit

The base deficit or excess is a useful tool in quantifying the metabolic components of an acid-base derangement. It can be defined as the amount of base (mmol) that must be added or removed to restore 1 L of whole blood to a normal pH, assuming normal values of PaO_2, $PaCO_2$, and temperature. A positive base excess signifies a metabolic alkalosis, a negative base deficit signifies a metabolic acidosis with a normal range between −2 and +2 mmol/L.

Metabolic acidosis and lactate in the trauma patient

Metabolic acidosis can be present in the trauma patient at all stages of the patient pathway—pre-hospital, resuscitation, in the operating theatre and intensive care unit. In the early stages of major injury (but not always) a metabolic acidosis is accompanied by a raised plasma lactate and reflects a state of patient shock due to inadequate tissue oxygen delivery.

Glucose is metabolized in the presence of oxygen to pyruvate, which is then metabolized to CO_2 and water, producing energy in the form of ATP. In the absence of oxygen pyruvate is metabolized to lactate via the enzyme lactate dehydrogenase. When production of lactate exceeds its metabolism and the buffering capacity of the blood, plasma lactate will rise. In solution lactate can dissociate and donate a proton, thus the pH of the blood will also fall in proportion to the increasing concentration of lactate in the plasma. The normal plasma lactate level is 1–2 mmol/L.

Management of lactic acidosis involves the identification and treatment of any precipitating cause and the restoration of adequate oxygen delivery to the tissues.

Acidosis as a predictor of outcome after trauma

Initial plasma lactate concentration has been shown to correlate well with injury severity, and can predict organ failure and survivors from non-survivors after major trauma. Alcohol and substance abuse does not seem to impair predictive accuracy. A base deficit of more than −6 in the first 24 h of admission after trauma predicts an increased risk of massive transfusion, ARDS, coagulopathy, and overall mortality. A significant abdominal injury is also more likely and a base deficit of −6 should be considered a strong indication for further diagnostic investigation, such as computerized tomography. In the setting of traumatic vascular injury, SIG has been shown to be a better predictor of mortality than plasma lactate.

Acidosis as a marker of resuscitation

Serum lactate, lactic acidosis and base deficit are useful as markers of successful resuscitation. An increased time to clear a lactic acidosis despite resuscitation is associated with an increased risk of organ failure and may suggest occult hypoperfusion. A worsening base deficit or lactic acidosis may suggest ongoing haemorrhage, and can be used to guide volume replacement or damage control surgery.

Venous bicarbonate may also provide a useful alternative predictive marker and guide to resuscitation in certain patients where arterial blood gas sampling is not possible or available, for example in children.

Hyperchloraemic acidosis

The use of large volumes of fluids containing excess chloride (0.9% saline, delivery solution for some colloids) for resuscitation after major trauma can cause an increase in plasma chloride out of proportion to the increase in plasma sodium and a dilution in the concentration of weak acids. Excess protons are generated to equalize the excess negative charge, leading to hyperchloraemic metabolic acidosis, which will compound a metabolic acidosis from another cause, such as unresuscitated shock. High and frequent doses of beta-lactam antibiotics may also result in the administration of high concentrations of sodium chloride.

Acidosis and coagulopathy

The clotting cascade involves a sequence of pH dependent reactions. A notable impairment of haemostasis ensues at a pH <7.1 or a base deficit of −12.5, by actions upon platelets, calcium-binding sites, and enzymatic function of the clotting cascade.

In a situation of coagulopathy due to haemorrhage and the massive transfusion of stored blood, the use of buffering agents such as sodium bicarbonate or THAM to correct a metabolic acidosis, may offer a potential benefit in a ventilated patient or a patient with normal respiratory function.

Administration of sodium bicarbonate should be of a dilute solution (1.26%) if administered through a peripheral venous route, increasing to a concentrated solution (8.4%) if administered through central venous catheter. Use of sodium bicarbonate should be titrated to serial blood gas measurements.

Acidosis and aging

The elderly trauma patient may have significant co-morbidity, which reduces the ability to tolerate significant periods of hypoperfusion and clear any subsequent lactic acidosis. Mortality in trauma patients over the age of 55 is associated with a reduced base deficit (25% mortality, base deficit −8 mmol/L) than in patients under 55 (25% mortality, base deficit −15 mmol/L).

Systemic inflammatory response and sepsis

Introduction

The classical trimodal distribution of death after major trauma, although recently challenged, describes a group of patients (up to 45%) who will die after surviving the initial injury and their immediate resuscitation and stabilization.

These deaths often occur days to weeks after admission in patients who subsequently remain in the intensive care unit. The vast majority of these deaths are due to severe sepsis and multiple organ failure (MOF). Patients with a more severe injury are more likely to generate a greater inflammatory response and suffer more frequent and severe infectious complications.

Definitions

Systemic Inflammatory Response Syndrome describes a non-specific whole body inflammatory response regardless of cause. SIRS is frequently seen in a variety of conditions; major trauma and tissue injury are potent stimuli. To diagnose SIRS, two of the following criteria must be present:

- Hypothermia (<36°C) or hyperthermia (>38°C).
- Tachycardia (heart rate >90/min).
- Tachypnoea (>20/min) or a $PaCO_2$ <4.3 kPa.
- Leucopenia (<4 x 10^9/L) or leucocytosis (>12 x 10^9/L).

Sepsis is a syndrome characterized by a systemic inflammatory response (SIRS) to an infection. An infection is the invasion of normally sterile tissues by micro-organisms or their toxins. To diagnose sepsis, the SIRS has to be present and infection has to be proven or highly suspected (Fig. 26.11).

Severe sepsis occurs when sepsis is associated with organ dysfunction, evidence of hypoperfusion, or hypotension. Hypoperfusion and perfusion abnormalities may include, but are not limited to lactic acidosis, oliguria, or acute alteration in mental status.

Septic shock is sepsis-induced hypotension (systolic <90 mmHg or a reduction in >40% from baseline in absence of other causes) refractory to adequate fluid resuscitation with the presence of perfusion abnormalities as above. Patients may be on vasopressors or inotropic agents and, therefore, not hypotensive at the time of assessment.

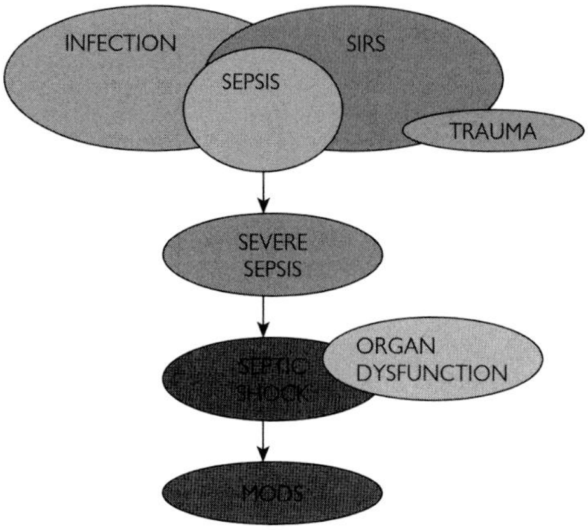

Fig. 26.11. The interrelationship between SIRS, sepsis, infection and trauma.

If left untreated then sepsis can progress to *multiple organ dysfunction syndrome (MODS)*, the presence of altered organ function in an acutely ill patient such that homeostasis cannot be maintained without intervention.

Incidence of SIRS and sepsis in trauma and intensive care patients

Severe sepsis is now a relatively common condition, and is a more common cause of mortality in the UK than lung cancer or breast and bowel cancer combined. In the past decade the incidence of sepsis has increased markedly as the population has aged. Intensive care units are dealing with an increasing proportion of patients with severe forms of sepsis and presenting with a greater number of organ dysfunctions. Within an ICU population the incidence of severe sepsis has been estimated at 10% (±4%), with a population incidence of 1(±0.5) cases per 1000 admissions. This may reflect the treated incidence, rather than the true incidence, and could be a reflection of the availability of critical care services. The true incidence may be much higher—Padkin *et al.*'s UK study in 2003 reported an ICU incidence of 27% and a population incidence of 0.51 cases per 1000.

Trauma has been shown to be an independent risk factor for the development of SIRS and severe sepsis with both injury severity and the incidence of MOF correlating well with plasma concentrations of measured inflammatory markers. The extent of systemic inflammation also shows a relationship with the risk of developing organ failure and subsequent mortality.

Patients with major injury after trauma are more likely to develop an ICU-related infection, with increasing age, injury severity, and multi-system trauma associated with a greater risk. Traumatic brain injury and spinal injuries are also associated with a higher risk of nosocomial pneumonia; burns over 20% of the body surface area are associated with an increased risk of MOD, sepsis, and death.

Despite the advances in medical technology the mortality of severe sepsis remains high (20–50%), although trauma patients may have a better outcome in comparison to non-traumatic patient groups.

Pathophysiology

The immune response to major injury is complex and involves interaction between the host's immune system, infecting organisms, and numerous pro- and anti-inflammatory mediators. This immune response follows a biphasic pattern, with an initial pro-inflammatory response causing SIRS followed by a compensatory anti-inflammatory response (CARS) or a mixed antagonist response syndrome (MARS), which leads to a period of immune paralysis and then recovery or death.

Bone *et al.* described a three-stage development of SIRS:

- In response to a significant insult such as trauma or infection local cytokines from activated monocytes, lymphocytes, and endothelial complexes are produced. This process activates an inflammatory response, which is designed to promote tissue repair and prevent further damage, by recruitment of the reticulo-endothelial system.
- Some of the cytokines are released into the systemic circulation to engage additional macrophages and

lymphocytes. This initial escalation (the acute phase response) is antagonized by anti-inflammatory mediators and the temporal reduction in the release of the pro-inflammatory mediators.

- If the inflammatory cascade becomes unbalanced, further systemic amplification can occur, leading to the release of further mediators. The effects of this *cytokine storm* are eventually to cause SIRS, and direct and indirect damage to the function of local and distant organ systems. A multi-hit theory that can occur in major trauma has been postulated—each individual or sequential insult produces an escalating abnormal and exaggerated response that is eventually overwhelming.

The cytokines thought to be particularly central to the development of SIRS are tumour necrosis factor alpha (TNFα), interleukin-1 (IL-1), interleukin-6 (IL-6) with TNFα, and IL-1 producing the systemic and metabolic features of SIRS and IL-6 the acute phase response.

Bacterial toxins

The inflammatory cascade can be initiated by various bacterial products including endotoxins and exotoxins. Endotoxin is a lipopolysaccharide found on the outer membrane of Gram-negative bacteria and, therefore, can still activate biological mediators even if the bacteria are killed. Exotoxins are antigenic proteins produced by the bacteria themselves. Bacteria can produce one toxin (tetanus, cholera), or several (*Staphyloccocus, Streptococcus*). Some can produce both endo- and exotoxins (e.g. *Pseudomonas*).

Immune dysfunction in trauma

As part of the host attempt to restore equilibrium to the pro-inflammatory reaction, an anti-inflammatory response is initiated. This can over-compensate and cause an immunosuppressed state, where the body cannot mount a further response to new injuries or insult, such as nosocomial infections. The mechanisms of immune suppression are thought to include the following.

A shift to secretion of anti-inflammatory cytokines

Activated CD4 helper cells reduce secretion of pro-inflammatory cytokines and begin to produce cytokines with anti-inflammatory properties such as interleukin-4 (IL-4) and interleukin-10 (IL-10). IL-10 is a potent inhibitor of monocyte function, and reduces production of TNFα and IL-6. Elevated levels of IL-10 have been associated with adverse outcomes in sepsis.

Anergy

Anergy is a state of unresponsiveness—the failure of a cell to secrete cytokines in response to their specific antigen. Patients with trauma or burns are known to have reduced levels of circulating T cells and these cells are anergic.

Death of immune cells

Sepsis is thought to promote immune cell apoptosis (programmed cell death), which potentiates the anergic state.

Trauma patients and sepsis—predisposing factors

Multiple and varied factors predispose the trauma patient to infection (Table 26.8). The integrity of barriers such as skin or mucosa can be breached and foreign or pathogenic matter introduced into sterile tissues. This breach may be caused during the act of injury itself or from an iatrogenic source such as endotracheal intubation or venous access.

Table 26.8. Factors increasing risk of infection in ICU trauma patients

Trauma factors	Patient and medical factors
Damage to host defences: • Penetration of sterile tissues • Damage to sterile tissues	Insertion of catheters, drains and indwelling lines
Compensatory anti-inflammatory response (CARS)	Endotracheal intubation and mechanical ventilation
Severity of injury	Age
Hyperglycaemia	Co-morbidity (e.g. diabetes and COPD)
Hypothermia	Nutritional deficiency
Stress ulcer prophylaxis	Changes and overgrowth of normal bacterial flora by more virulent pathogens (e.g. oropahyrnx and gut)
Administration of blood products	Genetics

The normal gut, skin, and orophayngeal flora of critically ill patients become colonized and overgrown with pathogenic and virulent bacteria, which can then predispose to nosocomial infections and bacteraemias. The risk of developing an infection is compounded by immunosuppression, catabolism and poor nutritional intake. Infections are more common in the elderly, and those more severely injured and with associated major co-morbidities. Current and ongoing research suggests that genetic profile may also determine susceptibility to death from an infectious disease, by determining the extent of the host's pro- or anti-inflammatory response to infection.

The most common sources of sepsis in trauma patients are the respiratory system, urinary system and primary bacteraemias (Box 26.8).

Manifestations of severe SIRS and septic shock

SIRS and sepsis have multi-system and multi-organ consequences.

Hypotension

Sepsis is associated with a marked reduction in systemic vascular resistance, resulting in hypotension despite an adequate or increased cardiac output. This is due to induction of the enzyme nitric oxide synthase, which causes an increase in the production of nitric oxide (NO), a potent endothelial, and smooth muscle cell vasodilator. Venodilatation also occurs, causing increasing venous capacitance and pooling of blood in the peripheries. A relative hypovolaemia therefore ensues due to a reduction in right heart pre-load.

Reduced myocardial function

Although sepsis is characterized by a hyper-dynamic circulation and an increased cardiac output, ventricular systolic, and diastolic function are impaired and the work of the heart is increased for a given stroke volume. Possible causes are myocardial depressant factors (MDF) related to sepsis, diminished coronary blood flow, pulmonary

Box 26.8. Common causes and sources of infection in ICU trauma patients

Site and type of infection

Respiratory
- Nosocomial pneumonia.
- Empyema.

Gastrointestinal
- Bacterial peritonitis.
- Antibiotic induced colitis.

Urinary
Urinary tract infections.

Dermatological infections
- Traumatic wound.
- Delayed closure of wound.
- Surgical infection.

Central nervous system
Meningo-encephalitis.

Primary bacteraemias
In-dwelling vascular access catheters.

hypertension, and beta-receptor down-regulation. Sepsis-induced myocardial depression can take many days to recover, even after recovery from sepsis.

Reduced oxygen utilization

Despite the increased cardiac output there are often signs of inadequate oxygen delivery and oxygen extraction (e.g. worsening lactic acidosis, high mixed venous oxygen saturation). Peripheral shunting of blood flow caused by abnormal autoregulatory mechanics in tissue beds, and cellular metabolic defects, can prevent effective delivery and utilization of oxygen by the cells. Maldistribution of oxygen delivery can be compounded by compression of capillaries from external oedema or capillary blockage by inflammatory cells or clot formation.

Coagulopathy

An imbalance in clotting activation, suppression of fibrinolysis and consumption of modulators of coagulation, such as activated protein C may manifest as microvascular thrombosis, contributing to multi-organ failure, or disseminated intravascular coagulopathy (DIC).

Increased capillary permeability

Increased endothelial permeability of capillary beds causes leakage of fluid from the intravascular space into the interstitium, which has systemic consequences:
- Interstitial and alveolar oedema with pulmonary hypertension and increased shunting can lead to hypoxia, ALI and ARDS.
- Translocation of pathogenic bacteria in the colonized gastrointestinal tract can cross the more permeable endothelium contributing to the septic response.
- Hypovolaemia from loss of vascular circulating volume can contribute to hypotension and shock.

Other mechanisms

The normal function of gastrointestinal, renal, and central nervous systems can also be affected (see Table 26.9).

Identification and diagnosis of the septic trauma patient

As SIRS and sepsis are part of a continuum of disease it can be difficult to distinguish between a non-infectious SIRS response due to trauma, or an infectious septic cause. The consequences of failing to recognize and treat an infection can be devastating, thus a high level of clinical suspicion is required.

A raised white cell count, pyrexia or cardiovascular deterioration should precipitate a thorough clinical examination of potential sources of infection. Microbiological culture of urine, skin, sputum, and blood should be performed routinely. The use of focused imaging techniques (ultrasound, computerized tomography, and X-ray) can help support or refute a diagnosis, and occasionally surgical intervention may be required even in the absence of conclusive evidence.

Biochemical markers may help support the diagnosis of sepsis over that of SIRS.

Procalcitonin

Procalcitonin (PCT) is a prohormone of calcitonin that is secreted from C-cells of the thyroid. Normally plasma levels are very low (<0.05 ng/L), but in the presence of bacterial infection PCT is induced and released from other sites in the body and significant concentrations can be measured in blood (up to 1000 ng/L). Plasma levels of greater than 10 ng/L are consistent with severe sepsis.

PCT has been shown to be a more sensitive and specific marker for bacterial infection than CRP, TNFα, IL-2, IL-6 and IL-8 levels, and can differentiate successfully between SIRS, sepsis, and severe sepsis. Improved diagnostic accuracy can reduce inappropriate antibiotic administration, diagnostic investigation and potential interventions.

Table 26.9. Systemic manifestations of SIRS and septic shock

Organ system	
Cardiovascular	Reduction in systemic vascular resistance
	Increase in venous capacitance
	Systolic and diastolic dysfunction
	Increased cardiac output
	Impaired and reduced oxygen extraction
Respiratory	Acute lung Injury
	Acute respiratory distress syndrome
Gastrointestinal	Ileus
	Bacterial translocation
Renal	Acute renal failure
Central nervous	Acute confusional state
	Depressed level of consciousness
Haematological	Coagulopathy
	Microvascular thrombosis
	DIC
Metabolic	Hyperglycaemia
	Catabolism
	Relative adrenal insufficiency
Hepatic	Cholestasis
	Jaundice

Management of sepsis

Immediate stabilization and resuscitation

The primary aim of resuscitation in a septic patient is to maintain oxygen delivery to the tissues, and the immediate priority is therefore to ensure patency of the airway and adequate ventilation. High flow oxygen should be administered and appropriate venous access secured. Intubation and mechanical ventilation may be necessary.

Early goal-directed therapy

Aggressive fluid resuscitation should be commenced as soon as possible to achieve measurable resuscitation goals within 6 h of the onset of sepsis. This has been shown consistently to reduce morbidity, mortality and hospital costs in severe sepsis. An example of an early goal-directed therapy (EGDT) protocol for sepsis can be seen in Fig. 26.12. EGDT has three progressive stages, which are used if resuscitation goals are not met:

- Aggressive fluid resuscitation to a CVP of 8–12mmHg.
- Vasopressors to restore MAP.
- Augmentation of oxygen delivery.

What type of fluid?

Both crystalloids and colloids expand the intravascular space and have been used to successfully resuscitate

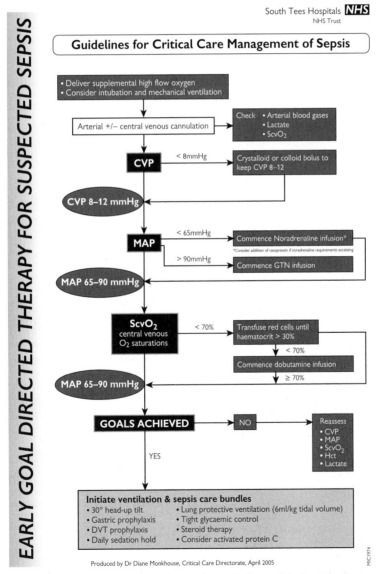

Fig. 26.12. Example of an early goal-directed therapy protocol in sepsis (reprinted with persmission from Diane Monkhouse).

shocked septic patients. Recent clinical trials have failed to show any superiority of one fluid over another, although a combination-based resuscitation strategy may offer the benefits of prolonged and quick plasma expansion with reduced oedema formation and drug side effects. There is no place for dextrose based solutions in the acute resuscitation situation.

There has been a great deal of interest in the use of hypertonic saline (7.5%) in resuscitation as this expands the plasma by up to 10 times the infusion volume, by redistribution of extravascular fluid down a concentration gradient. These solutions are often formulated with a colloid to prolong the intravascular volume effect and retain the osmotically-displaced water. Hypertonic saline may offer other benefits including improved microvascular flow and immunomodulation, although there is currently insufficient evidence to recommend its routine use in sepsis.

In conclusion, rapid attainment of resuscitation goals to improve oxygen delivery to the tissues is critical, irrespective of the type of fluid used. Resuscitation goals include improvement in blood pressure, urine output, and conscious level, a decrease in heart rate and a central venous pressure of 8–12 mmHg.

Vasopressors

If hypotension persists despite adequate fluid resuscitation, it is appropriate to commence vasoactive medication to restore tissue perfusion. Noradrenaline has pharmacological agonist effects at alpha-1 receptors, causing vasoconstriction and an increased mean arterial pressure (MAP). There may also be a mild increase in stroke volume at low doses due to a beta-1 agonist effect. Heart rate may fall due to reflex baroreceptor stimulation. The effect of an increase in MAP is to increase perfusion of vital organs, such as the heart and brain. When used with adequate volume resuscitation and oxygen delivery, noradrenaline is also thought to improve renal perfusion via an increased glomerular filtration rate and to maintain splanchnic perfusion.

Oxygen delivery

The majority of oxygen in the blood is carried by haemoglobin, thus the quantity of oxygen in the blood can be determined by the equation:

$$CaO_2 = Hb(g/L) \times SaO_2\% \times 1.31 \ (mlsO_2/gHb)$$

where 1.31 represents the amount of oxygen a gram of haemoglobin can carry.

The delivery of oxygen to the tissues is also dependent on cardiac output thus:

$$DO_2 = CO \ (L/min) \times CaO_2 \ (mL/O_2/min)$$

Any evidence of inadequate oxygen delivery, such as a worsening lactic acidosis or decreased central venous oxygenation (suggesting the need for increased oxygen extraction), can be treated by the transfusion of red cells, optimization of ventilation, or augmentation of cardiac output.

Inotropes

Dobutamine is a beta-1 receptor agonist, which causes increased contractility (inotropy) and increased heart rate (chronotropy). It also has mild beta-2 effects causing muscle bed vasodilatation. Dobutamine, when used in combination with noradrenaline in sepsis, increases oxygen delivery and splanchnic perfusion.

Cultures and source control

Persistent infection will continue to drive the SIRS response and prevent recovery from MOD. Septic foci should be aggressively sought and treated with medical or surgical measures.

Antimicrobials

Studies have shown a temporal relationship between the administration of antibiotics and mortality. Appropriate antibiotics should be given as early as possible in the illness. A general rule is if no pathogens have been isolated, antibiotic prescribing should initially be broad, to cover all potential pathogens and site of infection, then de-escalated to monotherapy if possible. Courses of antibiotics should be short and of adequate dose. Consultation with a clinical microbiologist can be invaluable in the intensive care patient.

Nutrition and immunonutrition

Trauma and SIRS induce an elevated basal metabolic rate, with elevated nutritional requirements in the face of a profound catabolic and nutritionally deplete state—protein and fat are metabolized to provide a source of glucose, causing reduced muscle mass, function, and hyperglycaemia.

In critically ill patients, malnutrition is associated with an increased risk of infection, impaired immunity, and prolonged ventilatory dependence. Adequate nutrition also improves wound healing, reduces the catabolic stress response, and gut function. This translates into reduced complications and improved clinical outcomes.

Early feeding (within 24–48 h) should be started in all critically-ill trauma patients, with a particular attempt to achieve early nutritional goals in the sub-group of patients with traumatic brain injury. Enteral nutrition is associated with lower rates of infection, hyperglycaemia and cost (when compared to total parenteral nutrition, TPN).

There has been considerable interest in the use of immunonutrition in trauma patients in an attempt to support the immune system during the period of immune dysfunction that occurs soon after injury. Immunonutrition is thought to exert its effects by improving cell functions and direct anti-oxidant and anti-inflammatory effects. Combinations of arginine, glutamine, and fish oils added to enteral feeds have been studied in both trauma and septic patient groups. Although some early studies have been encouraging and show potential benefit, a recent meta-analysis failed to demonstrate any advantage of immunonutrition over regular nutrition in the trauma population.

Selective decontamination of the digestive tract

Selective decontamination of the digestive tract (SDD) is a technique using combinations of topical and systemic antibiotics to eradicate carriage of potentially harmful gram negative bacteria in the oropharynx, stomach, and gut, reducing the rates of nosocomial infections. Trials have confirmed its efficacy, but ongoing concerns over resistance and applicability to a UK population have prevented its widespread use. Topical oral antisepsis using chlorhexidine-based products may offer an alternative approach.

Further supportive therapy

A number of further therapeutic measures may be undertaken to attempt to reduce the mortality of the septic trauma patient. The *Surviving Sepsis Campaign* (SSC) was created in 2004 by collaboration between international experts in intensive care and infectious diseases, representing 11 organizations in an attempt to improve outcome in severe sepsis and septic shock. The recommendations provide a good summary of the available evidence supporting the use of various interventions in sepsis.

A summary, including the level of evidence available, is outlined below:

- *Thromboprohylaxis*: both trauma and sepsis predispose to the formation of deep vein thrombosis. Low molecular weight heparin should be used (1A). If there is a contraindication a mechanical compression device should be used (1A).
- *Stress ulcer prophylaxis:* the incidence of significant upper GI bleeding has been shown to be reduced by the use of prophylactic measures in ICU patients. Stress ulcer prophylaxis should be given by either a proton pump inhibitor (1B) or a H_2 receptor antagonist (1A).
- *Protective lung ventilation:* where mechanical ventilation is undertaken, protective lung ventilation should be use to reduce ventilator induced lung injury (1A–C).
- *Glucose control:* hyperglycaemia in sepsis has been associated with a worse outcome. Insulin infusions should be used to treat hyperglycaemia (1A).
- *Steroids (2C):* adrenal insufficiency can be present in up to 75% of patients with severe sepsis, which can blunt the cardiovascular response of patients to catecholamines. Low dose physiological replacement (50 mcg qds) can be used in patients with shock unresponsive to fluids and vasopressors.

- *Vasopressin (2C)*: arginine vasopressin (anti-diuretic hormone, ADH) is an endogenous hormone stored and released from the posterior pituitary. In health the cardiovascular effects are marginal. In severe sepsis, the vasopressor effects become more pronounced and vasopressin levels are increased. In some patients with continued shock the vasopressin levels decrease, thus a state of relative vasopressin deficiency exists. There is currently no conclusive evidence that vasopressin alters outcome, and concerns have been expressed over the use of high doses which can cause splanchnic, cardiac, and digital ischaemia. Low dose vasopressin is therefore indicated as an adjunct to noradrenaline in refractory septic shock (0.03 U/min).
- *Recombinant human activated protein C (rhAPC) (2C)*: activated protein C (AP-C) is an endogenous anticoagulant which inactivates factors Va and VIIIa, prevents generation of thrombin, promotes fibrinolysis, and has direct anti-inflammatory effects. Reduced levels of AP-C are common is sepsis and are associated with a disordered inflammatory and coagulation response to infection. rhAPC has been shown to reduce mortality in patients with a high risk of death. There is an increased bleeding risk associated with the use of rhAPC.

Further reading

Balcı C, Sungurtekin H, Gürses E, Sungurtekin U, Kaptanoglu B. Usefulness of procalcitonin for diagnosis of sepsis in the intensive care unit. *Crit Care Med* 2003; **7**: 85–90.

Bagshaw SM, George C, Gibney RT, Bellomo R. A multi-centre evaluation of early kidney injury in critically ill trauma patients. *Ren Fail* 2008; **30**(9): 581–9.

Bilkovski RN, Rivers EP, Horst HM. Targeted resuscitation strategies after injury. *Curr Opin Crit Care* 2004; **10**: 529–38.

Bone RC, Balk RA, Cerra FB, Dellinger RP, Fein AM, Knaus WA, et al. Definitions for sepsis and organ failure and guidelines for the use of innovative therapies in sepsis. The ACCP/SCCM Consensus Conference Committee. *Chest* 1992; **101**(6): 1644–55.

Bone RC. Towards a theory regarding the pathogenesis of the systemic inflammatory response syndrome: what we do and do not know about cytokine regulation. *Crit Care Med* 1996; **24**(1): 163–72.

Brain Trauma Foundation Cerebral Perfusion Thresholds. *J NeuroTrauma* 2007; **24**(S1): 59–64.

Brain Trauma Foundation Indications for intra-cranial pressure monitoring. *J NeuroTrauma* 2007; **24**(S1): 37–44.

British Thoracic Society Standards of Care Committee. Non-invasive ventilation in acute respiratory failure. *Thorax* 2002; **57**: 192–211.

Cavalcanti M, Ferrer M, Ferrer R, Morforte R, Garnacho A, Torres A. Risk and prognostic factors of ventilator associated pneumonia in trauma patients. *Crit Care Med* 2006; **34**(4): 1067–72.

Chan EY, Ruest A, O Meade M, Cook DJ. Oral decontamination for prevention of pneumonia in mechanically ventilated adults: systematic review and metanalysis. *Br Med J* 2007; **334**: 889.

Cheatham ML, Malbrain ML., Kirkpatrick, Sugrue M, Parr M, De Waele J, et al. Results from the International Conference of Experts on Intra-abdominal Hypertension and Abdominal Compartment Syndrome. II Recommmendations. *Intens Care Med* 2007; **33**(6): 951–62.

Cheung KW, Green RS, Magee KD. Systematic review of randomised controlled trials of therapeutic hypothermia as a neuroprotectant in post cardiac arrest patients. *Canad J Emerg Med Care* 2006; **8**: 329-37.

Dellinger RP, Levy MM, Cartlet JM, Bion J, Parker MM, Jaeschke R, et al. Surviving Sepsis Campaign: International Guidelines for the management of severe sepsis and septic shock. *Crit Care Med* 2008; **36**(1): 296–327.

Dreyfuss D, Saumon G. Ventilator induced lung injury. *Am J Resp Crit Care Med* 1998; **157**: 294–323.

Dunne JR, Tracy KJ, Scalea TM, Napolitano LM. Lactate and base deficit in trauma: does alcohol or drug use impair their predictive accuracy? *J Trauma* 2004; **58**(5): 959–66.

Fitzwater J, Purdue GF, Hunt JL, O'Keefe GE. The risk factors and time course of sepsis and organ dysfunction after burn trauma. *J Trauma* 2003; **54**(5): 959–66.

Garfield MJ, Howard-Griffin RM. Non-invasive positive pressure ventilation for severe thoracic trauma. *Br J Anaesth* 2000; **85**(5): 788–90.

Gentilello LM, Pierson DJ. Trauma critical care. *Am J Respir Crit Care Med* 2001; **163**: 604–7.

Gunduz M, Unlugenc H, Ozalevli M, Inanoglu K, Akman H. A comparative study of continuous airway pressure (CPAP) and intermittent positive pressure ventilation (IPPV) in patients with flail chest. *Emerg Med J* 2005; **22**(5): 325–9.

Halter JM, Steinburg JM, Gatto LA, DiRocco JD, Pavone LA, Schiller HJ, et al. Effect of positive end-expiratory pressure and tidal volume on lung injury induced by alveolar instability. *Crit Care* 2007; **11**(1): R20.

Hedrick TL, Smith RL, McEearney ST, Evans HL, Smith PW, Pruett TL, et al. Differences in early and late ventilator associated pneumonia between surgical and trauma patients in a combined or trauma intensive care unit. *J Trauma* 2008; **64**(3): 714–20.

Heyland DK, Dhaliwal R, Drover JW, Gramlich L, Dodek P; Canadian Critical Care Clinical Practice Guidelines Committee. Canadian Clinical Practice Guidelines for Nutritional Support in Mechanically Ventilated, Critically Ill Adult Patients. *J Parenter Enteral Nutr* 2003; **27**(5): 355–73.

Hotchkiss RS, Karl IE. The pathophysiology and treatment of sepsis. *N Engl J Med* 2003; **348**(2): 138–50.

Kaplan LJ, Kellum JA. Initial pH, base deficit, lactate, anion gap, strong ion difference, and strong ion gap predict outcome from major vascular injury. *Crit Care Med* 2004; **32**(5): 1120–4.

Klompas M. Does this patient have ventilator associated pneumonia? *J Am Med Ass* 2007; **297**(14): 1583–93.

Kollef MH, Sherman G, Ward S, Fraser VJ. Inadequate antimicrobial treatment of infections: a risk factor for hospital mortality among critically ill patients. *Chest* 1999; **115**(2): 462–74.

Laudi S, Donaubauer B, Busch T. Low incidence of multiple organ failure after major trauma. *Injury* 2007; **38**(9): 1052–8.

Lausevic Z, Lausevic M, Trbojevic-Stankovic J. Predicting multiple organ failure in patients with severe trauma. *Can J Surg* 2008; **51**(2): 97–102.

Lazarus HM, Fox J, Lloyd JF, Evans RS, Abouzelof R, Taylor C, et al. A six year descriptive study of hospital-associated infection in trauma patients. Demographics, injury features and infection patterns. *Surg Infect* 2007; **8**(4): 463–73.

Lier H, Krep H, Schroder S, Stuber F. Preconditions of hemostasis in trauma: a review. The influence of acidosis, hypocalcemia, anemia, and hypothermia on functional hemostasis in trauma. *J Trauma* 2008; **65**(4): 951–60.

Linde-Zwirble WT, Angus DC. Severe sepsis epidemiology: sampling, selection and society. *Crit Care* 2004; **8**(4): 222–6.

Marik PE, Zaloga GP. Immunonutrition in critically ill patients: a systematic review and analysis of the literature. *Intens Care Med* 2008; **34**(11): 1980–90.

Martin MJ, FitzSullivan E, Salim A, Berne TV, Towfigh S. Use of serum bicarbonate measurement in place of arterial base deficit in the surgical intensive care unit. *Arch Surg* 2005; **140**(8): 745–51.

Meade MO, Cook DJ, Guyatt GH, Slutsky AS, Arabi YM, Cooper DJ, et al. Ventilation strategy using low tidal volumes, recruitment maneuvers, and high positive end-expiratory pressure for acute lung injury and acute respiratory distress syndrome: a randomized controlled trial. *J Am Med Ass* 2008; **299**(6): 637–45.

Morris CG, Low J. Metabolic acidosis in the critically ill: Part 1. Classification and pathophysiology. *Anaesthesia* 2008; **63**(3): 294–301.

MRC CRASH Trial Collaborators. Predicting outcome after traumatic brain injury: practical prognostic models based on large cohort of international patients. *Br Med J* 2008; 336: 425–9.

Muscadere J, Dodek P, Keenan S. Comprehensive evidence-based clinical practice guidelines for ventilator-associated pneumonia: diagnosis and treatment. *J Crit Care* 2008; **23**(1): 138–47.

National Trauma Research Institute. The DECRA Trial: Early decompressive craniectomy in patients with severe traumatic brain injury. Available at: http://clinicaltrials.gov/ct2/show/NCT00155987 (accessed 04 September 2008)

Padkin A, Goldfrad C, Brady AR, Young D, Black N, Rowan K. Epidemiology of severe sepsis occurring in the first 24 hours in ICU in England, Wales and Northern Ireland. *Crit Care Med* 2003; **31**: 2332–8.

Peterson K, Carson S, Carney N. Hypothermia for traumatic brain injury: a systematic review and meta-analysis. *J Neurotrauma* 2008; **25**: 62–71.

Rello J, Ollendoef DA, Oster G. Epidemiology and Outcomes of ventilator-associated pneumonia in a large US database. *Chest* 2002; **122**: 2115–21.

Rico FR, Cheng JD, Gestring ML, Piotrowski ES. Mechanical Ventilation Strategies in Massive Chest Trauma. *Crit Care Clin* 2007; **23**: 299–315.

Rivers EP, Coba V, Whitmill M. Early goal directed therapy in severe sepsis and septic shock: a contemporary review of the literature. *Curr Opin Anaesthesiol* 2008; **21**(2): 128–40.

Salim A, Martin M, Conatantinos C. Acute Respiratory Distress Syndrome in the Trauma Intensive Care Unit. *Arch Surg* 2006; **141**: 655–8.

Shafi S, Elliott AC, Gentilello L. Is hypothermia simply a marker of shock and injury severity or an independent risk factor for mortality in trauma patients? *J Trauma* 2005; **59**: 1081–5.

The Acute Respiratory Distress Network. Ventilation with lower tidal volumes as compared with traditional tidal volumes for acute lung injury and the Acute Respiratory Distress Syndrome. *N Engl J Med* 2000; **342**(18): 1301–8.

Tsuei BJ, Kearney PA. Hypothermia in the trauma patient. *Injury* 2004; **35**: 7–15.

World Society of the Abdominal Compartment Syndrome (WSACS) (2007) Intra-abdominal hypertension (IAH)/Abdominal Compartment Syndrome (ACS) management algorithm. Available at: http://www.wsacs.org/algorithms.php (accessed 18 March 2010).

Trauma retrieval

Trauma retrieval

We want a catch phrase that will fire the imagination.
Safety … safety … 'a mantle of safety'.
We shall cast our mantle of safety over the Inland.

[The Very Reverend John Flynn, Founder of the Royal Flying Doctor Service.]

Introduction: trauma systems

Trauma systems were developed following the experiences of American surgeons and the US military, first, in the first and second World Wars, and then in the Korean and Vietnam conflicts. The latter two wars demonstrated that straightforward retrieval of injured soldiers was much more difficult in the challenging terrain of the Far East than it had been in Europe, and the availability of helicopters contributed to management much more focused on rapid retrieval of patients to definitive surgical care, with 20,000 soldiers being evacuated from the combat zones by helicopter in Korea.

Mean times to transport patients from the battlefield to this surgical care fell from 240 min in WWII to 27 min in Vietnam, with associated reductions in mortality from 4.5 to 1.9%. Although helicopter retrieval gained prominence in the later conflicts, much of the increased survival may also be due to the other systematically organized elements, such as appropriate and well-prepared receiving facility, a short time to definitive surgical care and the availability of whole blood transfusion. The medical care system was designed, however, to ensure that no soldier was more than 25 min away from resuscitation and definitive trauma care.

In civilian practice, studies appeared to support the regionalization of trauma care, with West et al. showing that only 1% of deaths from a system in California based around a single trauma centre were judged to be preventable, whereas 73% of deaths were similarly categorized in a Californian system with 40 centres managing trauma. Reduction in time to definitive care, effective airway management, and haemorrhage control have been considered critical to outcomes in serious trauma.

A trauma system has been defined as that which encompasses a continuum of care that provides injured persons with the greatest likelihood of returning to their prior level of function and interaction within society. This continuum of care includes intentional and unintentional injury prevention, Emergency Medical Services (EMS), dispatch, and medical oversight of pre-hospital care, appropriate triage and transport, emergency department (ED) trauma care, trauma centre team activation, surgical intervention, intensive, and general in-hospital care, rehabilitative services, mental and behavioural health, social services, community reintegration plans, and medical care follow-up.

Systems

The organization of community health resources into trauma systems offers an opportunity to substantially improve health care outcomes for the severely injured. An important concept, which is fundamental to this approach to improvement, is that of a system. In one dictionary definition a system is defined as both 'a group of interacting bodies under the influence of related forces' and 'a group of body organs that together perform one or more vital functions'. What ties together these definitions is the idea of multiple individual elements forming a harmonious whole,

in order to serve a common purpose. If the goal of the system is to maximize the efficient delivery of trauma care, and all available evidence suggests that this is achieved by the most rapid delivery to definitive treatment, then the common purpose is to ensure this. Thus, we need to design our trauma systems to achieve a specific goal, which may usefully be thought of the best possible outcome for each individual patient suffering serious trauma.

The systems approach is often talked about, particularly in trauma, but it is often not achieved. This is frequently due to a lack of understanding, not only about the necessity to actively plan a system in the knowledge that the parts have to fit precisely together to form a functionally integrated whole, but also that even systems composed of simple parts often produce unexpected results once the simple parts begin to interact. This is called *emergent complexity*, and is a hallmark of complex systems. The requirement for the construction of trauma systems based on this thinking is not a recently identified need, and in 1973, John J. Hanlon, the Assistant Surgeon General and Coordinator for Public Health Programmes of the US Health Services Administration stated, 'an effective, efficient, and acceptable emergency medical service program must be built upon a comprehensive systems approach, and it must include the following … systematic planning, organization, administration, and operation … coordination of efforts and resources … uniform communications networks and dispatching procedures'.

It is evident that for a trauma system to work efficiently in the best interests of a seriously-injured patient, the planning must recognize that complexity within the system and between the elements of the system is unavoidable, and that there will always be emergent behaviours that arise from the functions and interactions of these component parts. There must be planning and harmonization on many levels for a trauma system to work well, including in areas such as education, training, and resource management. A common flaw in trauma treatment, for example, is the application of therapies that are performed because they *can* be done, rather than because they *should* be done. This is often seen in over-enthusiastic fluid resuscitation, which rather than optimizing the cardiac output and essential organ perfusion, whilst maintaining what vascular homeostasis is present, often is delivered with an aim to achieve a notional normal blood pressure, and may rather produce the consequences of coagulopathy, hypothermia, and acidosis with continued bleeding and organ failure as a result.

Roles and responsibilities

Trauma systems essentially consist of two poles, particularly in regions that encompass rural areas. There are the geographic and demographic catchment areas where injuries occur, with a varying degree of distance from a centre, and a central provision of peak levels of care, often referred to as definitive care. The goal of a mature trauma system is to match the needs of the injured patients to the capabilities of the trauma receiving facility, thus maximizing the chances for the best possible outcome.

Following the Vietnam model would mean that the system is designed to take every trauma patient and deliver them directly to definitive care within approximately half-an-hour; however, this is impossible in all but the most centralized of metropolitan trauma systems. There is, therefore, an unavoidable necessity to either delay the provision of definitive care (but with delivery of essential resuscitation and immediate life-saving management), followed by a transfer to the higher-level centre; or to design a system that has a large number of dispersed centres that are all able to deliver definitive levels of care.

The latter choice has not been shown to be practical, as the skills needed to deliver definitive care for trauma are essentially surgical, with allied specialties, such as anaesthesia, emergency medicine, and intensive care. Many countries do not have systems organized to train surgeons specifically for trauma management, and there is often no trauma surgical subspecialty defined as a specialist area of practice. In many areas, trauma surgery is delivered by general surgeons, with either an interest or experience in trauma, or with targeted training to allow them to provide a resource for a system.

A further essential component of the discussion about the roles of trauma centres within a system is centred on the concept of definitive care. If it is accepted that beyond airway management, resuscitation and diagnosis, trauma is essentially a surgical disease, in that the definitive interventions that may alter the prognosis of the severely-injured patient are those performed in the operating theatre, then the availability of immediate surgical competencies are key to these interventions.

Within the paradigm of damage control surgery, the need for advanced skills in both decision-making and surgical intervention means that the requisite competencies are more likely to be found in the hub hospital with a larger trauma load and dedicated surgical trainees. Discussions among trauma surgeons themselves have also suggested that a more distributed, regionalized, de-centralized model of trauma system may benefit the provision of definitive care, and also the clinicians themselves.

Essential components of trauma systems

It is generally accepted that delivery of the highest levels of trauma care will be in the setting of trauma centres or hospitals designated as the hub of the hub-and-spoke model (Fig. 27.1).

The provision of definitive care at the hub (of the hub-and-spoke model) has certain unavoidable consequences. The capability to recognize the severity of injury coupled with the provision of sophisticated imaging modalities, (but also allowing the ability to bypass these diagnostic refinements and take a patient straight from arrival in the ED to a waiting operating theatre complete with anaesthetic and surgical expertise) is concentrated in the hub hospital. This has benefits in that the volume of trauma cases in need of dedicated multidisciplinary trauma care is high and, therefore, the chances of developing staff expertise is similarly increased. It does, however, dilute the chances of smaller regional or rural hospital clinicians accumulating the opportunities to gain practical hands-on experience in trauma definitive care.

None of this means that these smaller hospitals stop seeing trauma, in fact, this is far from the case. Trauma centres remain only one part of many trauma systems, as patients stubbornly resist the attraction of only getting injured within the magic half-hour radius. Smaller rural hospitals serve a community that may be geographically extended and, therefore, may be the only rational choice for many injured patients. Although many ambulance services serving rural areas, particularly in locations such as Australia, have bypass protocols that allow continuing travel to the highest-level centre within a given time frame and, assuming some pathophysiological stability, this may not be useful in especially remote locations.

Trauma management in hospitals with small trauma caseloads and a lack of training in the management of time-critical injury may contribute to errors that lead to poorer

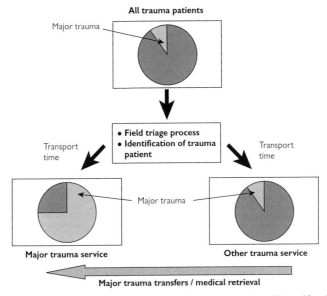

Fig. 27.1. Distribution of major trauma patients between major trauma and other trauma services. (Adapted from Evaluation of the Emergency and Clinical Management of Road Traffic Fatalities in Victoria 1997).

outcomes for patients; although some studies in smaller hospitals have suggested that good outcomes may be achieved in this setting. Some early studies suggested equivalent outcomes in the rural setting to that achieved by level 1 trauma centres, although the authors recognized that with a mean travel time to hospital of 4 h the patients with the highest ISS might have succumbed to their injuries, giving a selected group entering the hospital. Later studies suggested that categorization as rural trauma centres was not as relevant as early decision-making and prompt activation of a system to transfer patients. In the State of Victoria, Australia, a 1999 report entitled the Report of Trauma and Emergency Services (ROTES) was produced by the Ministerial Taskforce on Trauma and Emergency Services. This seminal report identified a number of system-wide deficiencies adversely impacting on outcomes for severely-injured patients. Examples of these are given in Table 27.1.

Table 27.1. Common management/system errors (adapted from Evaluation of the Emergency and Clinical Management of Road Traffic Fatalities in Victoria 1997).

Setting	Management/system errors
Prehospital	No paramedic/delay in arrival of senior paramedics
	Prolonged time at scene
	No 'scoop and run'
	Inadequate documentation/observations
	No/delayed intubation or definitive airway management
	Inadequate ventilatory resuscitation
	No/delayed/inadequate IV access and fluid resuscitation
	Failed intubation/IV access
	No/delayed chest decompression
	These problems largely related to decreased availability of ATLS officers, most commonly in rural areas
Emergency Department	Inappropriate reception by junior staff
	Delayed arrival of appropriate consultant
	No consultant general surgeon
	No/delayed neurosurgical consultation
	Inadequate documentation/observations
	No/delayed chest decompression
	Delayed/inadequate ventilatory resuscitation
	Inadequate fluid/blood resuscitation
	External haemorrhage control problems
	No/delayed CT investigation
	Appropriate investigations delayed/unavailable
	Infrequent ABG/O_2 monitoring
	No CVP/inadequate perfusion monitoring
	Inadequate management of hypothermia
	Inappropriate drugs/dosage
	Delay in despatch to theatre
	Delay in interhospital transfer
Intensive Care Unit, Ward/ High Dependency Unit	Insufficient/delayed fluids
	Insufficient/delayed blood transfusion
	Insufficient/delayed coagulation factors
	No JVP/CVP assessment
	Inadequate/inappropriate respiratory support
	Inadequate respiratory assessment
	Inadequate/inappropriate chest injury assessment
	Inadequate/inappropriate analgesia
	Delayed/inadequate chest drain
	Inadequate/delayed abdominal assessment
	Delayed/no general surgical consultation
	Delayed/no repeat CT brain
	No ICP monitoring
	Inadequate cerebral perfusion pressure
	Delayed/no neurosurgical consultation
	No DVT prophylaxis
	Fractures not fixed
	Delayed transfer to operating theatre
	Delayed transfer to ICU
Transfer	Delayed response of transport
	No medical escort/inappropriate escort
	Inappropriate form of transport
	Inadequate warming

Medical retrieval

Transfer of patients suffering from serious trauma has been shown to be associated with a poor outcome. One answer to this challenge is centred on the concept of medical retrieval. This concept refers to the practice of taking highly-qualified medical staff from either a hospital setting, or from a dedicated medical retrieval service, and transporting them to the patient to enable stabilization and lifesaving interventions with the degree of sophistication present in larger critical care clinical areas. This concept is distinct from two alternative models that have been used and continue to be used in many places. The model used by many ambulance services, that of employing paramedical personnel with a constrained set of skills and competencies, is seen all over the world and tends to work well in many primary trauma situations. It is not necessarily a useful model to utilize in the inter-hospital transport scenario, however, as the necessarily limited skill set of paramedic staff does not lend itself to the need for more complex interventions. A further model, which has traditionally been in operation for many years, is the junior medical model in which the most supernumerary member of medical staff is sent with a critically ill or injured patient transfer as they are the least needed in the hospital setting. This model has led to some significant errors in patient management, with predictable adverse outcomes.

One early study showed that incidents that could cause secondary brain damage were present in 61 of 150 comatose patients transferred after head injury, and that extracranial injuries were overlooked or inadequately treated in 21 of these patients. The commonest incidents were airway obstruction and hypotension. This early paper (Gentleman 1981) recommended a systematic approach to the transfer of head-injured patients that, combined with rapid transport to a neurosurgical unit, would minimize the hazards of transfer, and would reduce mortality and morbidity. These findings were replicated in a further study in 1990, which found that despite more patients having interventions such as endotracheal intubation, and despite more patients being accompanied in their transfer by doctors, 23% had a compromised airway, 15% were hypoxic, 7.5% had a seizure, and 2.5% suffered a respiratory or cardiac arrest.

A 1996 survey by the Royal College of Anaesthetists revealed that 78% of hospitals that received neurotrauma had to transfer these patients due to lack of on-site neurosurgery cover. 87% expected their senior house officer (who could be just over 1 year after medical qualification) to escort the critically-injured patients. In this group, although over 93% of hospitals were able to supply equipment to monitor ECG, blood pressure, and pulse oximetry, less than half were able to facilitate the monitoring of end-tidal carbon dioxide. Due to findings like these, in 1996 the Association of Anaesthetists of Great Britain and Ireland (AAGBI) in conjunction with the Neuroanaesthesia Society produced a set of guidelines for the inter-hospital transport of head-injured patients. Sample recommendations from these guidelines are given in Table 27.2.

In 1997, the Intensive Care Society released their own guidelines. In these, two attendants were specified, of which one was defined as a medical practitioner with appropriate training in intensive care medicine, anaesthesia or other acute specialty, competent in resuscitation,

Table 27.2. Recommendations for transfer standards

Category	Recommendation
Patients	Thorough resuscitation and optimization prior to transfer. Patients with altered consciousness should be transported intubated, sedated, and ventilated.
Administration	Designated consultants responsible for the conduct of transfers should be identifiable at the referring and receiving hospitals.
Personnel	Medical escort has ideally 2 years training in anaesthesia. A trained assistant is needed to help with the transfer.
Equipment	Monitoring during transfer should be of the same standard as that available on an intensive care unit. Paediatric transfers need separate equipment.
Insurance	Adequate medical indemnity and personal insurance for staff undertaking transfers.
Others	Maintain adequate records. Referring and receiving hospitals should liaise with one another. Recognition of a need for time spent in ensuring training and education.

airway care, ventilation and other organ support. Further detailed standards and guidance were detailed in areas such as whether to retrieve or send a patient, selection of transport mode, preparation for transport, and monitoring and management during transport. These guidelines are as applicable to the transfer of the critically ill and injured today as when they were written. In Australia collaborative guidelines have been authored and promulgated by the Australasian College for Emergency Medicine, the Joint Faculty of Intensive Care Medicine, and the Australian and New Zealand College of Anaesthetists.

Benefits of organized medical retrieval
Patient
Clinical management during transport must aim to be at least equal to the management at the point of referral, and must prepare the patient for admission to the receiving service.

Transport for a patient is a high-risk episode; their illness is either sufficiently severe or worsening to demand transport, but they have often been removed from adequate care and appropriate monitoring, and potentially managed by the most junior staff with the least training. The benefit for the patient of an organized retrieval system is to maintain the level of care at a constant level, or even to increase it by performing interventions that increase the ability to manage the critically ill or injured patient effectively. Fig. 27.2a illustrates the level of care in a poorly organized and managed transfer, often with insufficient equipment and inappropriate levels of training for escorting staff. Adequate planning, organization, equipment, training and competence should attempt to elevate the level of care through Fig. 27.2b to that illustrated in Fig. 27.2c, where there is no diminution of care at all.

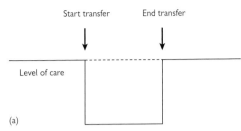

Fig. 27.2. (a) Decrease in level of care with patient transfer.

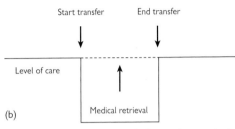

Fig. 27.2. (b) Impact of specialist medical retrieval team on level of care.

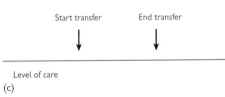

Fig. 27.2. (c) Patient transfer with consistent high level of care with specialist medical retrieval.

Furthermore, essential interventions, such as airway management through rapid sequence induction and endotracheal intubation, chest drain insertion, blood transfusion, and advanced monitoring techniques mean that a retrieval team composed of a critical care trained doctor and another attendant, often a specially trained paramedic, may be able to commence the management of shock and the effects of hypoperfusion, with rewarming, long before they arrive at the definitive care hospital.

System
The ideal trauma system may be based around the Vietnam model, where all patients are taken to a centre offering immediate, definitive care; however, although this is potentially closer to reality in some States in the USA or in some European countries, it is far from possible in most geographical areas. Countries such as Australia, although offering sophisticated and competent trauma systems based around the cities, is still ruled by the 'tyranny of distance'. Patients will always have to attend smaller centres with less trauma experience, by virtue of the fact that many people live in rural or remote locations. The irony is that the more urgent the need for transfer of an injured patient, the less stable they often are, and the greater the need for expert assistance. Medical retrieval acts as the integrator of the trauma system.

The benefits to the system are divided into those seen at a whole system level, and those seen in the local area from which the patient is drawn. The overall system benefits from an organized scheme of medical and trauma retrieval, especially when capabilities are in place to recognize the occurrence of serious trauma very early in the patient journey. This last issue has been addressed in calls to primary trauma with the London HEMS practice of allowing a HEMS paramedic to monitor calls to the emergency 999 number, to interrogate callers, and to task the doctor-paramedic team to respond as a primary resource.

Benefits of an organized retrieval system to the area from which the patient comes are often forgotten or underestimated. Notwithstanding the level of care that the patient may receive from clinicians without specialized trauma knowledge and training, allowing local ambulances with ad hoc medical cover from small hospitals to undertake transfers of critically-injured patients means that the limited, or potentially the only, resources available to a small community are removed for a period of several hours or more. Patients with other time-critical conditions may suffer from a lack of timely care as local medical, nursing and paramedical staff are not available.

The retrieval team
Personnel involved in transport of critically ill and injured patients must ideally be specifically selected and trained in the transport role; they must have training allowing competent management of the patient in the same manner as in hospital, but also must have training in the techniques and requirements for operating in an out-of-hospital environment. In keeping with the standards promulgated by the Intensive Care Society, the Australian College for Emergency Medicine, and others, most retrieval team members are drawn from emergency medicine, anaesthesia and intensive care backgrounds, where specialties have an expectation of expertise in the management of the acutely ill and of procedural capability. These doctors are subsequently trained in the out-of-hospital environment, which has distinctly different imperatives and pitfalls to hospital work. Many training schemes in these specialties allow accreditation for time spent working in retrieval as a senior trainee. Retrieval doctors are often accompanied by paramedics with extended training in critical care, including the operation of non-invasive and invasive monitoring devices, transport ventilators, and invasive vascular pressure monitoring. Critical care nurses are frequently involved in inter-hospital transfer of critically ill and injured patients, although this professional group need specific training in operating in potentially austere environments.

Equipment

Equipment for retrieval may be divided into two types, life support and monitoring, and clinical intervention equipment.

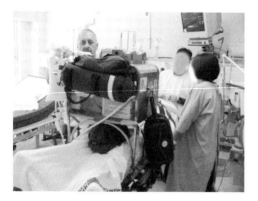

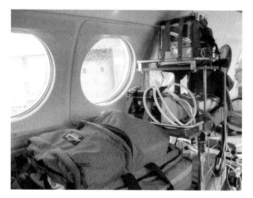

Figs. 27.3 and 27.4. Stretcher bridge with ventilator and monitoring equipment.

Life support and monitoring

Complex life support equipment, such as transport ventilator and syringe pumps, and monitoring equipment including ECG, pulse oximetry, end-tidal carbon dioxide, and both non-invasive and invasive intravascular pressure monitoring, are ideally organized and made stable on a 'bridge'. This arrangement has had many incarnations, but was described in 1990 as the CareFlight Stretcher Bridge, a compact, mobile intensive care unit. This is a multi-story tray, which locks on to the patient stretcher, and onto which essential equipment may be secured. These bridges also facilitate the provision of a single power supply to all equipment via the fabric of the bridge, and allow the mounting of an oxygen cylinder and a suction device.

Clinical intervention equipment

Clinical interventional equipment consists of similar equipment to that found in an emergency department or intensive care unit, but is often stored and transported in a dedicated, compartmentalized bag, which may be carried as a rucksack. This bag is often organized with sub-packs

within it, such as cannulation kits, intubation rolls and drug packs, to separate and make conveniently available equipment used for specific interventions (Fig. 27.5). Thus, there may be a collection of equipment for the purposes of airway management, including laryngoscopes, a collection of varying-sized endotracheal tubes, Magill forceps, stylettes and gum elastic bougies, lubricant gel and tube ties. A full list of the contents of a typical retrieval pack is given in Box 27.1. A full range of interventional drugs is also carried, listed in Box 27.2.

Other important aspects of the retrieval system are the transport platform and the organization of a bed at a trauma centre. Transport platforms for retrieval of critically ill and injured patients may take place using fixed wing (Fig. 27.6) or rotary wing aircraft, or potentially using road ambulance. Generally speaking, the factors that determine the mode of transport are geography, weather and urgency.

In countries with remote areas, fixed wing retrieval is common with services such as the Royal Flying Doctor Service. Helicopters have a shorter activation time, but a reduced radius of operation (Fig. 27.7). Fixed wing aircraft provide a relatively stable environment in which to manage a patient, although there are disadvantages of fixed wing transport, such as the need for a suitable landing strip, and the subsequent requirement for ambulance transport at either end of the flight. Much of the vulnerability for transferred patients is present at the times of transfer between one stable environment to another, although this definition may be relative, and therefore the number of extra transfers greatly increases the risk for the patient.

Helicopters alleviate many of the problems in terms of taking off and landing that make fixed wing retrieval problematic, but are often cramped, noisy environments, with little temperature control and challenging working

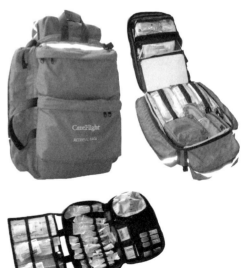

Fig. 27.5. (a,b,c) Retrieval and cannulation packs.

Box 27.1. Contents of medical retrieval pack

- Pre-cut white tapes, 0 silk ties (securing paediatric tube).
- Small plastic bags × 2.
- Lubricant sachets × 2.
- Magill forceps: adult × 1 and paediatric × 1.
- 20 mL cuff syringe.
- Laryngoscope handles × 2.
- Sterile laryngoscope blades: Macintosh size 2, 3, and 4.
- Sterile Miller blade size 1.
- Sterile bougies × 3 (adult 5 mm and paediatric 3.8 and 2 mm).
- Sterile ETT stylets adult and paediatric.
- Disposable scalpel with blade cover.
- Tracheal dilators one pair sterile.
- Roberts forceps one pair sterile.
- Sterile ET tubes: adult and paediatric.
- Laryngeal mask airways: sizes 4, 3, 2.5, and 2.
- Peep valve.
- Masks sizes 4, 3, 2, 0/1.
- Child resuscitator with reservoir bag.
- Airway manometer with tubing and 3-way tap.
- Nasopharyngeal airway 7 mm ID × 2.
- Guedel airway: sizes 100, 90, 70, 60 mm.
- Oxygen cylinder with integral regulator.
- Adult Laerdal bag complete with HME/gooseneck CO_2 sensor adaptor, and adult mask.
- Adult O_2 mask with reservoir (NRB).
- Paediatric mask.
- O_2 tubing.
- Y-suction catheters 14fg, 10fg, 6fg × 2 each.
- Lightweight volume cycled ventilator with circuit.
- Battery powered suction unit.
- Sharps bin and garbage bag.
- Cannulae: 14, 16, 18, 20, 22g × 2 each.
- Short IV extension (3-way tap).
- Needle free valves × 2.
- Dressing pack.
- Alcowipes.
- Bandaids.
- Steristrips.
- Opsite dressings.
- Gauze squares.
- Disposable razor.
- Marking pen.
- Tapes: 1 roll each Elastoplast, brown and silk.
- MicroShield hand gel.
- Adult multi-select C collar.
- Pedi-select C collar.
- Stethoscope.
- Aneroid BP and cuff (standard, large adult & paediatric).
- Steristrips x 2, Bandaids x 2, Alcowipes x 5.
- Cannulae 24g, 22g, 20g, 18g x 2, 16g, 14g.
- Opsite x 2, gauze swabs x 2.

- Tourniquet.
- Emergency pneumothorax set × 1.
- Needles: blunt × 3, 23g × 3.
- Needle free valves × 2.
- Combi-Stopper × 2.
- Syringes: 10 mL, 5 mL, 2 mL 1 each.
- 10 mm silk tape.
- Broselow paediatric tape.
- Shears on coil cord.
- Epistaxis catheters.
- 50-mL syringes Luer lock2 (IO infusions).
- Rapid infusion exchange catheters 7fr, 8.5fr.
- Needleholder.
- Toothed forceps.
- Scissors.
- Tube clamp forceps.
- Artery forceps straight × 2.
- Artery forceps curved × 2.
- Amputation kit.
- Gigli handle × 2.
- Blade × 2.
- Multifunction patient monitor with a minimum of oximetry with waveform, capnography with waveform, ECG, and non-invasive blood pressure.
- Defibrillator.
- Handheld ultrasound.
- Pelvic splint.
- Military tourniquet.
- Interosseous access device.
- Limb splints.
- Rigid arm splint.
- Wound dressing pack.
- Crepe bandages: 10 cm × 2.
- Large combine × 2.
- Multitrauma dressings × 1.
- Chest drain kit.
- Chest drains 28fg × 2, 20fg, 12fg.
- Portex emergency drainage bag.
- Portex emergency chest drainage bag (separate).
- Emergency pneumothorax sets.
- Procedural disposable kit.
- Dressing pack × 1.
- Disposable scalpel × 1.
- Chlorhexidine 5 mL × 2.
- Betadine swabs × 9.
- Sterile gloves size 7 and 8.
- Sutures: Vicryl ties, 0 nylon, 4/0 nylon, 1 Mersilene, 0 black silk.
- Nasogastric kit.
- Nasogastric tubes 16fr, 12fr, spigot.
- Lube sachet.
- Hartmann's 1 L, loaded onto pump set.
- 7.5% saline 250 mL loaded onto pump set.

Box 27.2. Contents of drug pack

- Adrenaline: 1:1000.
- Adrenaline: 1:10,000.
- Atropine.
- Bupivicaine plain.
- Calcium chloride.
- (Etomidate recommended in jurisdictions where it is licensed for use).
- Fentanyl 500 µg/intranasal preparation 900 µg.
- Glucose 50%.
- Ketamine.
- Lignocaine 1%.
- Metaraminol.
- Metoclopramide.
- Midazolam.
- Naloxone.
- NaHCO$_3$ 8.4%.
- Normal saline ampoules.
- Ondansetron.
- Rocuronium.
- Suxamethonium.
- Thiopentone.
- Water for injection.
- Syringe:10 mL × 4, 2 mL × 3.
- Blunt needles × 5.
- 20-mL syringes × 3.
- MicroPins × 2.
- Blunt drawing up needles × 2.
- Drug and additive labels.

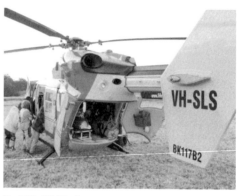

Fig. 27.7. BK117 helicopter on a trauma retrieval mission.

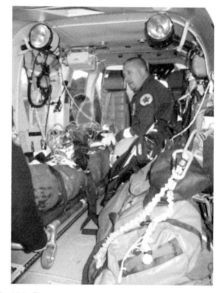

Fig. 27.8. The cramped interior of a medical retrieval helicopter.

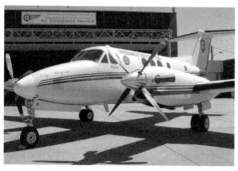

Fig. 27.6. Fixed wing air ambulance.

conditions (Fig. 27.8). Part of efficient and good quality medical retrieval relies on planning to identify the potential of these adverse conditions to affect the patient, and to prepare adequately to prevent these effects. Whilst managing a relatively stable patient in the rear of a small helicopter may be merely demanding, a cardiac arrest in the same situation may be catastrophic.

Road retrieval is often undertaken with a standard road ambulance, and in large cities this may occur much more often than helicopter or fixed wing retrievals. The disadvantage of road ambulance retrieval is the short distance over which it may operate in a given time frame.

The retrieval process

Inter-hospital patient transport generally occurs in two circumstances:
- *Emergency inter-hospital transport:* acute life-threatening illnesses and lack of diagnostic facilities or staff for safe and effective therapy.
- *Semi-urgent inter-hospital transport:* moving a critically ill or injured patient to a higher level of care or for a speciality service.

Retrieval of trauma patients may often occur when a seriously injured patient has been taken to a small hospital with little capacity to manage severe trauma.

Training in medical retrieval involves consideration of the approach to transporting patients who may be physiologically unstable and whose injuries may mandate particular care and stabilization, such as head or spinal injuries. Many experienced retrieval trainers will suggest that the novice imagines their worst nightmare that could occur with each patient, and then takes all reasonable precautions to minimize the likelihood of its occurring.

Recognition of the need for retrieval

The critical message is that retrieval should be initiated sooner, rather than later. For those working in a remote, rural, or even outer metropolitan hospital, that does not have the facility to manage serious trauma, the time to think about transferring a patient is when they arrive, not when their deterioration heralds disaster.

Many ambulance systems use a trauma triage tool based around the acronym MIST. In this instance, it stands for
- **M**echanism of injury.
- **I**njuries seen and suspected.
- **S**igns and symptoms.
- **T**reatment required/transport decisions.

These decision tools are used to sort trauma cases into their potential or actual severity, and their possible need for urgent intervention. Being aware of the scheme used by the ambulance service in your local area, or of a scheme such as the one shown below, will allow you to assess the need for help early. Awareness of the predictive value of mechanism of injury, the injuries that are seen and the abnormalities in physiological signs that may be present is very useful to help in making this decision. It is important to be aware that many patients, particularly children, compensate efficiently for injury and blood loss, and the severity of injury is often only recognized when their ability to compensate is eventually overwhelmed.

The principles of safe retrieval are expressed in the following list:
- *Right patient.*
- *Right time.*
- *Right people.*
- *Right place.*
- *Right transport.*
- *Right care.*
- Transport of patients is HIGH RISK.
- Planned transfer or retrieval DECREASES RISK.
- Possibly the most important parts of patient transfer and retrieval are to THINK EARLY and CALL EARLY.

Whatever the transport platform, the retrieval process for critically ill and injured patients builds in unavoidable delay (Fig. 27.9). As the pathophysiology of trauma starts at the time of injury, it is vital to the patient to minimize these phases as much as possible, whilst still maintaining the safety of patient and staff. The best periods to try to safely minimize in this timeline are before calling, i.e. call early on suspicion of need, rather than wait for obvious deterioration; and reducing patient preparation and packaging time. Although retrieval specialists will have their own practiced techniques, methods, and equipment, paying attention to adequate analgesia and splinting, making clear notes, collecting X-rays, and getting the results of blood tests will make the job of the team much easier and faster (Fig. 27.10).

Preparation for retrieval

The patient can be safeguarded from potential harm by planning ahead, communicating early, and performing meticulous preparation. Almost all potential mishaps or deteriorations may be prevented by painstaking preparation before transfer:
- Communication.
- Planning and organization.
- Patient evaluation and preparation.
- Monitoring.
- Transportation.
- Communication.

The first communication with the retrieval team may be to a medical retrieval co-ordinator, an ambulance controller, or a speciality trainee or consultant. All communications should be planned in advance, and it is important to find out who is the most appropriate person to talk to, not to

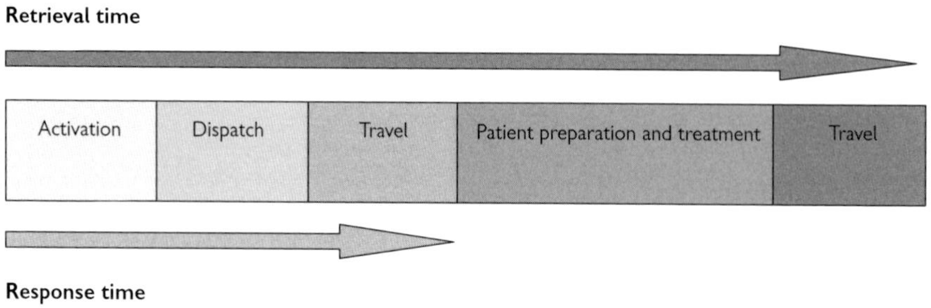

Retrieval time

Response time

Fig. 27.9. Retrieval timeline. Adapted from ROTES.

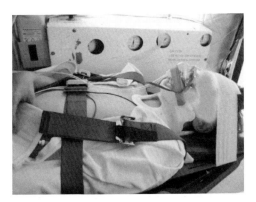

Fig. 27.10. Patient prepared for transport.

simply ring the first person you think of. Even as the person performing the retrieval the same principles of communication apply. The ubiquity of mobile phones means that there is usually a constant ability to maintain contact and to ensure all concerned are prepared, updated and aware of any changes in a patient's condition.

Intensive care transfers often have some central co-ordination, but the patient still needs a 'home team' to accept care, often a specialist team, such as neurosurgery or cardiothoracic surgery.

Notes must be made about the key issues in the patient's presentation and course, clearly and logically describing the need and reason for transfer. All appropriate test results must be to hand, but investigations must not delay transfer for inessential testing.

People who need to be consistently informed about a transfer are:
- Consultant responsible for current care.
- Consultant responsible for future care.
- Intensive Care Unit consultant.
- Relatives.
- Ambulance control or medical retrieval unit.

Key elements of this communication are:
- Who is calling.
- What the relevant patient details are.
- What the problem is.
- What has been done to address the problem.
- What is needed from the listener.
- What the level of urgency is.

Planning and organization

It is essential to think about the potential needs of the patient during transfer. Do they need an ambulance crew, a nurse escort, a medical escort, or a medical retrieval team? If there is no retrieval team available locally, will it be possible to organize transport? In which case, the appropriate person, rather than the most easily available person should be dispatched.

An estimate should be made of how long the transport will take, and discussed with nursing staff—it may be possible to wait for a shift change or to get staff from other areas. Ambulance availability and timing must be determined. Ambulance control will want to know perceived urgency—lights and sirens, immediate transport or delayed

transport. If a trauma patient is being transferred, it is likely that the patient will need more urgent, rather than less urgent transport.

Similar planning and organization is essential for the receiving clinician. This involves estimating the time required to complete the transport, envisioning potential hazards and pitfalls, and ensuring that all eventualities have been considered and prepared for, including timings, assistance needed, transport availability, power, medications, monitoring, temperature, noise, notes, and relatives.

Patient evaluation and preparation

This is a dynamic process, beginning with the initial patient contact, and involving elements of the primary and secondary survey. Requirements are an assessment of current physiological status, and awareness of previous trends and treatments, responses to therapy, current and planned interventions, and physical environment. It is important to minimize risk in all areas.

Retrieval of the critically ill or injured patient means that not only must there be an awareness of actual failure or compromise of anatomical and physiological systems, but also need to assess for:
- Potential airway compromise.
- Potential respiratory failure.
- Potential circulatory failure.
- Potential neurological failure.

It is vitally important to identify when any patient approaches the end of their ability to compensate for illness or injury, and it is important to realize that just because a clinical variable is normal does *not* mean that it still will be in 5 min time. It is much better for both patient and doctor to intervene early, for instance, by performing a rapid sequence induction and endotracheal intubation in the warmth and light of a resuscitation room, rather than trying to perform the same procedure in the back of an ambulance in the dark. Patient preparation, like so much else in patient care, is usefully implemented using ABCDE:

Airway
- Consider the need for intubation or replacement/repositioning of tube.
- If the patient is intubated, check security of ETT (always re-tie tube). Consider Leucoplast® 'trousers'.
- Add secondary fixation to ETT and ventilator tubing to prevent traction.
- Insert orogastric or nasogastric tube if intubated.

Breathing
- Assess ventilation using repeated primary survey components of effort, efficacy, and effectiveness, respiratory rate, oxygen saturation by pulse oximetry, venous (or arterial) blood gases, and chest X-ray.
- Assess whether the patient needs a chest drain before transport (e.g. for pneumothorax and positive pressure ventilation).
- If a drain is present, ensure it is well sutured, and apply secondary fixation.
- Change underwater seal drains for closed urinary drainage bags.
- If bleeding into drain, measure and record. More than 200 mL/h suggests the need for an urgent transfer for thoracotomy if not available at the sending hospital—consult surgeons urgently.

Circulation
- Assess need for further peripheral or central IV access, fluid boluses, inotropes, or vasopressors.
- Insert urinary catheter if needed. If a urinary catheter is already *in situ*, empty the bag, and note the volume. Apply secondary fixation to catheter tubing.
- Ensure at least two IV routes are available, are well secured, and have easy access, especially if transporting in cramped situations with poor patient access, such as in a helicopter.
- Ensure running maintenance fluid lines on both IV access points, with ports for medications. All running fluids should be administered via blood sets to enable volume resuscitation and prompt medication use.
- Intravenous lines, monitor leads, catheters, nasogastric tubes will all get tangled, will always catch on the end of the bed oxygen/suction/other obstacle, and may pull out the ETT, CVP or other very valuable tube!
- Cap off all unnecessary lines.
- Secondary fixation is very important for all tubes, and strong adhesive tape is needed (paper tape/IV dressings are not enough; see Fig. 27.11).

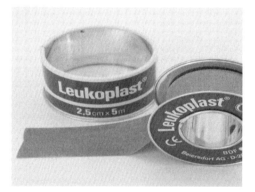

Fig. 27.11. Strong adhesive tape used for secondary fixation of all lines and tubes.

Disability (neurology)
- Check (and record) patient Glasgow Coma Scale. AVPU is too insensitive for trend monitoring in these circumstances.
- Check pupil reactivity and assess fundi if possible, especially in neurosurgical transfers.
- Perform focused neurological examination, concentrating on identifying deficits.

Drugs
- Estimate how much further medications and fluids will be necessary. Always be conservative and take too much, rather than too little.
- Get all essential infusions made up in syringes that can fit onto a syringe driver. Infusion pumps are heavy, awkward, and a recipe for disaster in transport, especially for those not adequately trained to use them.
- Sufficient sedation and paralysis for infusions, and for boluses if needed must be available. Although paralysis has associated problems, it is preferable to a patient pulling out an ETT in transit.

- If a patient is paralysed, it is vital to be very aware of the potential for apnoea/disconnection from the ventilator.
- Ensure spinal and limb immobilization is maintained when appropriate.

Everything else
- Develop a checklist for all equipment before connecting patient - e.g. ventilator checklist will include:
  - adequate oxygen;
  - secure connection to oxygen (cylinder key);
  - securely fitted tubing without leaks (cycle ventilator with patient end blocked; check airway pressure meter);
  - alarms functioning and audible/visible;
  - check battery life on ventilator/monitor/pumps
- 'Mummy wrap': use an insulating blanket or a sheet to wrap the patient from head to toe; held together with towel clips or artery forceps (Fig. 27.12).
- Remaining leads and tubes may be threaded through one end of the wrap nearest the monitors. Leads and tubes may also be fed through a split piece of ventilator tubing or 'umbilicus' to ensure safety.
- *Remember*—one line is always left out for immediate access.

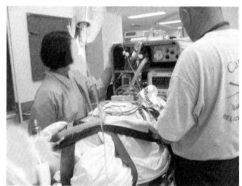

Fig. 27.12. Patient 'mummy wrapped' as part of preparation for transport.

Monitoring
- *End tidal CO_2*: essential in assessing ventilation and disconnection. Waveform shape may indicate spontaneous breathing.
- *Pulse oximetry*: attempt to place on well-perfused digit, use adhesive probes if possible. Do not tape on fingers as this may lead to pressure necrosis. If there is a well shaped waveform, the SpO_2 is likely to be reasonably accurate.
- *ECG.*
- Invasive and non-invasive blood pressure.

Transportation
- *Three phases:*
  - patient to vehicle;
  - vehicle, team, and patient to receiving unit;
  - patient from vehicle.
- Need to be thought about separately.
- Have a checklist and go through it prior to leaving.
- Most risk for patient when in transport.

Summary

Although minimizing the time to definitive care is essential, allowing experienced assessment, appropriate resuscitation and timely surgical intervention, this is frequently not possible in the context of the many geographically diverse health systems. By necessity, injured patients are often taken to local services where there may be an inconsistent level of training and experience in the management of the seriously-injured patient and, therefore, inter-hospital retrieval of these patients is necessary.

Inter-hospital retrieval of the seriously-injured patient requires timely recognition, not only of actual injuries and the pathophysiological responses to these, but of the potential for occult injury. To enable this, trauma systems need to put in place educational and operational infrastructures that give clear criteria for transfer, and make the processes of calling for assistance and of bed-finding straightforward and routine. A systematic method of patient assessment, the use of decision and triage aids such as MIST, and effective, structured handovers encompassing early and comprehensive communication, are needed to ensure system efficiency and effectiveness. There are few instances of this holistic system approach in evidence.

Adequate patient preparation and successful retrieval are based on an appropriate sense of urgency combined with the recognition that the period of inter-hospital transport is when dangers are at their highest. Success also rests on the principles of comprehensive planning, and of performing necessary pre-emptive interventions to ensure the opportunity for disaster never occurs.

Acknowledgements

Grateful acknowledgement to the Media Unit, Ambulance Service of NSW for the use of the photograph of the Air Ambulance King Air; and to Alan Garner and CareFlight for the use of the photographs of the retrieval pack and contents, and of the CareFlight equipment lists.

Further reading

Australasian College for Emergency Medicine, Joint Faculty of Intensive Care Medicine, Australian and New Zealand College of Anaesthetists. Minimum standards for transport of critically ill patients. *Emerg Med (Fremantle, W.A.)* 2003; **15**(2): 197–201.

Bartolacci RA, Munford BJ, Lee A, McDougall PA. Air medical scene response to blunt trauma: effect on early survival. *Med J Aust* 1998; **169**(11–12): 612–16.

Celso B, Tepas J, Langland-Orban B, Pracht E, Papa L, Lottenberg L, et al. A systematic review and meta-analysis comparing outcome of severely injured patients treated in trauma centers following the establishment of trauma systems. *J Trauma-Injury Infect Crit Care* 2006; **60**(2): 371–78.

Clark DE, Anderson KL, Hahn DR. Evaluating an inclusive trauma system using linked population-based data. *J Trauma-Injury Infect Crit Care* 2004; **57**(3): 501–9.

Deane SA, Gaudry PL, Woods WPD, Read CM, McNeil RJ. Interhospital transfer in the management of acute trauma. *Aust NZ J Surg* 1990; **60**: 441–6.

Demetriades D, Martin M, Salim A, Rhee P, Brown C, Chan L. The effect of trauma center designation and trauma volume on outcome in specific severe injuries. *Annl Surg* 2005; **242**(4): 512–17; discussion 517–19.

Fan E, MacDonald RD, Adhikari NK, Scales DC, Wax RS, Stewart TE, et al. Outcomes of interfacility critical care adult patient transport: a systematic report. *Crit Care* 2006; **10**(1): R6.

Garner A, Rashford S, Lee A, Bartolacci R. Addition of physicians to paramedic helicopter services decreases blunt trauma mortality. *Aust NZ J Surg* 1999; **69**(10): 697–701.

Gebremichael M, Borg U, Habashi NM, Cottingham C, Cunsolo L, McCunn M, et al. Interhospital transport of the extremely ill patient: The mobile intensive care unit. *Crit Care Med* 2000; **28**: 79–85.

Gentleman D, Dearden M, Midgley S, Maclean D. Guidelines for resuscitation and transfer of patients with serious head injury. *Br Med J* 1993; **307**: 547–52.

Gentleman D, Jennett B. Hazards of inter-hospital transfer of comatose head-injured patients. *Lancet* 1981; **2**(8251): 853–4.

Gray A, Bush S, Whiteley S. Secondary transport of the critically ill and injured adult. *Emerg Med J* 2004; **21**(3): 281–5.

Gray A, Gill S, Airey M, Williams R. Descriptive epidemiology of adult critical care transfers from the emergency department. *Emerg Med J* 2003; **20**(3): 242–6.

Intensive Care Society. Guidelines for the transport of the critically ill adult. 2002. Available at: http://www.ics.ac.uk/intensive_care_ professional/standards_and_guidelines/transport_of_the_ critically_ill_2002 (accessed 18 March 2010).

Jacobs LM, Bennett B. A critical care helicopter system in trauma. *J Nat Med Ass* 1989; **81**(11): 1157–67.

Kerr WA, Kerns TJ, Bissell RA. Differences in mortality rates among trauma patients transported by helicopter and ambulance in Maryland. *Prehosp Disaster Med* 1999; **14**(3): 159–64.

Knowles PR, Bryden DC, Kishen R, Gwinnutt CL. Meeting the standards for interhospital transfer of adults with severe head injury in the United Kingdom. *Anaesthesia* 1999; **54**(3): 283–8.

Kronick JB, Kissoon N, Frewen TC. Guidelines for stabilizing the condition of the critically ill child before transfer to a tertiary care facility. *Canad Med Ass J* 1988; **139**(3): 213–20.

Lee A, Lum ME, Beehan SJ, Hillman KM. Interhospital transfers: Decision-making in critical care areas. *Crit Care Med* 1996; **24**(4): 618–22.

Leppäniemi A. Trauma systems in Europe. *Curr Opin Crit Care* 2005; **11**(6): 576–9.

Markovchick VJ, Moore EE. Optimal trauma outcome: trauma system design and the trauma team. *Emerg Med Clin N Am* 2007; **25**(3): 643–54.

McDermott FT, Cordner SM, Tremayne AB. *Evaluation of the Emergency and Clinical Management of Road Traffic Fatalities in Victoria (1997).* Report of the Consultative Committee on Road Traffic Fatalities in Victoria. Melbourne: Transport Accident Commission, 1998.

Mock C, Joshipura M, Goosen J, Lormand JD, Maier R. Strengthening trauma systems globally: the Essential Trauma Care Project. *J Trauma-Injury Infect Crit Care* 2005; **59**(5): 1243–6.

Mullins RJ, Hedges JR, Rowland DJ, Arthur M, Mann NC, Price DD, et al. Survival of seriously injured patients first treated in rural hospitals. *J Trauma-Injury Infect Crit Care* 2002; **52**(6): 1019–29.

Nathens AB, Brunet FP, Maier RV. Development of trauma systems and effect on outcomes after injury. *Lancet* 2004; **363**(9423): 1794–801.

Advanced Life Support Group. *Advanced Life Support Group. Safe Transfer and Retrieval of Patients (STAR): The Practical Approach,* 2nd edn. London: BMJ Books, 2006.

Tall G, Manning R. *Adult Retrieval Clinical Guidelines.* Sydney: Medical Retrieval Unit, 2002.

Wallace PG, Ridley SA. ABC of intensive care. Transport of critically ill patients. *Br Med J* 1999; **319**(7206): 368–71.

Waydhas C. Intrahospital transport of critically ill patients. *Crit Care* 1999; **3**(5): R83–9.

West JG. Trunkey DD. Lim RC. Systems of trauma care. A study of two counties. *Arch Surg* 1979; **114**(4): 455–60.

Whitelaw AS, Hsu R, Corfield AR, Hearns S. Establishing a rural Emergency Medical Retrieval Service. *Emerg Med J* 2006; **23**: 76–8.

Wishaw KJ, Munford BJ, Roby HP. The CareFlight Stretcher Bridge: a compact mobile intensive care unit. *Anaesthesia & Intens Care* 1990; **18**(2): 234–8.

Zulick LC, Dietz PA, Brooks K. Trauma experience of a rural hospital. *Arch Surg* 1991; **126**(11): 1427–30.Fig. 27.3

Psychological aspects of trauma

Psychological aspects of trauma

Trauma comes in many guises, is occasioned by different causes, and has different psychological effects, in the long and short term. Traumatic events include individual trauma (e.g. road traffic, domestic, and criminal incidents) and major catastrophes, some of which are due to natural causes (e.g. earthquakes and tsunamis) and some due to human error or malevolence (the latter including terrorist activity). The impact of these events may extend from individuals to their families and even to their communities and whole culture. Even a single traumatic incident, such as a fatal road traffic incident, can trigger a 'ripple effect', whereby a number of individuals, with different kinds and degrees of exposure to the event, might be adversely affected. Such individuals could include the surviving driver and passenger (as 'primary victims'), passers-by who witnessed the death of a child passenger, the bereaved, and, finally, professional responders. A key message is, therefore, to be aware of possible 'hidden victims'.

Unless otherwise stated, 'trauma' will be used in a generic sense to embrace a wide constellation of incidents and circumstances. The key feature of the psychological aspects of trauma is that it overwhelms or threatens to overwhelm an individual's or community's ability to cope. The key precipitants include:
- (Perceived) threat to life and limb (of self and/or others).
- Exposure to dead, dying, and injured.
- Loss (often extensive, including bereavement).
- Extensive disruption of daily functioning (in the social, family, educational, and employment domains).
- An increased sense of personal vulnerability and insecurity.

Epidemiology

Prevalence rates across studies vary because of different intervals between trauma and assessment, different methods of assessment (self-report produces higher rates than clinical examination), and the type of trauma. It is sometimes difficult, therefore, to make meaningful comparisons between published prevalence figures. The following are rough guidelines.

Prevalence: traumatic events
- About 60% of men and 50% of women will experience at least one trauma in life.
- About 20% of men and 11% of women will experience at least three traumatic events.
- Men are more likely to experience violent assault (apart from rape), life-threatening events, and disasters; women are more likely to have experienced rape and childhood sexual abuse.

Prevalence: post-traumatic stress disorder
It must be noted that post-traumatic stress disorder PTSD in about 80% of cases occurs in the context of co-morbidity especially depression, anxiety, and substance misuse. Examples of incidences of PTSD following specific traumatic events include:
- Female rape... 50%.
- Road traffic incidents... 15%.
- Non-sexual male assault... 12.4%; female assault... 30.8%.
- Burn victims... 45%.
- Childhood sexual abuse about... 50%.
- Major disasters... 25%.
- Severely-injured survivors of terrorist attacks... 30%.
- Children after a ferry sinking... 15%.

Reactions to trauma
Normal

It is difficult to generalize across so many different possible types of trauma, but about 75% of survivors do not develop psychiatric symptoms, but display normal reactions. Resilience, rather than psychopathology is therefore the norm.

Post-traumatic symptoms can be divided into physiological, cognitive, social, and emotional.

Physical
- Insomnia (punctuated by nightmares).
- Headaches (often non-specific).
- Loss of appetite (sometimes 'comfort eating').
- Weight loss (sometimes weight gain).
- Reduced energy.
- General physical malaise.
- Hyperarousal (e.g. exaggerated startle response).

Cognitive
- Impaired memory (retrograde and anterograde).
- Impaired concentration.
- Confusion and disorientation (without clouding of consciousness).
- Hypervigilance (an exaggerated sense of being at risk).
- Intrusive images ('flashbacks'), memories, and thoughts of the trauma. Flashbacks may entail any or all sensory modalities.

Social
- Withdrawal (even from potential sources of support).
- Irritability.
- Avoidance of reminders of the trauma (including persons, places, and even talking about it).

Emotional
- Shock, numbness.
- Denial (partial or complete inability to accept the reality of the event).
- Helplessness and hopelessness.
- Guilt (at having survived when others died—'survivor guilt'—or guilt at not having done enough to help others in the incident—'performance guilt').
- Anger (commonly ill-directed in many directions—even at rescuers and caregivers).
- Anhedonia (loss of pleasure from previously pleasurable interests).
- Loss of personal confidence and self-esteem.
- Anxiety and fear (survivors should be reassured that being afraid is a normal response; it is not something to be ashamed of or to be viewed as a sign of weakness).
- Panic is not a common reaction. It is most likely to occur when:
  - individuals are trapped and helpless;
  - there is no effective leadership;

- resources (e.g. safety equipment) seem to be available only on a 'first come, first served' basis.

Whilst normal in themselves, some of the above reactions can lead to secondary problems. An important example is the use of alcohol to reduce autonomic hyperactivity. Similarly, social withdrawal may lead to the survivor depriving him or herself of the very sources of support that are needed.

Pathological responses

Most psychiatric diagnoses involve continua, rather than categories. There is, therefore, no absolute cut-off point between normality and abnormality.

Some cultures do not verbalize their emotional distress; rather they somatize it. Also, certain cultures do not have words, which represent our clinical terms, such as 'depression'. The features set out in Box 28.1 help to identify pathological reactions.

Box 28.1. Features of pathological reactions

- Excessively severe.
- Delayed onset.
- Impact renders the individual dysfunctional.
- Reactions endure well beyond several weeks.

Post-traumatic diagnoses

According to the ICD-10 International Classification of Mental and Behavioural Disorders (ICD-10, WHO, 1992) there are a number of conditions which may be triggered by traumatic stress, as shown in Box 28.2. It should be noted these are not identical to the criteria set out in the other major taxonomy, the Diagnostic and Statistical Manual (DSM-IV, American Psychiatric Association, 1994).

Box 28.2. Main post-traumatic diagnoses (ICD-10)

- Acute stress reaction (ASR) [F43.0].
- Post-traumatic stress disorder (PTSD) [F43.1].
- Adjustment disorders (ADs) [F43.2].
- Dissociative disorders (DDs) [F44.0].
- Enduring personality change (EPC) after catastrophic experience [F62.0].

Acute stress reaction

Acute stress reaction is characterized by initial shock and numbness, followed by a fluctuating picture of mixed emotions (e.g. depression, anxiety, anger, withdrawal, and hyperarousal). The onset is acute following exposure to the trauma and symptoms subside usually within a few days.

Post-traumatic stress disorder

A diagnosis of PTSD requires exposure to a 'stressful event or situation… of an exceptionally threatening or catastrophic nature which is likely to cause pervasive distress in almost anyone'. This is called the 'stressor criterion'. The key symptom is: 'intrusive re-experiencing of the trauma (through flashbacks, intrusive memories, and thoughts against, a background of feeling numb, emotionally blunted, detached from others, and a lack of pleasure from previously pleasurable events').

There is commonly fear and avoidance of reminders of the trauma, and individuals usually report hyperarousal and hypervigilance. Rarely, there may be dramatic outbursts of fear, panic, or regression.

PTSD, according to the ICD-10, should be diagnosed only if the symptoms have endured for several weeks. (The DSM-IV states after 1 month.) There can be cases of delayed onset, but the diagnosis is not usually made more than 6 months after the trauma.

Adjustment disorders

Adjustment disorders are states of distress and emotional upset following an adverse life event. They typically begin within about a month of the event and remit within about 6 months of it. 'Prolonged depressive reaction' is an exception that may endure for up to 2 years post-trauma. Personality factors seem to play a greater role in these conditions than in PTSD.

Dissociative disorders

These include functional amnesia, fugue states, and a loss of certain bodily functions, which may result in aphonia, paralysis, deafness, and gait disturbance. (These were commonly associated with 'shell shock' during World War I.) A noteworthy feature is that, despite the apparent severity of the physical symptoms, the patients often display a lack of concern. This is sometimes called 'belle indifference'. Characteristically, they have an acute onset and tend to

remit spontaneously after a few months once the stress has been removed.

Enduring personality change after catastrophic experience

Certain events are so dreadful they seem to have an almost permanent effect. Such events include being taken hostage, being tortured, or being exposed for a long time to some horrifying experience.

Their effects are:

- Persistent hostility and suspiciousness.
- Social withdrawal.
- Feelings of emptiness and hopelessness.
- Being constantly hyperaroused and 'on edge'.

This is sometimes seen to be the chronic unremitting end product of PTSD.

Risk and vulnerability

No single trauma, however objectively awful, is guaranteed to generate post-traumatic disorders in all those exposed. Our current state of knowledge does not allow us to predict with sufficient specificity and selectivity who will develop such conditions. However, there are useful guidelines that can be grouped under the following three headings.

Pre-trauma factors

- Female gender.
- Children, adolescents and the elderly.
- Childhood sexual abuse.
- Previous psychiatric history (including alcohol misuse).
- Socially, educationally, and economically disadvantaged.
- Particularly anxious personality.
- Previous trauma. The experience of previous trauma may have an inoculating effect, and help the individual to cope with the current one. However, if the individual has not come to terms with the first one there may be a cumulative effect. A key point seems to be whether or not the person believes he or she coped well with the previous trauma.
- Concurrent ill health and adverse circumstances.
- Increased concordance of PTSD in monozygotes.

Peri-trauma factors

- Proximity to the event (there is usually a dose-related effect).
- Multiple deaths, injuries (especially if children are the victims).
- (Perceived) threat to one's own life or loved ones.
- Prolonged exposure (e.g. being trapped at sea).
- Sudden and unexpected event (not allowing time for psychological or physical preparation).
- Man-made events (including acts of violence and terrorism).
- Severe physical injury to self or others. It may be the personal meaning of the injury that is important, rather than the surgical opinion or Injury Severity Score.

Post-trauma factors

These are probably more important in determining outcome than pre-trauma ones. This may be particularly pertinent in the case of demobilized troops:

- Subsequent adverse life events.
- Absence of social, family, and peer support.

At risk and vulnerability factors can underpin a 'screen and treat' strategy (as was used after the London terrorist bombings of 2005).

Children and adolescents

Normal reactions

In addition to the normal reactions described above, children may also display:

- Regressed behaviour.
- Marked loss of trust.
- Inability to tolerate separation.
- Increased need for security.
- (In the case of adolescents) increased use of alcohol and drugs.

They may be unable to express distress directly; it may be shown indirectly, for example, by what would otherwise be described as 'naughty behaviour'.

At risk and vulnerability factors

Whilst they can display remarkable resilience and fortitude, certain factors increase the vulnerability of children and adolescents. Additional risk factors include a young age and stage of development, the scale of other losses (home, pets, and loved ones) and unsupportive reactions from others around them.

Children may sometimes be too protective of their own parents (by shielding their parents from their own distress) and dysfunctional family relationships will worsen the effects of trauma on children. Over-exposure to the trauma (e.g. through the media) may also exacerbate problems.

Bereavement, grief, and mourning

Major trauma almost invariably entails loss of various kinds. Typical normal reactions are set out below. Patients and families may need reassurance that these are 'normal'.

Normal reactions

Emotional reactions include:
- Being stunned and in denial ('I just can't believe he's dead').
- Depression.
- Anxiety.
- Guilt ('If only I hadn't…').
- Envy (at those who are not bereaved).
- Anger (even at the deceased, themselves, rescue services, and healthcare staff).
- Loneliness and emptiness (particularly in the longer term).

These feelings often come in waves and can be triggered by reminders of the deceased.

Behavioural reactions include:
- Pining and searching for the deceased (probably related to denial).
- Agitation and restlessness.
- Crying.
- Apathy and loss of interest.
- Avoidance of reminders of the deceased (hiding away photographs and clothes).
- Using 'linking objects' (i.e. carrying or wearing objects symbolic of the deceased).
- Inability to part with possessions of the deceased.

Physical symptoms include:
- Weakness.
- Insomnia (sometimes with nightmares).
- Loss of appetite (sometimes 'comfort eating').
- Loss of weight (or sometimes weight gain).
- Loss of libido.
- Globus hystericus (a lump in the throat).
- Headaches.
- Sighing.
- Cardiovascular symptoms.

Physical symptoms may mask the underlying grief.

Cognitive symptoms include:
- Impairment of memory.
- Impairment of concentration.
- Disorientation and confusion (without impaired consciousness).
- Changed beliefs (including religious ones).
- Changed attitudes (e.g. about life values and priorities).

Social reactions include:
- Temporary withdrawal from social events.
- Shifting roles and responsibilities.
- Conflicts (e.g. about forging new relationships and being able to enjoy things again).

Perceptions include
- Misperceptions (e.g. a belief that one has heard or seen the deceased).
- A sense of 'presence' of the deceased.

Adjustment

Most adjustment takes place in the first 6 months. However, it can take up to 2 years and even longer in the case of traumatic deaths. Individuals may experience a resurgence of intense reactions at any anniversary associated with the death (e.g. the date of the death itself, the date of the wedding that never happened, and the birth of a child who never saw its parent).

At risk and vulnerability factors

Most individuals do not require professional help to adjust to a bereavement. They will gain sufficient support from family, friends, and colleagues, and through cultural and religious rituals. Normal grief should not be regarded as an illness. Certain factors do contribute, however, to make adjustment more difficult.

A number of risk factors are associated with an increased risk of adverse reactions.

Features of the death
- Sudden, unexpected, and untimely deaths (all children's deaths are untimely).
- The death of a child or spouse.
- A painful, horrifying, and mutilating death.
- A mismanaged death (e.g. due to alleged medical or other incompetence).
- The lack of a body (a body confirms the reality of the death and allows the bereaved to say 'goodbye', 'sorry', etc.).

Features of the bereaved individual
- Overly protected from earlier losses.
- Anxious, insecure, low self-esteem.
- Previous psychiatric history.
- Excessive anger at the death (it can become a 'cause célèbre').
- Excessively guilty (usually the guilt is unrealistic, but expert help may be required if the guilt is justified).

Features of their relationship with the deceased
- Highly dependent ('we lived for each other').
- Strongly ambivalent (the 'love/hate' relationship).

Circumstances of the bereaved
- Lack of family support.
- Concurrent life stresses (unrelated to the death).
- Inability to access statutory social and community support.
- Low socio-economic status.

General guidelines: caregivers dealing with the bereaved

Listening to is better than talking at the bereaved. It is important to avoid being judgemental; there are many successful ways of coping with grief. The bereaved should not be swamped with information (it should be remembered that they are likely to have impaired memory and concentration). It is important not to be afraid of the word 'dead' and clichés must be avoided (they can be hurtful and insensitive).

False promises and offers of help that cannot be fulfilled should not be made. Throughout the process it is important to emphasize the normality of the reactions, and to provide information where further help might be obtained (e.g. through CRUSE). Leaflets about procedural and legal matters are often helpful and reassuring.

General guidelines: parents dealing with bereaved children

Parents usually worry as to what to say or do in the case of grieving children. Some may be over-protective of their children from the realities of death. Children will often use parents as models for how they themselves should behave in terms of the meaning and significance of the death. There are some generally agreed principles about managing the grieving child:

- Children who express their feelings least after a parental death may be the most disturbed.
- Children do not need to be completely protected from the funeral and other important rituals.
- Accurate and honest information is usually helpful taking into account the age and development of the child.
- It is important to beware of ambiguous euphemistic language. The word sleep, as a euphemism for death, may create anxieties about the child not wakening up from their own sleep.

- Reassurance that there will be continuity of love and care is key.
- Parents do not need to be afraid of displaying their own tears, which confirms this is natural and purposeful.
- Routines relating to play, bed and feeding. Should be maintained, and permission given to talk about the impact of the loss and express feelings (young children sometimes blame themselves for the death of the loved one).
- It is necessary to beware of being overly protective by lowering standards of behaviour, morality, and discipline.

Major incidents

There are certain issues that are specific to major incidents. These are addressed below:

Myths and misconceptions about trauma

- *Disasters are rare:* they are frequent and regular.
- *Panic is common:* it is relatively uncommon (see above).
- *Disasters kill and cause suffering indiscriminately:* it is usually the poor and the disadvantaged who are the most common casualties.
- *People will flee in large numbers from the disaster zone:* the opposite is the case; individuals tend to converge on the area.
- *Looting is common after disasters:* it is relatively uncommon and mostly occurs when communities are already divided.
- *Unburied bodies represent a serious health hazard:* generally, this is not the case; the over-hasty burial of bodies without appropriate rituals may compromise grieving and mourning (particularly for certain cultures)

Chemical, biological, radiological and nuclear incidents

The UK has not yet had to contend with a CBRN event on any significant scale. Good preparation is, however, essential. Lessons can be learned from international terrorist incidents and industrial accidents.

Features of a CBRN incident

- The effects may be extensive and enduring.
- Some agents will not be identifiable through the usual sensory means.
- There may not be an identifiable low point (i.e. the point from which things will improve).
- There may be high risk of toxicity and infection.
- The scientific identification of the agent may take time.
- They can cause considerable inconvenience (Box 28.3).

Planning must be made to include the management of divided families.

Box 28.3. Inconveniences caused by CBRN incidents

- Barrier environments.
- Quarantine.
- Travel restriction.
- Mass immunization.
- Decontamination.

Mass psychogenic illness (MPI) and medically unexplained symptoms (MUS)

Major trauma can give rise to many victims sharing the same symptoms without an identifiable physical aetiology. It has been noted during wartime, after accidents (involving toxic substances), after terrorist incidents, and in schools.

Three groups of people have to be dealt with:

- Those genuinely affected by a toxic agent.
- Those genuinely affected by a toxic agent, but who also have concurrent unrelated psychiatric symptoms.
- Those who have not been genuinely affected by the toxic agent but fear they have (sometimes wrongly called the 'worried well').

The ratio of the last group to the other two can be as high as 400:1.

Guidelines for management

Mass psychogenic illness (MPI)/medically unexplained symptoms (MUS) patients should be kept separate from affected ones. Hyperarousal should be recognized and managed. It is important to encourage effected individuals to engage purposefully, and to eat, drink, and sleep appropriately. They should also be encouraged to re-engage with friends, colleagues, and family.

These individuals should not be treated as if they are mentally ill unless they do have genuine psychiatric symptoms. Scepticism should be avoided and reassurance offered that such symptoms are a normal reaction to a stressful event.

Rescuers, first responders, and healthcare trauma workers

Selection, training, experience, and motivation can be expected to create greater resilience in these personnel than among ordinary citizens. However, there is overwhelming evidence that such individuals are not completely immune to adverse effects of trauma work. They can have raised rates of PTSD, depression, anxiety, and alcohol misuse. Particularly, after major incidents (such as the Pakistan earthquake and the Asian tsunami), staff may themselves also be primary victims through losing their own homes, possessions, and loved ones.

Staff may be exposed to:
- Gruesome sights, smells, and other materials.
- On-site dangers and interpersonal violence.
- Distressing survivor stories.
- *Powerlessness:* being unable to help at the level they wish.

In addition, there may be some non-trauma specific sources of stress
- Lack of skills and equipment.
- Poor role definition and unclear expectations.
- Poor organization and leadership.
- Unnecessary bureaucracy.
- Lack of time for self care and recreation.
- Poor communication.
- Poor scheduling of workload and hours.

Employers and managers should be alert to
- The risk of cumulative exposure to trauma.
- Unexpected changes in work performances of their staff.
- Unexpected irritability and moodiness.
- Excessive denial of adverse effects and reactions.
- Excessive risk taking
- Excessive use of food, alcohol, tobacco and work.
- Preoccupation with the incident.
- The risk of 'compassion fatigue' and 'burn-out' (staff are dedicated and altruistic; they find it hard to stand themselves down. Good management is essential to counter this risk.).

Patients will have a number of frequently asked questions (Box 28.4) frequently asked questions

Box 28.4. Patients' frequently asked questions (FAQs)

What can individuals do to help themselves?
They should try to:
- Keep up normal routines.
- Talk, when they feel able, to those whom they trust.
- Find time for relaxation.
- Eat regular meals.
- Take physical exercise.
- Be aware of certain drugs and 'potions' (e.g. cold preparations), which may interfere with sleep.
- Develop good sleep habits.
- Avoid excessive use of alcohol.

What are the basic steps others can take to help survivors of trauma?
They should:
- Comfort and protect from further harm.
- Reduce the sense of helplessness.
- Re-introduce them to their normal routines.
- Re-establish a sense of order and control.
- Allow the expression of feelings (but do not force).
- Reassure them of the normality of their feelings.
- Provide accurate information.
- Re-unite with others (especially others who shared their experience).
- Identify sources of support (lay and professional).
- Avoid clichés (e.g., 'I know how you feel').
- Be realistic about recovery time and aims.
  Many of these steps are similar to Psychological First Aid.

When should individuals consider seeking expert help from mental health specialists?
Expert help should be sought in the event of:
- Symptoms worsening over a month or show no sign of easing.
- Regular carelessness at work and at home.
- Impaired work performance.
- Radical life changes.
- Excessive denial of any adverse effects.
- Over-indulgence (food, alcohol, work.).
- Risk-taking behaviour.

Non-mental health specialist help

There is a well established hierarchy of needs after trauma. The principal ones are those relating to safety, food, warmth, and rehydration. It is also important to help survivors to re-engage with their families, friends, and colleagues. All interventions should be guided by the Galenic principle, 'first, do no harm'.

Public health communication

This is likely to be particularly important in the case of a CBRN incident. Because most individuals do not panic, the public can be entrusted with information. The media can also be allies, as they are expert in disseminating information.

Information must be accurate, cast in terms that are intelligible to the general public, and consistently reported. The authorities will need to identify individuals who are credible, as the public may have some scepticism about what they are being told, depending on who is giving that information. The general principle is that individuals cope well when they know what it is they are required to deal with; what is hardest to cope with is uncertainty and a sense of being out of control.

Peer support

When an accident has occurred at work, colleagues can do a lot to assist. Attending first to physical needs is essential. Maintaining a sense of composure and reassurance eases the victim's distress. Peer support is not always readily available due to:

- Fear of breaches of confidentiality.
- Concern that admitting to being distressed will represent a black mark in their career plans.

Psychological first aid

This is not a treatment or single intervention, it is intended for use, particularly after major incidents, by those who have some basic skills and knowledge in relation to post-traumatic reactions, and does not require mental health specialists.

It comprises a number of basic elements. These include:
- Normalizing the reactions of individuals.
- Attending to basic needs (e.g. safety, warmth and food).
- Reducing physiological arousal.
- Providing *accurate* information and support.
- Psycho-education (e.g. what is normal and what is the likely natural history of reactions).
- Assessing needs and screening (to identify different needs).
- Monitoring the rescue and recovery environment.
- Fostering resilience, coping, and adjustment (see above).
- Subsequently conducting an outreach programme (as many survivors of trauma are often reluctant to ask for any help).
- Triage.

As was indicated above, a minority of individuals may require specialist help. The 'at risk and vulnerability factors' can help to identify them.

Critical incident stress debriefing (CISD)

Popular in the late 1980s and early 1990s, CISD was intended as a group intervention for the emergency services and the military as a means of reducing distress and preventing PTSD. Subsequent research has questioned its value. In particular, the National Institute for Health and Clinical Excellence has advised against mandatory one-off debriefings.

The main risk of CISD when it is mandatory, is that individuals may be required to re-experience (and listen to harrowing accounts of others) when they are not ready so to do. This does not mean that staff should not discuss informally with each other the events they have endured (as was indicated under Peer Support).

Trauma risk management (TRiM)

Initiated by the Royal Marines, this is based on the principle of trained peers assessing individuals about 3 days after a trauma and then again 28 days post-trauma, to identify those who might require more professional help.

TRiM has face validity, and is generally very well received. It does, however, require more rigorous research evaluation.

Counselling

The phrase 'a team of trained counsellors is standing by' is often reported in the media following trauma. It is questionable how many people really wish to be counselled in the immediate aftermath of an incident. Whilst there is a role for trained counsellors, the question is when are they most useful. Presumably, the best judges are the survivors and the bereaved themselves.

Survivors should be given information as to where counselling can be obtained, and allowed to make their own decisions. It certainly should not be a mandatory policy, and it is self-evident that counsellors should be trained.

Specialist interventions
Acute phase
Even in the acute phase, most individuals will not display the symptoms of an identifiable post-traumatic diagnosis. They will respond generally to reassurance, support and comfort. For those few who do develop an acute disorder (e.g. acute stress reaction), the short-term use of a benzodiazepine or beta-blocker may be helpful. There are concerns about the extended use of benzodiazepines due to the risk of inducing dependence, disinhibition, and depression.

Antipsychotics have no role except in cases of frank psychosis or grossly aggressive behaviour. Hyperventilation usually responds to re-breathing by means of a paper bag until the CO_2 level normalizes. Cardiorespiratory causes of anxiety and panic symptoms should be excluded. It is unlikely that mental health specialists will be required to treat individuals in the immediate aftermath other than as advisers to the authorities.

Watchful waiting
In the absence of the development of an acute disorder, for PTSD the National Institute for Clinical Excellence (8) recommends the strategy of watchful waiting for about 4 weeks before professional help is offered, in order that normal reactions have an opportunity to remit. It is important that professionals do not interfere with the natural healing processes and methods of coping used by individuals, families and communities.

Early symptoms should be monitored according to a screen and treat approach using the Trauma Screening Questionnaire.

Later post-traumatic symptoms

Enduring psychiatric symptoms, such as anxiety, depression, and substance misuse should be dealt with by mental health specialists. There is now a growing evidence base regarding psychological therapies and drug treatments for those in need of specialist help. However, whilst trauma-related conditions are amenable to evidence-based treatments they have the potential to become chronic and irreversible. As is the case with PTSD, psychological therapies are the first choice treatments. The two recommended by the National Institute for Health and Clinical Excellence, both of which should be conducted by competently trained mental health specialists, are:

- Trauma-focused cognitive behavioural therapy (TFCBT), the aim of which is to assist the survivors to modify their beliefs, thoughts, and attitudes in relation to the trauma. It may be administered in conjunction with other stress management procedures.
- Eye movement desensitization and reprocessing (EMDR), whilst causing dispute as to why this treatment should be effective, it certainly helps individuals, in particular to deal with disturbing flashbacks and memories in relation to trauma.

Medication can be used when psychological therapies have failed, the patient is for some reason not willing to undergo psychological therapy, symptoms are so severe that medication stabilizes the patient in order that he or she can then benefit from a psychological treatment or a lack of trained personnel to deliver psychological therapies. SSRIs are generally regarded as effective for anxiety and depression. For PTSD, NICE recommend the following agents:

- Paroxetine and mirtazapine (both antidepressants) for general use (e.g. by non-mental health specialists).
- Amitriptyline and phenelzine for use by mental health specialists.

Resilience

Generally, there is too much emphasis on the negative aspects of trauma, including post-traumatic conditions (PTSD being the worst offender). It is important to emphasize the resilience of individuals and their capacity to adjust even to the most adverse circumstances. Certain factors can compromise that resilience. These include:

- Over-dramatization of the incident.
- Medicalizing normal reactions.
- Creating negative expectations about outcome and health.
- Providing misleading and inaccurate information.
- Over-emphasizing the essential role of experts.
- Ignoring individual feelings and displaying indifference to them.

It is possible to have a genuine post-traumatic condition, as well as to display resilience.

Key tips

- Instead of just asking, prior to discharge, *'Have you anyone to go home to?'*, it is helpful to also ask *'What are you going home to?'* A patient's ability to cope with a trauma may be seriously compromised by other life stresses. It may be possible for medical and other authorities to help with these.
- Patients should not be encouraged to aim to get back to normal. After a major trauma this is unrealistic. The aims are to come to terms with and adjust to what has happened.
- Patients must not be made to feel they must talk about their experiences. There is a time and a place for talking; patients are usually the best judges of when and where. On the other hand, it is important to display a willingness to listen if they do wish to describe how they feel and what happened.
- Survivors and their families should be reminded that help is available in the community. Information about such help is available from www.stish.com.

Further reading

Alexander DA. Early mental health intervention after disasters. *Adv Psychiat Treat* 2005; **11**: 12–18.

Alexander DA, Klein S. Biochemical terrorism: too awful to contemplate, too serious to ignore: subjective literature review. *Br J Psychiat* 2003; **183**: 491–7.

American Psychiatric Association. *Diagnostic and Statistical Manual of Mental Disorders DSM-IV-TR*, 4th edn. Washington, DC: American Psychiatric Association, 1994.

Bartholomew RE, Wessely S. Protean nature of mass sociogenic illness: from nuns to chemical and biological terrorism fears. *Br J Psychiat* 2002; **180**: 300–6.

Brewin CR. Risk factor effect sizes. In: Cardeña E, Croyle K (eds). Acute Reactions to Trauma and Psychotherapy. New York: Haworth Medical Press, 2005, pp. 123–30.

ICD-10 International Classification of Mental and Behavioural Disorders. Available at http://www.who.int/classifications/icd/en/ (accessed 18 March 2010).

Jones N, Roberts P, Greenberg N. Peer-group risk assessment: a post-traumatic management strategy for hierarchical organizations. *Occup Med* 2003; **53**: 469–75.

Klein S. Post-traumatic stress disorder 1 & 2. In Smedley J, Dick F, Sadhra S (eds). Oxford Handbook of Occupational Health. Oxford: Oxford Medical Publications, 2007, pp. 352–5.

Klein S, Alexander DA. Good grief: a medical challenge. *Trauma* 2003; **5**: 261–72.

National Institute for Health and Clinical Excellence. *Post-traumatic stress disorder. The management of PTSD in adults and children in primary and secondary care.* London: Royal College of Psychiatrists, and Leicester: British Psychological Society, 2005.

Ursano RJ, Fullerton CS, Weisaeth L, Raphael B. *Textbook of Disaster Psychiatry.* Cambridge: Cambridge University Press, 2007.

Williams RJ. The psychosocial consequences for children of mass violence, terrorism and disasters. *Int Rev Psychiat* 2007; **19**: 123–30.

Support group: The Sudden Trauma Information Service Helpline <www.stish.org>.

Rehabilitation after trauma

Rehabilitation after trauma

Rehabilitation is the management of disorders that alter the function and performance of an individual. This alteration limits choices, and the aim of rehabilitation is to restore these choices to the individual. Disability is defined as the outcome or result of a complex relationship between an individual's health condition and personal factors, and of the external forces that represent the circumstances in which the individual lives. Impairments are defined as the problems in body function or structure, such as significant deviation or loss.

The immediate priority following trauma is to save life and reduce morbidity. Long-term outcome and rehabilitation potential will often be determined by decisions made during resuscitation and initial surgery, for example, the mobility of an amputee is dependent on the length of the residual limb and fashioning of a healthy stump. The rehabilitation process starts in the acute phase of treatment. Patients commence their rehabilitation while on acute wards, with input from the trauma team with their medical knowledge and insight into the nature of the injuries.

General principles of rehabilitation

Rehabilitation is different from most other clinical specialities. It involves problems that can occur to any patient with long-term ill health, but also those problems associated with acute illness. In a young man who has suffered multiple fractures, a plethora of problems may arise. Many of these are well recognized, including the medical risks of immobility, such as deep vein thrombosis, rapid loss of muscle mass, flexibility, and balance. Other factors may be less obvious, such as the effects of nutrition (either under or over-nourished), and mental state problems, such as anxiety or depression. Further issues may come to light as a result of the original incident or as a result of the treatment received. Relationships with the medical staff, nursing teams, and family and friends may be profoundly affected. If these issues can be predicted, identified, and addressed, the patient's long-term outcome may be improved.

Rehabilitation aims to minimize complications and restore physical, emotional, social, and intellectual function, even if the patient cannot return to full health. A patient with serious injuries will have a range of specific needs, including physical, psychological, functional, social, or financial. Due to the scope of many of these problems rehabilitation has developed a multi-disciplinary team (MDT) approach. Some of these problems are best dealt with by a doctor, but many are best dealt with by other health care professionals. The type and severity of the patient's injuries determine the structure and skills of a rehabilitation team. It will probably consist of medical and nursing staff, psychologists, occupational therapists, physiotherapists, speech, and language therapists and social workers. The team must have the facilities to seek assistance from other professions, such as the acute medical specialties, particularly in the early stages of rehabilitation and with patients with multiple injuries, where recurring problems arising from the original injuries may require attention.

The holistic care and problem-solving skills, due to the wide range of expertise, are the strengths of the MDT. However, the number of people involved and the complexity of the problems can cause the MDT to lose focus. For this reason, the team should be well led, meet regularly to discuss the patient's progress and set clear goals so that all of the members of the team and the patient know where to concentrate their efforts.

Rehabilitation is an active process. Each individual needs to be actively case-managed. This will help both in the short term by identifying any complications and in the long term to help with future planning of needs.

Goal setting is the process by which the team identifies the problems that are important, developing concrete strategies for dealing with them and reviewing the progress after a realistic period of time. A useful acronym is SMART:

- **S**pecific.
- **M**easurable.
- **A**ttainable.
- **R**ealistic.
- **T**imely.

Goals can be short or long term. As an example, in a tibial fracture, is that a short-term goal would be to control pain, while the long-term goal would be to run. After an initial period of assessment a treatment planning meeting should occur, which allows the treating team to propose the long-term goals and predicted outcomes.

Accurate and detailed notes must be kept, as for all areas of medicine, but it is particularly important for rehabilitation as patients may spend many months undergoing their treatment. It also facilitates good communication among the team members and reduces misinterpretation by the patient and family, as well as aiding review of the documentation in subsequent years as many patients will have ongoing legal and compensation cases.

For rehabilitation to be successful the patient must actively participate. It also requires good communication within the team to set appropriate goals. Most patients do not fully appreciate the significance of their injuries in the acute stages, particularly following a traumatic brain injury. To this end education and support is one of the key responsibilities so that the patient comes to accept the situation. Some MDTs will appoint a key worker to liaise and work more closely with the patient and family.

Many patients will respond better to a structured environment and routine (see Table 29.1 for an example of a day's timetable. Rehabilitation is an active process and requires that the patient is as occupied as they can cope with. It is important to include rest in the routine, as fatigue will be a major problem in the early stages of rehabilitation. Some patients respond to group work. Others, particularly those with a brain injury may require a distraction free environment.

The scope of the problem

An estimated 10% of the world's population experience some form of disability or impairment (WHO Action Plan 2006–2011), many as a result of chronic disease, malnutrition or infectious disease. In the UK there are approximately 15 million affected. The proportion due to trauma varies widely across the continents. Rehabilitation services are variable not only from country to country, but also on a regional basis (for example, in the United Kingdom).

Amputations

Approximately 10000 amputations are performed in the UK annually, with 50% referred to a limb fitting centre.

Table 29.1. An example of a day's timetable

Time	
08.00–08.30	Nursing ADL
08.30–09.00	Nursing ADL
09.00–09.30	Psychology
09.30–10.00	Rehabilitation workshops or computers
10.00–10.30	Rest
10.30–11.00	Break
11.00–11.30	OT treatment
11.30–12.00	SLT
12.00–12.30	Lunch
12.30–13.00	Lunch
13.00–13.30	Lunch
13.30–14.00	PyT
14.00–14.30	PyT
14.30–15.00	OT treatment
15.00–15.30	Break
15.30–16.00	Travel assessment
16.00–16.30	Rest
Evening activities	
Evening activities	

ADL = activities of daily living.
SLT = speech and language therapy.
PyT = physiotherapy.

Table 29.2. The level and proportion of lower limb amputations

Amputation level British Standard 1993	Proportion (%)
Transtibial (below knee)	50.6%
Transfemoral (above knee)	38.3%
Knee disarticulation	2.8%
Toes	2.3%
Partial foot	0.7%
Ankle disarticulation	0.6%
Hip disarticulation	0.6%
Hemipelvectomy (hind quarter amputation)	0.2%

3.9% reported as double lower limb amputation.
Taken from a series of 4584 lower limb amputees referred to limb fitting centres in England and Wales: NASDAB Steering group 1997/8.

Table 29.3. Aetiology of amputation in Western Society

Aetiology	Percentage
Vascular (PVD versus DM)	90 (60 vs 30)
Trauma	5
Neoplasm	1
Other causes including renal failure and infection following implant surgery	4

PVD = peripheral vascular disease.
DM = diabetes mellitus.

Within Western Society, trauma is a less common cause of amputation, but patients tend to be younger and their demands on limb fitting services are much greater.

96% of amputations performed in the UK involve a lower extremity (Table 29.2) and men outnumber women by 2.5:1, although this becomes closer to parity with increasing age (Table 29.3).

Spinal cord injury
In 2002, 666 new patients were admitted to Spinal Injury Centres in the UK, as a result of traumatic spinal cord injury (SCI), the majority of whom were young.

Falls from a height or down stairs are responsible for the majority of spinal cord injuries. Most of the road traffic collisions (RTCs) are on 4 or more wheels, although as a proportion motorcycle accidents do result in a higher incidence of SCI. Horse riding, diving, and altitude sports have a much higher prevalence for SCI than rugby (when examined per hour of participation; see table 29.4).

Traumatic brain injuries
The annual number of Traumatic Brain Injuries (TBI) in the UK is:
• 150,000—minor.
• 10,000—moderate.
• 4500—severe.

Table 29.4. Causes of traumatic spinal cord injury in UK

Cause	Percentage
Falls	41.7
Road traffic collisions	36.8
Sport	11.6
Knocked over/lifting	4.2
Assault/sharp trauma	2.7
Trauma not specified	3.3

More than 100,000 people are coping with the long-term effects of such injuries. Hospital Episode Statistics data for 2000/2001 indicate that there were 112,978 admissions to hospitals in England with a primary diagnosis of head injury. 75% of these were male and 33% were children under 15 years of age. 10–19% were aged more than 65 years.

Falls and assaults are the most common causes of a minor head injury, followed by road traffic collisions (about 25%), which account for a far greater proportion of moderate to severe head injuries. Alcohol is implicated in up to 65% of adult head injuries.

The annual incidence of disability in adults with head injuries admitted to hospital is 100–150 per 100,000 population. Survival with moderate or severe disability is common after mild (Glasgow coma score 13–15) head injury (47% of patients), and is similar to that after moderate (45%) or severe injury (48%). Moderate is defined as GCS 9–12 and severe as GCS less than or equal to 8.

Preventive measures to reduce the number of TBI and the subsequent impact include safer roads, barriers to prevent falls, and gun control legislation. In addition, bicycle and motorcycle helmets, seatbelts, airbags, and soft surfaces on playgrounds are effective at reducing injury.

Vocational rehabilitation

Work is central to many people's lives, and disability may deprive people of the ability to work. Vocational rehabilitation is the process of enabling individuals with either temporary or permanent disability to access, return to, or remain in employment. It may involve schemes to support those with illness or disability in the work place.

Vocational rehabilitation and return to work is often governed by legislation. There are also a number of other factors that determine the employability of an individual, including:

- Forces in the labour market.
- Social Security and Social Services systems.
- The individual's working environment.
- Personal factors: psychological, physical, and social.
- The availability of work support.

Many people will be able to return to work, but will require a period of a graduated return. This is often termed a period of work-hardening, which is best performed with the support of an appropriately trained occupational therapist or occupational health service. Often there are financial incentives for employers to retain, retrain, or take on disabled persons.

Prior to returning to employment it is important to remove any disincentives to return to work, including compensation and income replacement payments. These may be particularly important in trauma patients.

Preventing medical complications and promoting general health

In the acute stage following trauma it is important to prevent complications, which may have a detrimental bearing on outcome, and may delay the rehabilitation process or at least elements of it. Prevention is the key, as the treatment of these complications may take years:

- Pressure sores can be prevented by regular turning, pressure relieving mattresses and seat cushions, effective management of incontinence, good nutrition, and recognizing those at risk. The Waterlow score will indicate those at risk (Box 29.1). Seeking the experience of the tissue viability and vascular nurses is often the best way of managing a pressure sore.
- Nutrition in a trauma patient is frequently overlooked. Often trauma and acute illness are catabolic states further increasing energy demands. Early nutritional input is vital. This ensures not only the correct calorific intake, but also the right balance of protein,

---

Box 29.1. Grading of pressure sores

- *Grade 1:* the pressure ulcer is beginning to develop and the skin around the area will start to turn red. If a glass is pressed on the area the redness does not disappear as with healthy body tissue.
- *Grade 2:* the skin may break or blister, and the skin around it will look irritated and inflamed.
- *Grade 3:* damage to the body tissue begins to develop and the sore becomes more than a surface wound as it affects the tissue underneath the skin. At this stage the sore will have a crater-like appearance.
- *Grade 4:* the ulcer has eroded deeply, causing damage to body tissue, bone, muscle, tendons, and joints. The risk of infection is much higher at this stage.

---

carbohydrates, fat, and other nutrients. This may initially be intravenous, prior to the insertion of a nasogastric tube. A percutaneous gastrotomy feeding system is highly recommended for longer-term feeding particularly in the unconscious patient or those with a poorly protected swallow reflex. Good nutrition will reduce the risk of infection and pressure sores, and will help promote healing.

- Deep vein thrombosis (DVT) is avoidable and potentially lethal. The use of subcutaneous low molecular weight heparin for immobile patients is important, but must be balanced with the risk of further haemorrhage particularly after a TBI. Early mobilization will also be helpful. Preventing and treating dependant oedema will also reduce the risk of DVT. Flowtron devices and profiling beds can help displace dependant oedema.
- Prevention of infections, particularly of the urinary tract (UTI) and chest, is critical. The use of catheters may prevent urinary leakage but does increase the risk of UTIs. Other methods, such as convenes, pads, or bed protection may be used, but there is a trade off with skin care.
- Managing a trauma patient's bowel is equally important. The method may be determined by the type of trauma, a defunctioning colostomy may be necessary after an abdominal penetrating injury. Keeping the skin clean and dry will reduce the risk of pressure sores. Using aperients and ensuring good nutrition may help reduce the risk of constipation.

The role of the physician

Medical practitioners should ask the following questions to give some structure when assessing patients from the rehabilitation perspective. The last two questions, although not particularly medical, are of intense interest to the patient and are the main remit of the rest of the team.

- Is the diagnosis correct? Although the primary diagnosis may be clear, there may be other conditions that remain undiagnosed. Mild traumatic brain injury is a very good example of this in the context of severe trauma.
- Are there any secondary medical complications? For example pressure sores, urinary tract infection, poor nutrition, anaemia, and electrolyte disturbance. Neurological complications of spinal cord injury include

spasticity and contracture. Immobility leads to loss of muscle bulk, flexibility, and balance.

- What is the prognosis? This is very helpful to the patient and the team. In many instances, it is not immediately clear, but an honest assessment helps in setting appropriate goals.
- What are the disabilities resulting from the injury? In other words, what function has the patient lost?

Examples include walking, climbing stairs, or loss of short-term memory. Once identified, these problems may be overcome even if not reversible.

- What are the handicaps? In the longer term, what does the patient want to do with his life? Will a return to the original home be possible? Can they continue with their job? Will their relationships survive? Will they have enough money?

Amputation

Amputee care is a rapidly changing and improving field, stimulated by new technologies in prosthetic components, and in stump and socket care. The eventual function that an amputee can now expect is far better than a generation ago. However, during the acute phase, the principle of an experienced surgeon working closely with the rehabilitation team remains as important as ever.

This section discusses some of the more important factors that a surgeon should be aware of during the acute phase of treatment that can transform the eventual outcome. These include stump fashioning, choice of level and length of amputation, pre-operative preparation by the rehabilitation team, avoidance of chronic pain, and early mobilization.

All amputations should be performed by a surgeon experienced in amputation techniques. The surgery should be performed, where there are adequate prosthetic rehabilitation services. The surgery performed should also follow recognized operative techniques.

Within Western culture poor arterial circulation and diabetes mellitus-associated vascular disease are the main causes of amputation. Traumatic amputees tend to be young adults, particularly men, involved in road traffic and industrial accidents. Amputation is a truly life changing event for a young person. Worldwide, lower limb amputation as a result of residual ordnance (land mines) is increasingly common, with over 10,000 lost limbs a year.

Most traumatic amputations involve the lower limb and have vascular or neural damage with associated bone and soft-tissue injury. If damage is irreparable, primary amputation may be the best course of action, although it may be best to delay consideration of amputation until an accurate demarcation between the viable and non-viable tissues can be delineated. It is now clear that in the injured extremity, amputation does not necessarily have to be at the level of bone injury, as internal fixation of the fracture at a level of otherwise healthy soft tissue can allow amputation with a longer residual limb. Amputation surgery is prone to complications, particularly infection, haematoma and wound breakdown, and is, therefore, best performed by an experienced surgeon. Special care is necessary for the skin and when fashioning a muscle flap in the residual limb, as these will ultimately be the weight bearing structures.

Amputations are described by the level at which they are performed, but there is often confusion between the *level* and the *length* of amputation. Each level of amputation has advantages and disadvantages, but in general, more distal amputations require less energy for walking and have a more successful outcome long term (Table 29.5).

The transtibial amputation allows preservation of the anatomical knee joint, a comfortable prosthesis, a functional device and a cosmetically acceptable limb replacement. Ideally, the knee joint should be preserved, although through-knee disarticulations often walk earlier after surgery, and these patients are usually very satisfied with their results.

The length refers to the most distal segment of the residual limb. This has a significant bearing on outcome, functionality and cosmetic appearance. The residual limb

Table 29.5. Energy expenditure for different levels of amputation

Level of amputation	Mean O_2 consumption above normal at rest
Transtibial	9%
Transfemoral	49%
Hip disarticulation	125%
Bilateral transfemoral	280%
Crutch walking	45%

acts as the interface between the body and the prosthesis, and allows the transmission of force and sensory input. The length is often a compromise between a long lever (which reduces energy demands) and clearance for prosthetic components. However, a longer lever means there is less room available for the prosthetic components that have a minimum size and length.

If there is time, it is beneficial if the rehabilitation team can see the patient before surgery. From the physical point of view, amputation predisposes the patient to hip flexor contractures and weakness around the hip joint. These complications can be prevented by a simple exercise programme for the pre- and post-operative period. From the psychological point of view, it is very helpful for the patient to meet the team who they will be working with to regain function afterwards, including a clinical psychologist.

Good control of pain in the pre- and peri-operative periods reduces the incidence of chronic pain in the residual limb. There is growing evidence that local anaesthetic nerve infusions reduce the severity of phantom limb pain. Neuromas are unavoidable, but gentle traction and allowing the neuroma to form in the muscle reduces pain. As well as opiates and NSAIDs, neuromodulators such as gabapentin, pregabalin, and low dose tricyclic antidepressants are effective.

When considering which modalities of pain relief to prescribe, a distinction needs to be made between phantom pain, phantom sensations, and phantom limb. Without direct questioning patients will often call all of these symptoms phantom pain. Phantom limb phenomena may be distressing for the patient. They may be able to feel their lost limb in the position it was post-trauma and pre-amputation. They may also describe a process of telescoping as the distal part of the phantom limb progressively becomes more proximal.

An amputee should be mobilized as soon after surgery as the wounds and other injuries allow. There are a number of early walking aids (EWA) that can be used as early as 5–7 days after surgery and the evidence suggests that early mobilization encourages wound healing. The EWAs should only be used under the guidance of an appropriately trained specialist and are useful in assessing an amputee's suitability for later provision of a prosthesis.

A prosthesis consists of a socket, an interface between the socket and stump such as a silicone sleeve, a suspension system to keep the socket and stump together, and other components such as a joint. The type of prosthesis prescribed by the limb fitting team should be compatible with the function of the amputee. A young traumatic amputee will have very different functional expectations to an elderly dysvascular amputee. Many factors determine the success of limb fitting, but the most important is the interface between the residual limb and the prosthesis, which is why fashioning of the stump is so important. If the fit and comfort of the socket are not satisfactory the prosthesis will be unsuccessful. The components supplied should be consistent with the stage of the patient's rehabilitation. Cost is often an issue.

Other important factors affecting outcome include:

- *Age and fitness:* these may preclude the use of a prosthesis or limit functional outcome.
- *Gender:.* young women often find it harder to socialize following amputation.
- *Cause of amputation:* diabetic patients may well have reduced proprioception. This will make the use of a prosthetic limb very difficult.
- *Pre-existing medical conditions:* chronic medical conditions, such as lung disease or ischaemic heart disease will limit the patient's ability to mobilize following amputation.
- *Type of limb:* most amputees will use a lower limb prosthesis, even if only for assisted transfers. Less use is made of upper limb prostheses as the technology is less advanced and there are more ways to replace hand function.
- *Contra-lateral limb function:* if the contra-lateral limb is injured this will delay prosthetic rehabilitation and will also reduce the long-term potential outcome.
- *Provision of rehabilitation services:* limb fitting and rehabilitation tends to be regionalized. Some regions have a larger budget and are thus able to offer more intensive rehabilitation and more expensive prostheses.
- *Social circumstances:* if a patient lives in nursing or residential accommodation the mobility requirements are less than a young person living alone and in employment.
- *Mental state:* it is very difficult to teach someone with dementia or cognitive problems after a traumatic brain injury the techniques necessary to use prosthesis.
- *Family support:* people living alone will often need to use their prosthetic limbs to avoid social or economic isolation. Young amputees may suffer body image problems following an amputation and family support will be particularly important.

The level of function can be recorded using the SIGAM scale (Table 29.6). Unfortunately for young traumatic amputees it is an insensitive scale for measuring progress, as most will get to level E or F very rapidly.

Table 29.6. The SIGAM scale

Grade	Disability	Definition
A	Non-limb user	Those who have abandoned the use of an artificial limb or use only non-functioning prostheses
B	Therapeutic	Wear prostheses ONLY during transfer, to assist nursing, walking with the physical aid of another, OR during therapy
C	Limited or restricted	Walks up to 50 m on even ground with or without walking aids; a = frame, b = 2 crutches/sticks, c = 1 crutch/stick, d = no walking aids
D	Impaired	Walks 50 m or more on level ground in good weather with walking aids; a = 2 sticks/crutches, b = 1 stick/crutch
E	Independent	Walks 50 m or more without walking aids, expect to improve confidence in adverse terrain or weather
F	Normal	Normal or near normal walking

The SIGAM is not particularly helpful for monitoring progress for young amputees without associated morbidities. Other functional tests such as the distance walked in 6 min may be more helpful.

Traumatic brain injury

Traumatic brain injury (TBI) is part of an inclusive category of acquired brain injury (ABI). They are all rapid onset (acute) brain injuries. TBI can be devastating. Even an apparently trivial head injury may have long-term cognitive and functional sequelae. Rehabilitation services tend to be based on need, rather than diagnosis. The functional deficits arising from TBI depend to some degree on which area is damaged. The damage can either be focal or non-focal, diffuse or multi-focal. Trauma may result in focal injury from a direct blow or non-focal due to hypotension, raised intracranial pressure, hypoxia, or diffuse axonal injury.

The initial management of TBI involves prevention of secondary injury by maintaining oxygenation, controlling ventilation, optimizing perfusion, and control of intracranial pressure.

Brain injuries can be defined by their severity, which gives prognostic information both in the acute phase and for longer-term outcome. Depending on the severity and location of the injury a patient with TBI may present with a host of problems. These can be broadly divided into:

- *Physical:* these include motor deficits of paralysis, abnormal muscle tone, ataxia, and poor co-ordination. There may be loss of sensation, hearing, and vision. Dysphagia, seizures, headaches, and fatigue may persist.
- *Communicative:* expressive or comprehension deficits. Dysarthria, dyspraxia, dyslexia, and dysgraphia may be present.
- *Cognitive:* impairments of memory, attention, perception, problem solving (executive skills), insight, self monitoring, and social judgement.
- *Behavioural and emotional:* emotional lability, mood change, aggressive outbursts, disinhibition, poor motivation, and psychotic episodes can all be associated with TBI.

These deficits will limit a patient's ability to participate in physical and social activities depending on their severity. There may be long-term problems and restrictions with housing, living independently, work and education, mobility, and relationships.

As soon as a patient is medically stable, they should be assessed by a multi-disciplinary team and considered for transfer to a specialist rehabilitation unit. The rehabilitation process starts in the acute stages mainly focusing on reducing impairments. Long- and short-term goals should be set with regular reviews. The team works together to achieve these agreed goals.

A treatment planning meeting follows the initial assessment period, which will determine management and treatment duration. Appointing a key-worker as a point of contact for the patient and family may be done at this point. Patients with brain injury often respond better in structured environments free of distractions. Daily structured programmes with regular rest periods should be given to each patient.

Early and regular communication with the patient and family is important. Honesty, although difficult and often painful, is necessary when discussing long-term prognosis, as it is better to be wrong about a patient who makes a significantly better recovery than predicted than the converse. It is important to remember that the family will be involved in the patient's rehabilitation long after they have been discharged from all medical care. The mental capacity of the patient is also an important consideration. Depending on the severity of brain injury they may need the safety of being made a 'ward of the courts'.

There is often a variable period after TBI before functional memory and the ability to store new memories returns, known as post-traumatic amnesia (PTA). It has been used in the past as a measure of brain injury severity, although it is not currently used by most neurosurgical units. Loss of memory immediately prior to the injury is common (retrograde amnesia), which unlike PTA can recover to some degree. Incomplete recovery from TBI has significant long-term cognitive, emotional, behavioural, social, and economic effects.

The post-concussional syndrome refers to a syndrome of headaches, dizziness, poor concentration, memory impairment and personality change, which usually resolve after about a year, but can persist for longer. A period of education and reassurance is important to long-term recovery.

There are many ways of assessing outcome after TBI, of which the Glasgow Outcome Score is simple, validated, and probably the most well known (Table 29.7).

Table 29.7. The Glasgow Outcome Score

Good recovery	Able to resume pre-injury lifestyle
Moderate disability	Independent, but unable to resume full pre-injury activities
Severe disability	Dependent on the care of others for the activities of daily living
Vegetative	No sign of psychologically mediated responses
Dead	

The neurological recovery from TBI occurs over many months or years. In the initial stages, recovery tends to be more rapid. Patients will, as a result, require different services as they pass along their rehabilitation journey. This is best illustrated by the 'slinky model' of rehabilitation. Each stage requires planning to prevent deficits in the provision of specialist services to address each physical, psychological, medical, social, and vocational problem.

Spinal cord injury

Spinal cord injury (SCI) is a lifelong condition, affecting approximately 40,000 people in the UK. Following surgical stabilization, the greatest risks to a patient with SCI are the complications that immobility and loss of neurological function promote. Following surgery, the patient will probably spend several months in a rehabilitation unit. During this time, spinal shock will resolve and the degree of recovery of neurological function will become evident. The priority of a rehabilitation programme is to assess the risk of each of complication and put measures in place to prevent or treat them. Preventing complications is often much easier than treating them. The process of helping the patient to regain function can only be successful if this groundwork has been done.

The American Spinal Injuries Association (ASIA) scoring system provides a format for describing the level and degree of injury. It describes the degree of neurological deficit, and helps in predicting complications and the degree of disability that is likely to result from the injury. The level of SCI will determine long-term function and outcome. SCI is associated with reduced life expectancy mainly as a result of respiratory infections, pressure sores and renal failure.

Deep vein thrombosis (DVT) is common in the early stages following the injury because the muscles are flaccid while the cord is in shock. Most rehabilitation units have a formal policy of DVT prevention including the use of anticoagulants.

Once the spinal cord has recovered from spinal shock, spasticity is almost universal. Spasticity is an exaggeration of the normal stretch reflexes, and occurs when a muscle is stretched leading to an inappropriately strong contraction. In an able-bodied person, muscle stretch will stimulate the reflex arc, with inhibitory control from the brain via the spinal cord modifying the response of the muscle. In SCI, this inhibitory influence is cut off. Consequently, even slight stimuli such as a slight movement of the limb, or touching the skin can stimulate the reflex arc and lead to powerful muscle contractions, joint stiffness, loss of movement, muscle spasms, and contractures. The spasms are very painful and can be powerful enough to throw someone out of their wheelchair. Measures to control spasticity include stretching, postural management, and drugs, such as baclofen and tizanidine.

Muscle contractures can be prevented with regular stretching programmes, splinting and intramuscular botulinum toxin injections. Further denervation with phenol injections may be required, but has a permanent effect. These measures reduce the requirements for tendon lengthening procedures.

Pressure sores cause chronic infection and premature death. They occur in the skin over bony prominences. It is important to inspect the skin regularly because of its lack of sensation. Each patient's risk should be assessed and a care plan implemented. This plan should include the correct programme of moving and turning the patient, and cushions and mattresses that spread the pressure away from the vulnerable points.

Autonomic dysreflexia is a medical emergency and is a poorly appreciated problem. It can occur in any SCI above the level of T5 and occurs because of disruption to the sympathetic nervous system. The symptoms are directly attributable to loss of sympathetic control. They include hypertension, accompanied by pounding headache, a flushed face, red blotches on the skin, sweating above level of spinal injury, but a cold, clammy, pale skin with goosebumps below, nasal stuffiness, nausea secondary to vagal parasympathetic stimulation, and bradycardia (pulse <60 bpm). It can be triggered by any noxious stimulus, which would ordinarily act as a painful stimulus below the level of spinal injury.

The management is to identify and remove the offending stimulus, such as a blocked catheter, distended bladder, constipation, or a break in the skin. The patient should be sat up with frequent blood pressure checks until the episode has resolved. In the UK, sublingual nifedipine 10 mg is used to reduce blood pressure.

Denervation of the bladder can lead to incontinence, urinary retention and reflux, and the risk of renal impairment. Urodynamic studies and ultrasound scanning are used to assess bladder function. Bladder management may involve self-intermittent catheterization (SIC) or suprapubic catheterization, both of which reduce the risk of infection and renal failure. The preferred method is SIC as this allows the bladder to expand and then empty, rather than continuously drain. If an in-dwelling catheter is left *in situ* it does increase the risk of bladder cancer. Drugs such as oxybutinin and tolterodine may be required to reduce bladder pressures.

Loss of innervation to the lower bowel can lead to constipation and overflow incontinence. Transit times are increased. Patients are unable to sense the need to empty the bowel or control the complicated process of defaecation. An effective bowel care regime may include regular toileting, stimulation of the bowel using the gastro-colic reflex, manual evacuation, and the use of bulking agents and aperients. Advice should be given on diet to maintain good nutrition and to avoid obesity.

Most patients go through a very difficult time as the degree of the injury and the lack of recovery becomes clear to them. Early psychological support of the patient, family, and carers cannot be overstated.

Rehabilitation following musculoskeletal trauma

Following orthopaedic injury or operation there is often a considerable period of time when the patient is prescribed bed rest or is partially weight-bearing. This period of immobility leads to the risk of the same medical complications described above.

When planning a musculoskeletal rehabilitation programme, the following should be considered:

- The deficits that the primary injury has caused, the likely prognosis, and the need for reduced weight bearing or movement to facilitate recovery.
- The risk of secondary musculoskeletal complications, sometimes called deconditioning. These complications are primarily loss of joint mobility and flexibility, loss of strength and endurance, loss of balance and co-ordination, and loss of cardiovascular fitness. There is also the risk of loss of bone strength with very prolonged immobility.
- Levels of pain and anxiety.

As an example, a patient receiving conservative treatment for a pelvic fracture may need considerable time non-weight-bearing for fracture healing. This could lead to secondary loss of hip range of movement and the development of tight hip flexors, weak hip adductors, and loss of balance, all of which will adversely affect the patient's eventual ability to mobilize.

Ward-based musculoskeletal rehabilitation is usually primarily delivered by a physiotherapist, whose time is likely to be limited. There will be some time for some hands-on treatment for specific problems, but a great deal can be achieved by giving the patient a personal exercise programme from the very earliest stages.

An exercise programme usually contains the elements listed below. In the context of patients who have sustained significant injuries and are waiting for fractures to heal, the programme will probably start off at a very low level.

- Joint mobility exercises should take joints through their pain-free range of movement.
- All major muscle groups should be stretched at least four times a day. A stretch should be gentle, pain-free and last 30–40 s. In practice, a stretching programme consisting of two repetitions is done twice a day.
- Exercises for muscle power and endurance should be high repetition and low weight. In the very early stages, static exercises or movements in a horizontal direction that do not require resistance to gravity are used. Progression will involve movement against gravity and then the use of thera-bands or low weights.
- Balance and co-ordination exercises should be as close to the desired functional outcome as possible. In most cases, the return to weight bearing should be under the supervision of the physiotherapist.
- Cardiovascular fitness should be preserved as much as possible. It improves general health, avoids weight gain, and improves mood. Partial weight-bearing exercises, such as cycling are useful in the early stages.

The rehabilitation programme should begin as soon as possible after the injury. It should be designed to the specific injuries and abilities of the patient, and should start at a low level, with progression in a graded fashion as the surgical condition allows. Pain should be controlled and analgesia may need to be increased as the patient becomes more active. Poor progress should prompt a reassessment as it may be due to previously unrecognized injuries.

Conclusion

Rehabilitation is unlike most medical specialities. Many of the decisions made in the acute setting will determine long-term impairments. It is important to include a multi-disciplinary team in decision making. Rehabilitation is often a very slow process requiring patience from staff, patients and families. Good initial assessments, regular meetings and reassessments are the key to providing the best case management. Each case must be treated on its own merits. Knowledge of local services, both charitable and public, can aid transition from the acute services into post-acute rehabilitation. The family often plays a significant role in rehabilitation and should be included in the discussions. It is also important to remember psychological factors as important reasons for slow progress during rehabilitation.

Further reading

British Society of Rehabilitation Medicine. *Amputee and Prosthetic Rehabilitation Guidelines-Standards and Guidelines*, 2nd edn. London: BSRM, 2003.

British Society of Rehabilitation Medicine. *Chronic Spinal Cord Injury: Management of Patients in Acute Hospital Settings*. London: Royal College of Physicians/BSRM, 2008. http://www.who.int/classifications/icf/en/

British Society of Rehabilitation Medicine. *Musculoskeletal Rehabilitation*. London: BSRM, 2004.

Royal College of Physicians and British Society of Rehabilitation Medicine. *Rehabilitation Following Acquired Brain Injury: National Clinical Guidelines*. Turner-Stokes L (ed.). London: RCP/BSRM, 2003.

British Society of Rehabilitation Medicine. *Vocational Rehabilitation: The Way Forward*. London: BSRM, 2000.

Commonly missed injuries

Diagnostic errors

Diagnostic errors are an important cause of preventable morbidity and mortality in trauma, and a common cause for complaints and legal action. There is probably no injury that has not, at some time, by some person, been misdiagnosed and so this chapter cannot be comprehensive. It is based on the common and serious problems that occur as determined both from the literature and from the observations of practising clinicians

Diagnostic error usually covers:

- *Missed diagnosis:* an injury has been completely overlooked.
- *Misdiagnosis*: an injury is misdiagnosed as another (usually less severe) injury.
- *Delayed diagnosis.*

Diagnosis must also include an understanding of why the injury occurred. To diagnose the myocardial infarction that caused the accident may be more important than to diagnose the injuries. It is also important not to miss non-accidental injury in children, elder abuse, and domestic violence. Even the diagnosis of alcohol problems may enable interventions to prevent further injury.

While the importance of timely diagnosis of life and limb-threatening injuries is obvious, it is equally important to diagnose less serious injuries promptly. The prognosis of many injuries is improved by early management and this can only occur with early diagnosis. While definitive treatment of less serious injuries may be delayed, while severe injures are managed, late diagnosis does not allow the option of early management. A patient with major torso injuries may spend weeks in intensive care and eventually make a full recovery, but be prevented from returning to work by a missed finger dislocation that could have been reduced in seconds, had it been diagnosed early. Not only must the secondary survey be thorough, but it should be repeated the following day (tertiary survey) and at intervals until the patient is fully mobile and independent.

In addition to being aware of the injuries that are easily missed, it is also important to be aware of the situations that predispose to error.

Handover

At some stage there will be handover between one doctor going off duty and another taking over, or as a patient leaves one department and is transferred to another. It is easy to assume that the other person has done (or will do) some vital piece of the history taking, examination, or has requested or interpreted some test. Thus, it is important not make assumptions. Full documentation must be made, as well as a full verbal handover. On taking over a patient's care, it is mandatory to read or re-read the notes as well as receiving a verbal handover.

Fatigue

Errors will occur more often when staff are tired, towards the end of a shift.

Multi-tasking

Looking after several multiply-injured patients or trying to run a busy Emergency Department (ED), and looking at X-rays and ECGs, whilst advising junior doctors on the management of other patients will inevitably lead to in increased risk of clinical errors.

Wrong triage

When a patient is seen in the resuscitation room, clinicians are expecting to find significant injuries. Occasionally, patients with major injuries make their own way to hospital and if they are triaged to the 'minors' side of the department the assumption that they have a minor problem may lead to errors.

Communication difficulties

Inability to communicate with a patient, for example, due to dementia or language incompatibility, makes history-taking impossible and examination more difficult, and is an indication for taking more care.

Patient factors

If the patient sustained their injuries while committing a crime or is deliberately unco-operative or abusive, it is easy to (subconsciously) take less care. Professional standards must not be allowed to drop.

Rare injuries

Many injuries will be seen every day or every week. Others may be seen once a year or less often, and so a person working a normal duty rota may go many years without seeing them. Not surprisingly, such injuries may get missed, especially if the X-ray appearances are subtle or if the injury mimics a more common injury.

Team factors

Trauma teams (like other teams) will work best when members know each other and have trained and worked together. This is not always possible with rotation of personnel and employment of locum staff. Members of a team must be familiar with each other and each other's abilities. Given human nature, it is inevitable that from time to time, there will be some antagonism between individual members of the team. This can be very destructive and lead to error. It is essential that professionalism is maintained and the role of the team leader in prevention of this is vital.

Head injuries

Head injury

A depressed fracture is usually caused by a blow from a small hard object (for example, a golf club). This causes a localized force to the head, rather than a generalized force that causes a loss of consciousness. In the absence of concussive symptoms, a CT may not be requested. If the depressed fracture is compound and associated with a dural tear, there is a significant risk of cerebral abscess or meningitis. It is important to be aware of the mechanism of injury and to have a low threshold for CT. Scalp wounds should be inspected carefully; the presence of brain tissue in the wound is diagnostic of such an injury, but this is rare and its absence does not exclude the injury. If a gloved finger is put into scalp wounds to palpate the underlying skull before the wound is sutured, the fracture can often be palpated.

The diagnosis of an extradural haematoma must be made quickly to enable early evacuation. Diagnosis may be delayed by failure to appreciate the history. When faced with a deeply unconscious head-injured patient with fixed, dilated pupils, it is easy to assume that they have been unconscious since the time of injury and that this is a severe brain injury with a poor prognosis. If, however, they were initially alert, and then developed a headache and became unconscious, the probability is that the patient has a minor primary brain injury complicated by an extradural haematoma and this is a surgical emergency. Errors are particularly likely to occur when the patient is managed initially by one ambulance crew, but brought to hospital by helicopter accompanied by people who did not themselves talk to witnesses or see the patient initially.

Head injuries are occasionally missed if the decreased level of consciousness is attributed to another cause. Probably, the most common misdiagnosis is a head injury diagnosed as intoxication. The two do, of course, frequently co-exist. In an intoxicated patient with a head injury it is dangerous to attribute a decreased conscious level to intoxication. A raised blood alcohol level makes a serious head injury more likely, rather than less so, and a serious head injury should be assumed until it can be proven otherwise. A patient lying unconscious at the bottom of the stairs with a hemiplegia may have had a stroke that caused them to fall, but must be assumed to have had a head injury until proved otherwise. It is important to differentiate between a patient who has an epileptic fit that causes them to fall and hit their head, and the person who falls and hits their head, which is then complicated by a grand mal seizure. An accurate history is essential—every attempt must be made to speak to someone who witnessed the event.

It is also easy to make the opposite error and to assume that a decreased level of consciousness has a neurological cause. Shock causing decreased cerebral perfusion may also cause a decreased level of consciousness and patients have died of treatable intra-abdominal bleeding, while awaiting a CT scan of the brain.

Facial injuries

Good quality facial X-rays need to be taken and require that the patient remains still. X-rays taken in the middle of the night on an injured and intoxicated patient are often of poor quality and this may lead to fractures being missed. For this reason, it is often better to wait to perform the X-ray for such patients later when they are more alert and sober.

The roof of the orbit is thin and penetrating injuries of the orbit may easily penetrate the orbital roof and this too, may cause brain abscess or meningitis. It is essential to consider the possibility of a penetrating injury in all lacerations of the upper eyelid.

Fractures may not always be obvious and so it is important to take into consideration clinical and other radiological features of fractures, these include 'black eye', lateral subconjunctival haemorrhage with no posterior limit, 'steps' on palpation, diplopia, numbness of cheek and/or upper teeth. Other radiological features include opacity of maxillary antrum and surgical emphysema of orbit.

If no fracture can be seen on X-ray, but suggestive clinical features are present, the patient may need further investigation.

Blow-out fractures

A blow-out fracture is a fracture of the floor or medial wall of the orbit with some orbital contents (extra-ocular fat or muscle) herniated into the maxillary or ethmoid sinus. If there is an inferior blow-out, there will be decreased eye movement with pain and diplopia on upward gaze. In a medial blow-out these symptoms will occur on lateral gaze. This is a clinical diagnosis initially as X-rays may be normal (though in an inferior blow-out, there may be a 'tear-drop' appearance in the roof of the maxillary antrum on facial X-rays. CT will be required to confirm the injury

Eye injuries

These are not uncommon in association with head and facial injury. They are easily overlooked as the unconscious patient does not complain of visual impairment and swollen eyelids may make examination very difficult. The eye should be carefully examined and an ophthalmological opinion requested if the eye cannot be seen as a result of swelling.

Chest injuries

The resuscitation room is often noisy and the patient may be breathing shallowly. As a result clinical examination of the heart and lungs may not be reliable. For this reason a chest X-ray (CXR) must be performed early in the resuscitation phase.

Diagnostic-quality CXRs are, ideally, taken erect and PA, and with the patient taking a deep inspiration. In trauma they are (initially at least) taken supine, AP, and the patient may not be able to take and hold a deep breath. This means that the CXR is not always easy to interpret. Commonly missed injuries on a supine CXR are:
- Pneumothorax.
- Small haemothorax.
- Diaphragmatic rupture.

It is also important to note that the CXR under-estimates the degree of lung contusion or aspiration injury when it is compared with a chest CT

Many rib fractures will not be visible on a CXR. However, the finding of a rib fracture will not affect patient management—what is important is the degree of pain, disturbance to respiratory physiology, and disability that results from a chest wall injury, not whether there is a fracture.

Surgical emphysema may obscure all details of lung markings and make a pneumothorax impossible to see. However, the presence of surgical emphysema suggests that there is a pneumothorax and so if there is respiratory distress, a chest drain should be inserted anyway.

Flail chest is a clinical diagnosis, as the X-ray may be normal (particularly in an anterior flail, with fractures through the costal cartilages). It is important to stand at the foot of the bed to observe chest wall movement. The paradoxical respiration of flail chest and the 'see-saw' respiration of the tetraplegic patient are easily overlooked by the doctor standing at the patient's side.

If there is any doubt about the normality of a CXR, in the patient with significant injuries a CT is essential. In the less severely injured patient, it may be wise to repeat the CXR in the erect position once the spine has been cleared and the patient can sit up.

The chest X-ray may show incidental abnormalities, for example a bronchial carcinoma or a metastasis. Incidental abnormalities may also be seen on other X-rays. These are often missed or ignored.

Imaging of the chest will define anatomical injuries, but for many injuries, the injury itself is less important than the physiological abnormalities that it causes (e.g. a single rib fracture in a fit, healthy person may not even present to hospital, but the same injury may kill a person with COPD). It is therefore vital the diagnosis of chest injuries includes a diagnosis of the physiological abnormalities with pulse oximetry, blood gases, and, in ventilated patients, end-tidal CO_2 monitoring.

Rupture of the aorta is the commonest cardiovascular injury in blunt trauma. The most common radiological abnormality in this condition is a widened mediastinum, but this is difficult to interpret on a supine CXR.

Pericardial tamponade is common in penetrating chest trauma and so will be considered and hopefully not missed, but it is rare in blunt trauma. In addition, it may be difficult to diagnose and, therefore, easily missed. The signs of pericardial tamponade are shock, muffled heart sounds (which are likely to be impossible to hear in a noisy resuscitation room) and raised jugular venous pressure (which may not occur if the patient has haemorrhagic shock and may not be easy to see if the patient has a cervical collar). Ultrasound should give the diagnosis.

Cardiac injury is also rare in blunt trauma. A cardiac murmur or abnormality on ECG should raise the question as to whether this is related to the injury. Echocardiography should be requested.

A CXR is taken routinely in patients with major trauma, but it shows much more than the chest. Shoulder injuries including dislocations and fractures of the scapula will often be visible, but will be missed if one does not have a system for looking at the entire X-ray.

The abdomen

A major problem in the misdiagnosis of abdominal injury is the failure to detect the fact that occult bleeding has occurred or failure to appreciate the amount of bleeding.

The abdomen may be difficult to assess clinically. This is particularly true if there is bruising (and thus tenderness) of the abdominal wall resulting from fractures of the lower ribs or pelvis. The abdomen is impossible to fully assess clinically if the patient has a reduced level of consciousness (e.g. from a head injury or intoxication), if they have a spinal cord injury or if they are being ventilated for another injury. While repeated clinical examination may be reasonable for the alert patient with an isolated abdominal injury, anybody who is difficult to assess MUST have further evaluation and investigation.

It should also be noted that no investigation is 100% accurate (for example, the CT may need to be repeated if clinical suspicion is high). Retroperitoneal injuries (e.g. a ruptured duodenum) will also be difficult to detect clinically. It is important to be aware that a large spleen from whatever cause may rupture with minimal force (or even spontaneously).

It is also important not to forget that in penetrating trauma a chest wound may involve the abdomen and vice versa.

Spine

Cervical spine fractures are easily missed:

- Fractures of C1–C2 may not be easy to see on X-ray. Particular care should be taken with a low threshold for CT.
- Atlanto-occipital dislocations are uncommon, but may be overlooked on cervical spine X-rays.
- The cervico-thoracic junction is a common site of injury and, unfortunately, this may be a difficult area to image, and fractures and dislocations get missed if the top of T1 is not seen on plain X-rays.
- Cervical spine X-rays in older people are frequently difficult to interpret due to degenerative disease. 'Steps' in the cervical spine should never be attributed to degenerative disease and often require a CT to rule out acute injury.

Thoracolumbar spinal fractures are common, and clinical examination is not sensitive enough to exclude an injury in the patient with major trauma. If the mechanism of injury suggests the possibility of a fracture of the thoraco-lumbar spine, the whole spine must be imaged. If the patient is having a 'head to hip' CT the spine should be carefully examined by reformatting the CT images.

A patient with one spinal fracture has a 15% chance of having a second fracture—if one fracture is found, the whole spine should be imaged.

In less severe injuries, the site of the injury may have been localized to the thoracic or lumbar spine. The most common site of a fracture is the thoracolumbar junction and so any X-ray of the thoracic spine should include L1–2 and any lumbar X-ray should include T11–12.

Spinal deformity (e.g. extreme kyphosis or kyphoscoliosis) makes the plain X-rays difficult to interpret. CT may not be very helpful as the CT slices cannot be made in the usual planes. This makes it difficult to 'clear' the spine unless MRI is available.

Osteoporotic fractures of the spine are very common. If a patient presents with a back injury and an X-ray reveals several crushed lumbar spine bodies, it is usually impossible to determine which are new and which are long-standing. The diagnosis needs to be made from the history, examination findings and further investigation if necessary.

Fractures of the transverse process of the lumbar spine may be obscured by overlying bowel shadows. The injury itself is not important, but may be associated with renal injury (although this should be obvious on clinical and urine examination).

It is important to beware the patient with a partial spinal cord injury (the most common is a central cord syndrome) in the absence of a bony injury. The patient may walk into the department and these injuries are easily overlooked especially if the patient is intoxicated.

False positive diagnosis is often made. Congenital problems (e.g. fusions, hemivertebae) may cause confusion and other pre-existing problems, such as spondylolisthesis may be misdiagnosed as acute injuries. Children's spines are significantly different to adults. Pseudo-subluxation of C2/3 and C3/4 may be misdiagnosed as a dislocation and the ring epiphyses of the spinal bodies may cause confusion.

Limb injuries

In major trauma attention is initially directed at life-threatening head and truncal, and limb injuries may be overlooked. This section does not attempt to describe every injury that may be missed in the limbs of the walking wounded, rather points out a few common errors in the management of major trauma patients and a few reasons behind the pitfalls.

Common causes for diagnostic error

Referred pain
Pain is not always felt at the site of injury, but may be referred distally. The classical example is slippage of the upper femoral epiphysis, where the pain may be felt in the thigh or knee, but this can also occur with hip fractures, spinal problems, and in the upper limb. The joints above and below the apparently injured one must always be examined.

More than one injury
There is a cliché that the most commonly missed injury is the second one but, like all clichés, it is based on truth.

Distracting Injuries
One painful injury may distract attention from another, less painful, but possibly more serious injury either in the same limb or elsewhere in the body. The deformity of one injury (e.g. a fractured femur) may hide the typical deformity of another injury (e.g. dislocation of the hip), and so it is easy to overlook one injury.

Pain
A painful injury might prevent the rest of the limb being moved and examined. If a limb has one serious injury, the entire limb should be X-rayed.

Failure to correctly read X-rays
If one finds an abnormality on an X-ray, it is common to accept the diagnosis and to fail to examine the rest of the film properly, and thus miss the second (and possibly third) fracture that is visible on the film. This occurs not only in the multiply-injured patient, but also in the walking wounded. A fall onto the outstretched hand may cause fractures of the distal radius, the scaphoid, or the radial head. A small number of patients may have two fractures from one fall. Frequently, the radial fracture is diagnosed and the second fracture is missed. Once again, the need to examine the joint above and below the site of injury must be emphasized.

Bilateral Injuries
It is important to beware the bilateral injury. The patient with bilateral shoulder dislocation looks symmetrical and, with weakness of both arms and normal power in both legs, may be misdiagnosed as a central cord syndrome. Bilateral hip injury may be misdiagnosed as paraplegia.

Over-reliance on X-rays
If a clinical diagnosis is made of a fracture, but the X-ray appears normal, it is essential to consider the possibility that something has been missed. The patient and X-ray should be re-examined, and if necessary, a second opinion obtained

Errors with sides (right and left)
It is important to take care over the words 'left' and 'right'—injuries are occasionally missed because the wrong side is X-rayed. Many more have been prevented by observant radiographers. It is also remarkably easy to look at the wrong patient's X-rays.

X-ray interpretation pitfalls
When taking a limb X-ray, the expected abnormality should be in the centre of the film, with two views taken at right angles to include the joints above and below the fracture. It is often not possible to achieve this in the acutely traumatized patient as the patient is in a lot of pain, limbs may be deformed, and may be splinted or immobilized in plaster before being X-rayed. The X-rays may therefore be difficult to interpret and the plaster will obscure fine detail of the trabecular pattern of the bone. The films may need to be repeated when the patient is more stable.

Every X-ray must be taken out of the packet (or displayed on the computer)—the X-ray that is not looked at will undoubtedly be the X-ray that shows the abnormality. Every clinician must have a system for looking at X-rays. Finding one abnormality does not mean that there is not another one that must be carefully identified or excluded.

A system must be in place for ensuring that all the X-ray reports are checked.

Upper limb
Brachial plexus injuries may be difficult to diagnose if the patient has other injuries in the arm or is unconscious. Arm weakness may be thought to be due to a head injury.

Wrist fractures are not uncommon in car drivers who are holding onto the steering wheel as their car crashes. Minor fractures of the wrist are easily missed. Displaced fractures of the radius will not be missed, but may be thought of as a Colles fracture. The X-ray resembles a Colles fracture, but this is a more serious, high velocity injury with significant soft tissue injury and a risk of neurovascular injury.

In Monteggia and Galleazzi fracture dislocations, it is not uncommon for the fracture to be diagnosed, but for the dislocation to be missed. In fractures of any long bone, it is essential that the joint at either end of the bone is seen on the X-ray.

Lower limb
'Chip fractures' around the knee are not usually benign, but represent significant ligamentous avulsions. Foot and ankle injuries are not uncommon in car crashes if the foot is crushed under the pedals. Fracture of the neck of the fibula may be associated with an ankle fracture (Maissoneuve fracture). It will be missed unless specifically looked for.

Mid-tarsal dislocations may not be obvious on standard foot X-rays, but a lateral X-ray is often helpful. Dislocations of the tarsometatarsal joint (e.g. Lisfranc injuries) may show subtle abnormalities on X-ray, and these need to be specifically sought. The clue to the diagnosis of compartment syndrome in the leg (and elsewhere) is frequently severe pain. If the patient is not in a position to complain of pain due to coma, anaesthesia, spinal cord injury or peripheral nerve injury, the diagnosis may easily be missed. Suspect it and have a low threshold for measuring compartment pressures or performing a fasciotomy.

Conclusion

Missed injuries are common, but with care and diligence they can usually be avoided. For this reason, a key part of the assessment of the trauma patient is the tertiary survey.

Research in trauma

Introduction

This chapter will describe trauma scoring systems, the use of trauma databases, and some aspects of research in trauma. Some of the tools described can be used to predict outcome in trauma patients, and to compare trauma systems. Research can take many forms, and it is important to have an understanding of some of the terms used, such as audit, clinical trials, evidence-based guidelines, levels of evidence, quality of evidence, and grades of recommendations.

Audit

A classical audit involves setting a standard, measuring performance against the standard, intervening in the process to attempt to improve performance, then re-measuring to see if the intervention has had the desired effect. However, the loop is often not closed. Trauma audit is the term given to continuous monitoring of the performance of a trauma system. It has three stages:

- Observation and identification of patterns.
- Formation of a hypothesis.
- Experimentation to test the hypothesis.

The retrospective study

Retrospective studies look at data from patient charts or databases to test a hypothesis. Retrospective studies do have an important role to play in studying the natural history of a problem or condition, and in generating hypotheses, which can then be tested using a prospective trial. However, these studies have inherent weaknesses, the main one being the quality of the data that is available from retrospective analysis.

The prospective cohort study

The same hypothesis could be tested by using a prospective cohort study. The advantage in this is that the data required can be established beforehand, and a specific form designed, and data recorded as the patient is being assessed and treated. The group of patients being studied is known as a cohort. The trauma registry enables the accumulation of cases over a period of time.

Clinical trials

Clinical trials of therapeutic interventions are conducted to find better ways to prevent, diagnose, or treat a disease or conditions.

Guidelines

Evidence-based clinical practice guidelines are increasingly being developed, giving recommendations based on the best evidence currently available. The evidence from studies on which a recommendation is based can be graded on factors including the level and quality of evidence. Ideally, recommendations are based on the highest level of evidence, preferably a systematic review of high-quality randomized controlled clinical trials that measure relevant outcomes and demonstrate a strong, clinically important, beneficial effect of the intervention. As recommendations in clinical practice guidelines are often based on more than one study, many guidelines are now using a system to grade the quality of the evidence on which they are based.

Levels of evidence

The level of evidence refers to the study design used by investigators to minimize bias:

- *I*: evidence obtained from a systematic review of all relevant randomized controlled trials.
- *II*: evidence obtained from at least one properly designed randomized controlled trial.
- *III-1*: evidence obtained from well-designed pseudo-randomized controlled trials (e.g. alternate allocation).
- *III-2*: evidence obtained from comparative studies with concurrent controls and allocation not randomized (cohort studies), case control studies, or interrupted time series with a control group.
- *III-3*: evidence obtained from comparative studies with historical control, two or more single-arm studies, or interrupted time series without a parallel control group.
- *IV*: evidence obtained from case series or case reports.

History of trauma scoring

Homer recorded in *The Iliad* that there were 114 deaths among a group of 147 wounded men, giving an overall mortality of 77.5% among his legendary combatants. Military interest in the area has continued. Today data continues to be analysed from the Vietnam War and the ongoing conflicts in Israel, Iraq, and Afghanistan.

Interest in the description of civilian trauma developed from the 1960s with the belated recognition of the civilian trauma epidemic. The scientific study of any area of medicine requires a well-defined vocabulary and uniform system of measurement if interventions are to be evaluated and compared. The first trauma systems were developed for battlefield triage, primarily for victims of penetrating trauma. As more sophisticated trauma systems were introduced into civilian life in the late 1960s they were used to predict outcomes for victims of blunt trauma. By the early 1970s pooled data from various trauma severity scores coupled with outcome data formed the basis for the case arguing the need for stratification of trauma receiving centres.

Trauma scoring systems

Defining injury is fundamental to clinical trauma research. In order to compare results of trauma care in one centre over different time periods or between centres, scoring systems have been developed. These have been used for pre-hospital triage, description of injuries to single organs, description of multiple injuries and correlation with survival, patient care in the intensive care unit, and correlation with survival. Injury scoring is also applied to clinical decision-making, injury triage, billing, quality assurance, and epidemiological research. Despite this, trauma scoring systems remain poorly understood by the majority of clinicians.

Injury severity scales of proven reliability and validity are essential for the appropriate allocation of therapeutic resources, for evaluation of changes in status over time, for prediction of outcomes, and for the evaluation of the quantity and quality of trauma care in differing facilities. Trauma scoring systems may be classified into physiological, anatomical, and combined systems.

Physiological scoring systems

Glasgow Coma Scale

The Glasgow Coma Scale (GCS) was developed by Teasdale in 1974 (with only one minor modification in 1976) to standardize assessments of a patient's level of consciousness (LOC). Only three behavioural elements are evaluated with a score for eye opening, verbal response, and motor response. A higher score indicates a better prognosis. The minimum score is 3 (deep coma or death) and the maximum is 15 (no neurological deficit). The GCS is easy to use even in the pre-hospital setting and can be used to determine the urgency with which care is needed. The GCS has been modified for use with children producing the Paediatric Coma Scale for use with pre-verbal children. Only the verbal response subscale is different. A number of other scoring systems have incorporated the GCS into their formula.

Trauma Score

The Trauma Score (TS) was first described by Champion in 1981 for use as a field index of physiological derangement and was a modification of the Triage Index. The TS is essentially a field scoring system utilizing four physiological parameters—systolic blood pressure, capillary refill, respiratory rate, and respiratory expansion—combined with the Glasgow Coma Scale. Weighted values assigned to the variable are added to obtain the TS. It is generally understood that a person with a higher risk of death from injury requires a higher level and greater urgency of care. Thus, a primary use of the Trauma Score has been as a triage instrument in the field. Table 31.1 shows how to calculate the Trauma Score.

There are some deficiencies of the Trauma Score. Its sensitivity is only 80%, that is to say 20% of patients with severe injury will not be identified with this score usually because they have compensated physiologically for volume deficits or field response has been so rapid that physiological compromise has not been demonstrated.

The Trauma Score has a specificity of 75% and will overestimate severity of injury where physiological changes are related to factors other than hypovolaemia, cerebral oedema or hypoxia. It is not reliable in children less than 12 years. If the Trauma Score is combined with an index of severity based on known anatomical injury, the predictive value is greatly improved.

Revised Trauma Score

Two elements of the Trauma Score (degree of respiratory expansion and capillary refill) proved too difficult to reliably evaluate in the field and were removed. This led to the Revised Trauma Score (RTS).

The RTS is highly sensitive and a strong predictor of survival, and is easy to use in the field, although it is more cumbersome to calculate than the GCS. To begin the calculation the GCS is converted from a simple 3–15 summation to a 0–4 score. Next the physiological parameters of RR and SBP are fitted into specific ranges (each range has a score).

When used for field triage, the RTS is calculated by adding each of the coded values with a result range between 0 (death) to 12 (no physiological derangement).

The RTS can also be used to calculate probability of survival (Ps), when each sub-score is multiplied by a weighting factor, then the weighted scores are summed to produce a cohort probability of survival (Table 31.2). The weighted RTS can range from 0 to 7.84. Higher values are associated with a better prognosis.

Table 31.1. Trauma Score

Variable	Value	Score
Respiratory rate	10–24	4
	25–35	3
	>35	2
	0–9	1
Respiratory effort	Normal	1
	Shallow, retractive	0
Systolic BP	>90	4
	70–90	3
	50–69	2
	<50	1
	No carotid pulse	0
Capillary refill	Normal	2
	Delayed	1
	Absent	0
GCS	14–15	5
	11–13	4
	8–10	3
	5–7	2
	3–4	1
Trauma score	Total	

Table 31.2. Revised Trauma Score (RTS)

Glasgow Coma Score	Systolic BP	Respiratory rate	Coded value
13–15	> 89	10–29	4
9–12	76–89	> 29	3
6–8	50–75	6–9	2
4–5	1–49	1–5	1
3	No carotid pulse	No breathing	0

$RTS = 0.9368\ GCSc + 0.7326\ SBPc + 0.2908\ RRc$
where c refers to the coded value.

APACHE

The Acute Physiology and Chronic Health Evaluation (APACHE) score was developed in 1981 to measure injury severity in surgical intensive care unit patients. The APACHE I was designed to be scored within the first 24 h of SICU admission and is too cumbersome for most emergency department use. However, in 1981 it represented an advance in predicting injury outcome because it was the first system to take pre-injury health status into account.

The APACHE I evaluated 34 physiological elements, with 'normal' being assigned to the lowest scores. Unfortunately, because of its complexity APACHE I was abandoned. In 1985 the APACHE II modification was published. APACHE II retained 12 of the original 34 elements scoring each from 0 (normal) to 4 (severely abnormal), and added two additional elements. These were the inverse of the GCS, and age, which contributes one point per decade of age over 45 years to a maximum of six points. Chronic health status can contribute a maximum of 5 points. Elective postoperative patients receive 2 points, emergency admissions with chronic organ dysfunction are given a score of 5. Although theoretically the total score ranges from 0 to 71, no score above 55 has ever been reported.

APACHE II has been validated and has an interval linear relationship between score and mortality. It can be used to compare different treatments and their subsequent outcomes for similar injuries. The main limitation is its lack of anatomical component and, therefore, its limited accuracy in otherwise healthy patients. In 1990, a comparison of the index SICU patient to the national norm was added to APACHE II to create APACHE III.

CRAMS

The Circulation, Respiration, Abdominal/Thoracic, Motor and Speech Scale (CRAMS) is a simple and widely applicable physiological trauma scoring system. It scores five easily observable parameters (circulation, respiration, trauma to the trunk, motor, and speech) on a 0–2 scale (Table 31.3). A score of 0 indicates severe injury or absence of the parameter; a score of 2 indicates no deficit. Thus, the total possible score ranges from zero (death) to 10 (uninjured). Incorporating 0 as the score for death makes CRAMS more intuitive than the GCS, in which even a dead body can score 3. A CRAMS score of 8 or less indicates major trauma where a score of 9 or 10 indicates minor trauma. Although reliable for field triage, CRAMS is limited in its ability to predict the need for surgery.

Table 31.3. Circulation, Respiration, Abdominal/Thoracic, Motor and Speech Scale (CRAMS)

Component	Score
Circulation	
Normal capillary refill and BP >100	2
Delayed capillary refill or BP 85–100	1
No capillary refill or BP <85	0
Respiration	
Normal	2
Abnormal (laboured or shallow)	1
Absent	0
Abdomen/thorax	
Abdomen and thorax non-tender	2
Abdomen and thorax tender	1
Abdomen rigid, flail chest	
or penetrating trauma	0
Motor response	
Normal	2
Responds only to pain	1
No response (or decerebrate)	0
Speech	
Normal	2
Confused	1
No intelligible words	0

Anatomical scoring systems

Abbreviated Injury Scale (AIS)

Early work characterizing the severity of individual injuries was conducted by De Haven, at Cornell in the 1950s. The Abbreviated Injury Scale (AIS) was first introduced in 1971 by the American Medical Association and the Association for the Advancement of Automotive Medicine to provide researchers with a simple numerical method for ranking and comparing injuries by severity and to standardize the terminology used to describe injuries. The resultant AIS assessed injury severity on a scale from 1 (minor) to 6 (fatal) in each of the five body systems. Although a milestone in severity scoring using anatomic pathology, this system proved deficient in several areas including the description of multiple injuries.

Injury Severity Score (ISS)

The ISS is a summary score for multiple injuries and is the most widely used anatomical scoring system in the world. It was first introduced in 1974 as a method of comparing outcomes of patients with multiple injuries. Like the AIS, the ISS is not a quick score to calculate, as each injury must be coded first using the AIS system. However, the subsequent calculations are simple. Using the AIS system as a foundation, Baker et al. designed a method that was capable of expressing the cumulative effect of injury to several body systems. Each of six anatomical regions is scored with the highest AIS grade for any injury in that region. The AIS values of the three highest scoring body regions are squared and then summed. The maximum possible score is 25 + 25 + 25 = 75. A score of 6 in any body region incurs a maximum overall score of 75, indicating a fatal injury. ISS correlates better with mortality than the AIS, and is generally accepted as the standard for anatomic indices of injury severity. An ISS of 16 is predictive of 10% mortality and defines major trauma based on anatomical injury.

Both the AIS and the ISS, designed to quantify severity of injury due to blunt trauma sustained in motor vehicle collisions are deficient in appropriately scoring penetrating injuries, and require further revision to accurately identify major injuries in this population subset. Several revisions have attempted to address this deficiency, with further updates published in 1990 and 1998. The most recent version, AIS-2005, is much more complex, containing more specific anatomic descriptors, and it has a military version for scoring combat-related injuries.

The ISS is comprehensive and has good predictive power. Its disadvantages are that, at an early point in the care of the trauma victim, the nature of some injuries has not been fully determined. Also the ISS does not account for age or co-morbidities. Multiple injuries to the same body region are not weighted higher than a single injury to that area; for example, a patient with a combination of massive spleen, liver, and bowel injuries is scored the same as if that patient had just one of these injuries.

New injury severity score
The New Injury Severity Score (NISS) was developed in 1997 as a simple modification of the ISS. The NISS is defined as the sum of the squares of the AIS of each of the patient's three most severe AIS injuries, regardless of the body region in which they occur. NISS better predicts survival and is easier to calculate than ISS.

To demonstrate the differences between ISS and NISS scoring, take, for example, a driver in a car crash who sustains abdominal injuries. At laparotomy, a moderate liver laceration (AIS score = 3) is first discovered. The ISS is now 9, as is the NISS. Next, a small bowel perforation is discovered (AIS score = 3). The ISS remains 9, but the NISS increases to 18. In addition, a moderate pancreatic laceration with duct involvement is encountered (AIS score = 3). The ISS still remains 9, whereas the NISS increases again to 27. A bladder perforation is next discovered (AIS score = 4). The ISS now increases to 16, whereas the NISS continues its climb to 34. Next, a bi-malleolar ankle fracture (AIS score = 2) is discovered. The ISS increases to 20, but the NISS remains unchanged at 34.

The NISS therefore represents a more realistic trauma score than the ISS; as injuries increase in number, death becomes more likely, even if these injuries are accumulating in a single body region. Furthermore, adding a trivial injury (such as a fibular fracture) to a different body region should not significantly affect the likelihood of death. The main limitation of the NISS is that it does not account for physiological variables.

Anatomic profile
The anatomic profile (AP) classifies injuries by regional anatomical values into only four categories, but assesses every region separately Box 31.1. This increases the accuracy of assessment and helps to predict the outcomes of survival and length of hospital stay. All serious injuries (defined as an AIS score of >2) are grouped in anatomical regions A, B, or C. All minor injuries (those with an AIS score of 1 or 2) regardless of their anatomical location are classified as D.

Box 31.1. Anatomic profile (AP).

Body region and classification
- Head, brain spinal cord   A
- Thorax and front of neck   B
- All body regions other than A or B   C
- All non-serious injuries   D

Calculation formula
AP score = Σ of

$$\sqrt{[\text{Region A (injury 1)}^2 + \text{(injury 2}\dots n)^2]}$$
$$+\quad \sqrt{[\text{Region B (injury 1)}^2 + \text{(injury 2}\dots n)^2]}$$
$$+\quad \sqrt{[\text{Region C (injury 1)}^2 + \text{(injury 2}\dots n)^2]}$$

For example, a patient with two injuries in region A and the scores for those two injuries are 5 and 4, respectively, will receive a total score of $\sqrt{(25 + 16)} = 6.4$ for region A. If there are no other serious injuries to other body regions, the score for those regions will be zero (B = 0, C = 0, D = 0). As with most of the more accurate trauma scoring systems, this system is most useful in an in-patient setting or for retrospective analysis.

Combined physiological/anatomical systems
While physiological scoring systems are strong predictors of mortality, they fail to recognize the importance of site of injury on subsequent disability. The ISS and NISS, on the other hand, characterize the degree of anatomical disruption weighted by the importance of the site of injury, but fail to measure organ system derangements.

TRISS methodology and the Major Trauma Outcome Study (MTOS) aim to overcome these problems. The constituent components of TRISS are the Revised Trauma Score (RTS), the ISS, and the patient's age.

Trauma outcome evaluation

Much of our knowledge of trauma indices came from the Major Trauma Outcome Study (MTOS). MTOS began in 1982, and its aim was to refine the methods for injury severity scoring, to establish national normative outcomes for trauma and to provide trauma care institutions with objective evaluations of quality assurance and outcome.

Age

Cardiovascular morbidity associated with increasing age influences probability of survival. Among 23,000 patients studied in the Major Trauma Outcome Study, an age greater than 55 years, for comparable levels of physiologic derangement and anatomical injury severity, was shown to be associated with significantly increased mortality. For example, Trauma Scores and Injury Severity Scores resulting in a 10% predicted mortality for blunt trauma patients under 55 years of age have a predicted mortality of approximately 40% in patients over 55.

TRISS

TRISS methodology calculates the probability of survival. TRISS is based on RTS, ISS, age, and type of injury in a regression formula. Values for these factors are weighted and summed to yield a TRISS value between 0 and 1. Using TRISS methodology, the probability of survival for any one patient can be estimated from the following formula:

$$Probability\ of\ survival\ (Ps) = 1/(1+e^{-b})$$

Where

$$e = 2.7183\ (base\ of\ Naperian\ logarithms)$$
$$b = b_0 + b_1\ (RTS) + b_2\ (ISS) + b_3\ (Age\ Index)$$

The coefficients b0–b3 are derived from multiple regression analysis of the MTOS database. Age Index is 0 if the patient's age is below 54 years or 1 if 55 years and over. The coefficients are different for blunt and penetrating trauma. If the patient is aged less than 15 years then blunt coefficients are used regardless of mechanism.

Z-statistic

The Z-statistic, first described by Flora, is a statistic of outcome comparison between two subsets of a population (Box 31.2). The Z-statistic describes the difference between the actual number of deaths (or survivors) in the test (e.g. institution) subset, and the predicted number of deaths (or survivors) based on the baseline (the MTOS norm).

Box 31.2. Z-statistic

When considering mortality, the formula for calculating Z is:

$$Z = \frac{D - \sum Qi}{\sqrt{\sum PiQi}}$$

where D is the actual number of deaths; $Qi = (1 - Pi)$ predicted probability of death for patient i; $\sum Qi$ is the predicted number of deaths; and Pi is the predicted Ps for patient i (from baseline norm)

When mortality is studied, a negative Z value is the desired result since it indicates that the number of deaths predicted from the baseline exceeds the number observed in the test set. (A positive Z value would mean that more

deaths occurred than were predicted). To achieve a difference between the two groups (test and control) of statistical significance, the Z value needs to exceed a critical level, based on a standard normal distribution (Table 31.4)

Table 31.4. Statistical significance and critical value

Statistical significance (p)	Critical value
0.0001	3.29
0.005	2.81
0.010	2.58
0.025	2.24
0.050	1.96
0.100	1.65

M Statistic

Z values can be affected by the injury severity match between the study and the baseline patient sets. The M statistic is a measure of that match. Values for M range from 0 to 1, and the closer the value is to one the better the match of injury severity.

Limitations of TRISS

The Trauma Audit and Research Network (TARN), currently the largest trauma network in Europe, has been analysing outcome prediction using the TRISS methodology since 1989. Its database contains 200,000 hospital admissions from 110 hospitals in the UK. One of the limitations of the database is the amount of missing information. To improve some of the shortcomings of TRISS, a new model was developed, using the Glasgow Coma Score (GCS) instead of RTS to reduce the number of cases that could not be analysed due to missing data.

TRISSCAN

The TRISS method describes a means of determining probability of survival (Ps) utilizing current coefficients from the Major Trauma Outcome Study and Champion's original Trauma Score. Using these predetermined values, the TRISSCAN chart provides a visual display for close approximation of Ps. This is a quick and easy method of highlighting unexpected outcomes and also serves as an educational tool to emphasize the importance of the interrelationships of the variables representing physiological derangement (TS), anatomical injury severity (ISS) and age.

ASCOT

A Severity Characterization of Trauma (ASCOT) is a comprehensive anatomical and physiological scoring system that combines elements of the AP and RTS. Injuries are classified as blunt or penetrating, and patient age is assigned to five categories. The probability of survival is calculated according to a formula. Both ASCOT and TRISS are designed for in-patient use, and are particularly useful for patients requiring prolonged inpatient care.

The ASCOT score estimates the probability of survival (Ps). For example, a population-based probability of survival value of 30% indicates that only 30 of 100 patients with similar injuries would be expected to survive.

In general, the ASCOT Ps value is similar to the TRISS Ps among survivors, but there is a marked difference for non-survivors. Among the non-survivors the ASCOT score is usually lower than the TRISS. This is because ASCOT uses the more reliable AP instead of the ISS.

Ongoing development of trauma scoring

While the ISS is the international standard for comparison of trauma incidence and outcomes, it is not without its limitations.

Impairment and disability

The development of an injury outcome scale has recently become a priority. The Injury Impairment Scale (IIS) was based on the AIS severity code and assigned values from 1 to 6 for each injury descriptor with residual impairment one year following injury. This scale was superseded by the Functional Capacity Index (FCI) and it is anticipated that this will be integrated into the AIS dictionary.

ICDMAP

The International Classification of Diseases (ICD) is the most widely used hospital-based system in the world to characterize patient discharge diagnosis and for billing purposes for all hospital admissions for any cause. The ICDMAP was developed to convert the trauma related sections of the ICD. Work is underway to map AIS 2005 to both ICD9-CM and ICD10-CM

Summary

Injury classification systems provide the tools to document the frequency and severity of injuries by specific organ, anatomical structure, and body region. They provide a scientific basis for evaluating the effects of interventions and countermeasures on injury reduction. Indices for quantifying injury severity are integral to understanding the epidemiology of trauma and objectively judging the quality and results of treatment given both pre-hospital and during in-patient care.

The TRISS methodology is the most widely used combined scoring system in the world for outcome assessment and quality assurance in trauma care. TRISS offers a standard approach for tracking and evaluating outcome of trauma care. Anatomical, physiological, and age characteristics are used to quantify probability of survival in relation to severity of injury.

Trauma databases

A trauma registry collects uniform data elements that describe the injury event, demographics, pre-hospital information, diagnosis, care, outcomes, and costs of treatment for injured patients. The inclusion and exclusion criteria for trauma registries vary widely depending upon resources and the volume of trauma patients seen. This inconsistency makes accurate population-based data difficult to obtain.

The capacity to audit and improve injury management is a fundamental component of any trauma system. Trauma registries are used to collate detailed data on injured patients, which can provide the opportunity to improve the management of injured patients, and help in the planning of trauma services. They also inform injury prevention strategies, monitor changing patterns of injury and its management, and allow comparison of management across institutions.

Although the benefits of a comprehensive trauma registry are generally understood, they come at a cost. For good quality data there must be very specific inclusion criteria, and clear parameters and coding rules to determine what is being collected and what the data actually means. Good quality data does not come from sporadic collection by casual disinterested parties who have not been trained appropriately. Many hospitals want the information that the registry can provide, but do not adequately fund the resources necessary, such as a computerized database, and a designated person to manage the data, and ensure it is accurate and reliable.

Uses of a trauma registry

A trauma registry is useful for a range of purposes, including:
- Performance improvement.
- Public health.
- Injury prevention.
- Trauma systems.
- Outcome measurement.
- Resource utilization and cost analysis.
- Research.

The trauma registry is a rich source of data for researchers to examine important questions across the continuum of injury care. It is useful both within the institution as well and for multi-centre aggregated data, which can monitor and guide appropriate changes in practice.

Verification and designation

The process of trauma centre verification and designation requires that trauma centres document their volume, performance, and outcomes over time. In addition, the trauma centre must demonstrate an effective performance improvement programme. This verification process is mandatory in the USA, and voluntary in Australia and New Zealand.

Centralized trauma databases

Currently, all US trauma centres submit their patient data to National Trauma Data Bank (NTDB). In the UK, the Trauma Audit and Research Network (TARN) gathers and analyses data for hospitals to monitor their performance against past results and the performance of other hospitals. These databases have helped policymakers identify problems associated with various trauma systems.

Developing a trauma registry

Some hospitals have designed their own computerized registry; however there are several effective trauma registry software packages available commercially, which are designed to run on a personal computer or hospital computer system.

Data manager

Good data comes from accurate data collection, unambiguous criteria, and clinicians collecting data who have a clear understanding about what the data means and the questions the data will answer. The person responsible for entering and retrieving the data is an important member of the trauma team. This role may be performed by a registrar in the USA or data manager in Australia, or it may be a part of the role of the trauma nurse co-ordinator.

Confidentiality

Hospitals are required to maintain patient and hospital confidentiality. Appropriate measures must ensure confidentiality and protect against unauthorized uses, or disclosures of these data.

Inclusion and exclusion criteria

Unfortunately, inclusion and exclusion criteria for entry into a registry are not standardized. Some hospitals modify the inclusion and exclusion criteria to address specific needs of their population, and depending on the resources available to capture and enter the data. This makes comparisons problematic. While one hospital may collect some data on all patients admitted to the hospital another may only include those that meet criteria for trauma team activation and another hospital may include only those patients with ISS >15.

Data collection

There is a range of methods for collecting and entering data from the medical records. Most commonly, there is a paper form, which is later entered into a computer program. Portable computers and hand-held devices for data extraction and data entry are increasingly used, and data downloading from the hospital information system is expanding.

Typically one full-time equivalent employee dedicated to the registry will be needed to process 750–1000 patients annually.

Data quality and validation

Accurate data for the trauma registry comes from accurate coding and data entry. Strategies for monitoring quality of data are essential. These include internal validity rules within the registry to prevent data entry errors, a programme of inter-coder consistency, frequent review of data dictionary to eliminate ambiguous criteria and periodic re-checking of a proportion of patient records.

Report writing

Trauma registry reports support decision making and guide management. Most registry software enables generation of standard reports that summarize different ways to report specific questions or areas of concern.

Aggregated data

Participating hospitals contribute data to a central registry. Hospitals in England and Wales contribute to the Trauma Audit Research Network (TARN). Established in 2002, the

EuroTARN initiative consists of the regular participation of 14 countries and support from many others who have come together to develop an effective system to review the standards of trauma care across Europe and develop an effective method for future data collection.

The National Trauma Data Bank (NTDB) is the largest aggregation of trauma registry data ever assembled. It contains over 2 million records from trauma centres in the USA and Puerto Rico.

In Australia and New Zealand stakeholders have formed the National Trauma Registry Consortium (NTRC) with the aim of establishing a trauma registry to help monitor and improve the management of injured patients in Australasia. The project is ongoing.

Performance indicators

A performance indicator (PI) is a pre-determined standard of clinical care which can be measured against current performance. Any number of PIs can be tracked, although each must be clearly measurable. Performance indicators can be used to measure different phases of care, such as pre-hospital, resuscitation, definitive care, and documentation. One example of a pre-hospital PI is to limit on-scene time to less than 20 min, enabling rapid access to definitive treatment.

Role of the trauma nurse co-ordinator

Optimal management of the severely-injured patient requires a timely passage through appropriate diagnostic and treatment phases of care. The trauma nurse is responsible for a range of functions, which can be broadly categorized as clinical leadership, education, performance improvement, administration, and research.

The trauma nurse is responsible for data collection and entry, is involved in multidisciplinary rounds, assisting the coordination of clinical interventions and education.

Clinical leadership

The trauma nurse role can include working as a member of the resuscitation team on patient arrival, or monitoring the process to ensure quality of care and documentation. Typical functions are to ensure that the required team members are present and notifying relevant staff, such as operating room staff or radiology as necessary, as well as facilitating communication to ensure smooth and rapid patient flow through the system. Beyond the resuscitation phase, the nurse reviews patients in the intensive care unit and ward to ensure that the tertiary survey is completed, formal radiology results have been documented and appropriate referrals to specialty teams have been made and acted upon.

Performance improvement

Acting as advocate for the patient throughout the course of their stay in hospital, the trauma nurse will identify and track errors or system issues. Working with other clinicians they will develop, implement, and monitor strategies to solve or reduce the incidence of these errors. Part of this process may be the identification of cases for, and

facilitation of, peer review of all trauma deaths, and critical incidents.

Education

The trauma nurse is involved in orientation for new clinical staff and ongoing education of existing staff. Regular participation in teaching rounds and case audit is also typical of the trauma nurse role in the hospital. The trauma nurse can also provide education resources, and support to the patient and their family to aid recovery and adjustment to disability.

Tools

Items such as an injury and management list, spinal clearance, and positioning checklist, tertiary survey forms, and clinical pathways for specific injuries are examples of tools that may be used to facilitate trauma care. Networking with trauma nurses from other institutions provides the opportunity for support and the promulgation of useful tools.

Research

Because of the ongoing process of collecting and maintaining data for injured patients the trauma nurse is perfectly placed to identify trends in injury patterns or new treatment initiatives. The trauma nurse is integral to the capacity of an organization to conduct research due to their knowledge of what data is held in the trauma registry.

Further reading

Baker SP, O'Neill B, Haddon W, Long WB. *The Injury Severity Score: Development and Potential Usefulness*, 18th Proceedings, Lake Bluff, American Association for Automotive Medicine Publisher, 1974: pp. 58–74.

Boyd CR, Tolson MA, Copes WS Evaluating Trauma Care: The TRISS Method. *Journal of Trauma* 1987; **27**(4): 370–8.

Bull JP. Disabilities caused by road traffic accidents and their relation to severity scores. *Accid Anal Prevent* 1985; **17**(5): 387–97.

Champion HR, Copes WS, Sacco WJ, Frey CF, Holcroft JW, Hoyt DB, et al. Improved predictions from a severity characterisation of trauma (ASCOT) over Trauma and Injury Score (TRISS): results of an independent evaluation. *J Trauma* 1996; **40**(1): 42–9.

Champion HR, Copes WS, Sacco WJ, Lawnick MM, Keast SL, Bain LW Jr, et al. The Major Trauma Outcome Study: establishing national norms for trauma care. *J Trauma* 1990; **30**(11): 1356–65.

Champion HR, Sacco WJ, Copes WS, Gann DS, Gennarelli TA, Flanagan ME. A revision of the Trauma Score. *J Trauma* 1989; 29(**5**): 623–9.

Committee on Injury Scaling. Injury Impairment Scale 1994. Des Plaines: Association for the Advancement of Automotive Medicine; 1994.

Committee on Trauma American College of Surgeons. Optimal Care of the Injured Patient. Chicago: American College of Surgeons; 1990.

Copes WS, Champion HR, Sacco WJ, Lawnick MM, Gann DS, Gennarelli T, et al. Progress in characterising anatomic injury. *J Trauma* 1988; **30**: 1200–7.

Davis DP, Peay J, Sise MJ, Vilke GM, Kennedy F, Eastman AB, et al. The impact of prehospital endotracheal intubation on outcome in moderate to severe traumatic brain injury. *J Trauma* 2005; **58**(5): 933–9.

Fani-Salek MH, Totten VY, Terezakis SA. Trauma scoring systems explained. *Emerg Med* 1999; **11**: 155–66.

Flora JD. A Method for comparing survival of burns patients to a standardised survival curve. *J Trauma* 1978; **18**: 701–5.

Gennarelli TA, Wodzin E (eds). *Abbreviated Injury Scale*. Barrington: Association for the Advancement of Automotive Medicine Publisher, 2005.

Gustafsson H, Nygren A, Tingvall C. *Rating System for Serious Consequences (RSC) due to traffic accidents, risks of death or permanent disability*, Proceedings, 10th International Conference on Experimental Safety Vehicles, Oxford, 1985.

Lefering R. Trauma scoring systems for quality assessment. *Eur J Trauma* 2002; **28**: 52–63.

MacKenzie EJ, Damiano A, Miller T, Luchter S. The development of the Functional Impairment Scale. *J Trauma* 1996; **41**(5): 799–807.

Murray CJL, Lopez AD (eds). *The Global Burden of Disease: a Comprehensive Assessment of Mortality and Disability from Diseases, Injuries and Risk Factors in 1990 and Projected to 2020*. Boston: Harvard School of Public Health, 1996.

National Academy of Sciences National Research Council. *Injury in America: a Continuing Public Health Problem*. Washington, DC: National Academy Press, 1985.

Osler T, Baker SP, Long WB. A modification of the Injury Severity Score that both improves accuracy and simplifies scoring. *J Trauma* 1997; **43**(6): 922–5.

Teasdale G, Jennett B. Assessment of coma and impaired consciousness. A practical scale. *Lancet* 1974; **13**: 81–4.

Yates DW. ABC of major trauma. Scoring systems for trauma. *Br Med J* 1990; **301**(6760): 1090–4.

541

Bariatric trauma

Introduction

Definitions

Obesity is defined by the World Health Organization as:

abnormal or excessive fat accumulation that presents a risk to health.

The Body Mass Index (BMI) is frequently used to define obesity and is calculated by a patient's weight (kg)/the square of their height (m). Normal BMI ranges from 18.5 to 25. A BMI of 25–30 is considered overweight and obesity is defined as a BMI of more that 30. Morbid obesity is defined as a BMI of 40 or greater.

Incidence

Approximately 25% of adults in the United Kingdom are obese and 2% are morbidly obese. The incidence of obesity is increasing and an understanding of the specific challenges of managing the obese traumatized patient is vital for trauma clinicians.

Epidemiology

Obesity has been shown to be an independent risk factor for mortality and multiple organ failure (MOF) following major trauma. Additionally, injury patterns differ between obese and non-obese patients. Obese patients are more likely to sustain thoracic trauma, as well as pelvic and extremity trauma compared with non-obese patients. Obese patients have been shown to sustain fewer, and less severe head injuries compared with non-obese patients. It is also a risk factor for knee dislocation, even after relatively minor trauma.

Pathophysiology

The physiology of obese patients differs from non-obese patients in a number of ways:

Respiratory

Obese patients have compromised respiratory function with reduced lung compliance. Increased chest wall resistance and increased abdominal pressure also impairs respiratory function. Obese patients are at increased risk of ARDS and pulmonary complications following trauma.

Cardiovascular

Obese patients are frequently hypertensive with an increased cardiac output and circulating volume. Myocardial hypertrophy and decreased compliance make the obese patient particularly vulnerable to changes in cardiovascular status following trauma.

Metabolic response

Glucose intolerance, insulin insensitivity, and increased resting energy expenditure are common in obese patients. In the catabolic phase following trauma obese patients have a relative block to lipolysis and fat oxidation resulting in a preferential shift to protein catabolism. Despite their excess of fat reserves, obese patients are unable to utilize these reserves and are particularly susceptible to metabolic derangement.

Nutrition

Despite their excess of adipose tissue, obese patients frequently have nutritional deficiencies. This has important implications for wound healing.

Co-morbidities

Obesity is frequently associated with other co-morbidities, such as ischaemic heart disease and diabetes, which will affect the management of traumatised obese patients. Associated co-morbidities are one reason why obese patients have higher mortality following major trauma.

Principles of management

The traumatised bariatric patient presents unique difficulties to clinicians. Movement of the patient is difficult, equipment often does not fit, and assessment of injuries is more challenging.

Pre-hospital care

Control of exsanguinating external haemorrhage

Massive haemorrhage must be rapidly controlled. Tourniquets may not fit obese limbs. Direct external compression of haemorrhage relies on compression of bleeding vessels against bony structures. This may be impossible with excess overlying adipose tissue and direct pressure may be insufficient. Application of haemostatic agents will be harder to apply to bleeding vessels due to substantial layers of overlying fat.

Airway with cervical spine control

Airway management is more difficult in the obese patient. Simple airway manoeuvres, such as a jaw thrust are harder to perform. Obesity is associated with obstructive sleep apnoea, which will predispose the obese patient with reduced consciousness to airway compromise. Gastro-oesophageal reflux is also more common in the obese patient, making airway protection particularly important and challenging. Laryngeal masks may not fit the anatomy of the obese patient and intubation is more demanding. Oesophageal intubation may be harder to detect and definitive airway protection may have to be deferred until arrival at the trauma centre. Surgical airway management will be extremely challenging in the obese patient with excess soft tissues obscuring the normal airway anatomy.

Cervical collars are designed to fit a variety of neck sizes. The morbidly obese patient may be too large for standard cervical collars carried by ambulance personnel and alternative methods of protecting the cervical spine may have to be employed.

Breathing and ventilation

Examination and assessment of the thorax is more challenging. Breath sounds may be harder to hear due to overlying soft tissue, tracheal displacement impossible to feel and symmetrical chest expansion harder to assess. The diagnosis of flail chest will be hard to detect. Needle thoracocentesis using a standard intravenous cannula may not be possible due to the depth of soft tissue covering the chest, so the use of a longer needle, such as a 16G spinal needle, may be required. Thoracostomy will also be more challenging due to overlying soft tissues, as will insertion of an intercostal drain.

Increased chest wall resistance and raised intra-abdominal pressure require increased airway pressures to ventilate the unconscious obese patient. This may predispose these patients to iatrogenic barotrauma.

Circulation with haemorrhage control

The obese patient is at high risk of underlying cardiac disease making assessment and management of haemorrhage particularly difficult. Obese patients will frequently have underlying hypertension and relative tachycardia, and this should be considered when assessing circulatory status following trauma.

Equipment may be too small for the obese patient. Thigh tourniquets may have to be used on the upper limb. Poor peripheral vascular access will make peripheral cannulation difficult. Transport of the traumatized obese patient should not be delayed for prolonged attempts at obtaining intravenous access. Other techniques of peripheral venous access such external jugular vein cannulation may have to be used. Venous cut down is particularly useful in the obese patient as the saphenous vein remains relatively superficial at the ankle despite more adipose tissue. Insertion of central venous lines and arterial lines will be challenging for the same reasons and skin hygiene may also be difficult to maintain around vascular devices.

Disability

Obese patients should be assessed for neurological dysfunction in the same way as any other patient. As stated, airway compromise may occur with less impairment of consciousness compared with non-obese patients, due to underlying obstructive sleep apnoea. Patients should be log rolled as normal, although extra staff may be required to safely log roll the obese patient.

Exposure

Obese patients are as susceptible to hypothermia as non-obese individuals. Every effort should be made to maintain the patient's core temperature prior to arrival at hospital. Extrication and transport of the obese patient will be extremely challenging. Entrapped obese patients are more likely to have prolonged entrapment times than non-obese patients. Early consideration should be given to requesting medical personnel with advanced pre-hospital trauma skills.

Once extricated, the transport of obese patients, particularly morbidly obese patients, will require considerable numbers of personnel. The use of helicopter transport may be precluded by the size of the morbidly obese individual and liaising with the ambulance control early will help determine the most appropriate mode of transfer to the trauma centre. All personnel should be familiar with manual handling techniques. Use of these techniques will be particularly important to prevent injury to those charged with moving and transporting the morbidly obese patient. Forewarning the receiving emergency department about the patient's size will allow extra manpower to be made available on arrival to hospital and will allow suitable trolleys and equipment to be prepared for use.

Care in the emergency department

All emergency departments should have rapid access to bariatric trolleys suitable for managing the obese patient. Standard emergency department (ED) trolleys have a weight limit of around 160 kg, whilst bariatric trolleys can carry up to 300 kg. Moving the morbidly obese patient from the confined space of an ambulance to the resuscitation room will be difficult. The use of additional staff, such as hospital security, to assist in transferring these patients should be employed.

The diagnostic challenges of the obese patient

Management in the ED should follow the standard approach as for any other patient. The identification of life-threatening complications during primary survey is more challenging in the obese patient. As stated previously, maintaining and protecting the airway and cervical spine is particularly challenging. The use of fibreoptic equipment to aid intubation is particularly useful. Examination of the thorax may give limited signs of life-threatening complications—breath sounds may be masked, asymmetrical chest movements may not be apparent, flail chest may not be visible, and thoracic wounds may be obscured by skin folds. Adequate standard chest radiography may not be possible and several attempts may be required to view the entire thorax. Overlying adipose tissue may mask subtle radiographic changes. Obese patients are at particular risk of thoracic injuries and respiratory complications following trauma. The insertion of an intercostal drain (ICoD) is performed using standard techniques, but the use of an assistant will be invaluable and is strongly advised. Standard needles may not penetrate sufficient depth for the administration of local anaesthesia and longer needles, such as a 16G spinal needle should be available. Positioning the ICoD in a skin fold may make subsequent skin hygiene more difficult to maintain. Where possible the ICoD should be inserted away from skin creases.

Identifying the source of haemorrhage

The obese patient will show the same features of haemorrhagic shock as the non-obese patient. However, obese patients often have underlying hypertension and relative tachycardia. This should be considered when making decisions about their circulatory status. Vascular access will be more challenging and venous cut downs or central venous access may be required. The use of ultrasound to identify peripheral veins is particularly useful to avoid these measures.

The obese patient displaying signs of haemorrhagic shock presents a unique diagnostic challenge. Efforts to identify the source, or sources, of haemorrhage will be more difficult. Clinical signs of haemothorax will be masked. The chest radiograph may be inadequate and subtle signs of thoracic haemorrhage may be masked. Examination of the obese abdomen will be harder to interpret than the non-obese abdomen. Tenderness will be harder to localize and bruising may be less apparent. Examination of the pelvis and long bones will also be more difficult.

Haemorrhagic shock in the presence of a pelvic fracture should be treated with a pelvic splint. Commercially available splints may not fit around the obese patient and a sheet tied firmly around the greater trochanters may be used instead. Another sheet should be applied around the legs holding the limbs in internal rotation. Femoral fractures should be treated with traction. In the absence of a suitably sized Thomas splint then skin traction can be used instead. Significant external haemorrhage should still be easy to identify. External haemorrhage from upper limbs should be treated with elevation and direct compression. The use of a thigh tourniquet may be required for the obese upper limb. Massive lower limb haemorrhage should also be treated with a tourniquet and the absence of a suitably large tourniquet may require one to be improvised, such as with a pelvic splint.

The obese patient with severe unresponsive haemorrhagic shock should proceed directly to the operating theatre in the same way that a non-obese patient would. Early involvement of senior surgeons will facilitate the appropriate surgical strategy to be employed to control massive haemorrhage. Forewarning theatres of the patient's size, in addition to the usual information, is particularly important in organizing a bariatric surgical table and other equipment.

Patients displaying enough haemodynamic stability to be further investigated should have further radiographic imaging. Focused Assessment with Sonography for Trauma (FAST) is usually an accurate and rapid way to identify intraperitoneal haemorrhage in shocked patients. The thick layers of adipose tissue in obese patients may prevent accurate images being obtained. This may preclude the use of FAST scans, particularly in the morbidly obese patient.

Computed tomography (CT) scans are particularly useful in identifying sources of haemorrhage in patients with appropriate haemodynamic stability. Obese patients present a particular challenge. The maximum table weight of most CT scanners is around 210 kg. Some regional centres have CT scanners designed for bariatric patients, although the transport considerations in the context of acute trauma are likely to prevent this. If it is logistically possible for the obese patient to be scanned this should proceed as rapidly as possible, as it would for the non-obese patient. Extra personnel will be required to physically move the patient on to the CT scanner and this is likely to take longer than normal. This makes it particularly important that the trauma team should accompany the patient to the CT scanner.

In the event that the morbidly obese patient cannot logistically be scanned, consideration should be made for the use of diagnostic peritoneal lavage (DPL). Use of DPL in identifying intra-abdominal haemorrhage has been largely superseded by FAST and early CT scanning, but it may continue to have a role where CT scanning is not possible.

The obese patient with haemodynamic stability following trauma should have a secondary survey as usual. Injuries are harder to identify than in non-obese patients. Injuries frequently missed include carpal and finger fractures, and soft tissue knee injuries. A tertiary survey should be performed the following day to minimize the risk of delayed diagnosis of injuries.

Definitive management

As for all patients, planning the definitive management in the obese patient will depend largely on the injuries sustained. All injuries should be identified as early as possible and prioritized accordingly. In the context of multiple trauma, communication and planning between different clinical specialities is particularly important. Ideally, this multidisciplinary co-ordination should commence as soon as the patient arrives at hospital. The obese patient is likely to have other co-morbidities and less physiological reserve compared with non-obese individuals. Clinicians should have a low threshold for adopting a damage control approach to the management of these patients.

Multiply-injured obese patients are likely to require critical care support. Co-morbidities should be identified and addressed as soon as possible, if necessary liaising with the patient's general practitioner. Obese patients are likely to have poor respiratory function and are at higher risk of acute respiratory distress syndrome (ARDS) compared with non-obese patients. Adequate analgesia following thoracic trauma is particularly important in this patient group and early consideration should be made about the use of regional anaesthesia. The conscious patient should be able to cough up their sputum and respiratory physiotherapy is particularly useful in preventing respiratory complications. Such complications should be identified and treated as early as possible.

Obese patients are also at particular risk of venous thrombo-embolism, in part due to their relative immobility. Appropriate prophylaxis should be used, unless contraindicated. Early mobilization should be initiated wherever possible. The size of the obese patient presents a considerable challenge to nursing staff. Patients should be nursed on an appropriate bariatric bed. Obese patients are at particular risk of skin complications, particularly unconscious or immobile patients. Prevention, identification, and management of pressure sores are made more difficult by their physical size. At risk patients should be nursed on the appropriate mattresses and extra staff may have to be made available by ward managers to facilitate regular turning of patients.

Fracture management in the bariatric patient

The obese patient poses a particular challenge to the orthopaedic trauma surgeon. Surgical exposure of fractures is particularly difficult. Standard implant designs may not be strong enough to withstand the additional body weight of the obese patient. This is more likely if the obese patient is unable to keep their body weight off a lower limb fracture with the use of crutches. If surgical fixation of a fracture is necessary, implant selection should be influenced by the extra forces that the implant must withstand prior to fracture union. For example, a large solid nail may be preferable to a small cannulated nail. The obese patient is equally at risk of compartment syndrome and this complication should be actively excluded, particularly in the unconscious patient. Plaster casts are harder to apply and the obese patient is at particular risk of skin complications beneath the plaster. Care should be taken to pad skin areas at risk and folds and finger prints in the plaster avoided. Standard orthotic devices such as Thoracic-Lumbar-Sacral orthosis (TLSO) may not fit and alternatives may have to be sought.

Nutritional assessment.

Despite their normal dietary calorific excess, obese patients are at risk of malnutrition. This may influence wound healing following trauma. Following major trauma the obese patient has a relative block to lipolysis and fat oxidation resulting in a preferential shift to protein catabolism. The multiply-injured obese patient should have their nutritional status assessed as part of their definitive care and the involvement of a dietician may be particularly useful. Strategies for affecting long-term weight loss should also be considered when the patient is recovering from their injuries.

Key points

- The incidence of bariatric patients sustaining major trauma will increase in the next decade.
- Standard equipment may not fit the obese patient and appropriate bariatric equipment should be readily available to clinicians involved in trauma management.
- Forewarning colleagues of the patient's size allows appropriate equipment to be prepared.
- Management should follow established trauma protocols. However, it should be recognized that these patients present a significant diagnostic and therapeutic challenge to trauma practitioners. Timely senior clinical involvement is essential.
- Bariatric patients are more likely to have underlying co-morbidities and are at higher risk of morbidity and mortality following trauma. These risks should be identified and steps taken to minimize them following trauma.

Further reading

Belzberg H, Wo CCJ, Demetriades D, Shoemaker WC. Effects of age and obesity on hemodynamics, tissue oxygenation, and outcome after trauma. *J Trauma* 2007; **62**:1192–1200.

Bochicchio GV, Joshi M, Bochicchio K, Nehman S, Tracy JK, Scalea TM. Impact of obesity in the critically ill trauma patient: a prospective study. *J Am Coll Surg* 2006; **203**: 533–8.

Brown CVR, Neville AL, Rhee P, Salim A, Velmahos GC, Demetriades D. The impact of obesity on the outcomes of 1,153 critically injured blunt trauma patients. *J Trauma* 2005; **59**: 1048–51.

Brown CVR, Velmahos GC. The consequences of obesity on trauma, emergency surgery, and critical care. *Wld J Surg* 2006; **1**: 27.

Christmas AB, Reynolds J, Wilson AK, Franklin GA, Miller FB, Richardson JD, et al. Morbid obesity impacts mortality in blunt trauma. *Am Surgeon* 2007; **73**: 1122–5.

Ciesla DJ, Moore EE, Johnson JL, Burch JM, Cothren CC, Sauaia A. Obesity increases risk of organ failure after severe trauma. *J Am Coll Surgeons* 2006; **203**: 539–45.

Dossett LA, Heffernan D, Lightfoot M, Collier B, Diaz JJ, Sawyer RG, et al. Obesity and pulmonary complications in critically injured adults. *Chest* 2008; **134**: 974–80.

Duane TM, Dechert T, Aboutanos MB, Malhotra AK, Ivatury RR. Obesity and outcomes after blunt trauma. *J Trauma* 2006; **61**: 1218–21.

Jeevanandam M, Young DH, Schiller WR. Obesity and the metabolic response to severe multiple trauma in man. *Am Soc Clin Invest* 1991; **87**: 262–9.

Joffe A, Wood K. Obesity in critical care. *Curr Opin Anaesthesiol* 2007; **20**:113–18.

Neville AL, Brown CVR, Weng J, Demetriades D, Velmahos GC. Obesity is an independent risk factor of mortality in severely injured blunt trauma patients. *Arch Surg* 2004; **139**: 983–7.

Zhu S, Layde PM, Huse CE, Laud PW, Pintar F, Nirula R, et al. Obesity and risk for death due to motor vehicle crashes. *Am J Publi Hlth* 2006; **96**: 734–9.

Major incidents

Definitions and context

The Civil Contingencies Act 2004 defines a major incident in the United Kingdom as:

> An event or a situation which threatens serious damage to human welfare in a place in the UK, the environment of a place in the UK, or war or terrorism which threatens serious damage to the security of the UK.

In general, a health major incident is considered to be one where the location, number, severity, or type of live casualties requires special operational arrangements to manage the situation. This has evolved to encompass a much wider range of situations for response and the current Department of Health for England guidance defines one as:

> Any occurrence that presents serious threat to the health of the community, disruption to the service or causes (or is likely to cause) such numbers or types of casualties as to require special arrangements to be implemented by hospitals, ambulance trusts or primary care organizations.

In most minds, a major incident follows a sudden event such as an explosion or train crash. Using this broader definition, a much wider range of events need to be included:

- *Big Bang:* a significant transport incident or industrial explosion, the traditionally understood major incident.
- *CBRN (Chemical, Biological, Chemical, Nuclear):* an event where casualties have been contaminated.
- *Rising Tide:* a developing event such as an infectious disease epidemic, or a capacity or staffing crisis.
- *Cloud on the Horizon:* a serious threat such as a major chemical or radiation leak elsewhere that requires preparatory action.
- *Headline News:* public or media generated alarm about a threat to health.
- *Internal incident:* a fire, flood, or loss of utilities (electrical power or water) in a health facility.

There is a plethora of other ways to divide and categorize major incidents, depending on the purpose. An effort has been made to standardize such an approach using an Utstein style by the World Association for Disaster and Emergency Medicine (WADEM). Here, a number are outlined to give the reader a perspective on the different ways of considering such incidents.

Natural/man-made

Earthquakes and volcanic eruptions, whilst not typically a UK phenomenon, are at the extreme end of the natural spectrum. Also included are weather events such as hurricanes and flooding, and even a heavy snowfall may mandate a major incident response by the health system.

The man-made potential is far more wide ranging:

- *Transport:*
  - aeroplane crash;
  - ferry capsize;
  - train crash;
  - road traffic collision.
- *Industrial:*
  - mass gathering;
  - football stadium;
  - air show.

- Public demonstration.
- Terrorism.

Simple/compound

The health system is required to have a planned and prepared for response to a major incident and, if the response infrastructure remains intact, then the sequence of events should follow the expected 'simple' course.

In contrast, if the infrastructure is damaged in some way, then the incident is 'compound'. Examples might include disruption to part of the road network by flooding, radio communication failure, or even loss of hospital facilities, e.g. University Hospital New Orleans, USA (Fig. 33.1), 2005, or Musgrave Park Hospital bombing, Belfast, Northern Ireland, 1991.

Compensated/uncompensated

A compensated incident is one where, once the special arrangements are in place, the response is considered to be sufficient. The patient load can be managed by the capacity available.

In an uncompensated incident, the patient load exceeds the capacity that can be created. Under these circumstances, care standards will need to be adjusted and some injured may not be able to receive the care they would receive under normal circumstances. In an international natural catastrophe such as the Indian Ocean tsunami in 2004, this is something readily comprehended.

Size of incident

In many texts, the terms major incident, mass casualty incident, disaster, and catastrophe are used almost interchangeably.

In UK emergency planning terms, the numbers of people involved is specified (Table 33.1):

Considering the most significant major incidents in the UK to date, the numbers injured have never been on a scale that could be considered beyond 'Major' by this definition. Other countries have not been so fortunate; the Bali nightclub bombing (202 dead, 300 injured), the attack on the World Trade Centre (2993 dead, 8700 injured).

Surge capacity

This is defined as the ability of the health system to expand beyond its normal capacity to meet an increased demand for clinical care. Under these circumstances, the use of rationing in terms of the interventions that might be applicable, or the amount and duration of care that can be delivered may become necessary. There are some basic principles that apply to such a situation:

- The care that is given when resources and capability are finite should be maximized.
- The change to clinical standards should be incremental, and reflect both local demand and the resources available.
- The application of the plan should be consistent with the aim to preserve and maintain essential health services.
- The changes should be consistent with established and agreed ethical principles.
- The whole health system should be engaged in the management of the surge.

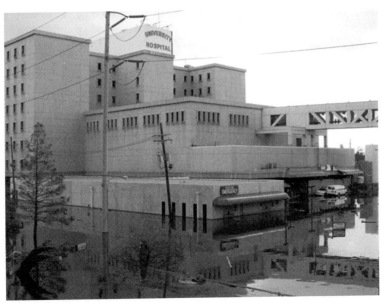

Fig. 33.1. University Hospital New Orleans, 2005. A compound incident.

Implicit in these principles is a strategic perspective on the health response and a decision on adjusting care standards needs to come from this level. The health command hierarchy is described later.

Any decision to implement a surge plan, together with its potential consequences, is likely to come under intense scrutiny at a later stage and so it is vital that the level of the altered standard of care is consistently applied, and that both the decision-making process and the identity of the decision makers is recorded. The information that was available to them at the time of the decision is key to justifying it.

Incident response and the 'science'

With the broad range of potential major incidents, most planning is now based on an All Hazards approach. Health major incident plans are generic and can be applied to any form of incident. Adaptation to specific circumstances will be necessary, but the core approach is always the same. In the UK, a Medallion Command System is applied and this will be outlined in the section to follow. In North America, the National Incident Management System (NIMS) is used.

Having made the generic All Hazard assertion, a number of incidents are still regarded as needing specific supplemental guidance. Examples include:
- Paediatrics.
- Critical care.

Table 33.1. NHS incident size definition

NHS level	Number of casualties
Major	10's
Mass	100's
Catastrophic	1000's

- Major burns.
- CBRN.

The current state of these examples illustrates the nature of major incident response planning. There has been little science involved in the design of major incident response; most aspects are based on previous experience and expert opinion. Case reports, the outcome of formal enquiries and the output from various levels of exercise are the best sources of information available. The WADEM Utstein template and the Haddon Matrix are examples of the efforts being made towards disaster science and its evolution. There will never be the possibility of carrying out randomized controlled trials for disaster response.

Legal and statutory oversight

Those that fail to plan, plan to fail.

The Civil Contingencies Act 2004 makes failure of organizations a criminal offence for their responsible officers. The Emergency Planning Guidance is quite clear that the Management Boards and Chief Executives of health organizations have a duty to ensure that their organizations are properly prepared to respond to a major incident. A live exercise should be carried out at least as often as every third year, a suitable table-top exercise should happen every year and a communication cascade assessment should take place every 6 months.

In terms of a license to operate as an NHS organization, the Performance Management Framework includes, as Core Standard 24, an assessment of the level of emergency preparedness, which states that the organization must 'protect the public by having a planned, prepared and, where possible, practised response to incidents and emergency situations which could affect the provision of normal services'. This was reported annually as part of the

Healthcare Commission review of each organization, but this has now transferred to the Care Quality Commission. It has since been toughened; the phrase 'where possible' has been removed and it is now explicitly stated that plans must be 'tested and practised'.

Phases of a major incident

A Major Incident can be considered to be in three phases:
• Preparation.
• Response.
• Recovery.

Preparation

This covers the planning and training of all responders for an event. Whilst the approach is All Hazard, there is an obligation to address specific local risks. If the catchment area of the particular organization includes an airport or an industrial complex then efforts to ensure that an appropriate response can be mounted to an event of this sort are expected. Exercises that specifically involve these risks are expected.

Response

When a major incident is declared, emergency plans are initiated. In the UK, the common parlance for response has evolved to consider the acronym CSCATTT:
• Command.
• Safety.
• Communication.
• Assessment.
• Triage.
• Treatment.
• Transport.

Each component is described in the sections to follow.

Recovery

The dramatic part of a major incident is typically quite short; major incident scenes in the UK over the last 30 years have been cleared of all live casualties within 4 h. The implications of the Recovery Phase for the health system may last weeks to months. The Coroners' Inquests, public inquiry, and legal proceedings may last for years after the event. The late psychological consequences to those involved as casualties and also as responders may be present for decades.

Scientific advice to the emergency services

In a major incident, the responding emergency services frequently need specialist scientific advice. There have been a plethora of acronyms for this centrally administered resource. The Joint Health Advisory Cell (JHAC) became the Health Advice Team (HAT). This has now been subsumed into the Science and Technical Advisory Cell (STAC).

This cell is formed to support and inform the higher echelons of the command system, at the Strategic Co-ordinating Centre. The composition will be tailored to the local event requirements, and will aim to provide scientific and technical advice. It will almost always include specialists in health, the environment, and site specific response concerns. Examples of the latter might include the Meteorological Office and the Health and Safety Executive in industrial incidents, and the Government Decontamination Service and the Food Standards Agency where there is contamination and a risk to food safety. Utility companies and transport operators may also need to be engaged. Many of these organizations are considered to be Category 2 responders under the Civil Contingences Act and have a statutory duty to support the incident response where appropriate.

Command and control

It is normal to consider the command and control issues in the context of a 'Big Bang' event. The structure and systems that apply can then be transferred to a more protracted 'Rising Tide' or potential 'Cloud on the Horizon' event.

By the very nature of a major incident, there is chaos and confusion during the first few minutes and the responding emergency services need to function on autopilot. This is managed by the presence of Action Cards in emergency plans. A detailed understanding is not required; a person adopts an identified role and follows the list of instructions in sequence.

The Achilles heel of any response is the recognition that a major incident has occurred. In retrospect, this is often very evident, but the sooner an incident is declared, the more rapidly systems can be mobilized and receiving facilities given sufficient time to prepare to receive an influx of injured. Action cards tend to have 'Declare a Major Incident' as the first action.

Command is a vertical transmission of authority and instruction. Whilst command is a clear concept to the Police and Fire Service, it is not a natural system in the health service where individual clinicians are typically accountable for their actions on a patient by patient basis. In the environment of a major incident, a command hierarchy is essential.

The first health resource responding is typically from the ambulance service. Action Cards for these personnel require them to take a command role and, rather than move into the scene and begin to care for the injured, begin to lay the foundations of an organizational framework for dealing with the incident. This includes assuming the title of 'Ambulance Incident Commander' or AIC, and liaising with their counterparts in the other responding services, the Police Incident Commander and Fire Incident Commander.

Medallion command system

The UK incident command system is based on a medallion structure. In the latest guidance, these titles have been altered to reflect their specific role:
- Gold = strategic.
- Silver = tactical.
- Bronze = operational.

Strategic command

Gold is 'Strategic' command and has overall command of the resources from their own organization, and is usually remote from the scene of the incident. Local decisions are delegated to the 'Tactical' (Silver) command at the scene of the incident. In a complex or large scale incident there is a need to ensure that there is co-ordination of the wider health response, recruitment of mutual aid from adjacent health providers, maintenance of logistic supply to the scene, and also maintaining the business continuity of services to other areas, whilst the system is focused on responding to the local events (Fig. 33.2)

The civil response to an incident may require the integration of a much wider group of organizations than the emergency services, including the Local Authority, Environment Agency, and even Utility Companies. This Strategic Co-ordinating Group (SCG) is brought together and typically chaired by the Police. It operates on a geographical basis, often defined by the Police Constabulary boundary. If an event is of sufficient magnitude that a number of SCGs are formed, then a Regional Civil Contingencies Committee (RCCC) will convene to oversee this.

In turn, this will communicate vertically to the Major Incident Co-ordination Centre (MICC) at the Department of Health Emergency Planning Division and, through them, to the Cabinet Office Briefing Room (COBR) and the Civil Contingencies Committee (CCC).

Military aid

In the event of a major incident where there is considerable threat to life, the emergency services can call upon the support of the military through arrangements termed Military Aid to the Civil Community (MACC). A decision to request this support belongs to the SCG.

There are some core principles that apply to the request for Military Aid to the Civilian Authority (MACA).
- Mutual aid capacity and civil resources are anticipated to be insufficient or have been exhausted e.g. regional flooding.
- The Civil Authority lacks the capability, e.g. explosive ordnance disposal.
- There is capability but the speed with which it is required cannot be met, e.g. search and rescue and logistic supply.

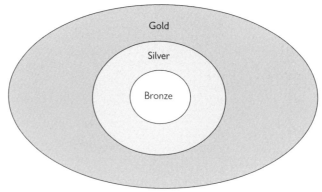

Fig. 33.2. Command circles.

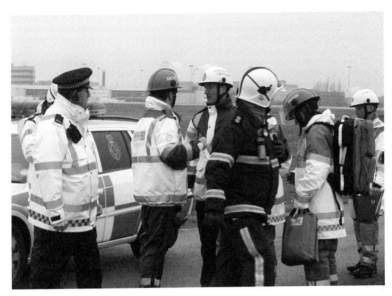

Fig. 33.3. Scene command team.

Tactical command

The term Tactical or Silver is used to define the command level that will attend the scene of the incident, take charge, oversee, and be responsible for managing the local plan. They will usually be supported by a command vehicle and specific resources for this role.

The Tactical Commanders for the attending emergency services should act together as a Scene or Incident Command Team, identify the cordons for security and safety, and determine the flow in and out of the scene area for responding vehicles. The flow direction for evacuation and management of casualties should also be defined. Whilst the detail will be defined by local geography, such as the availability of buildings and the nature of the road network, the structure is fairly clear.

The tactical commander for health is the Ambulance Incident Commander or AIC. He or she should be supported by a Medical Incident Commander (MIC). This person should be a clinician who is trained for the role, and is able to give a perspective on the clinical needs of the casualties, understands the resource limitations of the environment, and can advise the AIC on appropriate management and evacuation planning.

While specific training for such a command role is a requirement for the other emergency services, such formal training and accreditation for the health response is not yet available. The appointments are usually a consequence of the officer's experience and local knowledge. This is currently an area for competency determination and educational development.

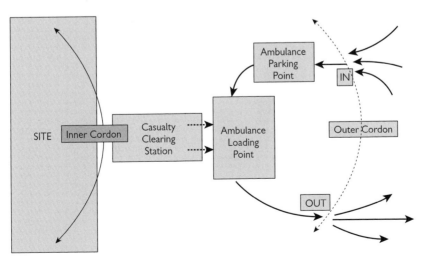

Fig. 33.4. Cordons at a major incident.

Operational command

The AIC and MIC roles are hands-off positions (Fig. 33.3). An incident may be divided into a number of different sectors, such as individual train carriages in a rail incident, and a command element may be needed to move forward into the scene to inform the command structure. These Forward AICs will deliver the tactics defined by the Scene Commanders.

There are a number of other operational ambulance command appointments that help to manage the response. In purely operational terms, an Ambulance Parking Officer manages the parking and flow of the ambulances, an Ambulance Loading Officer oversees the evacuation of the casualties from the Casualty Clearing Station. There is typically a Health and Safety Officer to ensure that all reasonable steps to mitigate the risk of further injury are being taken.

At the Casualty Clearing Station there should be an officer overseeing the on-going triage and delivery of clinical care to the injured, whilst awaiting evacuation. This is likely to be the base for the majority of the medical assets working at scene and often a medical officer is required to support this element of the command structure and ensure that only appropriate clinical interventions are provided.

Safety

The scene of a major incident will be an environment with inherent hazards that pose a risk to rescuers. Basic pre-hospital emergency medicine principles apply; the Safety 1-2-3. Personal safety must be considered, then that of the scene, before finally addressing the safety of the survivors (both casualties and the involved, but not injured).

Personal safety

Employers have an obligation under Health and Safety legislation to minimize the risk to their staff in the pursuance of their duties. The effect of this can be seen through the evolution of PPE worn by staff entering an environment over the last few years (Fig. 33.5).

A reflective jacket was all that was considered necessary 25 years ago. Now a responder would not be allowed to enter an emergency scene without (Fig. 33.6):

- Kevla® type protective helmet.
- Face visor.
- High visibility jacket.
- Flame retardant overall.
- Rubber gloves and debris gloves.
- Steel toe-capped and chemical resistant boots.
- Personal issue radiation detector/dosimeter (when applicable).

Whilst the level of equipment that ought to be worn is subject to a dynamic risk assessment, where the member of staff makes a judgement about the level of personal protection that they should be wearing, the responder should be able to achieve the full level of protection that might be necessary.

Where a hazard, such as a toxic environment, potentially exists, the expectation and the basic training is to withdraw to a safe position and call for a higher level of protection. The 'Stay Out, Get Out, Call HART' principle, where HART is the Hazardous Area Response Team, is the norm.

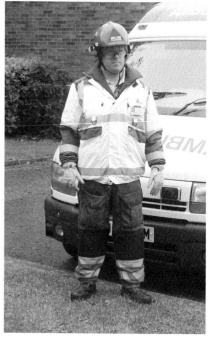

Fig. 33.6. New style PPE.

Scene safety

As part of the command assessment of the scene and the planning for management by the Scene Command Team, a security (Silver) cordon and a safety (Bronze) cordon are defined and entry to each is controlled. If there is a fire,

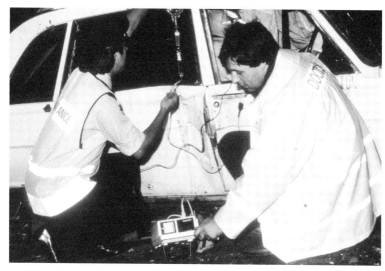

Fig. 33.5. Old style PPE.

chemical, or radiation hazard, the Inner Cordon will be secured by the Fire Service; in a terrorist or firearms incident the Police may control the cordon.

Once it has been deemed safe to enter the incident scene, the rescuers can begin to attend to those involved.

This description assumes that the scene can be contained. In a terrorist explosion, for example, those involved and still able to walk will self-evacuate and scatter in all directions. It is unlikely that a cordon to contain a large number of people could be drawn in sufficient time to control the event. Those with injuries may move directly to a local hospital and the receiving staff will need to make a judgement about levels of contamination, and whether it is safe to approach and treat those involved without decontamination at the point of contact.

Casualty safety

Those casualties involved in a major incident may be affected by a number of unknowns. To date, there have been many examples of chemical contamination affecting both casualties and rescuers. Bio-hazards, including body fluids from those injured or deceased, and spread by an explosive force, and the contents of toilets on trains or aircraft, are a theoretical risk to all. To date, there has not been a significant issue with radiation contamination, but it is surely only a matter of time before this occurs and decontamination of all involved may become necessary.

Communication

Communication both within the scene between different levels of command and between the emergency services at a major incident, and from the scene to the remote command chain is vital to the smooth running of a 'simple' major incident response. This is also includes communication from the scene to the identified receiving hospitals.

There have been serial examples of communication systems failing at the scene of a major incident. Radio systems are often overwhelmed by the volume of traffic and do not have universal coverage. Whilst the standard VHF and more local UHF radio systems have been the standard for several decades, a new digital radio network, termed Airwave, is currently being introduced by all the emergency services in the UK. Based upon the TETRA (TErrestrial Trunked RAdio) standard, it has been designed with multiple layers of redundancy and, once fully operational, should allow full inter-service communication.

As part of this evolution, well-known communication black-spots, such as tunnels, are also being addressed. Over the summer of 2009, a system that allows Airwave radio communication throughout the London Underground system was introduced.

In recent years, the emergency services have become increasingly dependent upon the use of mobile phone cellular technology. Since familiarity with radio procedure and comfort with this form of slightly cumbersome communication is a time consuming skill, the emergency services have become quite dependent on mobile telephone technology. Telephone conversation is far less taxing for the communicator.

The danger of this dependency has been shown serially in the analysis of communication difficulties in a major incident. The mobile phone network is limited in the amount of communication traffic that it can carry and becomes overloaded. Under these conditions, mobile phones are unable to access the network and communication is not possible.

A system was developed, termed ACCOLC (ACCess Over-Load Class), where specified mobile phone cell areas could be closed to all but pre-registered (and so priority) mobile phone traffic. This option was managed centrally and, because rather clumsy, has never really been shown to work effectively in practice. The system is being changed to MTPAS (Mobile Telecommunications Privileged Access System) where there is more local control of the priority SIM cards for the Entitled Organizations by the Local Resilience Forum.

In any event, the technological solutions can fail and the old style runner system may be required. To avoid the Chinese Whispers phenomenon, messages should ideally be written.

Public messages

Megaphone delivered messages to groups of newly arrived responders, gatherings of survivors, and to the general public may be an effective means of conveying information. It should be remembered that this method does run the risk of miscommunication and misunderstanding.

The media

The 24-h news organizations have become incredibly effective at communicating details of an evolving emergency situation over the airwaves, both by radio and television (Fig. 33.7). It is quite possible that news reporting, particularly live from the scene, may give vital information to the more remote commanders and to the wider health response before the normal communication channels can generate a properly informed report.

While responders tend to shy away from the media, if not given access to the information that they feel they need, the media will find its own way of getting news. All access to the media should be handled by the command hierarchy and through the Police. Any statements or information given out should be checked for accuracy and approved in advance. Allowing free questioning of the spokesperson may be unwise until the full facts are known.

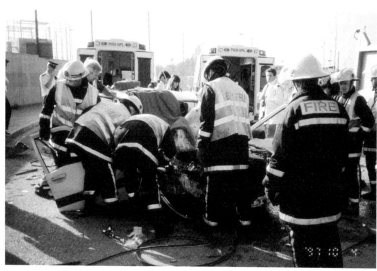

Fig. 33.7. Real time images via the media.

Assessment

Initial report

On arrival at the scene of a major incident, an assessment of the nature and scale of the incident needs to be made. This will determine the response mounted by the emergency services. There are two commonly used acronyms: METHANE and CHALET.

- M: Major incident declared or standby.
- E: Exact location.
- T: Type of incident.
- H: Hazards present and potential.
- A: Access, the direction of approach.
- N: Numbers of casualties, with nature and type.
- E: Emergency services present and required.

- C: Casualties.
- H: Hazards.
- A: Access.
- L: Location.
- E: Emergency services range and commitment.
- T: Type of incident.

The most important aspect of using such an acronym is that it is comprehensive, and both the sender and recipient of the message understand the structure of the report. Sending this information as a first report from scene will allow the system to determine an appropriate and proportionate response.

Report refinement and cascade

As the response becomes established, more information becomes available about the scale and type of the incident, and more experienced and trained commanders arrive at the incident scene, a more detailed analysis of the situation will be made.

The level of resources to be brought to the scene will depend on the nature of the event and number of people involved. The AIC and MIC will need to decide how the casualties are going to be managed and to where they are to be evacuated. Hospitals will be notified and information sought on the numbers of injured that can be received.

Local knowledge by the commanders of the capability and specialist skills of the surrounding hospitals will be important in determining how far the activation process radiates from the scene. In an incident involving major burns, the cascade may need to go as far as the National Burn Bed Bureau, beginning the search for dedicated burn

bed capacity around the UK. A similar process may be necessary if there are significant numbers of critically injured children through the intensive care networks.

Medical asset roles

Traditionally, a Mobile Medical Team might have been brought to the scene from the local Emergency Department. The latest emergency planning guidance recommends that a dedicated medical asset, administered by the ambulance service, termed a MERIT (Medical Emergency Response Incident Team), drawn from across the region rather than from a specific location, is mobilized. These personnel should be familiar with the pre-hospital environment, have trained for it, and come both equipped and prepared for the environment of the Casualty Clearing Station and possibly forward into the scene of the incident as deemed necessary by the Tactical Commanders, the AIC and MIC.

The number and type of response from the MERIT will need to be determined by the nature of the incident. There are a number of different potential roles:

- *Casualty clearing station:* medical and nursing staff to assist the ambulance crews with the delivery of care in a relatively controlled environment.

- *At the scene:* pre-hospital emergency medicine skilled medical staff to go forward to support the paramedics in the wreckage with the management and extrication of the injured.

- *Clearing from scene:* not all those involved in a major incident are physically injured and so do not need transfer to hospital. Clinical review and discharge from scene to the care of the Police may be an appropriate disposition.

- *Diagnosis of death:* it may be necessary for a doctor to be assigned to work with a Police Officer and officially diagnose death on those who have perished in the major incident, ensuring that the time of determination and location are properly recorded.

- *Special teams:* the National Burn Plan calls for specialist skills in the form of a BAT (Burns Assessment Team) to be made available. This team of specialist practitioners may be best deployed to the designated receiving hospitals, but there may be circumstances where their deployment to support the medical staff in the CCS may be beneficial, allowing for the direct transfer of seriously burned patients directly to burn units around the country.

Triage

The sorting of casualties into priority for both treatment and evacuation is necessary in a resource constrained environment. When there are more injured people needing assistance than there are resources to provide care, then some form of prioritization is necessary. It is a dynamic process, in that the operational situation and the clinical state of the casualties involved are constantly changing; the process must retain the flexibility to accommodate these changes. The process should occur serially; at the incident scene, at entry into the Casualty Clearing Station (Front Triage), out of the CCS (Rear Triage) and again on arrival at the hospital entry point.

Triage sieve

There are many ways that triage can be achieved. To be acceptable, it is important that it can be done quickly, reliably, and reproducibly. A number of systems have been described, but the Sieve and Sort approach (described by the MIMMS programme) where an initial screen is applied at the point of first contact, and then a second and more detailed review of status is performed at a later stage, has become the UK standard.

The current first look, primary triage (or Sieve) is based upon START (Simple Treatment and Rapid Triage; Fig. 33.8).

This is based on a principle that each patient can be reviewed in under 30 s, and a rapid feel for the number and severity of the injured provided for the incident command team, to allow them to make decisions about resources required to respond to the incident and begin to make plans for the evacuation.

There are a variety of documentation systems for labelling the casualties and there is a danger of the process losing sight of its purpose in discussion about the best way to do this. Examples of these include the use of coloured clothes pegs, the SMART tag, and the Cambridge Cruciform System (Fig. 33.9). Each has an increasing level of complexity, but the principle is the same.

Children and triage

In terms of children, there is a need to accommodate the weight or size of the child, and the differences in their physiology. This is difficult to do in a hurry and from recall. The generally accepted approach is to use the standard START algorithm, but with a sizing tape (Fig. 33.10) with different physiological parameters for respiratory rate and pulse rate for different sizes of children marked on it.

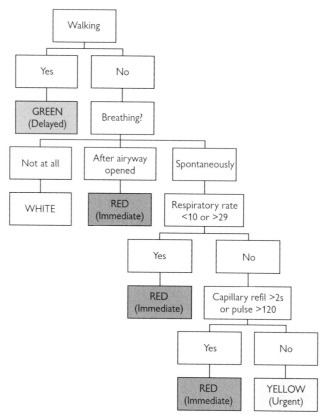

Fig. 33.8. Triage Sieve based on START.

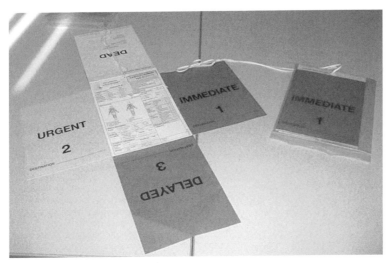

Fig. 33.9. Cambridge Cruciform triage label.

T1 hold

In the military context, an additional category of 'Immediate, but no intervention' has been described. In principle, this is for those circumstances where there are too many critically-injured for the system to cope and the 'Immediate' category needs to be subdivided. Essentially, this means 'too sick to receive treatment at the current time' and so these casualties are put to one side in the evacuation chain. In a civilian environment this is contrary to all the current principles of clinical practise, and has never been formally used or tested in a Coroner's Court. While the concept is a useful one to consider, any decision to introduce such a category needs to come from the senior command level within the incident and is certainly not one for the operational personnel within the scene.

Triage sort

Once the casualties have had an initial screen, and the numbers and severity of injured have been determined, a more detailed and clinically informed process can be applied.

There are various systems for determining severity of injury. Some are anatomical in origin; these tend to be used *post-hoc* when the full details of the injuries are known. The Injury Severity Score (ISS) is one such method. At the scene of an incident the casualty's physiological status at that point is a more available source of information and can be used to inform decision-making. There are different systems, but all are based on the use of simple physiological parameters; the pulse rate, respiratory rate, systolic blood pressure, Glasgow Coma Scale (GCS), and also, sometimes, the oxygen saturation as determined by pulse oximetry. Each variable has a different predictive value for severity of injury and the different systems weight them to allow for this. The more common ones all use the respiratory rate, systolic blood pressure and GCS. In the UK, the most common form is the TRTS (Triage Revised Trauma Score; Table 33.2).

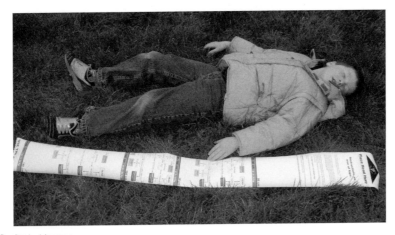

Fig. 33.10. Paediatric sizing tape.

Table 33.2. Triage Revised Trauma Score

Physiological variable	Measured value	Score
Respiratory rate	10–29	4
	>29	3
	6–9	2
	1–5	1
	0	0
Systolic blood pressure	>90	4
	76–89	3
	50–75	2
	1–49	1
	0	0
Glasgow Coma Scale	13–15	4
	9–12	3
	6–8	2
	4–5	1
	3	0

This table can then be used to assign a more refined triage category to each casualty (Table 33.3).

Triage to this extent is a laborious process at a time when clinicians are at full stretch trying to provide care to the injured. The need to leave one patient to attend to another who is more severely injured is difficult for carers, but the use of an objective tool can make it easier for them to make the decision.

Table 33.3. TRTS category

Priority	TRTS
T1	1–10
T2	11
T3	12
Dead	0

Triage inaccuracy

The reality is that emergency responders understand the principles of triage, but often fail to follow the process, allowing other factors to influence their decision-making. The less injured casualties will often not comply with evacuation decisions, preferring to stay with their friends and relatives who may be more severely injured. It is not reasonable to expect a parent to leave their more severely injured child to follow the predetermined evacuation chain. This requires the system to rigorously apply the triage decisions, but allow for some flexibility in terms of the nature and timing of the evacuation.

Over the last 20 years that the triage principle has been established in emergency plans as a clinical approach to a major incident, there have been few occasions where the system has been consistently and reliably applied. In the 1990s, responders rarely applied the system, although more recently triage has been shown to take place and influence the evacuation decisions. Analysis has shown that there is consistent over-triage, where responders put the injured in a more urgent category than warranted.

The use of a 2 × 2 Triage Table (Table 33.4) allows for sensitivity and specificity analyses to take place between both different triage systems and different incidents. For example, START based on capillary refill has a sensitivity of 85% and a specificity of 86% but using the Manchester Triage System Sieve with pulse rate the sensitivity is 45% and specificity 88%.

Inaccurate triage potentially means that resources are not distributed in an optimal manner and, further down the evacuation chain, people are evacuated to hospital in an order that may not benefit the most severely injured.

Likewise, analysis of incidents shows how significant field triage decisions can be in a potentially resource constrained environment. An over-triage rate of 64%, as happened in some locations of the London bombings in 2005, would potentially cause major issues if hospital resources were overwhelmed.

Table 33.4. 2 × 2 Triage Table

	Critically injured	Non-critically injured
Higher priority	Correct high triage	Incorrect high triage (OVER-TRIAGE)
Lower priority	Incorrect low priority (UNDER-TRIAGE)	Correct low triage

Treatment

Care provided at the scene of a major incident is, by the nature of such an incident, relatively limited. There are various levels of care:

- Bystander first aid.
- Simple treatment at the scene.
- Casualty clearing station interventions.

Many members of the public have received some level of training, and often health care providers are involved, but not injured; both groups will begin to provide assistance to the injured. Simple interventions such as opening the airway of an unconscious patient or applying a pressure dressing to a bleeding wound in the first few minutes can be life-saving.

Once the emergency services begin to arrive and the incident organizational structure begins to form, the injured will be moved to the CCS. The treatment in this environment is designed to be a holding measure, but part of this, as described above, is a more detailed triage process designed to identify those who have occult injuries. In addition, there are interventions that may adjust the triage category, often lowering the priority and allowing a more intelligent sieving of those who cannot be stabilized in the field.

Treatment in the CCS

The level of intervention in the CCS depends on the clinical skill set of those staffing it. Historically this was provided by a Mobile Medical Team (MMT) drawn from the local hospital. As response systems became more evolved, it was recognized that this would deplete the medical resources in the nearest hospital at the time of greatest need and so the resource was to be taken from a facility further away. The level of skill and experience was still potentially highly variable.

Under the Emergency Planning Guidance 2005, the concept of a MERIT was introduced. Whilst some personnel will come from the local facility, others will come from around the region and, as decided by the incident command team, form a scalable and ultimately substantial resource for the AIC and MIC, but without significantly compromising any single institution. The staff are drawn from the local BASICS schemes, hospital emergency departments, the air ambulance network and even non-front line carers with a special interest and willingness to volunteer.

Whilst casualties with a compromised airway or severe chest injuries are likely to have succumbed in the first minutes before they can be evacuated, a number may reach the CCS. Establishment of a definitive airway or the insertion of a chest drain may significantly adjust a casualty's physiology and allow a lowering of the evacuation priority. Control of haemorrhage, beyond that which might have been done as part of the first aid response and establishment of vascular access with the provision of fluid resuscitation can temporarily improve a shocked patient and allow re-ordering of priority for evacuation. The application of a traction splint to a fractured femur will significantly reduce haemorrhage, but there is little that can be done to manage a person with concealed intra-abdominal injury in the field. In terms of intelligent evacuation, treatment at this level will aid the decision-making process. It highlights the need for senior clinical input at Rear Triage.

The purpose of treatment in a CCS is to carry out critical interventions with the aim of stabilizing or temporizing the clinical picture sufficiently to allow safe and directed evacuation to a place for definitive care.

Treatment in the scene

Working in a major incident scene requires a skill set that is increasingly recognized as a unique environment, and needs special training and experience. Medical assistance for the Fire Service and Ambulance personnel in extrication of a casualty from a complex environment and the safe administration of analgesia for this purpose can significantly improve the speed and efficiency of the process. The presence of an experienced clinician who can work with the paramedics and other rescue personnel to risk assess the interventions being proposed and, with the rescuers, determine the process of extrication, can create a significant momentum.

Within the MERIT structure, there will be people who are purely able to work in the CCS and others who are sufficiently experienced to move forward into the incident scene. The need for this will be determined by the command team.

Discharge from scene

Many people at the scene of a major incident will have no or only very minor injuries. Depending on the nature of the incident, many may not actually require hospital treatment. The use of experienced health assets to assess the triage category Green casualties, including those involved, but not injured, discharging them from the scene, can significantly reduce the burden for transport and allow focused use of resources.

Diagnosis of death

The diagnosis of death is an important legal step in the management of an incident scene. Whilst a lower priority than the care of the injured, at some point it will be required.

The initial triage sieve will identify those who are already deceased. The labelling process includes a time of identification of death, but leaves the body *in situ*. Since the location of a deceased person is important to the incident investigation and possibly also identification of the dead, in general there are only two reasons to move a body:

- To gain access to a living person who is trapped within the incident.
- To prevent destruction of the deceased body, such as in an incident fire.

The Police manage the remains and under their guidance, once the living have been evacuated from the scene, will guide the recovery of the dead to a mortuary facility where formal identification will take place.

Public evacuation

There are some major incidents, particularly of the 'Rising Tide' and 'Cloud on the Horizon' type where a significant displacement of the population is required. Examples might include a river flooding an urban area, or an industrial incident with the potential for a toxic leak. If such an evacuation is required, most people will be able to self-evacuate, but there are residential facilities, such as Nursing Homes, where assistance will be required. Primary Care Trusts are required to maintain a record of all those who are potentially vulnerable within their community so that they can be identified and their specific needs met during an evacuation.

Local Authorities have a responsibility to establish care facilities for their displaced population, frequently involving the use of public buildings, such as sports facilities and schools. Many of the population will not have brought their regular medications and a primary care treatment facility together with a pharmacy will be necessary to accommodate the re-provision needs. Whilst most able-bodied people can sleep on a camp bed and live from a communal resource for a brief period of an emergency, the more highly care dependent, in particular the elderly, will require more specialized support.

The emergency services are required to provide support to this sort of facility, but Primary Care and the Voluntary Aid Societies come into their own in this situation.

Transport

In a conventional incident, the evacuation of the injured from the scene to hospital is the final stage in the clinical response to a major incident.

Evacuation

There have been occasions where the involved have self-evacuated to hospital and there has been little management or control of this. In the Manchester terrorist bombing in 1996, many of the injured took themselves to the local hospitals. There have been other incidents where the emergency services have, without any real co-ordination or planning, evacuated the injured to hospitals in an unmanaged manner resulting in even greater confusion. The Ramstein Air Show disaster in Germany in 1988 resulted in the uncontrolled evacuation of the injured to over 50 health facilities across northern Europe.

In planning terms for evacuation to hospitals, the science of emergency preparedness has adapted the concept of surge capacity and, in a major incident, this equates to the number of injured persons and the severity of the injuries that can be accommodated at any particular time.

Allowing for the time delay between a hospital receiving notification of the declaration of a major incident and the arrival of the first injured by ambulance, it is expected that a hospital should be able to largely empty its Emergency Department, creating a capacity equivalent to the number of resuscitation bays for Red (T1, Immediate) casualties and the number of trolley bays for the Yellow (T2, Urgent) casualties. For a large ED, this might equate to 6 Reds and 16 Yellows in the first instance; for a smaller department, this may only be 2 Reds and 6 Yellows.

After this initial influx, there will be a smaller, but continuing demand as the first injured are managed and moved onwards into the hospital. This continuing demand is expected to be of the order of half the initial wave per hour for up to 4 h. The exact detail will depend on the nature of the injuries, but this might equate to 18 Reds and 48 Yellows for a large hospital, and 6 Reds and 18 Yellows for a small hospital. This would certainly stretch the services that are available, but should not exceed their capacity in major incident mode.

The role of the AIC-MIC command system is to manage the flow to try to ensure that no location is completely overwhelmed. This will require communication between the hospitals and the control team. The number of hospitals utilized in the response and the flow of the injured to these should be actively managed.

As an additional complexity, if there are injuries requiring specialist treatment, they should ideally be moved directly to a facility with those specialist services available on site, reducing the need for secondary transfer at a later time, Examples of such injuries might be neurosurgical injury, burn injury, and complex orthoplastic injury.

An effective evacuation process is complex and the Rear Triage role is key to this. Experienced clinical judgement with a knowledge of the facilities of the surrounding hospitals, properly informed by the physiological Triage sort and a clinical assessment of the injuries sustained can allow intelligent disposition. This will require a relatively senior clinician, but should only be undertaken under the direction of the command team.

Mode of transport

Conventionally evacuation is done by ambulance. Old style ambulances used to have capacity to carry two stretchers, one being the normal transport trolley, and a second that formed the sideways facing seats, but could be used if necessary. Ambulance design and safety issues have now removed this capacity and each ambulance is only able to transport a single stretcher patient. One ambulance for one patient is now the rule.

The management of any scene requires careful coordination and the creation of a flow system is essential to avoid blocked roads and undue congestion (Figs 33.11 and 33.12).

Around the scene of a major incident, the traffic network will often become log-jammed as a result of road closures. Given time, the police will create blue light routes

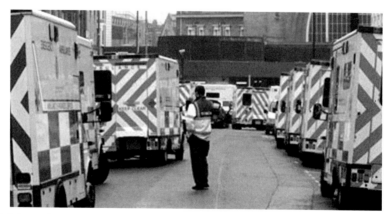

Fig. 33.11. Ambulance parking.

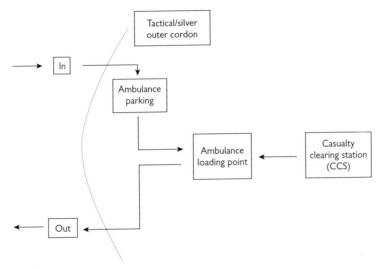

Fig. 33.12. Evacuation flow.

through this congestion to allow free movement to the local hospitals from the Casualty Clearing Station.

A significant number of the casualties may be only mildly injured, and other forms of transport and facilities might be available to treat them. Depending on the number, in some incidents, public transport such as buses have been commandeered to transport the minor injuries to a hospital a distance from the scene to keep the nearer hospitals for the more significantly injured. There may also be alternative treatment locations, such as walk-in centres that can provide simple dressings and treatment.

Once screened and discharged from the scene, those with no or minimal injury may not require transport to hospital at all. These people will need to be processed by the Police for investigation and documentation purposes. Emergency plans typically have a Survivor Reception Centre, and transport by non-emergency vehicle to such a location may be an appropriate disposition.

Helicopters

Over the last few years, a network of charitable and independent UK national air ambulances has developed and, with military Search and Rescue helicopter assistance, there is now sufficient air capacity to significantly impact on a major incident. The transport of resources into an incident scene and potentially also the movement of patients to specialist regional centres directly from the scene, is a realistic possibility (Fig. 33.13).

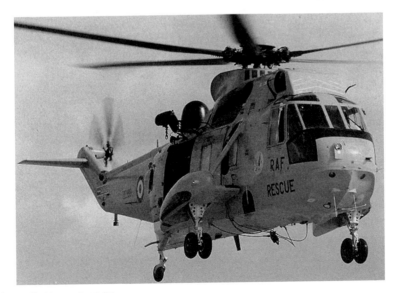

Fig. 33.13. Large patient transport capacity.

There is such potential, particularly in more remote environments, that some ambulance service emergency plans now have a specialist Air Movement Officer, as well as an Ambulance Parking Officer to try manage the air traffic.

Voluntary aid societies

Capacity is frequently a limiting factor in mounting a sufficient response to a large major incident. Although the lead-in time to a significant *de novo* response can be rather prolonged for the Voluntary Aid Societies, some incidents occur at pre-planned events, such as sports events or other forms of public gatherings. As part of the license from a Local Authority to hold such an event, there must be pre-positioned patient care assets scaled to the size of the event. The capacity may range from a small number of first-aiders from the St. John Ambulance (Fig. 33.14), Red Cross or, in Scotland, the St. Andrew's Ambulance at a village fete, through a small delegation with one or two vehicles from a private ambulance provider at a regional showground, to a full field hospital at a military air show.

The statutory Ambulance Service has primacy in terms of mounting a health response to such an incident, but these assets can be considerable and, properly directed and focused, can significantly support a major incident response, particularly with respect to the management of the minor injuries and those who have no significant physical injury.

These organizations also have access to a number of sufficiently equipped and identifiable emergency vehicles that can be used to transport the injured. The scope of clinical practice of the volunteers and even their capacity to travel under emergency conditions can be limited, but they are a resource that should not be overlooked in a constrained environment.

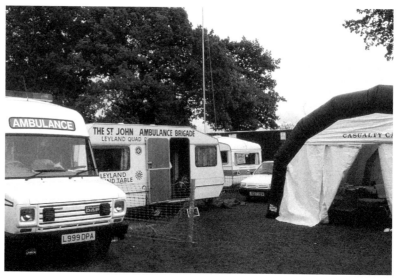

Fig. 33.14. St. John Ambulance facility.

Further reading

Advanced Life Support Group. *Major Incident Medical Management and Support*. 2nd edn. London: BMJ Books, 2002.

Aylwin C, Konig T, Brennan N, Shirley P, Davies G, Walsh M, Brohi K. et al. Reduction in critical mortality in urban mass casualty incidents: analysis of triage, surge, and resource use after the London bombings on July 7, 2005. *Lancet* 2006; **368**: 2219–25.

Barnett DJ, Balicer RD, Blodgett D, Fews AL, Parker CL, Links JM. The application of the Haddon Matrix to public health readiness and response planning. *Env Hlth Perspect* 2005; **113** (5): 561–6.

Champion H, Sacco W, Copes W, Gann D, Gennarelli T, Flanagan M. A revision of the Trauma Score. *J Trauma* 1989; **29**(5): 623–9.

Civil Contingencies Act 2004.

Department of Health, Emergency Preparedness Division. *NHS Emergency Planning Guidance 2005*. London: NHS, 2005.

Department of Health. Emergency Preparedness Division. *NHS Emergency Planning Guidance 2005—Mass Casualties Incidents: A Framework for Planning—Best Practice Guidance: A Consultation*. London: DoH, 2007.

FEMA. *National Incident Management System*. Washington DC: US Department of Homeland Security, 2009.

Garner A, Lee A, Harrison K, Schultz C. Comparative analysis of multiple casualty incident triage algorithms. *Annl Emerg Med* 2001; **38** (5): 541–8.

Sundnes KO, Birnbaum ML. Health Disaster Management Guidelines for Evaluation and Research in the Utstein Style. *Prehosp Disaster Med* 2003; **17**(Suppl): 3.

Index

Page numbers in *italics* denote figures or tables.